Hepatitis B in India
Prevention and Management

Hepatitis B in India
Prevention and Management

Edited by

S K Sarin MD, DM
Professor and Head
Department of Gastroenterology
GB Pant Hospital, New Delhi

A K Singal MD, DM
Consultant
Department of Gastroenterology
King Fahd Central Hospital,
Jizan, Saudi Arabia

CBS PUBLISHERS & DISTRIBUTORS
NEW DELHI • BANGALORE

Hepatitis B in India: Prevention and Management

ISBN: 81-239-1060-6

First Edition 2004

© Editors & Publisher
All rights reserved. No part of this publication may be reproduced, stored in a retrieval system, or transmitted in any form, or by any means—electronic, mechanical, photo-copying, recording or otherwise, without the prior permission of the editors and publishers.

Published by:
Satish K. Jain for CBS Publishers & Distributors
4596/1A, 11, Darya Ganj, New Delhi-110 002 (India)
E-mail : cbspubs@del3.vsnl.net.in
Website : http://www.cbspd.com

Branch Office:
Seema House, 2975, 17th Cross, K.R. Road,
Bansankari 2nd Stage, Bangalore - 560070
Fax : 080-6771680, E-mail : cbsbng@vsnl.net

Production Director : Vinod K. Jain

The author and publishers have made efforts to ascertain the authenticity of the material provided by the contributors and to trace the copyright holders for borrowed material. If any omissions have occurred, the editors and publishers will be pleased to make the necessary arrangements at the first opportunity.

Laser typesetting by:
NS Computers, New Delhi

Printed at:
Chaman Enterprises, New Delhi

Foreword

Hepatitis B infection is on rise in India with about 43 million people being infected with this virus. The virus is considered 100 per cent more infectious than AIDS. I earnestly appreciate the sincere efforts being done by authors in putting together the knowledge available on this infection in India. Written by scholars who have been actively involved in investigating this problem against the background of world scenario, the attempt definitely deserves all the appreciation. All the issues covered in this book have been addressed to by the scientists who have been actively involved in carrying out research in this particular area.

From natural history studies it is estimated that 1% of all deaths among adults in the country are HBV related. It is also clear from Indian studies that horizontal transmission is a dominant mode of transmission of HBV, rather similar to that seen in Africa and Middle East and unlike that seen in other parts of South East Asia and Pacific basis. There are effective vaccines now available which can provide long lasting immunity against the disease. However, the high cost of this vaccine has been a major deterring factor in inclusion of this vaccine in the Expanded Program of Immunization. Hence, at this juncture needs a careful review. It is heartening to note that the prevention strategies have been dealt with in a great detail in this book. This section of the book describes in detail, the universal precautions for prevention of HBV infection in endoscopy units, dialysis units and discuss some of the policy issues related to health care workers. The treatment options available to the patient today exceeds far more than what was available ten years back. Use of steroids, interferon, nucleoside analogous and gene therapy have already revolutionized the treatment of HBV infection. There are undoubtedly many gaps in our knowledge regarding the transmission, pathology, immunology and genetics of this infection. The lack of knowledge on the diagnosis of HBV mutants and reactivation of HBV infections, in particular, complicate diagnosis and subsequently the treatment of hepatitis B infection. Considerable amount of research efforts are being invested in looking at treatment options for HBV infection in the Indian system of medicine. All the research being carried out in this area is quite satisfactory.

HBV infection is health priority in India. India can no longer sweep the HBV problem under the carpet. Time is essence in public health. The cost factor has so far influenced India's decision to take the position of recommending hepatitis B vaccination in high risk groups only. While this practice is appropriate to control individual risk, it will not control hepatitis B in India. With declining of cost of hepatitis B vaccine and with India in a definite stage of producing its own hepatitis B vaccine, the situation calls for policy formulation for prevention of this condition. The chapters on the topics like "Economic burden of hepatitis B on the quality of life" bring into broader light the economic losses that an individual incurs owing to the HBV infection and its impact on the nation. The state of art on various aspects of hepatitis B problem in India depicted in this book ought to serve as the knowledge base for policy formulation in the prevention of this condition.

Prof. N.K Ganguly
Director General
Indian Council of Medical Research
New Delhi

Preface

Unlike in the developed and several developing countries, hepatitis B virus (HBV) infection remains a major public health challenge in India. The clinical manifestations are variable; with an asymptomatic 'chronic HBV infection' at one end and an advanced cirrhosis and hepatocellular carcinoma (HCC) at the other end of the spectrum. It is now known that the subjects with chronic HBV infection not only have the risk of developing serious consequences such as chronic hepatitis and cirrhosis, but also have a potential of transmitting the virus to others.

The effective control and management of any infection requires a thorough understanding of its epidemiology, the natural history of infection, and the available pharmacological agents and vaccines. Our previous book (1996) entitled *Hepatitis B in India: Problems and Prevention* provided the information on prevention of hepatitis B after critical analysis by leading experts. In the last decade, there has been a tremendous increase in awareness and knowledge on different aspects, particularly the treatment of hepatitis B, the development of new drugs, drug resistance, combination therapy, gene therapy, etc. The availability of the immense literature has also raised many questions and issues.

To deliberate all these issues related to prevention and management of hepatitis B in India, 2nd National Symposium on "Hepatitis B in India: Therapeutic Options and Prevention Strategies" was organized in 2000 under the auspices of the Indian Association for Study of the Liver (INASL). The aims of the symposium were two fold: (a) to review and put into perspective advances in our understanding of prevention and management of hepatitis B, and (b) to derive consensus opinion and formulate guidelines for prevention and management of hepatitis B in context with Indian scenario. We were fortunate to have participation of leading experts mainly from India but also from abroad including Hongkong, Thailand, UK, Australia, and Germany. The deliberations were discussed in seven sessions and these contribute the seven different sections of the book. The present title, "Hepatitis B in India: Prevention and Management" is another step in our continuous efforts at INASL to accomplish (a) better management of patients with chronic hepatitis B (CHB) and (b) formulating prevention strategies for eradication of this serious infection from our country.

In the first section, on the "Epidemiology of hepatitis B virus infection in India" the emphasis has been given on the prevalence of HBV in the general population (comparing pre-1995 vs. 1995-2000), on the newer high risk groups such as injecting drug users (IDU's), transmission of HBV by blood which is already screened for HBsAg. A separate chapter on the transmission in patients with hematological and lymphoproliferative disorders has been added. In the second section entitled "Pathogenesis, clinical presentation, and diagnosis" a chapter has been incorporated on the incidentally detected asymptomatic HBsAg positive subjects (IDAHS), an important emerging group of subjects with chronic HBV infection. The emphasis has once again been on deleting the term 'carrier' and replacing it with 'chronic HBV infection'. The chapter on clinical spectrum of HBV infection highlights on the pre-core or HBeAg negative mutant related chronic hepatitis B in the backdrop of relevant techniques of laboratory diagnosis and new information on the mechanisms of immune injury by HBV. A few important clinical presentations have been discussed in separate chapters, e.g. acute-on-chronic liver disease, reactivation of chronic HBV infection, and extrahepatic manifestations of HBV.

A separate section on hepatocellular carcinoma has been added. The first chapter incorporates the epidemiological data on HBV-related HCC in India and role of co-factors like aflatoxins, HCV, alcohol, etc. The discussion on screening for HCC highlights the screening modalities, their cost-efficacy and ideal screening strategies for chronic HBV patients. Various levels of prevention of HCC have been provided in a separate chapter. Pathogenesis of HBV related HCC highlights about the absence of p53 mutation in India, role of HBx protein and the potential of HBV to cause HCC directly bypassing the cirrhotic phase. The surgical and non-surgical treatment options have been discussed in brief and a write up is added on the need and potential of liver transplantation facilities in India.

One of the important sections of the book is on "General measures for prevention of hepatitis B in India". This section deals with the use of universal precautions and proper handling of hospital waste in preventing the spread of HBV. Prevention in high-risk areas like nephrology units and endoscopy units have been dealt with separately. Two controversial issues on the 'Need for routine HBV screening before surgery' and 'Policy for HBsAg positive health care worker' have been deliberated. The fifth section deals with the prevention of HBV infection by more specific means, i.e. vaccination. Apart from the issues of pre- and post-vaccination screening, need for boosters, vaccination in health care workers, patients with end-stage renal disease (ESRD) and chronic liver disease (CLD), etc. have been provided. The ideal schedule for vaccinating newborns and how this can be modified in a practical setting is discussed in the following chapter. The economic analysis of this approach has been discussed in detail and compared with the economic burden of treating chronic hepatitis B patients in India. One of the important issues affecting the results of any EPI programs is the vaccine failure because of vaccine escape mutants and host genetic factors. These have been discussed at length by one of the pioneers in the field.

The last two sections are devoted to the therapy of chronic HBV infection. The two drugs officially approved for use are interferon and lamivudine. The response rate to IFN alone is lower (30–40%), and moreover the drugs are not free of side effects. The factors responsible for the response to IFN are discussed separately. The role of steroid priming has been discussed at length in the next chapter. Lamivudine, when used on a long-term basis, has a potential of producing mutants in the HBV (YMDD) which may have the potential of inducing hepatitis flare. Mechanisms and treatment options for these therapy-induced mutations have been discussed separately. Role of alternative treatment modalities like ribavirin, herbal drugs and gene therapy have been discussed by the respective experts. The future of hepatitis B therapy lies in combination of nucleoside analogues or combination of immunomodulators and nucleoside analogues. This has been discussed in a separate chapter. The last section deals with the management of hepatitis B in special groups like children, patients with ESRD, patients with HIV co-infection, dual (HBV+HCV) infection and post-liver transplantation recurrence of hepatitis B. Two separate chapters have been added on the 'Assessment of the impact of treatment on the quality of life by specific questionare based instruments' and 'Role of nutrition in the management of patients with acute and chronic liver disease'. In addition, we feel honoured that Prof. N.K. Ganguly, Director General, Indian Council of Medical Research, has very kindly written the Foreword to the book.

This volume is unique in its conception and presentation since it not only provides new information, but also a balanced analysis and rational approach to the overall diagnosis and management of hepatitis B. An effort has been made to avoid duplication in the different chapters and also to provide updated, comprehensive and authentic information.

The editors of this book, working in two different countries of the Asian continent, hope that the postgraduates, physicians, gastroenterologists, surgeons, microbiologists, basic scientists and people working in the field of preventive medicine round the world, would find the information contained in the book to be useful in practical situations while handling patients with chronic hepatitis B. We sincerely hope that the book shall also serve as a useful reference manual to the policy makers of our country for calculating the disease burden and evolving strategies for the implementation of vaccination programs. It is hoped and believed that through these continuing efforts we shall be able to contribute in our own little way in achieving the eventual goal of containing and eliminating hepatitis B viral infection in India.

Shiv K Sarin   **Ashwani K Singal**

List of Contributors

Dr Philip Abraham, MD, FCPS, DNB, FICP
Professor and Head
Department of Gastroenterology
KEM Hospital
Mumbai, India

Dr Anju Agarwal, MD
Specialist
Department of Pediatrics
ESI Hospital, Basai Darapur
New Delhi, India

Dr Sanjay K Agarwal, MD, DNB
Additional Professor
Department of Nephrology
AIIMS
New Delhi, India

Dr Sri R Agarwal, MD, DM
Senior Research Associate
Department of Gastroenterology
GB Pant Hospital
New Delhi, India

Dr Vineet Ahuja, MD, DM
Assistant Professor
Department of Gastroenterology
AIIMS
New Delhi, India

Dr Deepak N Amarapurkar, MD, DM, DNB
Consultant Gastroenterologist
Bombay Hospital and Medical Research
Centre
Mumbai, India

Dr Narender K Arora, MD, MAMS
Additional Professor
Department of Pediatrics
AIIMS
New Delhi, India

Dr Mark Atkins, MBBS, MRC (Path)
Director, Clinical Development (antivirals)
Department of Microbiology
Glaxo Wellcome
UK

Dr Sethu Babu, MD, DM
Consultant Gastroenterologist
Hyderabad, India

Dr Pechamuthu Balakrishnan, PhD
Research Fellow
Department of Microbiology
Dr ALM PGIBMS
University of Chennai
Chennai, India

Dr Angelin Bartholomeusz,
Senior Scientist,
Victorian Infectious Diseases Reference Laboratory,
WHO Collaborating Centers for Virus Reference and Research Biosafety,
North Melbourne, Australia

Dr. Anil K Bhalla, MD DM
Consultant
Department of Nephrology
Sir Ganga Ram Hospital
New Delhi, India

Dr Rajesh Bhatia, MD
Ex Director
National Institute of Biologicals
Noida, UP, India

Dr Rajesh Bhojwani, MS
Department of GI Surgery
GB Pant Hospital
New Delhi, India

Dr Hubert E Blum, MD
Professor and Chairman
Department of Medicine II
University Hospital Freiburg
Freiburg, Germany

Dr Shobha Broor, MD
Professor
Department of Virology
AIIMS, New Delhi, India

Dr George M Chandy, MD, DM, PGDHA
Professor and Head
Department of Clinical Gastroenterology and Hepatology
Christian Medical College and Hospital
Vellore, Tamilnadu, India

Dr Pantipa Chatchatee, MD
Lecturer
Immunology and Allergy Unit
Faculty of Medicine
Chulalongkon University
Bangkok, Thailand

Dr Adarsh Chaudhary, MS
Professor and Head
Department of GI Surgery
GB Pant Hospital
New Delhi, India

Dr Kishore Chaudhary, MD, DNB
Deputy Director
Indian Council of Medical Research
New Delhi, India

Dr Sujit Chaudhuri, MD
Medical Officer
Department of Gastroenterology
SSKM Hospital, IPGMER
Kolkata, India

Dr Yogesh Chawla, MD, DM
Professor and Head
Department of Hepatology
PGIMER
Chandigarh, India

Dr Virender Chauhan, MD
Senior Resident
Department of Gastroenterology
PGIMER
Chandigarh, India

Dr Voranush Chongsrisawat, MD
Lecturer
Viral Hepatitis Research Unit
Faculty of Medicine
Chulalongkon University
Bangkok, Thailand

List of Contributors

Dr Gourdas Choudhuri, MD, DM, MNAMS, FICP, FACG
Additional Professor
Department of Gastroenterology
Sanjay Gandhi Post Graduate Institute of Medical Sciences
Lucknow, India

Dr Ved P Choudhry, MD, FIAP, FIMSA, FIACM
Professor and Head
Department of Hematology
AIIMS
New Delhi, India

Dr Anuchit Chutaputti, MD
Professor
Section of Digestive Diseases
Department of Medicine
Pramongkutklao Hospital
Angkok, Thailand

Dr Bhudev C Das, PhD, FNASC
Deputy Director and Chief
Department of Molecular Oncology
Institute of Cytology and Preventive Oncology
Indian Council of Medical Research
New Delhi, India

Dr Julie C Dent, PhD
Senior Clinical Program Head
Hepatitis Development Group
Smith Kline R&D
Greenford, UK

Dr Hiralal G Desai, MD, PhD, DSc
Honorary Gastroenterologist
Jaslok Hospital Research Centre
Mumbai, India

Dr Radha K Dhiman, MD, DM
Associate Professor
Department of Hepatology
PGIMER
Chandigarh, India

Dr Elumalei Dhevahi, PhD
Senior Research Fellow
Department of Microbiology
Dr ALM PGIBMS
University of Madras
Chennai, India

Dr. Anand Dotihal, DM
Senior Resident
Department of Gastroenterology,
GB Pant Hospital,
New Delhi, India

Dr. Ajay Duseja, DM
Assistant Professor
Department of Hepatology
PGIMER
Chandigarh, India

Dr Ranjana Gondal, MD
Professor
Department of Pathology
GB Pant Hospital
New Delhi, India

Dr Vivekanandan Gopalakrishanan, PhD
Lecturer
Department of Microbiology
University of Malaysia
Kualalampur, Malaysia

Dr Debendra N Guhamazumder, MD
Ex-Professor and Head
Department of Gastroenterology
IPGMER
Kolkata, India

Dr. Ashwani Gupta, MD, DM
Consultant
Department of Nephrology
Sir Ganga Ram Hospital
New Delhi, India

Dr Raj C Guptan, MBBS, Mch
Senior Research Associate
Department of Gastroenterology
GB Pant Hospital
New Delhi, India

Dr Mohammed A Habeeb, MD, DM
Assistant Professor
Department of Gastroenterology
Osmania General Hospital and Research Center
Hyderabad, India

Dr Chitoor M Habibullah, MD, DM, FACG, FAMS, FNASC
Director
Center for Liver Diseases
Deccan College of Medical Sciences and Allied Hospitals
Hyderabad, India

Dr Ashok K Jain, MD, DM
Professor and Head
Department of Gastroenterology
Institute of Medical Sciences
Banaras Hindu University
Varanasi, India

Ms Preethi Jayakumar, MSc
Senior Research Fellow
Department of Microbiology
Dr ALM PGIBMS
University of Madras
Chennai, India

Dr Sannadi Jayaram, PhD
Assistant Professor
Department of Microbiology
Govt. Medical College
Pondicherry, India

Dr Yogendra K Joshi, MD, PhD
Additional Professor
Department of Gastroenterology and Human Nutrition
AIIMS
New Delhi, India

Dr Antony G Joyee, MSc
Senior Research Fellow
Department of Microbiology
Dr ALM PGIBMS
University of Madras
Chennai, India

Dr Lalit Kant, MD, PhD
Senior Deputy Director General
Indian Council of Medical Research
New Delhi, India

Dr Premasheesh Kar, MD, DM
Professor
Department of Gastroenterology
Lok Nayak Jai Prakash Narain Hospital
New Delhi, India

Dr Rajesh Kashyap, MD
Assistant Professor
Department of Hematology
AIIMS
New Delhi, India

Dr Mohammad N Khaja, MSc, PhD
Research Scientist
Center for Liver Research and Diagnostics
Hyderabad, India

List of Contributors

Dr. Dinesh Khullar, MD, DM (Nephro)
Consultant
Nephrology Department
Sir Ganga Ram Hospital,
New Delhi, India

Dr Rakesh Kochhar, MD, DM, MNAMS
Professor
Department of Gastroenterology
PGIMER
Chandigarh, India

Dr Praveen Kumar, MD
Surveillance Medical Officer
World Health Organisation
Patna, India

Dr. Rakesh Kumar, DM
Senior Resident
Department of Gastroenterology
GB Pant Hospital
New Delhi, India

Dr Ching L Lai, MD
Professor and Chief
Division of Hepatology
Department of Medicine
Queen Mary Hospital
University of Hongkong
Hongkong, SAR, China

Dr George K Lau, MD
Professor
Division of Gastroenterology
Department of Medicine
Queen Mary Hospital
University of Hongkong
Hongkong, SAR, China

Dr Stephen Locarnini, MD
Professor
Research and Molecular Development
Victorian Infectious Diseases Reference Laboratory
WHO Collaborating Centers for Virus Refrence and Research Biosafety
North Melbourne, Australia

Dr Xunrong Luo, MD
Resident in Internal Medicine
Department of Medicine
New York Prebyterian Hospital
New York, USA

Dr Govind K Makharia, MD, DM, DNB, MNAMS
Senior Research Officer
Department of Gastroenterology
AIIMS
New Delhi, India

Dr Veena Malhotra, MD
Professor and Head
Department of Pathology
GB Pant Hospital
New Delhi, India

Dr Anandita Mandal, MD
Professor and Head
Department of Microbiology
GB Pant Hospital
New Delhi, India

Dr. Prashant Mathur, DM
Pool Officer
Department of Pediatrics,
AIIMS
New Delhi, India

Dr Ketha Venkatakrishna K Mohan, PhD
Senior Research Fellow
Department of Microbiology
Dr ALM PGIBMS
University of Madras
Chennai, India

Dr K M Mohandas, MD, DNB
Professor and Head
Department of Digestive Diseases and
Clinical Nutrition
Tata Memorial Hospital
Mumbai, India

Dr Daurius Moradpour, MD
Assistant Professor
Department of MedicineII
University Hospital Freiburg
Freiburg, Germany

Dr Kailapuri G Murugavel, PhD
Staff Scientist
YRG, CARE
Chennai, India

Dr Sita Naik, MD
Professor
Department of Immunology
Sanjay Gandhi Post Graduate Institute of
Medical Sciences
Lucknow, India

Dr Subhash R Naik, MD, FNASC
Professor and Head
Department of Gastroenterology
Sanjay Gandhi Post Graduate Institute of
Medical Sciences
Lucknow, India

Dr Maniyalath Narendranathan, MD, DM, MPH
(Clinical Epidemiology)
Professor and Head
Department of Gastroenterology
Medical College
Thiruvanathapuram, India

Dr. Wolf B Offensperger, MD
Professor
Department of Medicine II
University Hospital Freiburg
Freiburg, Germany

Dr Viral Patrawala,
Lecturer
Department of Gastroenterology
JJ Group of Hospitals
Mumbai, India

Dr Ashok K Patwari, MD, DCH, MNAMS, FIAP
Professor
Department of Pediatrics
Kalawati Saran Children Hospital
New Delhi, India

Dr Shajan Peter, MD, DM
Lecturer
Department of Clinical Gastroenterology
and Hepatology
Christian Medical College
Vellore,
Tamilnadu, India

Dr Yong Poovorawan, MD
Professor
Viral Hepatitis Research Unit
Faculty of Medicine
Chulalongkon University
Bangkok, Thailand

List of Contributors

Dr. Mohan Prasad
Senior Consultant
Gastroenterologist
Coimbatore, India

Dr Amrinder S Puri, MD, DM
Associate Professor
Department of Gastroenterology
GB Pant Hospital
New Delhi, India

Dr Magaral R Rajasekar, MS, MD, FRCS
Senior Consultant
Department of Hepatobiliary Surgery and
Liver Transplantation
Apollo Hospital
New Delhi, India

Dr Paramasivam Rajendran, PhD
Professor
Department of Microbiology
Dr ALM PGIBMS
University of Madras
Chennai, India

Dr Devender S Rana, MD, MNAMS
Senior Consultant
Department of Nephrology
Sir Ganga Ram Hospital
New Delhi, India

Dr Surinder S Rana, MBBS
Post Graduate Resident
Department of Medicine
Division of Gastroenterology
Maulana Azad Medical College
Lok Nayak Jai Prakash Narain Hospital
New Delhi, India

Dr Suma Ray, PhD
Senior Research Fellow
Department of Microbiology
AIIMS
New Delhi, India

Dr Puja Sakuja, MD
Associate Professor
Department of Pathology
GB Pant Hospital
New Delhi, India

Dr Vinay Sakhuja, MD, DM
Professor and Head
Department of Nephrology
PGIMER
Chandigarh, India

Dr Shubhangi Saraswat, MBBS, PhD
Consultant Pathologist
Department of Transfusion Medicine
Ecorts Heart Institute and Rsearch Center
New Delhi, India

Dr Vivek Saraswat, MD, DM
Additional Professor
Department of Gastroenterology
Sanjay Gandhi Institute of Medical Sciences
Lucknow, India

Dr Shiv K Sarin, MD, DM
Professor and Head
Department of Gastroenterology
GB Pant Hospital
New Delhi, India

Ms Nandini Saxena, MSc (Nutrition)
Senior Research Fellow
Department of Gastroenterology
AIIMS,
New Delhi, India

Dr Sharad Shah, MD, MRCP, RCPS, FACG
Senior Consultant
Department of Gastroenterology
Jaslok Hospital
Mumbai, India

Dr. Manoj K Sharma, MD
Senior Resident
Department of Gastroenterology
GB Pant Hospital
New Delhi, India

Dr Mahesh P Sharma, MD, DM, FICP, FAMS
Professor
Department of Gastroenterology
AIIMS
New Delhi, India

Dr Anupam Sibal, MD
Consultant
Department of Pediatrics
Apollo Hospital,
New Delhi, India

Dr Ashwani K Singal, MD, DM
Consultant
Department of Gastroenterology
King Fahd Central Hospital,
Jizan, Saudi Arabia

Dr Kartar Singh, MD, DM, MNAMS
Professor and Head
Department of Gastroenterology
PGIMER
Chandigarh, India

Ms Namrata Singh, MSc
Department of Gastroenterology and
Human Nutrition
AIIMS, New Delhi, India

Dr Surinder Singh, MD
Scientist Gr I
National Institute of Biologicals
Noida, UP, India

Dr Saroj K Sinha, MD, DM
Assistant Professor
Department of Gastroenterology
PGIMER
Chandigarh, India

Dr Arvinder S Soin, MS, FRCS, FRCS (Transplantation)
Consultant
Department of Hepatobiliary Surgery and
Liver Transplantation
Apollo Hospital,
New Delhi, India

Dr Sanjay K Somani, MD
Senior Resident
Department of Gastroenterology
Sanjay Gandhi Institute of Medical Sciences
Lucknow, India

Dr Rakesh K Tandon, MD, PhD, FAMS
Professor and Head
Department of Gastroenterology
AIIMS
New Delhi, India

Dr Sameer Taneja, MD
Senior Resident
Department of Hepatology
PGIMER
Chandigarh, India

List of Contributors

Dr Archana Thakur, MD
Professor
Department of Microbiology
GB Pant Hospital
New Delhi, India

Dr Sadras P Thyagarajan, MSc, PhD, DSC
Professor and Head
Department of Microbiology
Dr ALM PGIBMS
University of Madras
Chennai, India

Dr Mark Thursz, MD, MRCP
Senior Lecturer
Department of Internal Medicine
Imperial College of Technology and Medicine
St Mary's Hospital
London, UK

Dr Subramanian Venkataraman, MD
Registrar
Department of Clinical Gastroenterology and Hepatology
Christian Medical College
Vellore, Tamilnadu, India

Dr Durairajan Vijayrajkumari, MS, FRCS
Consultant
Department of Hepatobiliary Surgery and Liver Transplantation
Apollo Hospital, New Delhi, India

Dr. Fritz V Weizsacker, MD
Professor
Department of Medicine II
University Hospital Freiburg
Freiburg, Germany

Dr Surender K Yachha, MD, DM
Associate Professor
Department of Pediatric Gastroenterology
Sanjay Gandhi Institute of Medical Sciences
Lucknow, UP, India

Dr Man Y Yuen, MRCP
Honorary Clinical Assistant Professor
Fellow of Division of Hepatology
University of Hongkong
Queen Mary Hospital,
Hongkong
SAR, China

Contents

Foreword — v

Preface — vii

List of Contributors — xi

Section I : Epidemiology of hepatitis B virus infection in India

1. Prevalence of hepatitis B virus infection in general population of India — 3
   Sadras P Thyagarajan, Raghu Hari, Kailapuri G Murugavel, Antony G Joyee, Pechamuthu Balakrishnan, Paramasivam Rajendran

2. Modes of transmission of hepatitis B virus — 15
   Ajay Duseja, Yogesh K Chawla

3. Transmission of hepatitis B virus in neonates — 22
   Ashok K Dutta, Praveen Kumar

4. Transmission of hepatitis B virus in children — 29
   Narendra K Arora, Lalit Kant, Prashant Mathur

5. Intrafamilial transmission of hepatitis B virus — 46
   Sadras P Thyagarajan, Raghu Hari, Sannadi Jayaram, Kailapuri G Murugavel, Ketha Venkatakrishna K Mohan, Elumalei Dhevahi

6. Transmission of hepatitis B virus in injecting drug users — 52
   Lalit Kant

7. Transfusion-associated hepatitis B after transfusion of blood negative for hepatitis B surface antigen — 58
   Shubhanghi Saraswat, Vivek A Saraswat

8. Transmission of hepatitis B virus infection in patients with hematological disorders — 72
   Ved P Choudhri, Rajesh Kashyap

Section II : Pathogenesis, clinical presentation and diagnosis of hepatitis B

9. Immunopathogenesis and mechanisms of persistence of hepatitis B virus 83
   Shobha Broor, Suma Ray

10. Incidentally detected asymptomatic HBsAg positive subjects 93
    Amrinder S Puri, Sri R Agarwal

11. Clinical spectrum of hepatitis B virus infection in India 99
    Anand Dotihal, Shiv K Sarin

12. Extrahepatic manifestations of hepatitis B 111
    Mahesh P Sharma, Govind K Makharia

13. Hepatitis B virus mutants: clinical presentation, diagnosis and management 127
    Stephen Locarnini, Angeline Bartholomeusz

14. Acute-on-chronic liver disease in reference to hepatitis B 148
    Saroj K Sinha, Kartar Singh

15. Reactivation of hepatitis B virus infection 161
    George K Lau, Xunrong Luo

16. Kinetics of hepatitis B virus and its relevance to the clinician 170
    Mark Thursz

17. Hepatitis B virus genotypes: an overview 175
    Varsha Thakur, B Bariar, Shiv K Sarin

18. Diagnosis of hepatitis B virus infection 193
    Ashwani K Singal

19. Liver biopsy in chronic hepatitis B 215
    Veena Malhotra, Puja Sakuja, Ranjana Gondal

Section III : Hepatocellular carcinoma and hepatitis B virus infection

20. Pathogenesis of hepatocellular carcinoma in hepatitis B virus infection 235
    Bhudev C Das

21. Epidemiology of hepatitis B asssociated hepatocellular carcinoma in India 244
    K M Mohandas

22. Screening for hepatocellular carcinoma in patients with chronic hepatitis B virus infection 250
    Ashok K Jain

23.	Prevention of hepatocellular carcinoma in reference to hepatitis B virus *Maniyalath Narendranathan*	262
24.	Surgical resection in hepatitis B virus related hepatocellular carcinoma *Adarsh Chaudhary, Rajesh Bhojwani*	275
25.	Newer non-surgical modalities for the treatment of hepatocellular carcinoma *Ching L Lai, Man F Yuen*	281
26.	Liver transplantation in the developing world *Magaral R. Rajasekar, Arvinder S. Soin, Anupam Sibal, Durairajan Vijayarajkumari*	287

Section IV: Prevention of hepatitis B virus infection in India

27.	Universal guidelines for health care workers in prevention of hepatitis B *Archana Thakur*	301
28.	Disposal of waste in hospitals with special reference to hepatitis patients *Anandita Mandal*	311
29.	Prevention of hepatitis B in the endoscopy units *Vineet Ahuja, Rakesh K Tandon*	318
30.	Prevention of hepatitis B in the nephrology units *Sanjay K Agarwal*	327
31.	Routine screening for hepatitis B virus before surgery or intervention *Chitoor M Habibullah, Mohammed A Habeeb, Mohammed M Hussain, Mohammed N Khaja, Viral Patrawala, Sharad Shah*	342
32.	HBsAg positive health care worker: the rational policy? *Subhash R Naik*	349

Section V: Hepatitis B vaccination

33.	Standardization and efficacy of hepatitis B vaccines in India *Surinder Singh, Rajesh Bhatia*	351
34.	Hepatitis B: who should be vaccinated? *Philip Abraham*	360
35.	Hepatitis B vaccination: are boosters needed? *Premashish Kar, Surender S Rana*	368
36.	Post-vacccination screening: for whom and why? *Virender Chauhan, Yogesh K Chawla*	373

37.	Hepatitis B vaccination policy for health care workers *Hiralal G Desai, Ashwani K Singal*	378
38.	Hepatitis B vaccination in patients with chronic renal failure *Devender S Rana, Dinesh Khullar, Ashwani Gupta, Anil K Bhalla, Ashwani K Singal*	389
39.	Vaccination against hepatitis A and B in patients with chronic liver disease *Vivek A Saraswat, Sanjay K Somani*	397
40.	Post-exposure prophylaxis of hepatitis B virus infection *Premashish Kar, Surinder S Rana*	412
41.	Ideal schedule for vaccinating children against hepatitis B in India *Anju Agarwal, Ashok K Patwari*	419
42.	Economic burden of hepatitis B in India *Kishore Chaudhary, Shiv K Sarin*	424
43.	Hepatitis B vaccine failure *Yong Poovorawan, Pantipa Chatchatee, Voranush Chongsrisawat*	431

Section VI: Treatment of chronic hepatitis B

44.	Treatment of chronic hepatitis B: current trends and Indian perspectives *Shiv K Sarin, Rakesh Kumar, Manoj K Sharma*	447
45.	Mechanisms of non-response to interferon in chronic hepatitis B *Sita Naik*	471
46.	Nucleoside analogues for the treatment of chronic hepatitis B *Julie C Dent, Mark Atkins*	477
47.	Incidence and profile of lamivudine resistance *Deepak N Amarapurkar*	489
48.	Mechanisms and treatment options for lamivudine resistance *Ching L Lai*	493
49.	Steroid priming before interferon therapy for chronic hepatitis B *Debendra N Guhamazumder, Sujit Chaudhuri, Sethu Babu*	498
50.	Ribavirin in the management of chronic hepatitis B *V G Mohan Prasad*	504

51.	Current status of *Phyllanthus amarus* and other herbal drugs in the treatment of chronic hepatitis B *Sadras P Thyagarajan, Raghu Hari, Sannadi Jayaram, Vivekanandan Gopalakrishnan, Preethi Jeyakumar*	512
52.	Combination therapy for chronic hepatitis B *George K Lau, Xunrong Luo*	522
53.	Gene therapy for hepatitis B *Daurius Moradpour, Wolf B Offensperger, Fritz V Weizsäcker, Hubert E. Blum*	530
54.	Instruments for assessment of impact of treatment for chronic hepatitis B on quality of life *Rakesh K Kochhar*	539

Section VII: Management of special groups with chronic hepatitis B

55.	Management of chronic hepatitis B in children *Surender K Yachha*	549
56.	Management of chronic hepatitis B in patients with end-stage renal disease *Vinay Sakhuja*	556
57.	Management of chronic hepatitis B in HIV patients *Gourdas Choudhuri*	563
58.	Role of antivirals and immunomodulators in acute hepatitis B *Anuchit Chutaputti*	571
59.	Antivirals in hepatitis B virus related decompensated cirrhosis *Radha K Dhiman, Sameer Taneja, Ashwani K Singal*	577
60.	Hepatitis B virus infection and liver transplantation *Subramanian Venkataraman, Shajan Peter, George M Chandy*	585
61.	Nutrition in the management of acute and chronic liver disease *Yogendra K Joshi, Namrata Singh, Nandini Saxena*	598
	Abstracts	611
	Index	629

Section I
Epidemiology of hepatitis B virus infection in India

1

Prevalence of hepatitis B virus infection in general population of India

Sadras P Thyagarajan, Raghu Hari, Kailapuri G Murugavel,
Antony G Joyee, Pechamuthu Balakrishnan, Paramasivam Rajendran

Humans are the only reservoir for the transmission of hepatitis B virus (HBV) infection. It is estimated that there are 350 million people in the world who are chronically infected with HBV, of which about 47 million are in India alone.[1] The term chronic HBV infection is defined as the persistence of hepatitis B surface antigen (HBsAg) in the serum of an individual for six months or longer as a marker of persisting HBV infection in the liver.[2] Chronic HBV infection gets established when the immune response that normally clears the infection fails to operate or is too weak to be effective. Thus, in neonates, HBV exposure leads to chronic infection in 80–90%, whereas, in adults the infection becomes chronic in 5–10% of individuals. Between these two extremes are immunocompromised individuals such as intravenous drug users, hemodialysis patients, or transplant recipients who are more likely to develop chronic infection as compared with healthy adults (10–60%).[3] The basic requirement for evolving a national policy decision on prevention and control of an infectious disease is to document its epidemiology in the given country.[4–31] This chapter highlights the prevalence pattern of HBV infection in India as in the year 2000.

Any epidemiological analysis becomes easier if there exists a network of reporting system. An alternative option could be to conduct a meta-analysis of all the reported data. A typical meta-analysis should include (a) a wide literature search so as to include all the data, (b) inclusion criteria for studies in the meta-analysis formulated, (c) first/second stage meta-analysis worked out based on identified criteria, and (d) statistical methods are to be adopted for data extraction from the available reports like sample size, comparable methodologies, statistical weightage to derive 95% confidence interval, publication bias assessment, and heterogenicity assessment, etc.

The analysis of epidemiology of hepatitis B in India is hampered by the non-availability of a national level network of reporting system and hence one has to resort to the meta-analysis approach. Although a significant number of published reports from India could be gathered through all the available literature retrieval facilities, they could not be subjected for an ideal meta-analysis due to enormous variables in the reports like (a) incomparable design of studies, (b) sample size differences, (c) incomparable methods adopted by investigators from different parts of the country, and (d) compelling need for indexing HBV prevalence in each and every part of India to obtain the national scenario necessitating inclusion of even poorly designed studies over the years with smaller sample size.

Of the 27 reports which were taken up for the meta-analysis of HBsAg positivity rate in the general population, a range of 1.1–12.2% was observed. The analysis of the HBsAg prevalence showed that Jammu and Kashmir and Kerala came below 2% zone; Karnataka, Maharashtra, Delhi, Haryana, Himachal Pradesh, West Bengal had a prevalence of 2–4% while Tamil Nadu, Pondicherry, Andhra Pradesh, Madhya Pradesh, Uttar Pradesh and Arunachal Pradesh belonged to high HBsAg prevalence zones of above 4%. However, the mean HBsAg prevalence rate for India from these reports is 3.34%. This means that, as on today, there are about 34 millon subjects chronically infected with HBV in India. The point to be remembered besides the formidable pool of HBV infected population is the significant regional variation of chronic HBV infection (Table 1).

Table 1. Prevalence of HBsAg among general population in different regions of India

Place/author	Number	Method	HBsAg positivity (%)	Year
North India, Delhi				
Nanu et al[6]	1,32,093	ELISA	2.5	1997
Singal et al[6a]	1,944	ELISA	2.1	2000
Irshad et al[7]	20,435	ELISA	2.6	1994
Dutta & Mohammed[8]		IEOP	2.65	1972
Chandigarh				
Pal et al[9]	1001	IEOP	2.2	1973
Kashmir				
Makroo et al[10]	7900	RPHA	1.1	1989
Uttar Pradesh – Lucknow				
Nagaraju et al[11]	605	Dot blot	9.9	1994
Choudhury et al[12]	313	ELISA	2.2	1998
Himachal Pradesh				
Thakur et al[13]	1012	RPHA	3.26	1990
West Bengal – Calcutta				
Roy Choudhury et al[14]	–	ELISA	1.79	1989
Chakraborthy et al[15]	–	CIEP	2.8	1977
Maharastra – Mumbai				
Joshi et al[16]				
Maruthas	–	ELISA	5.92	1983

(Contd.)

(Contd.)

Place/author	Number	Method	HBsAg positivity (%)	Year
Nava-Buddhas	–	ELISA	2.62	1983
Scheduled castes	–	ELISA	1.63	1983
Elavia et al[17]	3095	ELISA	3.68	1985
Elavia et al[17]	3883	ELISA	2.03	1986
Elavia et al[17]	3455	ELISA	2.02	1987
Elavia & Banker[18]	NG	ELISA	2.02	1991
Satoskar et al[19]	3104	ELISA	4.7	1992
Poona				
Kelkar et al[20]	420	AGD	1.49	1973
Aurangabad				
Kotuwal et al[21]	625	IEOP	4.0	1973
Madhya Pradesh				
Tribal population				
Joshi et al[22]	1314	RPHA	12.26	1990
Arunachal Pradesh				
Tribal population				
Prasad et al[23]	755	CIEP	5.58	1983
Prasad et al[23]	296	RPHA	8.45	
South India – Vellore				
Singhvi et al[24]	35395	ELISA	2.16	1990
Chennai				
Sumathy et al[25]	530	ELISA	7.17	1993
Mohan et al[26]	1036	ELISA	3.76	1998
Thyagarajan et al[5] (community population)	1856	ELISA	5.7	1998
Madras				
Tamil Nadu Tribal population				
Althaf Hussain et al[27]	227	ELISA	24.5	1991
Kerala – Trivandrum				
Shanmugham et al[28]	475	CIEOP	1.50	1978
Shangmugham et al[29]	240	CIE	2.5	1981
Jayaprakash et al[30]	8085	CIEP	1.25	1983
Shanmugham et al[31]	10,600	CIEP	1.3	1984

The 18 publications that were analysed for HBV prevalence in the ante-natal pregnant women has shown it to be between 1–12.3% with the mean prevalence of 4.22%. Rajasthan came under the <2% zone; Maharashtra and Tamil Nadu as the intermediate zone of 2–4%; Karnataka, Kerala, Delhi, Haryana and Uttar Pradesh as above 4% zones. Again, regional variation is observed significantly (Table 2). Community prevalence studies are considered as better denominators for assessing the disease burden in a country than the blood donor screening data representing general population. Literature search has revealed two such HBV

Table 2. Prevalence of HBsAg in antenatal pregnant women in India

Place / author	Number	Method	HBsAg positive No. (%)	Year
Rajasthan				
Vyas et al[32]	500	CIE	5 (1.0)	1983
Gupta et al[33]	1000	CIE	22 (2.2)	1985
Chandigarh				
Sehgal et al[34]	4137	ELISA	109 (2.6)	1992
Biswas et al[35]	1000	ELISA	23 (2.3)	1989
Gupta et al[36]	2337	ELISA	58 (2.5)	1992
Delhi				
Tandon et al[37]	837	ELISA	30 (3.6)	1986
Nayak et al[38]	8575	ELISA	322 (3.7)	1984
Panda et al[39]	8431	ELISA	191 (2.6)	1991
Mittal et al[40]	850	ELISA	54 (6.3)	1996
Sharma et al[41]	157	RPHA/ELISA	16 (10.0)	1996
Maharashtra – Mumbai				
Panda et al[39]	1276	RIA	8 (0.6)	1991
Gill et al[42]	2000	ELISA	100 (5.0)	1995
Uttar Pradesh – Varanasi				
Khatri et al[43]	400	RPHA	19 (4.8)	1980
Karnataka				
Kulkarni et al[44]	400	RPHA	20 (5.0)	1988
Kerala – Trivandrum				
Shanmugham et al[28]	400	CIE	12 (3.0)	1978
Shanmugham et al[29]	260	CIE	12 (4.6)	1981
Maheswari et al[45]	300	ELISA	37 (12.3)	1985
Tamil Nadu – Chennai				
Thyagarajan et al[46]	400	ELISA	17 (3.9)	1993

community prevalence studies from India.[4,5] The HBsAg prevalence was 5.3% in the West Bengal study by Choudhury et al, and 5.7% in the Tamil Nadu study by the Thyagarajan et al (Table 3).

Table 3. Community prevalence of chronic HBV infection in three districts of Tamil Nadu[5]

Districts	Number	HBsAg positive	%	95% CI
Thanjavur	573	21	3.7	2.34–5.45
Ramnad	650	62	9.5	7.45–11.98
Dindigul	633	23	3.6	2.37–5.31
Total	1856	106	5.7	2.9–7.6

The replicative status of HBV in the general population as denoted by HBeAg positivity based on the seven reports revealed a range of 2.6 to 56.1% with a mean rate of 24.22%. Similar to HBsAg prevalence, HBeAg prevalence also showed regional variation within India, with Maharashtra having below 10%; Delhi between 10 and 20% while Tamil Nadu, Kerala and Andhra Pradesh showing the HBeAg positivity of more than 20% (Table 4). The antenatal pregnant women revealed HBeAg positivity range of 7.8–47.8% (mean: 24.01%) based on seven different studies from India. Geographic variation within India became discernible in

Table 4. Prevalence pattern of HBeAg positive (replicative) and HBeAg negative (non-replicative / integrated) HBsAg positive subjects in India

Category/place	Author/year	HBsAg positive tested sera	HBeAg positive No. (%)	HBeAg negative No. (%)	Method
Pregnant women					
Chandigarh	Biswas et al (1989)[35]	23	11 (47.8)	12 (52.2)	ELISA
Delhi	Nayak et al (1984)[38]	322	25 (7.8)	297 (92.2)	ELISA
Delhi	Panda et al (1991)[39]	191	24 (12.5)	167 (87.5)	ELISA
Delhi	Mittal et al (1996)[40]	54	10 (18.0)	44 (82.0)	ELISA
Bombay	Gill et al (1995)[42]	100	12 (12.0)	88 (88.0)	ELISA
Trivandrum	Shanmugham et al (1983)[47]	32	13 (40.6)	19 (59.4)	ID
Madras	Thyagarajan et al (1992)[46]	17	5 (29.4)	12 (70.6)	ELISA
Blood donors and general population					
Delhi	Tandon et al (1979)[48]	10	1 (10.0)	9 (90.0)	ELISA
Bombay	Joshi et al (1983)[16]	38	1 (2.6)	37 (97.4)	CIE
Trivandrum	Shanmugham et al (1983)[47]	65	16 (24.6)	49 (75.4)	ID
	Shanmugham et al (1994)[49]	60	17 (28.3)	43 (71.7)	ELISA
Madras	Thyagarajan et al (1980)[50]	20	5 (25.0)	15 (75.0)	Rheophoresis ELISA
	Thyagarajan et al (1997)[51]	146	82 (56.1)	64 (43.9)	Rheophoresis ELISA
	Mohan et al (1998)[26]	39	9 (23.0)	30 (77.0)	ELISA

these groups of data also with Delhi and Maharashtra exhibiting intermediate HBeAg positivity of 10–20%. Kerala, Tamil Nadu and Haryana belonging to high HBeAg prevalent states (Table 4). In the two community based data from India, the HBeAg prevalence was 3.9% in the West Bengal study, while, it was 23.4% in the Tamil Nadu study (Table 5).

This again shows the pattern of geographic variation as seen in the data derived from blood donors representing the general population.

Table 5. Replicative (HBeAg positive) status of HBV in general population at the community level in West Bengal and Tamil Nadu

Region	Author/year	Number tested	HBsAg positive no. (%)	HBeAg positive no. (%)	Anti-HBe positive no. (%)
West Bengal	Choudhury et al (1999)[4]	960	51 (5.3%)	2 (3.9%)	ND
Tamil Nadu	Thyagarajan et al (2000)[5]	1856	106 (5.7%)	25 (23.4%)	81 (76.4%)

The risk of exposure to HBV infection in the high-risk groups in India ranges between 1.4 and 45% in different regions approximately 5 to 20 times more common than in the general population. The highest incidence is seen in hemodialysis patients, thalassemics, family contacts of HBsAg positive subjects, injecting drug users, STD patients, professional blood donors, truck drivers, etc. (Table 6).

Table 6. Prevalence of HBsAg status in high-risk groups in India

HRG/place	Author/Year	Number tested	HBsAg positive (%)	Method
Professional blood donors				
Delhi	Irshad et al (1992)[52]	1800	11.7	ELISA
Calcutta	Roy Choudhary et al (1989)[14]	–	5.84	ELISA
Calcutta	Ahmed et al (1984)[53]	–	5.0	ELISA
Trivandrum	Shanmugham et al (1983)[54]	154	13.1	ELISA
Vellore	Hill et al (1973)[55]	1546	3.80	CIE
Madras	Thyagarajan et al (1978)[56]	1100	4.9	CIE
Hospital personnel				
Chandigarh	Lalit Kant (1995)[57]	202	4.0	ELISA
Delhi	Irshad et al (1994)[7]	1313	1.4	CIE
Delhi	Joshi et al (1996)[58]	318	4.4	ELISA
Delhi	Lalit Kant (1995)[57]	83	10.9	ELISA
Delhi	Lalit Kant (1995)[57]	184	8.2	ELISA
Shimla	Thakur et al (1990)[13]	200	8.0	RPHA
Shimla	Lalit Kant et al (1995)[57]	250	16	ELISA
Bombay	Elavia & Banker (1992)[18]	863	10.0	ELISA
Bombay	Lalit Kant (1995)[57]	114	7.9	ELISA
Bombay	Lalit Kant (1995)[57]	606	6.6	ELISA
Ahmed Nagar	Jain et al (1992)[59]	188	2.7	RPHA
Pune	Chobe et al (1991)[60]	510	3.12	ELISA
Trivandrum	Shanmugham et al (1983)[54]	60	6.6	ELISA
Madras (Dental)	Thyagarajan et al (1986)[61]	224	14.2	RPHA
Madras (Medical)	Thyagarajan et al (1981)[62]	127	16.5	RPHA
Madras (Medical)	Mohan et al (1997)[26]	78	6.4	ELISA

(Contd.)

(Contd.)

HRG/place	Author/Year	Number tested	HBsAg positive No. (%)	Method
Family contacts				
Poona	Dhorje et al (1985)[63]	193	11.3	ELISA
Poona	Arankalle et al (1990)[64]	–	39.0	ELISA
Madras	Jayaram et al (1992)[46]	22	41.5	ELISA
Madras	Thyagarajan et al (1996)[65]	140	24.2	ELISA
STD patients				
Bombay	Kura et al (1998)[66]	182	8.8	ELISA
Shimla	Thakur et al (1990)[13]	1193	9.55	RPHA
Madras	Thyagarajan et al (1991)[67]	135	10.37	ELISA
Haemodialysis and renal transplant patients				
Multicentric	Study group (1997)[68]	540	8.1	ELISA
Madras	Mani et al (1994)[69]	1339	7.7	ELISA
Madras	Mohan et al (1997)[26]	165	35.1	ELISA
Thalassemic patients				
Bombay	Amrapurkar et al (1992)[70]	40	45	ELISA
Bombay	Jolly et al (1992)[71]	250	15.5	ELISA
Calcutta	De et al (1990)[72]		22.1	ELISA
Injecting drug users (IDUs)				
Calcutta	Panda et al (1998)[73]	103	20.0	ELISA
Madras	Mohan et al (1998)[26]	177	24.8	ELISA
Manipur	Saha et al (2000)[74]	77	100	ELISA
Commercial sex workers				
Delhi	Irshad et al (1994)[7]	635	3.6	ELISA
Truck drivers				
Delhi	Irshad et al (1994)[7]	217	5.0	ELISA

Much has been written during the last decade on all the aspects of hepatitis B infection and an enormous bibliography has accumulated on the complex epidemiological patterns of hepatitis B. Reliable information on the incidence and long-term trend of hepatitis B is available from few western countries only. However, the worldwide pattern of HBV infection has been categorized epidemiologically as high HBsAg prevalence zones (8–20%); intermediate prevalence zones (2–8%) and low prevalence areas (below 2%). While this general pattern is true, it is rather an oversimplification as individual countries may encompass several populations or groups with widely different infection rates. For example, in Australia, the rate of HBsAg positivity among people of British origin is about 1 per 1000 (0.1%) compared with 2–3% among migrants from Southern Europe and upto 15% in migrants from South East Asia, Australian aborigines (Maori population) and Torres Strait islanders.[75]

Although, India is categorised under intermediate prevalence zone, a similar picture of variability of mean prevalence rate of HBV infection in general population within different states of India has been observed in the present analysis with higher HBsAg prevalence in Uttar Pradesh (6.05%), Karnataka (5.0%), Tamil Nadu (4.69%), Maharashtra (3.1%), Himachal Pradesh (3.26%), Delhi (2.58%), Chandigarh (2.4%), West Bengal (2.29%), Rajasthan (1.6%), Kerala (1.39%) and Kashmir (1.1%). Similar variations have also been observed in the HBeAg positivity (Tables 1 and 2).

The replicative status of the virus not only increases the rate of HBV transmission, but also the progression of liver disease. It is an accepted view that the risk of HBV transmission depends, besides the host factors, on the survival and persistence of HBV in the population, prolonged shedding of the virus, and the hygienic conditions of the environment.

The overall picture of HBV infection when analysed in the background of this information underscores the following factors as responsible for the variability in its prevalence pattern even within the geographic regions of India: (a) The relative prevalence rate of infective HBV subjects as denoted by HBeAg positivity in antenatal women, newborns, children and general population seem to have influenced the higher prevalence of HBV in symptomatic acute and chronic liver diseases including hepatocellular carcinoma and (b) literacy of the population in the respective regions like Kerala, Kashmir, Delhi, Chandigarh who by better health awareness of keeping satisfactory personal and environmental hygiene might maintain a low HBV prevalence in these areas by restricting horizontal transmission. The fact that prolonged healthy carriage of HBsAg is not always a benign phenomenon, but frequently associated with the development of chronic liver disease and/or primary hepatocellular carcinoma has been fully established by the prospective study of 22,000 civil servants by Beasley and Huang in Taiwan followed up for 10 years. This study has clearly shown that the subjects with chronic HBV infection had 200 times increased risk of developing chronic hepatitis or hepatocellular carcinoma than the matched control subjects.[76] Asia and Africa have previously been classified as areas of high endemicity for hepatitis B virus (HBV), but in some countries highly effective vaccination programs have shifted this pattern towards intermediate or low endemicity. Thus, China is now the only country in Asia where HBV endemicity is high. Countries with intermediate endemicity include India, Korea, Philippines, Taiwan and Thailand, and those with low endemicity include Japan, Pakistan, Bangladesh, Singapore, Sri Lanka and Malaysia. Most countries in Africa have high HBV endemicity, with the exceptions of Tunisia and Morocco, which have intermediate endemicity. Zambia has borderline intermediate/high endemicity. In the Middle East, Bahrain, Iran, Israel and Kuwait are areas of low endemicity; Cyprus, Iraq and the United Arab Emirates have intermediate endemicity; and Egypt, Jordan, Oman, Palestine, Yemen and Saudi Arabia have high endemicity. All of these Middle East countries reach a large proportion of their population with hepatitis B vaccination, which is reducing the infection rate, particularly in Saudi Arabia. The vaccination program in Taiwan has also greatly reduced the HBV infection rate. Future vaccination programs must take into account the mode of transmission of HBV, the health care infrastructure to deliver vaccination, and the socioeconomic and political factors in each individual country to determine the most cost-effective way of infection control.[77,78]

REFERENCES

1. Thyagarajan SP, Jayaram S, Mohanavalli B. *Prevalence of HBV in general population in India. In:* Sarin SK, Singal AK. Eds. Hepatitis B in India: Problems and Prevention. CBS Publishers & Distributors, New Delhi, 1996; pp. 5-16.
2. Evans AA, London WT. *Epidemiology of hepatitis B. In:* Zuckerman AJ, Thomas HC. Eds. *Viral Hepatitis*: Harcourt Brace & Co. Ltd. London, United Kingdom, 1998; pp. 107-14.
3. Hyams KC. Risk of chronicity following acute hepatitis B infection. *Clin Infect Dis* 1995;20:992-1000.
4. Chowdhury A, Santra A, Chaudhuri S, Ghosh A, Banerjee P, Majumder DN. Prevalence of hepatitis B infection in the general population: a rural community based study. *Trop Gastroenterol* 1999;20: 75-7.
5. Thyagarajan SP, Jayaseelan KT, Rajendran P, Hari R, Krishnamurthy P, Sudhakar K. High community prevalence of STD/Hepatitis B/HIV in Tamilnadu. *Lancet* 1998 (submitted).
6. Nanu A, Sharma SP, Chatterjee K, Jyoti P. Markers for transfusion–transmissible infections in north Indian voluntary and replacement blood donors: prevalence and trends: 1989-1996. *Vox Sang* 1997;73: 70-3.
6a. Singal AK, Kaur V. Prevalence of HBsAg in population referred to a hospital in North Delhi. *Indian J Gastroenterol* 2000;20(suppl 3):C75-6.
7. Irshad M, Joshi YK, Acharya SK, Tandon BN. Prevalence of hepatitis B virus infection in healthy persons in north India. *Natl Med J Ind* 1994;7:210-2.
8. Dutta RN, Mohammed GS. Incidence of Australia antigen in voluntary and professional blood donors and also in cases of viral Hepatitis. *Ind J Med Res* 1972;60:1774-8.
9. Pal SR, Dutta DV, Choudhary S, Jolly JG, Deodhar SD, Samant AKS, Chitkara NL, et al. Serum hepatitis (SH) antigen HBsAg among patients with liver diseases and voluntary blood donors–prospective study. *Ind J Med Res* 1973;61:1784-98.
10. Makroo RN, Hasan G, Koul A, Shah GN. Incidence of HBsAg in Kashmiri blood donors. *Ind J Med Res* 1989;89:310-3.
11. Nagaraju K, Misra S, Saraswat S, Choudhary N, Hasih B, Ramesh V, Naik S. High prevalence of HBV infectivity in blood donors detected by the dot-blot hybridisation assay. *Vox Sang* 1994;67:183-6.
12. Choudhury N, Ramesh V, Saraswat S, Naik S. Effectiveness of mandatory transmissible diseases screening in Indian blood donors. *Ind J Med Res* 1995;105:229-32.
13. Thakur TS, Goyal A, Sharma V, Gupta ML, Singh S. Incidence of Australia antigen (HBsAg) in Himachal Pradesh. *J Commun Dis* 1990;22:173-7.
14. Roy Choudhry A, Bhattacharya DK. Incidence of hepatitis B carriers in Calcutta, West Bengal. *J Assoc Phys Ind* 1989;37:160.
15. Chakraborthy MS, Mukherjee KK, Mithra KK, Ghosh S, Chowdhary SK, Kundu S. Association between Australia antigen and leprosy in Calcutta. *Bull Cal Sch Trop Med* 1977;25:19-21.
16. Joshi SH, Baxi AJ, Mukherjee BN, Malhotra KC, Kate SL. Incidence of hepatitis B antigen among three communities in western Maharashtra, India. *India Hum Hered* 1983:33:231-6.
17. Elavia AJ, Banker DD. Prevalence of HBsAg and its subtypes in high-risk group subjects and voluntary blood donors in Bombay. *Ind J Med Res* 1991;93:280.
18. Elavia AJ, Banker DD. Hepatitis B virus infection in hospital personnel. *Natl Med J Ind* 1992;5: 265-8.

19. Satoskar A, Ray V. Prevalence of HBsAg in blood donors from Bombay. *Trop Gegr Med* 1992;44: 119-21.
20. Kelkar SS, Niphadkar KB, Khare PM. Titres of Australia (hepatitis-associated) antigen in healthy carriers, leprosy, cirrhosis of liver and acute hepatitis. *Ind J Med Res* 1973;61:684-8.
21. Kotwal SF, Kelkar SS. Hepatitis B antigen in endemic hepatitis at Aurangabad. *Ind J Med Sci* 1973;27: 856-60.
22. Joshi SH, Gorakshakar AC, Mukherjee M, Rao VR, Sathe MS, Anabhavane SM, Bhatia HM. Prevalence of HBsAg carriers among some tribes of Madhya Pradesh. *Ind J Med Res* 1990;91:340-3.
23. Prasad SR, Rodrigues FM, Dhorje SP, Ramamoorthy CL. Prevalence and subtypes of HBsAg in the tribal population in Arunachal Pradesh, India. *Ind J Med Res* 1983;78:300-6.
24. Singhvi A, Pulimood RB, John TJ, Babu PG, Samuel BU, Padankatti T, Carman RH. The prevalence of markers of hepatitis B, HIV, malarial parasites and microfilaria in blood donors in a large hospital in South India. *J Trop Med Hyg* 1990;93:178-82.
25. Sumathy S, Thyagarajan SP, Latif R, Madanagopalan N, Raghuram K, Rajasambandam P, Gowans E. A dip stick immunobinding enzyme linked immunosorbent assay for serodiagnosis of hepatitis B and delta virus infections. *J Virol Methods* 1992;38:145-9.
26. Mohan KVK, Hari R, Murugavel KG, Balasubramanian J. Prevalence of HBV/HCV markers in blood donors and high-risk groups. PhD thesis, University of Madras, 1997.
27. Althaf Hussain I, Rajendran P, Thyagarajan SP. HBsAg and HIV antibody in tribal populations of Tamilnadu, India. *Virus Inf Exch New Lett* 1991:8:62.
28. Shanmugham J, Balakrishnan V, Venugopalan P, Sukumaran C. Prevalence of HBsAg in blood donors and pregnant women from southern Kerala. *Ind J Med Res* 1978;68:91-6.
29. Shanmugham J, Molly Thomas, Jasper Daniel, Jayaprakash PA. Detection of HBsAg by CIEP and RPHA techniques in healthy individuals and cardiac patients. *Ind J Med Res* 1981;73:543-7.
30. Jayaprakash PA, Shanmugham J, Hariprasad D. Hepatitis B surface antigen in blood donors. An epidemiologic study. *Transfusion* 1983;23:346-7.
31. Shanmugham J, Molly Thomas, Jeyaprakash PA. Serological markers of hepatitis B virus among HBsAg carriers from Kerala state – south India Hepatitis Scientific Memoranda, 1984;3:45.
32. Vyas KK, Mathur AK, Vyas RK. A study of prevalence of HBsAg among pregnant women. *J Obstet Gynae India* 1983:33:778-81.
33. Gupta ML, Sharma U, Saxena S, Sharma ML, Pokharna DS. Vertical transmission of HBsAg from asymptomatic carrier mothers. *Indian Pediatr* 1985;22:339-42.
34. Sehgal A, Gupta I, Sehgal R, Ganguly NK. Hepatitis B vaccine alone or in combination with anti-HBs immunoglobulin in the perinatal prophylaxis of babies born to HBsAg carrier mothers. *Acta Virol* 1992;39:359-66.
35. Biswas SC, Gupta I, Ganguly NK, Chawla Y, Dilawari JB. Prevalence of hepatitis B surface antigen in pregnant mothers and its perinatal transmission. *Trans Royal Soc Tropical Med and Hyg* 1989;83: 698-700.
36. Gupta I, Sehgal A, Sehgal R, Ganguly NK. Vertical transmission of hepatitis B in north India. *J Hyg Epid Microbiol Immunol* 1992;36:263-7.
37. Tandon BN, Joshi YK, Gandhi BM, Irshad I, Gupta H, Gupta ML. Epidemiology of HBsAg carriers in India. A holistic approach to control of hepatitis B reservoir. *J Gastroentrol Hepatol* 1986;1:39-43.
38. Nayak NC, Panda SK, Zuckerman AJ, Bhan MK, Guha DK. Dynamics and impact of perinatal transmission of hepatitis B virus in north India. *J Med Virol* 1984;21:137-45.
39. Panda SK, Ramesh Rajagopal, Rao VS Kanury. Comparative evaluation of the immunogenicity of yeast derived (recombinant) and plasma-derived hepatitis B vaccine in infants. *J Med Virol* 1991; 35:297-302.

40. Mittal SK, Rao S, Rastogi A, Aggarwal V, Kumari S. Hepatitis B potential of perinatal transmission in India. *Trop Gastroenterol* 1996;17:190-2.
41. Sharma R, Malik A, Rattan A, Iraqi A, Maheswari V, Dhawan R. Hepatitis B virus infection in pregnant women and its transmission to infants. *J Trop Pediatrics* 1996;42:352-4.
42. Gill HH, Majumdar PD, Dhunjibhoy KR, Desai HG. Prevalence of hepatitis B e antigen in pregnant women and patients with liver disease. *J Assoc Phys India* 1995;43:247-8.
43. Khatri JV, Kulkarni KV, Vaishnav PR, Merchant SM. Vertical transmission of hepatitis B. *Indian Pediatr* 1980;27:957-62.
44. Kulkarni ML, Reddy PV. Prevalence of HBsAg in asymptomatic carrier mothers and vertical transmission in south India. *Am J Dis Child* 1988;142:124-5.
45. Maheswari TR, Devi RS, Shenoy KT, Sathiavathy N, Balakrishnan V. A Study of hepatitis B antigenemia in pregnant females and the risk of transmission to babies. *Indian J Gastroentrol* 1985;4:83.
46. Jayaram S, Thyagarajan SP. Prevalence of HBV markers in different age groups in Madras. Ph.D. thesis on "Prevention and control of Hepatitis B in Tamilnadu". Univ. of Madras, 1992.
47. Shanmugham J, Balakrishnan V, Molly Thomas, Jayaprakash PA. Prevalence of HBeAg and anti-HBe in Asymptomatic HBsAg carriers and patients with liver disease. *Ind J Pathol Microbiol* 1983; 26:1-5.
48. Tandon BN, Krishnamurthy L, Gandhi BM. HBeAg and anti-HBe in acute and chronic liver diseases. *Ind J Med Res* 1979;70:102-6.
49. Shanmugham J, Naseema K, Mathai J. HBeAg and anti-HBe among healthy HBsAg carriers from Kerala state–detection by micro-elisa. *Ind J Virol* 1994;10:67-71.
50. Thyagarajan SP, Subramanian S, Solomon S, Madanagopalan N. Pattern of HBeAg and anti-HBe among blood donors and patients with liver diseases in Tamilnadu. *Ind J Med Res* 1980;71:309-12.
51. Thyagarajan SP, Jayaram S, Panneerselvam A, Malathy S, Madanagopalan N. Characterisation of healthy hepatitis B surface antigen (HBsAg) carriers in Tamilnadu, India. *Ind J Med Microbiol* 1997; 15:163-6.
52. Irshad M, Singh YN, Acharya SK. HBV status in professional blood donors in north India. *Trop Gastroenterol* 1992;13:112-4.
53. Ahmed A, Chakraborthy MS, Mukherjee MK, De PN. Incidence of hepatitis B surface antigen (HBsAg) in liver diseases in Calcutta. *Cal Med J* 1984;81:86.
54. Shanmugham J, Balkrishnan KG, Hariprasad D. HBsAg detection by Micro-enzyme lanked immunosorbent assay (ELISA) technique. *Ind J Pathol Microbiol* 1983;26:121.
55. Hill PG, Jacob John T, Shanmugam RV, Carman H. Australia antigen in blood donors in Vellore. *Ind J Med Res* 1973;61:378-401
56. Thyagarajan SP, Subramanian S, Sundaravelu T, Madanagopalan N. Incidence of HBsAg and hepatitis B surface antibody in patients with liver diseases, blood donors and leprosy patients – A preliminary report. *Ind J Med Res* 1978;67:528-34.
57. Lalit Kant. Frequency of HBsAg positivity in health care workers in India. ICMR Report, 1995, as quoted by Joshi YK in *"Prevalence of hepatitis B in health care workers" In*: Hepatitis B in India – Problems and Prevention: Sarin SK, Singal AK, Eds. CBS Publishers & Distributors, New Delhi, 1996;pp. 33-8.
58. Joshi YK. *"Prevalence of hepatitis B in health care workers"*. In: Hepatitis B in India – Problems and Prevention: Sarin SK, Singal AK, Eds. CBS Publishers & Distributors, New Delhi, 1996;pp. 33-8.
59. Jain RC, Bhat SD, Sangle S. Prevalence of HBsAg among rural population of Loni area in Ahmednagar district of Western Maharashtra. *J Assoc Phys Ind* 1992;40:390-1.
60. Chobe LP, Chadha MS, Arankalle VA, Gogate SS, Banerjee K. Hepatitis B infection among dental personnel in Pune & Bombay, India. *Ind J Med Res* 1991;93:143-6.

61. Thyagarajan SP, Jayalakshmi M, Subramanian S, Suniti Solomon, Gnanasundaram M. Hepatitis B virus markers in dental personnel, dental patients and their dental specimens. *J Ind Dent Assoc* 1986;58:181-5.
62. Thyagarajan SP, Subramanian S, Sundaravelu T, Sivakumar S, Prasad PR, Thiruvengadam KV. Hepatitis B surface antigen carriers among hospital personnel (A sero-study in Govt. General Hospital, Madras). *J Assoc Phys Ind* 1981;29:941-5.
63. Dhorje SP, Pavri KM, Prasad SR, Sehgal A, Phule DM. Horizontal transmission of hepatitis B virus infection in household contacts, Pune, India. *J Med Virol* 1985;16:183-9.
64. Arankalle VA, Chadha MS, Banerjee K. Necessity to vaccinate spouses of hepatitis B patients and carriers. *J Assoc Phys Ind* 1990;36:517.
65. Thyagarajan SP, Jayaram S, Hari R, Sridhar G, Rani E, Paneerselvam A. Familial clustering of HBV among HBsAg carrier and non-carrier family members in India. *Biomedicine* 1996;16:21-7.
66. Kura MM, Hira S, Kohli M, Dalal PJ, Ramnani VK, Jagtap MR. High occurrence of HBV among STD clinic attenders in Bombay, India. *Int J STD & AIDS* 1998;9:231-3.
67. Thyagarajan SP, Kantharaj K, Parthasarathy S. Incidence of HBsAg among patients attending the STD clinic. Proceedings – International Union against general Diseases and Treponematoses conference – Christ Church, New Zealand. 1991; pp. 11-3.
68. The living non-related Renal Transplant Study Group. Commercially motivated renal transplantation: results in 540 patients transplanted in India. *Clin Transplant* 1997;11:536-44.
69. Mani MK, Bhaskaran S, Prakash KC. A study of hepatitis B surface antigen positive patients on hemodialysis and following transplantation. *J Assoc Phys Ind* 1994;42:363-5.
70. Amrapurkar DN, Kumar A, Vaidya S. Frequency of hepatitis B, C and D and human immunodeficiency virus infection in multi-transfused thalassemics. *Indian J Gastroenterol* 1992;11:80-3.
71. Jolly JG, Agnihotri SK, Choudhury N, Gupta D. Evaluation of hemotherapy in thalassemias (20 years of Indian experience). *J Ind Med Assoc* 1992;90:7-9.
72. De M, Banerjee D, Chandra S, Bhattacharya DK. HBV and HCV in multi-transfused hemophilacs and thalassemics in eastern India. *Ind J Med Res* 1990;91:63-6.
73. Panda S, Chatterjee A, Bhattacharjee S, Ray B, Saha MK, Bhattacharya SK. HIV, Hepatitis B and sexual practices in the street recruited injecting drug users of Calcutta: risk perception versus observed risks. *Int J STD & AIDS* 1998;9:214-8.
74. Saha MK, Chakrabarti S, Panda S, Naik TN, Manna B, Chatterjee A, Detals R, et al. Prevalence of HCV and HBV infection among HIV sero positive intravenous drug users and their non-injecting house wives in Manipur, India. *Ind J Med Res* 2000;111:37-9.
75. Gust ID. *Epidemiology of hepatitis B in Australia.* In: Lam SK, Lai CL, Yeoh EK, Eds. Viral Hepatitis B infection, World Scientific Singapore, 1984;pp.19-22.
76. Beasley RP, Li CC, Hwang LY, Chien SS. *Risk of hepatocellular carcinoma in HBV infections: a prospective study in Taiwan.* In: Szmuness W, Alter HJ, Maynard. Eds. Viral hepatitis. The Franklin Institute Press, Philadelphia, 1981;261-70.
77. Andre F. Hepatitis B epidemiology in Asia, the middle east and Africa. *Vaccine* 2000;18(suppl 1): S20-2.
78. Tandon BN, Acharya SK, Tandon A. Epidemiology of hepatitis B virus infection in India. *Gut* 1996;38(suppl 2):S56-9.

2

Modes of transmission of hepatitis B virus

Ajay Duseja, Yogesh K Chawla

Hepatitis B Virus (HBV) is a partially double-stranded DNA virus that belongs to the family of Hepadnaviruses.[1] No important animal reservoir of this virus is known and humans themselves are the only important source for human infection. Some non-human primates are known to be the reservoir of this virus but are unlikely to infect the humans in view of the intimate contact required for the transmission of this virus.[2] Although, HBsAg has been detected in urine, bile, tears, sweat, vaginal secretions, breast milk, cerebrospinal fluid, and synovial fluid; only serum, saliva and semen are reported to be infectious from chimp studies. The concentration of HBsAg is low in secretions other than serum. HBV may be detected in feces only when the patient has had a gastrointestinal bleed.

Most HBV infections result from parenteral route and sexual route but uncommonly non-parenteral routes of transmission of HBV have also been described.[2] The methods of spread of hepatitis B virus vary according to the geographic region.[3] In developing countries with a high prevalence of HBsAg, perinatal transmission from mother to infant occurs at or soon after birth, or horizontal transmission may occur later in infancy or early childhood. In developed nations, however, majority of infections are acquired in adolescence and adulthood.[3] For HBV transmission to occur, there should be a source, mode, and a susceptible host.

SOURCE

The source of spread is usually blood from chronic HBsAg positive subjects having a high level of virus in the blood. These subjects are usually asymptomatic, unaware of their potential infectivity which could vary from <10 virions/ml to >10^8 virions/ml. Patients who are HBeAg positive have levels more than 10^6 virions/ml, while anti-HBe positive patients have lower levels of virus concentration. This explains the higher incidence of transmission from HBeAg positive than anti-HBe positive subjects. Thus, all HBsAg positive blood is infectious, more so, when HBV-DNA and HBeAg are positive in the blood. A needle-stick exposure of HBeAg positive blood may transmit HBV as even 0.001 ml of plasma has levels of more than 10^3 virions/ml. Transmission has also been reported with HBsAg negative but anti-HBc positive blood representing low levels of infection.

MODES OF SPREAD

Parenteral

Parenteral routes of transmission of HBV include injection drug use, receipt of blood products and organs, and occupational exposure.[1] Other forms of parenteral spread are tattooing, ear-piercing, acupuncture, sharing needles and less frequent sources include hemodialysis and iatrogenic transmission.[4]

Drug abuse

This is an important cause in developed countries due to sharing of drug paraphernalia, which may be eliminated by use of disposable syringes and needles. The risk of infection is directly proportional to the duration of drug abuse, the incidence being higher if it is used for more than 5 years. Data from India also favors this as a source of infection in injecting drug users. In an explosive outbreak of HBV in Sirsa, Haryana, majority of patients with acute hepatitis B had received therapeutic injections before their illness.[5] Similarly, reuse of needles by medical and paramedical practioners for administering antileishmanial drugs to patients with Kala-Azar in Bihar, resulted in high prevalence of HBV (13.2%) in these patients.[6] Male spouses of 77 Manipuri couples, who were intravenous drug abusers and HIV positive, were found to be infected with HBV as well.[7]

Transfusion of blood and blood products

This is a less important mode of spread in countries where HBsAg screening is done in the donor's samples. It accounts for <1% of cases of HBV in USA, UK, and Ireland. Blood transfusion in India has its own problems, priorities and practicalities because of economic constraints, which limit screening and safety.[8] In a study on transfusion transmitted diseases in hemophiliacs from western India, 24 out of 400 (6%) were found to be positive for HBsAg.[9] Attack rate depends on the number of units transfused; administration of blood derivatives like commercially prepared plasma fractions including clotting factor concentrates, cryoprecipitates and fibrinogen. This transmission may have serious consequences like chronic liver disease in hemophiliacs and thalassemics. Recently, dry or wet heating and affinity purification of proteins and use of donors with a safe pedigree has further decreased the risk of hepatitis B. Risk still persists and these products should be used in patients who have received the HBV vaccine. There have been reports of HBV transmission by factor VIII concentrates that were negative for HBsAg and HBV-DNA indicating that heat treatment is not effective in eradicating HBV and suggests that low levels of HBV-DNA may transmit hepatitis.

Hemodialysis

Transmission via contamination has been most clearly implicated in hemodialysis units.[2] The prevalence of HBV in dialysis population in India[10] is reported to range from 3.4% to 42%. Numerous investigators have demonstrated that widespread blood contamination in such units, and transfer of virus from contaminated surfaces to nurses' hands and then to other patients can occur. Implementation of routine screening and isolation of HBV positive subjects and strict rules against sharing of all dialysis equipment breaks the cycle and decreases the disease transmission.

Health care workers

Transmission may also occur from doctors and health care workers to patients and vice-versa.[11] Three factors have been critical for transmission to occur: (i) if the health care worker is highly infectious (HBeAg positive), (ii) the worker performs traumatic procedure or surgery on patients, (iii) if the worker has dermatitis or traumatic lesions of the skin during work which allows his blood to be introduced percutaneously into the patient. A needle stick exposure of HBeAg positive blood may transmit HBV as even 0.001 ml of plasma has levels of more than 10^3 virions/ml. As compared to HCV and HIV–1, HBV has the maximum risk of transmission after a needle-stick injury. HBV has risk of getting transmitted in 30% of exposures compared to 3% in HCV and 0.3% in HIV–1 after a needle-stick injury.[12]

Materno-fetal transmission

In Taiwan, it has been estimated that 40–50% of chronic HBsAg positive subjects acquired their infection in the perinatal period[13] with only 5–10% of these infected in-utero (transplacental), majority getting infected at the time of delivery or in the first few months or years of life by contact with their infected mothers or siblings. Maternal milk may also be the source of infection. It is estimated that about one third of adult asymptomatic chronic HBsAg positive subjects in India evolve directly from perinatal infection, while the majority become infected during childhood or adulthood.[14]

A recent study[15] analysed the risk factors of transplacental transmission of HBV and found a significant association between the intrauterine HBV transmission and HBV infection in villous capillary endothelial cells (VCEC) in the placenta. The other significant risk factors of transplacental HBV transmission were maternal serum HBeAg positivity and history of threatened preterm labour.[15] Mutations in the C gene of HBV have also been associated with vertical transmission.[16] To prevent vertical transmission of HBV, lamivudine was used in a mother but could not prevent the perinatal transmission to the newborn in spite of HBV-DNA suppression in the mother.[17]

Organ transplantation

1. Liver transplantation from a HBV positive donor to a negative recipient can transmit the virus to the recipient. In a recent study, a liver transplant recipient who was negative pre-transplant for all HBV markers, became positive for HBsAg, six months after the transplantation.[18] The liver was obtained from a donor who was negative for HBsAg but positive for anti-HBs and anti-HBc.
2. There are case reports where HBV was suspected to have been transmitted by penetrating keratoplasty. In a recent study, 29 corneas of 17 donors seropositive by ELISA for HBsAg and 27 corneas of 14 donors seropositive by ELISA for anti-HCV were evaluated.[19] The organ culture media and the sera were screened for the presence of HBV-DNA or HCV RNA by PCR. Viral genomes of HBV could not be detected in the organ culture media by PCR (detection limit 100–1000 copies/ml) in any of the corneas, thereby signifying that the transmission through this route is low.[19]

Insects

The transmission through insects may be important in tropical countries. HBsAg has been detected in mosquitoes[2] and bedbugs. Virus does not replicate in insects but persists for several weeks after the insects have been fed HBV artificially. In South Africa, HBsAg was detected in 25 out of 29 pools of blood-fed mosquitoes caught in an institution for black children.

Other forms of parenteral spread

Tattooing and acupuncture with sharing of non-sterile needles, instruments and dye have occasionally accounted for large outbreaks of HBV infection. In one of the studies[20] there was significant association between the increasing number of tattoos and HBV infection and also an association between having non professional tattooing and testing positive for one of the transfusion transmitted diseases. For acupuncture, risk is related to the number of acupuncture needles.[21] With less than 150 needles, the attack rate was 9% and with more than 450 needles, the rate was 33%. In Israel, an outbreak related to the use of multiple dose vials of heparin and normal saline flush solution contaminated with HBsAg has been reported.

Occult HBV infection

Problem of silent HBV infection has been recently recognized, when the person has either very low level of replication, hence negative for all HBV markers but positive for HBV-DNA by sensitive techniques like PCR or has surface or core gene mutations. The role of occult HBV infection in causing liver disease has not been well established. The occult HBV infection has importance in the setting of blood donation and organ transplantation where the donor is negative for all screening tests of HBV but still transmits the virus to the recipient due to low replicating virus (HBV-DNA positive).[22] Although theoretically possible, in practice this is not a major problem. We recently analysed occult HBV infection in 100 healthy blood donors with negative HBsAg, by doing PCR for HBV-DNA. None of the donors was found to be positive for HBV-DNA (unpublished).

Sexual

In most developed countries, the major mode of spread of HBV is through sexual route. This accounts for a high rate of hepatitis B among male homosexuals and in promiscuous heterosexuals.[23] Spread occurs when primary patient has acute hepatitis B or is an asymptomatic chronic HBsAg positive subject, due to the presence of HBV in semen and a breach in skin/mucous membrane of susceptible host (hence more common in anal intercourse).[24] HBV is more easily transmitted by sexual spread than HCV and HIV. Risk increases with the duration of heterosexual activity. In a data from our department, 33.8% of HIV patients were found to be infected with HBV. Males were more commonly coinfected and all except one acquired infection through heterosexual route.[25] Transmission can also occur after artificial insemination, hence screening of semen donors is recommended.

Non-overt parenteral route

Although blood and blood products are the best documented sources of transmission of hepatitis B virus, presence of HBsAg has also been demonstrated in other body secretions like feces, urine, bile, sweat, tears, saliva, semen, breast milk, vaginal secretions, CSF, synovial fluid and cord blood.[2] Out of these serum, saliva, and semen have been shown to be infectious.[26] The concentration of the HBsAg, though in all these fluids is shown to be much lower than in the serum, infectious material coming in contact with open skin breaks or mucous membranes can result in transmission of the virus. Since HBV is quite stable virus, the transmission of the virus can occur after infectious material comes in contact with open skin or mucous membranes through articles like toothbrushes, toys, utensils, razors, hospital equipment such as respirators, endoscopes, and other laboratory instruments. In a study from Pune, household contacts of hospitalized patients were found to acquire the infection through horizontal transmission.[27] In one outbreak, computer cards which became contaminated with blood and which caused paper cuts in workers were implicated as the vehicle of HBV transmission. Direct blood contact with oral or ocular mucosa can also transit infection in the work setting. Contact through pipetting accidents and splash exposures could occur in the clinical laboratory, dental office or emergency room.

Non-parenteral route

Unlike the hepatitis A virus (HAV) and hepatitis E virus (HEV), HBV infrequently causes epidemics of hepatitis. This may be because there are no important environmental reservoirs like water or food, as are involved in the transmission of HAV or HEV.[2] Still uncommonly, the infection of HBV after oral intake of infectious material has been reported. However, the dose of virus needed for infection through oral route appears to be much higher than via the parenteral route and the infection probably occurs through small breaks in the oral cavity rather than through the intestinal tract.

REFERENCES

1. Lee WM. Hepatitis B virus infection. *N Engl J Med* 1997;337:733-45.
2. Robinson WS. *Biology of human hepatitis viruses. In:* Zakim D, Boyer TD, Eds. Hepatology–A textbook of Liver Disease, Vol. II, IIIrd edn. Philadelphia: WB Saunders, 1996: pp. 1146 1206.
3. Alter MJ, Mash EM. Epidemiology of viral hepatitis. *Gastroenterol Clin N Am* 1994;23:437-54.
4. Harpaz R, Von Seidlein L, Averhoff FM, Tormey MP, Sinha SD, Kotsopoulon K, Lambert SB. Transmission of hepatitis B virus to multiple patients from a surgeon without evidence of inadequate infection control. *N Engl J Med* 1996;334:549-54.
5. Singh J, Gupta S, Khare S, Bhatia R, Jain DC, Sokhey J. A sever and explosive outbreak of hepatitis B in a rural population in Sirsa district, Haryana, India: unnecessary therapeutic injections were a major risk factor. *Epidemiol Infect* 2000;125:693-9.
6. Singh S, Dwivedi SN, Sood R, Wali JP. Hepatitis B, C and human immunodeficiency virus infections in multiply infected Kala – azar patients in Delhi. *Scand J Infect Dis* 2000;32:3-6.
7. Saha MK, Chakrabarti S, Panda S, Naik TN, Manna B, Chatterjee A, Detels R, Bhattacharya SK. Prevalence of HCV and HBV infection amongst HIV seropositive intravenous drug users and their non-injecting wives in Manipur, India. *Ind J Med Res* 2000;111:37-9.
8. Wake DJ, Cutting WA. Blood transfusion in developing countries: problems, priorities and practicalities. *Trop Duct* 1998;28:4-8.
9. Ghosh K, Joshi SH, Shetty S, Pawar A, Chipkar S, Pujari V, Madkaikar M, et al. Transfusion transmitted diseases in hemophilics from Western India. *Ind J Med Res* 2000;112:61-4.
10. Saha D, Agarwal SK. Hepatitis and HIV infection during hemodialysis. *J Ind Med Assoc* 2001;99: 194-9.
11. Lewis TL, Alter HJ, Chalmers TC. A comparison of the frequency of hepatitis antigen and antibody in hospital and non-hospital personnel. *N Engl J Med* 1973;289:647-9.
12. Lauer GM, Walker BD. Hepatitis C virus infection. *N Engl J Med* 2001;345:41-52.
13. Beasley RP, Trepo C, Stevens CE, Szmuness W. The e antigen and vertical transmission of hepatitis B surface antigen. *Am J Epidemiol* 1977;105:94-8.
14. Nayak NC, Panda SK, Zuckerman AJ, Bhan MK, Guha DK. Dynamics and impact of perinatal transmission of hepatitis B virus in North India. *J Med Virol* 1987;21:137-45.
15. Xu DZ, Yan YP, Choi BC, Xu JQ, Men K, Zhang JX, Lin ZH, Wang FS. Risk factors and mechanism of transplacental transmission of hepatitis B virus: a case control study. *J Med Virol* 2002;67: 20-6.
16. Wang S, Jiang P, Peng G. Detection of C gene mutation strain in vertical transmission of hepatitis B virus and its significance. *Zhonghua Yu Fang Yi Xue Za Zhi* 2000;34:37-8.
17. Kazim SN, Wakil SM, Khan LA, Hasnain SE, Sarin SK. Vertical transmission of hepatitis B despite maternal lamivudine therapy. *Lancet* 2002;359:1488-9.
18. Sugauchi F, Orito E, Ohno T, Kato H, Suzuki T, Hashimoto T, Manabe T, Ueda R, Mizokami M. Liver transplantation-associated de novo hepatitis B virus infection: application of molecular evolutionary analysis. *Intervirology* 2002;45:6-10.
19. Sengler U, Reinhard T, Adams O, Gerlich W, Sundmacher R. Testing of corneoscleral discs and their

cultural media of seropositive donors for hepatitis B and C virus genomes. *Graefes Arch Clin Exp Ophthalmol* 2001;239:783-7.
20. Nishioka S de A, Gyorkos TW, Joseph L, Collet JP, Maclean JD. Tattooing and risk for transfusion-transmitted diseases: the role of the type, number and design of the tattoos, and the conditions in which they were performed. *Epidemiol Infect* 2002;128:63-71.
21. Kent GP, Brondum J, Keenlyside RA. A large outbreak of acupuncture-associated hepatitis B. *Am J Epidemiol* 1988;127:591-8.
22. Chemin I, Jeantet D, Kay A, Trepo C. Role of silent hepatitis B virus in chronic hepatitis B surface antigen (–) liver disease. *Antiviral Res* 2001;52:117-23.
23. Szmuness W, Much WM, Prince AM. On the role of sexual behaviour in the spread of hepatitis B infection. *Ann Intern Med* 1975;83:489-91.
24. Deitzman DE, Harnisch JP, Ray CG, Alexander ER, Holmes KK. Hepatitis B surface antigen (HBsAg) and antibody to HBsAg: prevalence of homosexual and heterosexual men. *JAMA* 1977;238:2625-6.
25. Sud A, Singh J, Dhiman RK, Wanchu A, Singh S, Chawla Y. Hepatitis B virus coinfection in HIV infected patients. *Trop Gastroenterol* 2001;22:90-2.
26. Alter JH, Purcell RH, Gerin JL. Transmission of hepatitis B to chimpanzees by hepatitis B surface antigen – positive saliva and semen. *Infect Immun* 1977;16:928-30.
27. Dhorje SP, Pavri KM, Prasad SR, Sehgal A, Phule DM. Horizontal transmission of hepatitis B virus infection in household contacts. *J Med Virol* 1985;16:183-9.

Transmission of hepatitis B virus in neonates

Ashok K Dutta, Praveen Kumar

Hepatitis B is one of the most prevalent infectious diseases of the world. There are approximately 300 million subjects chronically infected with hepatitis B all over the world, out of which approximately 43 million are in India alone.[1]

Hepatitis B virus (HBV) infection acquired during infancy and early childhood predisposes to persistent HBV infection. About 70–90% of infants develop chronic HBV infection if they acquire the infection during the perinatal period, compared to only 20–50% of children acquiring infection in early childhood (<5 yrs). The risk of primary hepatocellular carcinoma (HCC) or cirrhosis is related to the duration of chronic HBV infection. Infants who become chronically infected have an estimated 25% lifetime risk of cirrhosis or primary hepatocellular carcinoma in comparison to 15% lifetime risk if HBV infection is acquired in adults. Perinatal transmission of the hepatitis B virus usually results in development of a chronic hepatitis B surface antigen (HBsAg) positive state, making this one of the most important routes of transmission world wide.

PREVALENCE OF HBsAg IN PREGNANCY: RISK OF NEONATAL TRANSMISSION

The risk of neonatal hepatitis B virus infection in any community will be directly related to the prevalence of infection in the pregnant women. The prevalence rate of HBsAg positivity in pregnant women varies (0.6–5.0%) in different parts of our country (Table 1).

Most of the asymptomatic HBsAg positive pregnant women, continue to be persistent carrier for a prolonged period of time. This is a potential source of perinatal infection. Shanmugam and Nair[3] found that 85.7% of HBsAg positive pregnant mothers to be positive for a period ranging from 4 months to 5 years or more after delivery.

Maternal 'e' antigenemia: an additional risk for neonatal transmission

Maternal 'e' antigenemia is strongly related to the transmission of hepatitis B virus in the

Table 1. Prevalence of HBsAg positivity in pregnant women

Place	Authors	Year	Method	HBsAg+ve/total	%
Mumbai	Khatri et al[2]	1980	CIEP/RIA	8/1276	0.6
Trivandram	Shanmugam et al[3]	1982	CIEP	38/1475	2.6
Jodhpur	Vyas et al[4]	1983	CIEP	5/500	1.0
Jaipur	Gupta el al[5]	1985	CIEP	22/1000	2.2
Delhi	Nayak et al[6]	1987	ELISA	332/8575	3.7
Devengere (Karnataka)	Kulkarni et al[7]	1988	RPHA	20/400	5.0
Chandigarh	Sehgal et al[8]	1992	ELISA	100/4137	2.6
Chandigarh	Gupta et al[9]	1992	ELISA	58/2337	2.5
Delhi	Mittal et al[10]	1994	LATEX	39/850	4.58
Delhi	Singal et al[12]	2000	ELISA	—	2.1

neonates. Beasley et al[11] in their study from Taiwan found that 85% of babies were HBsAg positive whose mothers were HBeAg positive whereas only 31% of babies acquired HBsAg if mothers were HBeAg negative.

Nayak et al[6] from Delhi found HBeAg in 7.8% of chronic HBsAg positive females and transmission was most frequent (87.5%) if the mother was HBeAg positive as compared to 17.5% for anti-HBe positive and 9.6% for only HBsAg positive mothers. Infants of mothers who are positive for both HBsAg and HBeAg not only become infected early in life, mostly by 3–5 months of age, but are also more likely to have persistence of the virus. In infants born to women carrying either HBsAg alone or HBsAg with anti-HBe, transmission is uniformly spread throughout the first six months of life and the infection is relatively transient.

HBeAg is not known to enhance transmission directly but is a marker of active viral replication. HBV-DNA is a more direct measure of infectivity and also correlates with the likelihood of perinatal transmission. Why infants of HBsAg and HBeAg positive mothers are more likely to develop chronicity is not well understood. Immaturity of the infant immune system is the probable reason for inability of the infants to clear the HBV infection.

Modes of Transmission

Perinatal transmission

Perinatal infection has been reported to be the most important route of transmission of HBV from chronic HBsAg positive mothers to their newborn infants. During the perinatal period, infants are exposed to maternal blood through placental tears, trauma related to birth, and contact of conjuctiva and mucous membranes with blood and other body fluids during the labour and delivery.[13]

Infants born to mothers with chronic HBV infection who are also HBeAg positive have a risk as high as 60–90% of acquiring HBV infection during the perinatal period and as many as 90% of the infected infants become chronically infected with HBsAg (Table 2). However, if the mother is HBsAg positive and HBeAg negative or anti-HBe positive, the infant has only 10–15% chance of becoming infected. Cesarean section has not been shown to eliminate the risk of perinatally acquired HBV infection.

Table 2. Transmission pattern in infants born to chronic HBsAg positive mothers

Place	Duration of follow-up (months)	Mother's antigenic status (no. of mothers)	HBsAg+ve infants (%)
Jaipur[5]	12	HBsAg+(16)	3 (18.7)
Delhi[6]	16	HBsAg+(115)	11 (9.6)
		HBsAg+ HBeAg+(16)	14 (87.5)
Chandigarh[8]	12	HBsAg+(23)	3 (13.0)
		HBsAg+(15) HBeAg+	11 (73.3)
		HBsAg+(11) anti-HBe+	1 (9.0)

Transplacental or intrauterine transmission

HBV can also be transmitted to the fetus during the gestation period. Intrauterine or transplacental transmission has been suggested in 3–8% of infants born to HBeAg positive and HBsAg positive mothers. Transmission of HBV *in utero* is related to the placental leakage, although, it is difficult to demonstrate this in every case.[14] Anti-HBc IgM and HBeAg in the umbilical cord blood were not found to be useful for predicting intrauterine infection from 16 HBeAg positive mothers.[14]

Others

Neonates can also be infected by accidental contact with HBsAg positive blood during delivery and by transfusions. Patil et al[15] from Mumbai have reported HBV infection in neonates through exchange transfusion.

CLINICAL FEATURES

The majority of the infected infants remain asymptomatic. Clinical course is usually mild but long-term prognosis is not so good as they have increased risk of chronic liver disease and hepatic carcinoma. Berry et al from Delhi reported HBV in 58% of chronic liver disease, 52.9% of chronic hepatitis, 65.6% of cirrhosis, and 33% of the hepatocellular carcinoma patients.[16] HBsAg usually appears between 6 weeks and 5 months after birth. Tandon et al observed in their study that the babies who had perinatal infection expressed HBsAg in the serum after an incubation period of 4–12 weeks. One baby who was HBsAg positive at the age of 4 days probably acquired transplacental infection (Table 3).[17]

Table 3. HBsAg and anti-HBs status in pre-school children[17]

Age in months	HBsAg status		Anti-HBs status	
	Number tested	Number +ve	Number tested	Number +ve
0–1	108	1 (0.9%)	59	10 (17%)
2–6	89	2 (2.3%)	85	11 (12.9%)
7–12	123	5 (4.1%)	114	21 (18.4%)
13–36	353	8 (2.3%)	309	44 (14.2%)
37–60	309	5 (1.6%)	271	37 (13.7%)

However, a small number of infants with hepatitis B develop fulminant hepatitis. Infants of chronic HBeAg positive mothers usually result in a chronic HBsAg positive state, possibly by induction of immunologic tolerance to HBeAg *in utero*. On the other hand, babies born to HBeAg negative mothers are more likely to clear the virus and more frequently present with a severe clinical course of HBV infection, including neonatal fulminant hepatitis B. Sterneck et al in their study concluded that neither the emergence of a particular mutant strain nor infection with replicating HBV variants is necessary for the development of neonatal fulminant hepatitis B.[18]

MANAGEMENT AND PREVENTION

Once chronic HBV infection has developed, it is difficult to manage it by currently available drugs. Thus, prevention is most important for the control of HBV infection. Hepatitis B vaccine alone or in combination with hepatitis B immunoglobulin (HBIg) has been used for immunoprophylaxis. Hepatitis B vaccination strategies targeted at high-risk groups had limited impact in reducing the incidence of hepatitis B and in preventing infection. As the practice of vaccinating only the high-risk groups did not decrease the HBV prevalence significantly, American immunization advisory groups have recommended routine infant immunization with hepatitis B vaccine. World Health Organization (WHO) also proposed inclusion of hepatitis B vaccine as the seventh vaccine in the national Expanded Program of Immunization (EPI) of all member countries which fall in the high or intermediate endemicity for HBV prevalence.

Both plasma derived and recombinant vaccines have been found to be effective (Table 4). Ideal schedule of hepatitis B vaccination for the new born children is either 0, 1 and 6 months or 0, 1, 2 and 12 months. Unfortunately in India, 90% of the births occur at home and it is

Table 4. Immunogenicity of hepatitis B vaccine as per different schedules

Authors (Year)	Dose (μg)	Schedule	Seroprotection (%)	GMT (mIU/ml)
Goldfarb et al (1994)[19]	10	0, 1, 6 months	96	3142
Goldfarb et al (1996)[20]	5	0, 1, 6 months	98	3732
	10	0, 1, 6 months	98	8062
Greenberg et al (1996)[21]	10	2, 4, 6 months	99	1914
Mittal et al (1995)[10]	10	0, 6, 14 weeks		
		0, 1, 2 months	96	–
			100	–
Kumar et al (2000)[22]	10	6, 10, 14 weeks	100	2643
Gomber et al (2000)[23]	10	6, 10, 14 weeks	97	224

not generally possible to vaccinate them within 48 hours of delivery. Moreover, both schedules do not coincide with visits for EPI vaccines which are usually given at 6, 10, 14 weeks, and 9 months. Thus, these schedules will require additional visits which would lead to higher drop out rates and decreased compliance. In cases where vaccination cannot be initiated at birth, it may be more practical and convenient if hepatitis B vaccine could be given at the same time as the other EPI vaccine, i.e., at 0, 6 and 14 weeks or at 6, 10 and 14 weeks. However, the latter schedule would not prevent vertical transmission effectively which is responsible for about 50% cases of chronic infection. Studies which were conducted to find out feasibility of hepatitis B vaccination combining with other EPI vaccines have shown encouraging results.[21-23]

Following scheme of passive–active immunization is currently recommended: All infants born to HBsAg positive mothers should receive hepatitis B vaccine at birth or as soon as possible after birth, irrespective of the maternal HBeAg or antibody status.[24-26] If mother does not have anti-HBe, then hepatitis B immunoglobulin (200 IU) should be given intramuscularly within 24–48 hrs of birth along with the first dose of hepatitis B vaccine followed by three more doses of the vaccine at 1, 2 and 12 months. This provides a protective efficacy of almost 97%. However, due to some reasons, if it is not possible to administer HBIg, then hepatitis B vaccine alone in the above schedule should be given within 12 hr of birth and this gives a protective efficacy of about 92%.[10, 27]

ROUTINE ANTENATAL SCREENING FOR HBsAg

Most developing countries including India, do not have routine antenatal screening for HBsAg in pregnant mothers. Antenatal screening for HBsAg will allow the physician and the family to decide whether to use HBIg in addition to hepatitis B vaccine or not. Moreover, it is important to generate epidemiological data even after introduction of the vaccine in the routine immunization practice. Unfortunately, because of the cost of performing the screening test, non-availability of the screening test in smaller set up and large number of domicillary births, its practical utility in India at present is limited only to some selected centers and those who can afford it. Even if hepatitis B vaccine is introduced in the EPI program, screening practices should ideally be continued.

REFERENCES

1. Tandon BN. *Dimensions and issues of HBV control in India*. In: Sarin SK, Singal AK, Eds. Hepatitis B in India : Problems and Prevention. CBS Publishers & Distributors, New Delhi. 1996; pp.1-5.
2. Khatri JV, Kulkarni KV, Vaishnov PR, Merchant SM. Vertical Transmission of hepatitis B. *Indian Pediatr* 1980;27:957-62.
3. Shanmugam J, Nair SR. A three and half year follow-up study of HBsAg carrier state in asymptomatic mothers. *Indian J Pathol Microbiol* 1982;25:273-8.
4. Vyas KK, Mathur AK, Vyas RK, Mathur S. A study of prevalence of hepatitis B surface antigen among pregnant women. *J Obs and Gynae India* 1983;33:778-81.
5. Gupta ML, Sharma U, Saxena S, Sharma ML, Pokhara DS. Vertical transmission of hepatitis B surface antigen from asymptomatic carrier mothers. *Indian Pediatr* 1985;22:339-42.
6. Nayak NC, Panda SK, Zuckerman AJ, Bhan MK, Guha AK. Dynamics and Impact of perinatal transmission of hepatitis B. *J Med Virol* 1987;21:137-45.
7. Kulkarni ML, Reddy PV. Prevalence of HBsAg in asymptomatic carrier mothers and vertical transmission. *Am J Dis Child* 1988;142;124-5.
8. Sehgal A, Gupta I, Sehgal R, Ganguly NK. Hepatitis B vaccine alone or in combination with anti-HBs Immunoglobulin in the perinatal prophylaxis of babies born to HBsAg carrier mothers. *Acta Virol* 1992;38:247-51.
9. Gupta I, Sehgal A, Sehgal R, Ganguly NK. Vertical transmission of hepatitis B in north India. *J Hyg Epidemiol Microbiol Immunol* 1992;36:263-7.
10. Mittal SK, Rao S, Kumari S, Aggarwal V, Prakash C, Thirupuram S. Simultaneous administration of hepatitis B vaccine with other EPI vaccines. *Indian J Pediatr* 1994;61:183-8.
11. Beasley RP, Trepo C, Stevens CE, Szmunes W. The e antigen and vertical transmission of hepatitis B surface antigen. *Am J Epidemiol* 1997;105:94-8.
12. Singal AK, Kaur V. Prevalence of HBsAg in population referred to a hospital in North Delhi. *Indian J Gastroenterol* 2000;20(suppl 3):C75-6.
13. Shapiro CN. Epidemiology of hepatitis B. *Ped Infect Dis J* 1983;12:5:433-7.
14. Ohto H, Lin HH, Kawana T, Etoh T, Tohyama H. Intrauterine transmission of hepatitis B virus is closely related to placental leakage. *J Med Virol* 1987;21:1-6.
15. Patil RS, Wadgaonkar P, Joshi SH, Merchant RH, Gupta SC. Viral infections in newborns through exchange transfusion. *Indian J Pediatr* 1998;65:723-8.
16. Berry N, Chakravati A, Kar P, Das BC, Santhanam A, Mathur MD. Association of hepatitis C virus and hepatitis B virus in chronic liver disease. *Ind J Med Res* 1998;108:255-9.
17. Tandon BN, Irshad M, Raju M, Mathur GP, Rao MN. Prevalence of HBsAg and anti-HBs in children and strategy suggested for immunization in India. *Ind J Med Res* 1991;93:337-9.
18. Sterneck M, Kalinina T, Otto S, Gunther S, Fischer L, Burdelski M, Greten H, et al. Neonatal fulminant hepatitis B: structural and functional analysis of complete hepatitis B virus genome from mother and infant. *J Infect Dis* 1998;177:1378-81.

19. Goldfarb J, Baley J, Medendorp SV, Seto D, Garcia N, Toy P, Watson B, et al. Comparative study of immunogenicity and safety of two dosing schedules of Engerix–B hepatitis B vaccine in neonates. *Pediatr Infect Dis J* 1994;13;18-22.
20. Goldfarb J, Medendorp SV, Nagamari Y, Buscarino C, Krause D. Comparative study of the immunogenecity and safety of 5 micro gram and 10 micro gram dosages of recombinant hepatitis B vaccine in healthy children. *Pediatr Infect Dis J* 1996;15:768-77.
21. Greenberg DP, Vadheim CM, Wong VK, Marey SM, Partridge S, Greene T, Chiu CY, et al. Comparative safety and immunogenicity of two recombinant hepatitis B vaccines given to infants at two, four and six months of age. *Pediatr Infect Dis J* 1996;15:590-6.
22. Kumar TS, Abraham P, Raghuraman S, Cherian T. Immunogenicity of indigenous recombinant hepatitis B vaccine in infants following 0, 1 and 2 month vaccination schedule. *Indian Pediatr* 2000;37:75-80.
23. Gomber S, Sharma R, Ramachandran VG, Talwar V, Singh B. Immunogenicity of hepatitis B vaccine incorporated into expanded program of immunization schedule. *Indian Pediatr* 2000;37:411-3.
24. Beasley RP, Hwang LY, Lee GC, Lan CC, Roan CH, Huang FY, Chen CL. Prevention of perinatally transmitted hepatitis B virus infection with hepatitis B immunoglobulin and hepatitis B vaccine. *Lancet* 1983;2:1099-102.
25. Mazel JA, Schalm SW, de Gast BC, Nuijten ASM, Heijtink RA, Botman MJ. Passive–active immunization of neonates of HBsAg positive carrier mothers. Preliminary Observations. *Br Med J* 1984;288:513-5.
26. Paul Y. Hepatitis B vaccine and pregnancy. *Indian Pediatr* 2001;38:301.
27. Lolekha B, Warachit B, Hirunyachote, A, Bowonkiratikachoru P, West DJ, Poerschke G. Protective efficacy of hepatitis B vaccine without HBIg in infants of HBeAg-positive carrier mothers in Thailand. *Vaccine* 2002;20:3695-701.

4

Transmission of hepatitis B virus in children

Narendra K Arora, Lalit Kant, Prashant Mathur

It is estimated that over 1 billion individuals worldwide are exposed to hepatitis B virus (HBV) and that there are approximately 300 million who are chronically infected with the virus. Most of the positives are from East Asian countries and sub-Saharan Africa.[1] The term "healthy carriers" should preferably be avoided, as such individuals still harbor the risk of developing chronic liver disease, including hepatocellular carcinoma.[2] Thus "chronic hepatitis B virus infection without significant liver disease" is the preferred description.

The age at the time of primary HBV infection is perhaps the best-established determinant of its chronicity. In highly endemic countries, the majority of infections occur from infected mother to child either at birth or during early childhood. As majority of such infections are asymptomatic, the infected children remain undetected and unwittingly serve as ready reservoir of the infection. In contrast, acute HBV infection is symptomatic in 30–50% adults and only 1–5% acquire chronic HBV infection.[3] Understanding the dynamics of HBV transmission in the community would be useful for planning preventive strategies, particularly the timing and schedule of hepatitis B vaccination in the community.

MODES AND DETERMINANTS OF HBV TRANSMISSION

The major pathways for the transmission of HBV include parenteral exposure to blood or other infective body fluids, transmission from mother to infant, sexual transmission, and transmission to infants or young children from close contact with infected persons.[4] The pattern of HBV infection in any community seems to be dependent upon the per capita rate of infection and the risk of acquiring chronic infection. Both these are age-dependent processes. In developing countries with high endemicity of HBV infections, both these processes tend to decline non-linearly with increasing age.[5]

HBV has been found in the skin lesions and wound exudate of chronically infected persons. Environmental sampling in homes with an HBsAg positive subject showed the presence of

HBsAg on a number of surfaces and objects. Environmental contamination and transfer of the virus by fomites has been accepted as a primary pathway for disease transmission in hemodialysis units. Hence, in a home where an HBsAg positive subject lives, susceptible contacts are at risk of infection.[6] Yet, 20–30% of HBV infected patients do not have an identifiable risk factor for transmission.[7] Nosocomial transmission of HBV infection is prevalent in settings of inadequate infection control practices.

Perinatal transmission and hepatitis B e antigen (HBeAg) status

All HBsAg positive persons are considered potentially infectious. The relative degree of infectivity can be gauged by the presence or absence of HBeAg or anti-HBe. HBeAg positivity has a variable duration after an acute infection in different populations. Epidemiological studies have shown that the major determinant of risk of acquiring infection is HBeAg positivity in the mother or the sibling.[8,9] The rate of infection and outcome of infants born to HBV positive mothers is dependent upon the maternal HBeAg/anti-HBe status. If the mother is HBeAg positive, 85% of babies become persistently infected, whereas those born to anti-HBe positive mothers usually do not become chronically infected. Approximately 6% of these babies would develop fulminant liver failure or acute hepatitis B by 2–3 months of age. There are enough data to say that most mother to infant transmission occurs during the perinatal period rather than *in utero*. Recently, Wang et al[10] have demonstrated that HBV can cross human placenta and infect the fetus *in utero*.

A meta-analysis was done to look at the epidemiological relationship between HBV transmission, age at infection, and prevalence of HBsAg positivity in East Asian countries and Sub-Saharan Africa.[11] The analysis included published literature from 12 surveys that measured the HBsAg, HBeAg, anti-HBs, and anti-HBe status in their communities. Perinatal transmission was compared between Sub-Saharan Africa, East Asia and developing countries (Table 1).

Table 1. Prevalence of HBsAg and HBeAg among women and risk of perinatal transmission of infection over the first year of life[11]

Parameter	Sub-Saharan Africa	East Asia	Other developing countries	Developed countries
Mean prevalence of HBsAg in pregnant women	10.6% (7.4–15.0)*	9.5% (5.8–15.0)	3.6% (2.1–6.3)	–
Mean prevalence of HBeAg amongst HBsAg pregnant women	11.6% (4.9–24.8)	45.8% (22.2–71.5)	10.5% (3.1–30.4)	–
Risk of perinatal transmission in HBeAg in pregnant women	27.9% (9.2–59.6)	87.5% (62.6–96.7)	81.6% (46.7–95.8)	73% (25–95.5)

* 95% Confidence Interval

In this meta-analysis, the authors have defined perinatal transmission as infection of the infant during the first year of life. The areas studied had high prevalence of HBsAg (3.5–37.3%) and high rates of transmission in childhood (the age at which half the population was infected, A50, ranged from 1.5–18 years). Areas with low values of A50 (high transmission) had on average a greater proportion of HBV infected subjects in the population than areas with higher values of A50 (low transmission).

The incidence of perinatal transmission would depend upon the HBsAg prevalence rate in pregnant females, and the risk of transmission of virus from mother to her infant. From the above table it appears that the prevalence of HBeAg rate is higher in East Asia (45.8%; 95% CI:22.2–71.5) than sub-Saharan Africa (11.6%; 95% CI:4.9–24.8) though the HBsAg positivity rate is similar. The risk of perinatal transmission in East Asia is four times (87.5%; 95% CI:62.6–96.7) as compared to data from Sub-Saharan Africa (27.9%; 95% CI:9.2–59.6) and similar to that seen in other developing countries like India (81.6%; 95% CI:46.7–95.8) and developed countries (73%; 95% CI:25–95.5). There was, however, no evidence of significant geographic differences when the data from HBeAg negative mothers were analysed. The differences in HBeAg positivity and risk of perinatal transmission of infection between Sub-Saharan Africa and East Asia are not clear. One of the explanations might be the differences in perinatal practices in the two geographic regions. The authors also suggest that acquisition of perinatal infection would be associated with a slow clearance of HBeAg in infants and thus perhaps would explain the higher HBeAg rates in pregnant females in East Asian countries. The role of improving environment and social conditions in reduction of HBeAg positivity has also been suggested from some countries. In Taiwan[12], over a period of 5 years there was a significant reduction in the HBeAg positivity rate in pregnant mothers per calendar year per pregnancy.

Serological data from developed countries indicate that 70–75% of infants of acutely infected mothers acquire HBV infection within 3 months of birth, whereas only 0–27% infants are infected by mothers with chronic HBV infection in a similar time period. Studies have suggested that acutely infected mothers were 7 times more infectious than mothers with chronic HBV infection. But since chronically infected mothers remain so for an average of 30–40 years, this offsets the time duration advantage over acutely infected mothers and thus, overall constitute more important source for HBV transmission in the community.[13, 14]

Age

Areas with lower mean age at infection irrespective of the route of transmission is likely to have high prevalence of chronic asymptomatic HBV infected individuals in the community, because of the age dependent nature of acquiring chronic infection. These areas can, therefore, be expected to have a higher force of infection (as positive are responsible for the majority of transmission) and hence a lower average age of infection.[4] Data from most developing countries including India show a clear trend for the force of infection to be greatest in infants and young children followed by a steady decline throughout childhood. Among infants who do not acquire infection at birth, almost 40% of them born to mothers who are hepatitis B e antigen (HBeAg) positive will become infected before the age of 5 years (unless vaccinated) because of continued close contact with the mother and other infected persons within the household.[15]

In China[16], the highest HBsAg prevalence rate was found among children under 3 years of age, and the highest annual increase in HBsAg to anti-HBs positivity was also seen in children aged 3 years or less, who were therefore at the highest risk of infection and thus of acquiring chronic HBV infection. Asians acquire HBV infection during neonatal period or by 3 years from mothers or close contacts whereas Caucasians acquire the infection during adolescence or adulthood through sexual or parenteral routes.[17]

Horizontal transmission of HBV

It commonly denotes transmission of HBV infection from infectious individuals to susceptible 'close contacts'. Thus, horizontal transmission is defined as unrelated to recognized perinatal exposure and excluding sexual infection.[18] In high endemicity regions, the force of infection is highest during early childhood and declines in late childhood only to have a second peak in adults (presumably due to sexual transmission).[4] In these areas perinatal transmission would explain the high infection rate in infancy, but thereafter continued close contact transmission between the mother and the child accounts for the increasing number of subjects with chronic HBV infection. These observations are supported by data from high endemic areas in Africa and East Asia including Singapore.[4,19]

Childhood infection by HBV is primarily due to horizontal transmission in developing countries, and, therefore, the rate or force of infection in this age group is measure of the rate of horizontal transmission.[4] In low endemicity countries such as North America and Western Europe, where perinatal transmission is negligible, the use of safe disposal systems and safe injection practices have reduced the horizontal transmission rate. Hence, in these areas, the transmission of HBV remains mainly through sexual route.[11]

According to a nation wide epidemiological survey in 1979 to 1980 in China, the prevalence of HBsAg among children under 1 year of age was comparatively low (3.2%). From one to four years of age, however, it increased to 8.9% reaching > 10% among five to nine year of age. This pattern of age distribution suggested that horizontal transmission is an important route of HBV infection during early childhood.[20] In a large cross sectional study in China,[21] children born to HBsAg positive mothers had a relative risk ratio of 5.3 to acquire chronic infection as compared to those born to HBsAg negative mothers. This increased risk could be attributed to the combined effects of horizontal and perinatal transmission. It was estimated that the proportion of chronic HBsAg carriage attributable to perinatal transmission ranged from only 13% to 19.6%. Horizontal transmission, therefore, seems to outweigh perinatal transmission as a risk for HBV infection in China. Younger children with chronic HBV infection have higher prevalence of HBeAg and consequently higher infectivity, making them a more likely source of HBV transmission than adults.[22] Vequente et al[23] pointed out that the chronicity rate was significantly higher among children (73.4%) than adults (35.6%) in household horizontal transmission.

Goh et al[24] showed that asymptomatic subjects with chronic HBV infection are the main source of acute HBV infection. Spouses and parents of acute cases had a significantly higher prevalence of HBV infection than other members of the families. Factors associated with the risk of transmission of HBV included sharing various personal and household articles such as tooth brush, towel, handkerchief, clothing, razor, comb, bed, and bedding, etc. Sleeping in the same bedroom, eating together, and sharing of eating and drinking utensils were not associated with increased risk of transmission of infection. In Ghana, Martinson et al[25] identified sharing of bath towels (OR=3.4; 95% CI:2.1–4.5), chewing gum or partially eaten candies (OR=3.4; 95% CI:2.3–5.0), dental cleaning material (OR=2.5; 95% CI:1.3–4.6) and biting of finger nails in conjunction with scratching the back of chronically infected subjects (OR=2.5; 95% CI:1.6–4.3) as the most strongly associated risk factors of horizontal transmission of HBV infection.

HBV mutants and transmission

The important issues associated with HBV mutants are conditions in which mutants emerge/selected, their infectivity and pathogenecity, transmissibility, and routes of transmission. The global frequency of HBV variants is not known and their biologic implications are more speculative. HBV mutants can broadly be of three types. (a) hepatitis B surface antigen mutants, (b) core gene deletion mutants, and (c) pre-core mutants. In the study by Hsu et al,[26]: examination of maternal serum and serial serum samples from their infants who developed acute or chronic HBV infection despite immuno prophylaxis showed that in 16 of 22 (73%), the HBV inoculum transmitted from the mother to the infant was generally the wild type strain. S-variants with mutations within the "a" determinant emerged or were selected later under the immune pressure generated by the host *per se* or by HBIg plus subsequent hepatitis B vaccination in a smaller proportion (6/22; 27%). In another study also, there was no evidence of horizontal transmission of such mutants to other vaccinated siblings, or to older siblings with chronic HBV infection, nor to their fathers with natural immunity.[27] However, horizontal transmission of S-mutant from an infected infant to his Singaporean mother with chronic HBV (wild type) infection was recorded.

In a long-term follow-up study from Taiwan,[28] core gene deletion mutants were found in 18 of the 365 HBV infected children (4.9%). Most cases (83%) with deletion mutants heralded HBeAg sero-conversion phase. Deletion mutants were not associated with high liver enzymes. Core gene deletion mutants appeared preferably in children acquiring HBV by horizontal transmission and could appear as early as the age of 5 years.

A few anti-HBc positive patients remain viremic with active liver disease. This discrepancy is explained by the finding of stop-codon mutation in the precore region of HBV that prevent HBeAg secretion but still permit HBV replication and HBeAg production. These precore stop-codon mutants may be detected in patients with fulminant hepatitis and also in asymptomatic subjects. Akarca et al[29] studied 53 index patients and 89 HBsAg positive family members. They found that pre-core HBV mutants can be detected in 33% of asymptomatic individuals with chronic HBV infection, in 24% of HBeAg positive vs. 55% of HBeAg negative family members (p=0.002) and 34% family members with normal vs. 21% those with increased ALT levels (p=0.05). Thus, these mutants are not necessarily associated with acute liver disease. M1 mutant is infectious and is usually present *ab initio*. In contrast, M2 mutant appears to emerge from wild type later in the course of infection. Clustering of M0 and M1 mutants in family members indicated intra-familial or horizontal transmission.

INDIAN SCENARIO

Prevalence of HBeAg in HBsAg positive pregnant women

The importance of HBV carriage in pregnant women is well recognized and is responsible for the vertical transmission of hepatitis B from asymptomatic mothers with chronic HBV infection to their newborn children.[30-32] Several studies have been conducted in India to investigate the prevalence of HBsAg in pregnant women. Studies using second generation tests showed prevalence rates ranging between 1.0% to 3.9%. The results suggest that HBsAg positivity rate among pregnant women using the 3rd generation tests ranged between 0.6 and 5.0%, and the weighted average was 2.8% (95% CI:2.6-3.1).

Perinatal transmission is highly dependent on HBeAg status of pregnant women. However, very few studies have investigated the HBeAg and anti-HBe (using ELISA based tests) status in subjects with chronic HBV infection in India (Table 2).

The proportion of HBsAg positive mothers having 'e' antigen vary considerably in available studies (Table 2) and, because of small numbers have wide confidence intervals. There is no data from several regions of the country. Socio-cultural factors besides geographic and ethnic factors may also influence the prevalence of HBV markers.

A recent community based survey for estimating prevalence of HBV markers in Tamil Nadu (K Thomas et al, personal communication) showed that the life-time risk of exposure to hepatitis B infection was 27.4% and 5.4% individuals were HBsAg positive. HBeAg was positive in 23.6% of HBsAg positive subjects (25 of 106; 95% CI:15.8–32.8).

Perinatal transmission

In a study conducted at the PGI Chandigarh, 20 babies born to HBV mothers with chronic HBV infection were followed up for 6–18 months. Seven of the 10 babies born to mothers

Table 2. Prevalence of HBV markers in women with chronic HBV infection

Place	HBsAg+ve alone+ve/ total	% 95% CI	HBsAg+ve and HBeAg+ve/ total	% 95% CI	HBsAg+ve and antiHBe+ve/ total	% 95% CI
Delhi[33]	200/322	62.1 (56.7–67.5)	25/322	7.8 (4.8–10.8)	97/322	30.1 (25.0–35.2)
Delhi[34]	88/191	46.0 (38.9–53.3)	24/191	12.5 (7.8–17.4)	79/191	41.4 (34.2–48.5)
Chandigarh[35]	7/23	30.4 (11.3–49.6)	11/23	47.8 (27.0–68.7)	5/23	21.7 (4.5–38.9)
Delhi[36]	32/39	82.1 (66.5–92.5)	7/39	17.9 (7.5–33.5)	ND	

ND – Not done

positive for both HBsAg and HBeAg had persistent HBsAg in their blood as compared to 2 of the 10 babies born to mothers positive only for HBsAg. Transmission rate was therefore 70% and 20% respectively. None of the mothers or babies had anti-HBe.[35]

In a more detailed study conducted at the PGI Chandigarh during 1987-88, 49 infants born to HBsAg positive mothers were followed up till one year for determination of rate of acquiring chronic HBV infection[37] (Table 3). The risk of transmission was highest (73%, 95% CI: 50.5–96.2) if the mother was positive for both HBsAg and HBeAg and lowest (9.0%, 95% CI: 0.0–32.1) if she was anti-HBe positive. The relative risk (RR) for a child to get infection if mother was both HBsAg and HBeAg positive was 8.1, and if she was only HBsAg positive, the RR was 1.44.[37]

High circulating virus load has also been implicated in breakthrough perinatal transmission inspite of both active and passive immunoprophylaxis given at birth. Interestingly, it has been

Table 3. Transmission pattern in children born to mothers with chronic HBV infection

Follow-up (age in months)	Maternal antigen status and transmission rates		
	HBsAg +ve only (n=23) (%)	HBsAg and HBeAg +ve (n=15) (%)	HBsAg and anti-HBe (n=11) (%)
3	4 (17.4)	8 (53.3)	1 (9.0)
6	3 (13)	10 (66.6)	1 (9.0)
12	3 (13)	11 (73.3)	1 (9.0)

demonstrated that lamivudine (150 mg) when given to pregnant mothers from 36 weeks of gestation until delivery with a HBV-DNA load of more than 1.2×10^9 geq/ml reduced DNA levels significantly and their off-springs did not develop persistent HBV infection as evidenced by loss of HBsAg and appearance of anti-HBs antibodies. All these babies also received immunoprophylaxis at birth.[38] However, in a recent report Kazim et al from New Delhi have shown that lamivudine therapy does not prevent perinatal transmission of precore mutant HBV infection to the newborn.[39] Despite immunoprophylaxis and vaccination, the newborn developed biochemical and histological evidence of chronic hepatitis.

In a study conducted at the AIIMS, Delhi[33], 188 children born to HBsAg positive mothers and 328 children born to HBsAg negative mothers were followed-up. Results of the first six months follow-up indicated that the transmission was most frequent (87.5%) if the mother was HBeAg positive and was less so, if she was positive for anti-HBe (17.5%) or for HBsAg alone (9.6%). However, 10 (3%) children born to HBsAg negative mothers were also positive for HBsAg at 6 months. The study demonstrated that mechanisms other than vertical transmission were operative in the first six months of life in our community.

In a recent study from Aligarh, eight infants out of 16 born to HBsAg positive mothers were found to have HBsAg in their cord blood, indicating 50% perinatal transmission. In 15 out of 16 mothers, HBsAg was tested positive during third trimester. In 25% of these mothers there was evidence of acute HBV infection as indicated by positive IgM anti-HBc. Interestingly, seven out of eight neonates (87.5%) had IgM anti-HBc antibody indicating *in utero* transmission of the virus. The study indicated high transmission rate of HBV if the infection was acquired during pregnancy.[40]

Prevalence of HBV markers in children and adults

A limited number of studies in India have assessed the prevalence of HBsAg and anti-HBs in different age groups. In a multi-center study (Table 4), 982 children of either sex below the age of 5 years from well-baby clinics of four centres (Kanpur, Mysore, New Delhi and Secunderabad) were investigated for HBsAg and anti-HBs using mELISA.[41] The data from this multicenter study showed that the overall HBsAg prevalence rate in the preschool age group was 2.1% (21/982). Almost 15% (209/1396) children below the age of five years were also carrying anti-HBs antibody. Thus, it was evident that HBsAg positivity rate was built up in early childhood and major exposure to HBV occurred in the pre-school age group. A closer examination of the data revealed that the prevalence amongst children under one year (2.5% 95% CI: 1.1–4.9) was almost equal to those between one and five years (1.96%, 95% CI: 0.9–3.0). Thus, it appeared that bulk of the infection pool was acquired during infancy and continued throughout childhood.

A WHO collaborative study on hepatitis B in twenty countries had a center in Pune, India.[42] RIA was used to determine HBsAg on sera collected from apparently healthy individuals of

Table 4. Prevalence of hepatitis B markers in children under 5 years of age in a multi-center study, 1991

Age (yr.)	HBsAg +ve/total	% (95% CI)	anti-HBs +ve/total	% (95% CI)
<1	8/320	2.5 (1.1–4.9)	42/249	16.9 (12.4–22.1)
1–3	8/353	2.3 (1.0–4.4)	44/309	14.2 (10.5–18.6)
4–5	5/309	1.6 (0.5–3.7)	123/838	14.7 (12.3–17.3)

both sexes. The results of the study are shown in Table 5. The HBsAg positivity rate amongst children below the age of 15 years was 4.9% (7/144, 95 % CI:1.3–8.5), and in adults was 6.5% (36/556, 95% CI:4.4–8.6). The difference was statistically not significant (chi-square=0.52, p=0.472). The anti-HBs prevalence rate was 12.9% (23/179, 95% CI:7.9-17.9) in children as compared to adults 32.2% (213/661, 95% CI:28.6–35.9). This difference was significant (chi-square=26.17, p=<0.001). The prevalence of HBsAg among males was 7.2% (26/367) and 5.2% (17/333) in females. Seven percent (17/244) of the rural population and 5.3% (24/456) of the urban population were positive for HBsAg, while 26.7% (151/566, 95% CI:23.0–30.4) of the rural population, and 30.4% (83/274, 95% CI:24.7–35.8) of the urban population were anti-HBs positive. These differences were not significant. There was a trend for increasing HBsAg prevalence rate from below 5 years of age to 5–9 and 10–14 year age categories. Anti-HBs antibody levels increased significantly with advancing age, particularly beyond 20 years.

In another study conducted at New Delhi, healthy children and adults were screened for markers of HBV (SK Panda et al, personal communication). About 10% of children under

Table 5. Prevalence of markers of HBV in different age groups, Pune, 1980

Age (yr.)	HBsAg +/total	% (95%CI)	anti-HBs +ve/total	% (95% CI)
0–4	0/6	0 (0–0)	1/9	11.1 (0.0–32.0)
5–9	1/50	2.0 (0.0–6.0)	8/62	12.9 (4.4–21.4)
10–14	6/88	6.8 (1.4–12.2)	14/108	13.0 (6.5–19.4)
15–19	7/107	6.5 (1.8–11.3)	15/131	11.5 (5.9–17.0)
20–29	5/130	3.8 (0.5–7.2)	40/159	25.2 (18.3–32.0)
30–39	9/122	7.4 (2.6–12.1)	47/147	32.0 (24.3–39.7)
40–49	9/101	8.9 (3.2–14.6)	54/115	47.0 (37.7–56.3)
>49	6/96	6.3 (1.3–11.2)	57/109	52.3 (42.7–61.9)

15 years (77/739, 95% CI:8.2–12.7) were HBsAg positive as compared to 3.7% (353/9549, 95% CI:3.3–4.1) among adults. The difference was highly significant (chi-square-77.41, p=<0.001). Anti-HBs positivity rate amongst children was 20.5% (88/429, 95% CI:16.6–24.4), and of adults 22.9% (223/972, 95% CI:20.3–25.6). The findings indicated that a major portion of the exposure to HBV took place in children below 15 years of age, and a large proportion (27.4%) were under 5 years of age. Anti-HBc was also measured among adults in this study. It was 24.6% (283/1151, 95% CI:22.1–27.1), highest being in the age group of 16–25 years. There appears to be a decline of this antibody with age (Table 6). It could be argued that the older people have a reduced exposure or at-risk activities or this was an artifact because of difference in the socio-economic status and differential health care access of the populations in different age groups.

Table 6. Prevalence of HBV markers in different age groups, Delhi, 1993

Age (yr)	HBsAg	% (95% CI)	anti-HBs	% (95% CI)	anti-HBc	% (95% CI)
1-5	18/148	12.2 (7.4–18.5)	31/113	27.4 (19.5–36.6)	ND	
6-15	59/591	10.0 (7.7–12.7)	59/316	18.7 (14.5–23.4)	ND	
16.25	33/1303	2.5 (1.7–3.5)	94/480	19.6 (16.1–23.4)	200/659	30.3 (26.9–34.0)
26-35	260/7036	3.7 (3.3–4.2)	96/363	26.4 (22.0–31.3)	65/363	17.9 (14.1–22.2)
36-45	57/1160	4.9 (3.7–6.3)	28/95	29.5 (20.6–39.7)	15/95	15.8 (9.1–24.7)
>45	3/50	6.0 (1.3–16.5)	5/34	14.7 (5.0–31.1)	3/34	8.8 (1.9–23.7)

* ND – not done

A population based study was conducted at Madras (Thyagarajan SP, personal communication). The HBsAg prevalence rate was 8.9% (27/304, 95% CI:5.6–12.1) among children below 15 years and 5.4% (34/633, 95% CI:3.6–7.2) among adults. The difference was significant (chi-square=4.16, p=0.0141). The prevalence rate was highest in children below the age of 5 years. Anti-HBs prevalence was about 29.3% (89/304, 95% CI:24.1–34.5) amongst children under 15 years of age and 19.4% (123/633, 95% CI:16.3–22.6) in adults. Further, it was observed that children below one year of age showed an HBsAg prevalence of 12.5%, suggesting a high perinatal transmission rate. Due to small sample size and wide confidence interval (2.9% to 22.1%) there was unreliability of the estimate. The higher prevalence of anti-HBs detected was also probably of maternal origin (Table 7).

Table 7. Prevalence of HBV markers in different age groups, Madras, 1993

Age (yr.)	HBsAg+ve/total	% (95% CI)	Anti-HBs+ve/total	% (95% CI)
<1	6/48	12.5 (2.9–22.1)	21/48	43.7 (29.4–58.1)
1.5	12/128	9.4 (4.2–14.5)	40/130	30.8 (22.7–38.9)
6–10	4/64	6.3 (0.2–12.3)	15/62	24.2 (13.3–35.1)
11–15	5/64	7.8 (1.1–14.5)	13/64	20.0 (10.3–30.4)
16–25	9/202	4.5 (1.6–7.4)	40/202	19.8 (14.2–25.4)
36–45	8/125	6.4 (2.0–10.8)	21/125	16.8 (10.1–23.5)
>45	2/52	3.9 (0.0–9.2)	9/52	13.3 (6.8–27.8)

Population-based studies

Recently, two populations based studies were published (Tables 8, 9): one from urban population in two South Indian cities[43] and another conducted among rural subjects in West Bengal.[44] Appropriate sampling techniques were adopted and hence were likely to be reasonable estimates of the true picture of HBV infection in the community. Both studies more or less confirmed the previous observations that most of the HBV infection pool built up below the age of 15 years, specifically before five years of age. In the study by Singh et al, three of 57 infants (5.3%; 95% CI:1.1–14.6) (i.e. <1 yr. age group) in Bangalore and Rajahmundry had acquired HBsAg.[43] In the study by Chaudhary et al,[44] number of subjects below five years was less; and hence the 95% confidence intervals of the estimate was wide (0.03–7.2). In both these population based studies, chronic HBsAg positivity rates increased from below five years to above five years, though the differences were not significant. Unfortunately, in neither of these population-based studies, HBeAg status was determined.

Table 8. Prevalence of HBsAg in different age groups in urban Rajahmundry and Bangalore, Karnataka[43] (population-based data)

Age categories (yr.)	Number of persons tested	Number postive for HBsAg	% (95% CI)
0–4	620	25	4.0 (2.6–5.9)
5–9	285	14	4.9 (2.7–8.1)
10–14	189	4	2.1 (0.6–5.3)
15–29	190	8	4.2 (1.8–8.1)
20–39	244	6	2.5 (0.9–5.3)
≥ 40	25	1	4.0 (0.1–20.4)
Total	1553	58	3.7 (2.8–4.8)

Table 9. Prevalence of HBV markers in different age groups in a rural community of West Bengal[44] (population based data)

Age categories (yr.)	No. tested	No. +ve	HBsAg % (95% CI)	Anti-HBc %
< 5	75*	1	1.3 (0.03–7.2)	8.2
5–9	117	8	6.8 (3.0–13.0)	9.8
10–19	204	13	6.4 (3.4–10.7)	10.4
20–39	405	23	5.7 (3.6–8.3)	11.9
40–59	113	6	5.3 (2.0–11.2)	19.7
≥ 60	46	0	0 (0–7.7)	27.8
Total	960	51	5.3 (4.0–6.9)	13.2

* Only 15 children below one year

Horizontal transmission

In a study from Jaipur,[45] 236 family members of 70 index HBV associated liver disease patients were studied for markers of HBV infection. HBV markers were positive in at least one member of the index patients (46/70; 65.7%). Probability of HBV infection amongst the family members of HBeAg positive index patients (63%) was significantly more than those of HBeAg negative index patients (32%). The most common probable mode of spread in family members was horizontal (72%) followed by vertical transmission (14%) and sexual route (14%).

A sero-epidemiological study was conducted in an orphanage in Pune, among children 5–16 years of age.[46] The HBsAg prevalence was 15.3% (13/85) while 56.5% (48/85) were positive for anti-HBs. The overall exposure to HBV infection was 71.8% (61/85), as compared to 8.0% of general school going population. The prevalence was higher among boys living there for more than three years as compared to those with a shorter stay. In another study, 193 household contacts of 40 HBsAg positive hepatitis patients and 103 contacts of 27 HBsAg negative hepatitis patients were screened for the presence of markers of HBV.[47] The family contacts of HBsAg positive patients had a significantly higher prevalence of HBV infection [HBsAg 22/193 (11.34%) and anti-HBs 49/193 (25.3%)] as compared to those with HBsAg negative hepatitis [HBsAg 4/103 (3.8%) and anti-HBs 14/103 (13.5%)]. However, the absence of IgM anti-HBc in the HBsAg positive contacts indicates that they had most probably acquired the infection prior in the past. These two studies underscored the role of horizontal transmission of the infection in Indian settings.

Tribal populations

Murhekar et al[48] carried a survey for hepatitis B prevalence in four out of six primitive tribes in Andaman and Nicobar islands. The overall prevalence of HBsAg in the Nicobarese tribe was 23.3% (267/1144; 95% CI:21.0–25.9) with males being positive more than females (28.4% vs. 18.9%, p< 0.0001 respectively). The prevalence was 9.4% in 5–10 years age group and increased with age with a peak at 21–30 years (31.8%) and was common in all age groups. HBsAg positivity was also high in the non-Nicobarese tribes viz. Shompens (37.8%) and Onges (31.0%). It was interesting to note that ratio of HBsAg positivity to anti-HBs positivity was nearly one in almost all age categories. This pattern is usually described for infancy when most of HBV infection results in chronic infection. But this alone does not explain progressive increase in carriage state after 10 years of age. There might be other host and genetic factors in these tribes which predispose to the risk of developing persistent infection despite advancing age. This is contrary to observations in studies from other parts of the country. Limited number of adults in this population were tested for anti HBc antibodies and almost all (94.7%) were positive. The message of a high proportion of anti-HBc positivity in the absence of other markers raises the possibility of circulating surface mutants in the population. There appears to be regional variation amongst tribal populations. Other tribes in the country where studies have been done do not demonstrate such high HBsAg prevalence as reported in the earlier study. The HBsAg prevalence rates have been reported in tribes from Arunachal Pradesh (5.5–8.4%),[49] Madhya Pradesh (4.4%),[50] and Maharashtra (6.8–11.8%).[51]

CURRENT PERSPECTIVES

Transmission of hepatitis B virus from mother to infants during the perinatal period is of concern for several reasons. During the perinatal time, infants are exposed to maternal blood through trauma related to birth and contact of conjunctiva and mucous membranes with blood and other body fluids during labour and delivery. *In utero* infection occurs rarely. As indicated in the study by Sharma et al, *in utero* transmission was more likely if HBV was acquired during pregnancy.[40] The presence of HBsAg in cord blood does not necessarily indicate *in utero* infection, since it may represent transient maternally derived antigenemia. Infants born to HBeAg positive mothers have a risk as high as 60–90% of acquiring HBV infection.[31] However, if the mother is HBsAg positive but HBeAg negative or anti-HBe positive; the infant has only 2–15% chance of becoming infected[32]. The relative importance of perinatal route thus varies with HBV endemicity and frequency of HBeAg positivity among HBsAg positive mothers. Secondly, the risk of chronic infection is believed to be highest (70–90%) for infants who acquire the infection during the perinatal time, and many would eventually develop cirrhosis of liver or hepatocellular carcinoma.[3]

One to nine percent (95% CI) of pregnant women in the various studies in India were positive for HBsAg (weighed average: 2.8%, 95% CI:2.7–3.1), and between 4.8 to 68.7% (95% CI) of them also showed HBeAg, while 4.5 to 48.5% (95% CI) had anti-HBe. The large confidence intervals, because of small sample sizes, therefore make precise estimation difficult. From the available studies, the transmission rates worked out to be 70–87% among HBsAg positive mothers who are also positive for HBeAg, 9–20% in those who have only HBsAg positivity, and 9–17% in those who were positive for anti-HBe.

The reported prevalence in pregnant females varies widely in different parts of the world.[52] It has been reported to be high in several Asian countries: Taiwan 15.2%, Korea 9.8%, Burma 6.8%, China 5.4% and Japan 2.5%, the figure for UK was 0.1% and Germany 0.8%. Approximately 40% of the chronic HBsAg positive women of child bearing age in East Asia are estimated to be HBeAg positive. In Africa, approximately 10% women are HBsAg positive but only about 12% of them are HBeAg positive.

There is only a single study[33] which has systematically looked at the issue of relative contribution of perinatal and horizontal transmission. Accordingly in North India, where HBeAg positivity was 7.8%, risk of perinatal transmission was 18.6% from HBsAg positive mothers and horizontal transmission during the same period (6 months) was 3% among infants of HBsAg negative mothers. When modeling was done with this data, only 14% of the total pool of HBsAg positive infants could be attributed to vertical transmission. Most of the remaining transmission would be due to horizontal mode. If one does sensitivity analysis for varying prevalence of HBeAg among HBeAg positive population, the proportion of vertical and horizontal transmission does not change much. If we assume in the same data, HBeAg positivity was 20% and 25% instead of 7.8%, the positive pool due to vertical transmission will be 22.3% and 24.9% of the total pool respectively. Hence most of the HBV transmission occurring in the country is due to horizontal mode.

It is equally important to note that there is evidence of significant transmission of HBV occurring in first year of life. In the above mentioned study[33], 3% infants (95% CI:1.4–5.5) born to HBsAg negative mothers developed chronic HBsAg positive state by 6 months. Hence, attributing all HBV infection in the first year of life to vertical transmission is erroneous.

Cross-sectional surveys estimating prevalence of HBV in different age categories will have to be interpreted in the light of above discussion. Almost all studies from across the country have consistently shown that force of HBV infection is maximum in the first five years of life and the chronic HBsAg positivity rates are similar among those younger than one year and 1–5 year old. Recent population based studies from rural and urban areas of Karnataka[43] do provide some indication of increasing HBsAg positivity rate from 0–5 yr. to 5–10 year age groups, reflecting contribution of horizontal transmission. In the overall assessment it appears that the cross-sectional surveys will continue to give an ambivalent picture regarding mode of transmission because of a significant rate of horizontal transmission occurring in the first year of life. If further confirmation of relative contribution of vertical and horizontal transmission to the over all HBsAg positive pool is required, we need one year follow up of infants born to either HBsAg positive or HBsAg negative mothers for risk of HBsAg positivity at different time intervals. Such studies can be carried out in different parts of the country to take into account variations in HBeAg status of chronic HBV infected subjects.

To reduce the burden of HBV infection in our country, universal immunization has been recommended as the most cost effective strategy[53]. In our country 30–60% of the pregnant women get antenatal care and only 10–15% infants are born at health centers. Even in the capital city of Delhi, only 30–35% of the deliveries are institutional. If the focus of universal immunization is to interrupt all HBV transmission including vertical, then all newborns will have to be vaccinated within 48 hours of birth. This clearly is not feasible in foreseeable future. On the other hand, integration of HBV immunization with DPT and OPV vaccines starting at 6 weeks of life appears to be a pragmatic and reasonably efficient way of initiating the process[54]. Most of the horizontal transmission of HBV can be effectively interrupted by this strategy. Babies born at health centers can be given an additional dose of HBV vaccine to avail the opportunity of interrupting vertical transmission in this subgroups. However, as the health facilities improve in future all new borns can be vaccinated soon after birth.

REFERENCES

1. Maynard JE. Hepatitis B: global importance and need for control. *Vaccine* 1990;8(suppl 1):S18-20.
2. Naik SR. Hepatitis B virus: infected or just carrying? *Indian J Gastroenterol* 2000;19:130-2.
3. Maddrey WC. Hepatitis B: an important public health issue. *J Med Virol* 2000;61:362-6.
4. Edmunds WJ, Medley GF, Nokes DJ. The transmission dynamics and control of hepatitis B virus in the Gambia. *Stat Med* 1996;15:2215-33.
5. Edmunds WJ, Medley GF, Nokes DJ, Callaghan CJ, Hall AJ, Whittle HC. The influence of age on the development of the hepatitis B virus (HBV) carrier state. *Proceedings of the Royal Society (London), Series B.* 1993;253:197-201.
6. Peterson NJ, Barret DH, Bond WW, Berquist KR, Favero MS, Bender TR, Maynard JE. Hepatitis B surface antigen in saliva, impetigous lesions, and the environment in two Alaskan villages. *Appl Environ Microbiol* 1976;32:572-4.
7. Lemon SM, Thomas DL. Vaccines to prevent viral hepatitis. *N Engl J Med* 1997;336:196-204.
8. Beasely RP, Hwang LY. Post-natal infectivity in hepatitis B surface antigen carrier mothers. *J Infect Dis* 1986;147:185-90.
9. Toukan AU, Sharaiha ZK, Abdul-El-Rob OA. The epidemiology of hepatitis B virus among family members in Middle East. *Am J Epidemiol* 1990;132:220-32.
10. Wang JS, Zhu QR. Infection of the fetus with hepatitis B e antigen via the placenta. *Lancet* 2000;355:989.
11. Edmunds WJ, Medley GF, Nokes DJ, Callaghan CJ, Whittle HC, Hall AJ. Epidemiological patterns of hepatitis B virus (HBV) in highly endemic areas. *Epidemiol Infect* 1996;313-25.
12. Lu SN, Liu JH, Wang JH, Lu CC. Secular trends of HBeAg prevalence among HBsAg-positive delivery mothers in a hepatitis B endemic area. *J Trop Pediatr* 2000;46:121-3.
13. Prince AM. An antigen detected in the blood during the incubation period of serum hepatitis. *Proc Natl Acad Sci USA* 1968;60:814-21.
14. Schweitzer IL, Mosley JW, Ashcavai M, Edwards VM, Overby LB. Factors influencing neonatal infection by hepatitis B. *Gastroenterology* 1973;65:277-83.
15. Ghendon Y. WHO strategy for the global elimination of new cases of hepatitis B. *Vaccine* 1990;8:129-33.

16. Yao GB. Importance of perinatal versus horizontal transmission of hepatitis B virus infection in China. *Gut* 1996;38(suppl 2):S19-42.
17. Yuen MF, Lai CL. Towards control of hepatitis B in the Asia-Pacific Region: Natural history of chronic hepatitis B virus infection. *J Gastroenterol Hepatol* 2000;15(suppl)E20-4.
18. Hsu SC, Chang MH, Ni YH, Hsu HY, Lee CY. Horizontal transmission of hepatitis B virus in children. *J Pediatr Gastroenterol Nutr* 1993;16:66-9.
19. Tan CC, Guan R, Yap I, Tay H, Kang JY. Horizontal or vertical transmission of hepatitis B virus? A serological survey in family members of hepatitis B carriers in Singapore. *Trans Royal Soc Trop Med Hyg* 1991;85:656-9.
20. Qu ZY. An epidemiological study on the distribution of HBsAg and anti-HBs in China. *Chinese J Microbiol Immunol* 1986;6 (Suppl):S20-40.
21. Xi LF, Xu ZY, Shen YD. The horizontal and perinatal transmission of hepatitis B virus infection. *Chinese J Virol* 1991;7(Suppl):S21-4.
22. Chang MH, Sung JL, Lee CY, Chen CJ, Chen JS, Hsu HY, Lee PI, et al. Factors affecting clearance of hepatitis B e antigen in hepatitis B surface antigen carrier children. *J Pediatr* 1989;115:385-90.
23. Vegnente S, Lorio R, Guida S, Cimmino L. Chronicity rate of hepatitis B virus infection in the families of 60 hepatitis B surface antigen positive chronic carrier children: role of horizontal transmission. *Eur J Pediatr* 1992;151:181-91.
24. Goh KT, Ding JL, Monteiro EH, Oon CJ. Hepatitis B in households of acute cases. *J Epidemiol Comm Health* 1985;39:123-8.
25. Martison FEA, Weigle KA, Royce RA, Weber DJ, Scuhindran CM, Lemon SM. Risk factors for horizontal transmission of hepatitis B virus in a rural district in Ghana. *Am J Epidemiol* 1998;147(5):478-87.
26. Hsu HY, Chang MH, Ni YH, Lin HH, Wang SH, Chen DS. Surface Gene mutants of hepatitis B virus in infants who develop acute or chronic infections despite immunoprophylaxis. *Hepatology* 1997;26:786-91.
27. Oon CJ, Tan KL, Harrison T, Zuckerman A. Natural history of hepatitis B surface antigen mutants in children. *Lancet* 1997;349:1105.
28. Ni YH, Chang MH, Hsu HY, Chen HY. Long term follow up study of core gene deletion mutants in children with chronic hepatitis B virus infection. *Hepatology* 2000;32:124-8.
29. Akarca US, Greene S, Lok ASF. Detection of precore hepatitis B virus mutants in asymptomatic HBsAg positive family members. *Hepatology* 1994;19:1366-70.
30. Syndman DR. Hepatitis in pregnancy. *N Engl J Med* 1985;313:1398-1401.
31. Beasley RP, Hwang LY, Lee GCC. Prevention of perinatally transmitted hepatitis B infection with hepatitis B immunoglobulin and Hepatitis B vaccine. *Lancet* 1983;322:1099-102.
32. Margolis HS, Alter MJ, Hadler SC. Hepatitis B. Evolving epidemiology and implications for control. *Semin Liver Dis* 1991;11:84-92.
33. Nayak NC, Panda SK, Zuckerman AJ, Bhan MK, Guha DK. Dynamics and impact of perinatal transmission of hepatitis B virus in North India. *J Med Virol* 1987;21:137-45.
34. Panda SK, Ramesh R, Rao KV, Gupta A, Zuckerman AJ, Nayak NC. Comparative evaluation of the immunogenicity of yeast derived (recombinant) and plasma-derived hepatitis B vaccine in infants. *J Med Virol* 1991;35:297-302.
35. Biswas SC, Gupta I, Ganguly NK, Chawla Y, Dilwari JB. Prevalence of Hepatitis B surface antigen in pregnant mothers and its perinatal transmission. *Trans Royal Soc Tropical Med Hyg* 1989;83:698-700.
36. Mittal SK, Rao S, Rastogi A, Aggarwal V, Kumari S. Hepatitis B – Potential of perinatal transmission in India. *Tropical Gastroenterol* 1996;17:190-2.
37. Gupta I, Sehgal A, Sehgal R, Ganguly NK. Vertical transmission of hepatitis B in North India. *J Hyg Epid Microbiol Immunol* 1992;36:263-7.

38. Nunen AB, Man RA, Heijtink RA, Niesters HGM, Schalm SW. Lamivudine in the last 4 weeks of pregnancy to prevent perinatal transmission in highly viremic chronic hepatitis B patients. *J Hepatol* 2000;32:1040-1.
39. Kazim SN, Wakil SM, Khan LA, Hasnain SE, Sarin SK. Vertical transmission of hepatitis B virus despite maternal lamivudine therapy. *Lancet* 2002;359(9316):1488-89.
40. Sharma R, Malik A, Rattan A, Iraqi A, Maheshwari V, Dhawan R. Hepatitis B virus infection in pregnant women and its transmission to infants. *J Trop Pediatr* 1996;42:352-4.
41. Tandon BN, Irshad M, Raju Manikya, Mathur GP, Rao MN. Prevalence of HBsAg and anti-HBs in children and strategy suggested for Immunization in India. *Ind J Med Res* 1991;93:337-9.
42. Sobeslavsky O. Prevalence of markers of hepatitis B virus infection in various countries: a WHO collaborative study. *Bull WHO* 1980;58:621-8.
43. Singh J, Bhatia R, Khare S, Patnaik S, Biswas S, Lal S, Jain D, Sokhey J. Community studies on prevalence of HBsAg in two urban populations of Southern India. *Indian Pediatr* 2000;37:149-52.
44. Chowdhury A, Santra A, Chaudhuri S, Ghosh A, Banerjee P, Guha Mazumder D. Prevalence of hepatitis B infection in the general population: a rural community based study. *Tropical Gastroenterol* 1999;20:75-7.
45. Rai RR, Sharma, Jain NK, Mathur A, Nijhawan S. Intra familial transmission of hepatitis B. *Indian J Gastroenterol* 2001;20(suppl 2):A92.
46. Sehgal A, Arankalle V, Gadkari D, Pavri K. Hepatitis B infection in an orphanage. *Ind J Med Res* 1983;78:607-10.
47. Chorje SP, Pavri KM, Prasad SR, Sehgal A, Phule DM. Horizontal transmission of hepatitis B virus infection in household contacts, Pune, India. *J Med Virol* 1985;16:183-9.
48. Murhekar MV, Murhekar DD, Arankalle VA, Sehgal SC. Prevalence of hepatitis B infection among the primitive tribes of Andaman & Nicobar Islands. *Ind J Med Res* 2000;111:199-203.
49. Prasad SR, Rodrigues FM, Dhorje SP, Ramamoorthy CL. Prevalence & subtypes of hepatitis B surface antigen in the tribal population of Arunachal Pradesh, India. *Ind J Med Res* 1983;78:300-6.
50. Reddy PH, Tedder RS. Hepatitis virus markers in the Baiga tribal population of Madhya Pradesh, India. *Trans R Soc Trop Med Hyg* 1995;89:620.
51. Mukherjee M, Joshi SH, Rao VR, Gorashakar AC, Sathe MS. Prevalence of hepatitis B surface antigen among some tribes of Madhya and Maharashtra. *J Ind Anthorp Soc* 1990;25:68-72.
52. Shaprio CN. Epidemiology of hepatitis B. *Pediatr Infect Dis J* 1993;12:433-7.
53. Miller M. Routine hepatitis B immunization in India: Cost effectiveness assessment. *Indian J Pediatr* 2000;67:299-300.
54. Arora NK, Agadi SN. Hepatitis B immunization–a practical approach for India. *Indian J Paediatr* 1998;65(suppl):S72-4.

5

Intrafamilial transmission of hepatitis B virus

Sadras P Thyagarajan, Raghu Hari, Sannadi Jayaram, Kailapuri G Murugavel, Ketha Venkatakrishna K Mohan, Elumalei Dhevahi

Chronic hepatitis B virus (HBV) infection continues to be a significant public health problem all over the world. Current data projects that there are 350 million people infected with HBV in the world.[1] Of these about 47 million subjects are in India alone, keeping 4.7% as the prevalence of HBV infection in our country.[2] These human reservoirs not only facilitate the maintenance of the HBV pool but are also potential source of transmission of HBV to the healthy population. Since HBV is a blood-borne virus, the most important modes of transmission are sexual, transfusion of blood and blood products, injuries with infected needles or sharing of needles in intravenous drug users, or from infected mothers to newborns. In spite of stringent criteria for analysis, HBV transmission studies have revealed that the source of HBV infection was not traceable in about 20-25% of cases. The horizontal/intrafamilial spread is the most likely mechanism of HBV transmission in those cases. An understanding of the transmission of HBV in a given country is necessary to initiate prevention and remedial measures in HBV control.

HISTORICAL PERSPECTIVES

Bancroft et al in 1971[5] reported for the first time the occurrence of the family clustering of HBV with in the family of a 5½ year old child with giant cell hepatitis wherein three of the four family members were found to be having asymptomatic chronic HBV infection. The first family study to characterize intrafamilial spread of HBV was reported by Reeves et al[6] in 1975 which involved 255 Panamanian Guaymi Indians representing 48 families and 32 living units. It was observed that the infection rate in the families of HBsAg positive index cases was 0.64 in contrast to 0.19 in families without the infection (p < 0.001). Their results indicated that families with chronic HBV infected subjects had higher HBV infection rate than families without such subjects.

Subsequently, many studies from USA,[7,8] European countries,[9,10] Australia,[11] Newzealand,[12] Africa,[13] and Asian countries[14,15] including India[16] have been reported. Following is the summary of observations made in these studies:

(a) Intrafamilial spread is a possible means of HBV transmission,[17]
(b) there is increased risk of acquiring HBV infection by living with a subject with chronic HBV infection on a long-term basis,[18]
(c) prevalence of HBV markers is significantly higher among the contacts of more than one HBsAg positive subject (75.9%) than among those with only one HBsAg positive subject (26.0%),[19]
(d) horizontal, non-parenteral[20] transmission of HBV among siblings played a major role in the families of HBsAg positive cases,
(e) the family clustering was striking in all populations where the genealogies were known,[11]
(f) viral markers were detected more frequently in blood relatives than in non-blood relatives of index HBsAg positive cases,[21]
(g) the subjects in the group without clustering had a higher rate of HBeAg negativity than the group with clustering. Of the original HBeAg negative subjects, the group without clustering had less damage to the liver than the groups with clustering.[22]

In an epidemiological study by Toukan et al[23] among family members in the Middle East, a history of contact with a jaundiced person and socio-economic status were independent risk factors for HBsAg positive status. On the other hand, contact with a jaundiced person, rural background, and age were independently related to HBV infection. There was a trend towards an association of HBsAg positive children with HBsAg positive mothers. Postnatal early childhood horizontal transmission among children of poorer and larger families probably accounted for the high endemicity of HBV in that region. Wang[24] adopting HBV subtyping in a family clustering study showed that familial transmission was classifiable into six types, namely, generational, horizontal, recessive, intra- and extra-familial, non-familial and undetermined ones. Yao[25] suggested that in China, horizontal transmission is an important route of HBV infection during early childhood, and the proportion of chronic HBsAg positivity attributable to perinatal transmission has been estimated at only 13–20%.

An African study by Karim et al[13] hypothesised that low socio-economic status, living in crowded conditions with an average of seven people in a house with one or two bedrooms, might provide an appropriate milieu for the spread of HBV infection.

Indian studies on intrafamilial transmission of HBV are scanty. In one study Dhorje et al[16] compared the household contacts of HBsAg positive subjects with those of HBsAg negative subjects, in Pune, India. The risk of HBV infection was significantly higher in the former group with 80% positivity for HBV markers than in the latter group, which had only 48.1% HBV markers positivity.

In all these studies conducted across the globe, the possibility of family clustering and intrafamilial HBV transmission has been authenticated.[5-26] The actual mechanism of this intrafamilial transmission of HBV is not always known. However, sexual transmission or inapparent percutaneous exposure through shared razors, tooth brushes, etc. are frequently suspected. The impact of replicative HBV status in determining HBV transmission rate within families gives credence to the hypothesis, that a consistent, cumulative exposure of family members to one or more HBeAg/HBV-DNA positive persons, blood contaminated body fluids especially saliva has to be thought of as the principal source of horizontal transmission.

Interestingly, the analysis of the pre-1995 (Tables 1, 2, 3 and 4) and post-1995

Table 1. Family clustering of HBV in chronic HBsAg positive and negative families

Group	Families analysed	No.	HBsAg positive No.	%
Chronic HBsAg positive	60	140	34[a]	24.2
HBsAg negative	24	90	4[b]	4.4

a vs. b p < 0.001

Table 2. Pedigree analysis of HBsAg status among families of indexed chronic HBsAg positive subjects (*n*=60)

	Family members analysed	No. +ve for HBsAg	% HBsAg positive
Total HBsAg positivity	140	34	24.2
HBsAg positivity in mother only	10	5	50.0
HBsAg positivity in father only	20	7	35.0
HBsAg positivity in mother & father	5	3	60.0
HBsAg positivity in spouses	43	4	9.3
HBsAg positivity in brother & sister	12	6	50.0
HBsAg positivity in children	21	3	14.2

Table 3. Rate of HBV transmission within families of HBeAg positive and negative subjects

Family member pattern	No. tested positive	No. HBsAg positive	No. HBeAg positive
HBeAg positive subject family (*n*=20)	43	18 (41.9%)[a]	10 (55.5%)
HBeAg negative subject family (*n*=40)	97	16 (16.6%)[b]	7 (43.7%)

a vs. b p < 0.001

Table 4. Analysis of risk factors for acquiring chronic hepatitis B virus infection

Factor	Pre-1995 (% positive)	1995–2000 (% positive)
Previous history of jaundice	20.5	30.6
Blood transfusion	4.1	8.0
History of surgery	5.1	17.0
History of prolonged hospitalization	6.9	8.8
History of series of injections	11.6	2.9
Unprotected sexual contact with high-risk groups / convalescing jaundice patients	2.7	7.9
None of the above	59.5	24.8

(Tables 5, 6, 7 and 8) family clustering data from our Chennai studies strongly suggest that the rate of intrafamilial transmission of HBV is on the decrease in this geographic region. This could most probably be due to (i) increasing awareness about HBV among the general

Table 5. Family clustering of HBV in Chronic HBsAg positive and negative families

Group	Families analyzed	No. of individuals	HBsAg positive n (%)	HBeAg positive n (%)	Anti-HBs positive n (%)	Anti HBc positive n (%)	HBV markers n (%)
Chronic HBsAg positive	81	264	48 (18.1)[a]	17 (35.4)	42 (16.2)	29 (11)	119 (45.3)
HBsAg negative	28	102	4 (4.4)[b]	1 (25)	5 (5.1)	8 (7.9)	17 (17.4)

a vs. b $p < 0.01$

Table 6. Pedigree analysis of HBsAg positive status among families of index chronic HBsAg positive subjects

	Family members analysed	HBsAg +ve Number	%
Total HBsAg positivity	264	48	18.1
HBsAg positivity in mother only	83	18	21.68
HBsAg positivity in father only	68	11	16.17
HBsAg positivity in mother and father	20	5	25
HBsAg positivity in spouses	43	3	6.9
HBsAg positivity in brother and sister	12	5	41.6
HBsAg positivity in children	38	6	15.78

Table 7. Rate of HBV transmission within families of HBeAg positive and HBeAg negative index case

Index case	No. tested	HBsAg +ve n (%)	HBeAg +ve n (%)
HBeAg positive (n=26)	96	28 (19.16)[a]	10 (10.14)
HBeAg negative (n=55)	168	16 (9.5)[b]	7 (4.1)

a vs. b $p < 0.01$

Table 8. Impact of HBeAg status on contacts within families in Tamil Nadu (n=1856)

HBV status	HBeAg contact in family		Negative family control		Total	
	No.	%	No.	%	No.	%
HBsAg positivity	28	50.8	78	43	106	57

public, and (ii) the increasing practice of vaccinating HBV negative family members of known HBsAg positive subjects. It is to be strongly recommended that all HBsAg negative family members of known HBV infected individuals should be routinely administered with the hepatitis B vaccine.[27]

REFERENCES

1. Seeger C, Mason WS. Hepatitis B virus biology. *Micro and Mol Biol Reviews* 2000;64:51-68
2. Thyagarajan SP, Jayaram S, Mohanavalli B. *Prevalence of HBV in General population of India.* In: Sarin SK, Singal AK, Eds. Hepatitis B in India: Problems & Prevention. CBS Publishers & Distributors, New Delhi 1996; pp.5-16
3. Thyagarajan SP, Jayaram S, Hari R, Sridhar G, Rani E, Paneerselvam A. Familial clustering of HBV among HBsAg carrier and non-carrier members in India. *Biomedicine* 1996;16:21-7.
4. Thyagarajan SP, Jayaram S, Pannerselvam A, Malathy S. Characterisation of healthy hepatitis B surface antigen (HBsAg) carriers in Tamilnadu, India. *Ind J Med Res* 1997;15:163-6.
5. Bancroft WH, Raphael L, Warkel, Anthony AT. Russell PK. Family with hepatitis associated antigen. *JAMA* 1971; 217:1817-20.
6. Reeves WC, Peters CJ, Moon TE, Purcell RH. Familial clustering of hepatitis surface antigen among Panamanian Indians. *J Infect Dis* 1975;131:67-70.
7. Peters CJ, Purcell RH, Lander JJ, Johnson KM. Radio immunoassay for antibody to hepatitis B surface antigen shows transmission of hepatitis B virus among household contacts. *J Infect Dis* 1976; 134:218-23.
8. Mazzur S, Jones N. Limited family clustering of hepatitis B surface antigen in a Melanesian population. *Am J Epidemiol* 1977;105:113-7.

9. Hess G, Born M, Dormeyer H, Zoller B, Arnold W, Knolle J. Hepatitis B virus markers among family contacts of asymptomatic HBsAg carriers. *Scand J Gastroenterol* 1979;14:373-8.
10. Pastore G, Dentico P, Angarano G, Lapedota E, Schiraldi O. Infectivity markers in HBsAg chronic carriers and intrafamilial spread of hepatitis B virus infection. *Hepatogastroenterology* 1981;28:20-2.
11. Barrett EJ. Hepatitis B in Australian aborigines and Torres Strait Islanders: Geographical, age and familial distribution of antigen subtypes and antibody. *Aust NZ J Med* 1976;6:106-11.
12. Powell E, Duke M, Cooksley WGE. Hepatitis B transmission within families: potential importance of saliva as a vehicle of spread. *Aust NZ J Med* 1985;15:717-20.
13. Abdool Karim SS, Thejpal R, Hoosen M Coovadia HM. Household clustering and intra household transmission patterns of hepatitis B virus infection in South Africa. *Int J Epidemiol* 1991;20:495-503
14. Sung JL, Chen DS. Clustering of different subtypes of hepatitis B surface antigen in families of patients with chronic liver diseases. *Am J Gastroenterol* 1978;69:559-64.
15. Tong MJ, Weiner JM, Ashcavai MW, Vyas GN. Evidence for clustering of hepatitis B virus infection in families of patients with primary hepatocellular carcinoma. *Cancer* 1979;44:2338-44.
16. Dhorje SP, Pavri KM, Prasad SR, Sehgal A, Phule DM. Horizontal transmission of hepatitis B virus infection in household contacts, Pune, India. *J Med Virol* 1985;6:183-9.
17. Tan HZ. (Family clustering analysis of HBV infection). *Chung Hua Yu Fang I Hsueh Tsa Chih.* 1989;23:135-8.
18. Perrillo RP, Gelb L, Campbell C, Wellinghoff W, Ellis FR, Overby L, Aach RD. Hepatitis B e Antigen, DNA polymerase activity and infection of household contacts with hepatitis B virus. *Gastroenterology* 1979;76:1319-25.
19. Porres JC, Carreno V, Bartolome J, Gutiez J, Castillo I. A dynamic study of the intrafamilial spread of hepatitis B virus infection: relation with the viral replication. *J Med Virol* 1989;28:237-42.
20. Craxi A, Tine F, Vinci M, Almasio P, Camma C, Garofalo G, Pagliaro L. Transmission of hepatitis B and hepatitis delta viruses in the households of chronic hepatitis B surface antigen carriers: A regression analysis of indicators of risk. *Am J Epidemiol* 1991;134:641-70.
21. Tong MJ, Weiner JM, Ashcavai MW, Redeker AG, Comparini S, Vyas GN. A comparative study of hepatitis B viral markers in the family members of Asian and non Asian patients with hepatitis B surface antigen positive hepatocellular carcinoma and with chronic hepatitis B infection. *J Infect Dis* 1979;140:506-12.
22. Habu D, Monna T, Saithoh S, Kuroki T, Kobayashi K. Relationship between the condition of the liver in-patients and carriers with hepatitis B virus (HBV) and whether there is intrafamilial clustering of HBV. *Nippon Shokakibyo Gakkai Zasshi* 1991;88:1545-53.
23. Toukan AL, Sharaiha ZK, Abu-el-Rub OA, Hmoud MK, Dahbour SS, Abu-Hassan H, Yacoub SM, et al. The epidemiology of hepatitis B virus among family members in the middle east. *Am J Epidemiol* 1990;132:220-32.
24. Wang Q. Application of HBV gene subtyping method in study on familial transmission. *Chung Hua Liu Hsing Ping Hsueh Tsa Chih* 1993;14:199-203.
25. Yao GB. Importance of perinatal versus horizontal transmission of hepatitis B virus infection in China. *J Hepatol* 1997;2:221-7.
26. Pazdiora P, Brejcha O, Kubatora A, Moravkova I, Ovradova R, Prechora M, Turkov D, et al. 33-years study of family contacts of HBsAg positive individuals. *Cas Lek Cesk* 2001;140:397-401.
27. Staff MP, Angel PA. Vaccination among household contacts of chronic hepatitis B carriers by general practitioners. *Aust Farn Phys* 2002;31:491-3.

6

Transmission of hepatitis B virus in injecting drug users

Lalit Kant

Parenteral administration is one of the quickest ways to reach any drug into the blood and this holds true for many infections. Use of contaminated needles is a well-known route of transmission for various blood-borne infections, especially the hepatitis (notably B and C) and the human immunodeficiency viruses. The route is well recognized but like the injecting drug users often marginalized. Injecting drugs for non-medical purposes, mostly illicit drugs, appears to be on the rise and calls for a concerted multi-pronged effort towards its control.

INJECTING DRUG USE IN INDIA

There are no firm numbers of the injecting drug users (IDUs) in India,[1,2] but a review published by the Asian Harm Reduction Network under the auspices of the United Nations estimates that there are around 3 million heroin users, plus a large population which uses pharmaceuticals. The state of Manipur has about 25,000–40,000 injecting drug users out of a population of 1.8 million.[2]

India is an important producer of legal narcotics (gum opium), pharmaceuticals such as buprenorphine and propoxyphene, and some illicit narcotics. It is also a cross-road for international trafficking. In 1985, prohibition was clamped on cannabis and opium, and since then the heroin based "brown sugar" appears to be domestic drug of choice. In Manipur and Nagaland injectable heroin is preferred.[1,2] Brown sugar heroin is usually inhaled by 'chasing', but there appears to be a recent trend towards injecting, particularly in metropolitan cities of Mumbai and Chennai.[3] Transition to drug injecting has also been facilitated by scarcity of heroin and increased availability of buprenorphine.

RISK BEHAVIOUR OF IDUs

Sharing patterns of needles and syringes

Two studies have been chosen to illustrate about the risk behaviour of IDUs. Though disposable needles and syringes are available over the counter without prescription all over the country, the injecting drug users tend to share them. In a study conducted in Chennai,[4] it has been observed that many IDUs disposed of their needles only when they became blunt. Needles and syringes are often stored in house corners, wrapped up in cloth. Only about one-third did not share needles or syringes with others. Of those who shared, the average size of sharing pool was four to five. Whereas in Calcutta,[5] the number of needle/syringe sharing partners ranged 1–12, with an average of three. IDUs also had a tendency to withdraw blood a few times into the syringes and push in back in the belief that it enhanced euphoria. The needle coming in contact with blood was cleaned by licking with saliva or sucking it off. In Chennai[4] most users reported using water to clean the syringe, a few cleaned with saliva. Use of bleach or boiling of glass needle/syringe in water is quite uncommon.

Sexual behaviour

Unprotected multi-partner sexual activity appears to be quite common among IDUs. In two studies from Chennai[4] and Calcutta[5] nearly one-third had history suggestive of sexually transmitted diseases. Thirty-three to 73% of the subjects visited commercial sex workers. In addition, 15% of the subjects from Calcutta indulged in homosexual activities. Regular condom use was very infrequent in both the studies.

Hepatitis B among IDUs

Not many investigators having studied the prevalence of HBV in injecting drug users. The new findings of some of the major studies are summarized in Table 1.

In several countries world over, high rates of infection with hepatitis B among injecting drug users have been reported. Prevalence rates vary from 51–88% in USA to 38–89% in Europe.[8] A cross-sectional study among street youths in Montreal to study behaviour for hepatitis B infection showed that those having injected drugs were 3.5 times (95% CI: 1.5–8.3) more likely to have HBV infection.[9]

Table 1. Hepatitis B markers among injecting drug users, India

Place (yr.)	HBsAg	Anti-HBs	Anti-HBc	Group
Chandigarh[7] (96)	2.9	10.4	–	NS
Calcutta[5] (98)	19.0	–	–	NS
Calcutta[8] (97)	8.0	–	–	IDUs in jail
Chennai[4] (99)	32.0	–	–	NS
Manipur[6] (2000) (HIV+ve IVDUs)	100.0	–	100.0	HIV+ve

HBsAg sub-type distribution has been studied in Spain among 670 samples from subjects belonging to various epidemiological risk groups. Similar frequencies of *d* and *y* sub-type determinants were found among non-risk normal HBsAg positive subjects. In contrast the *ay* subtype was clearly predominant (79–87%) among intravenous drug users.[10] In a study from Sweden, genotype D (among 58% of IDUs) was the predominant[11] genotype. Whether subtypes have a preference for a particular route of transmission needs to be further investigated.

In Budapest, the prevalence of hepatitis B virus infection in intravenous and non-intravenous drug users is the same as in general population. Risk of HCV infection was nearly 13 times higher in subjects sharing needles vis a vis disposable needle users (38% vs. 3%).[12] The study underscores the important role played by needle sharing in transmission of HCV infection.

Among the IDUs, sharing of needles/syringes and high-risk sexual behaviours are common. The group shares two routes of transmission of hepatitis viruses, viz., through injection or through sex. Therefore, it becomes imperative not only to study and associate demographic variables such as age and duration of drug use with HBV markers, but also patterns of drug injection and sexual behaviours. This would help to draw inferences regarding relative importance of these alternative routes of transmission. Equally important is to study all the important sero-markers (HBsAg, anti-HBs and anti-HBc) to draw inferences regarding particular HBV serologic marker profiles among injecting drug users.[13]

Prevention policies

Steps to prevent hepatitis B infection in India must include guidelines for injecting drug users. Needle sharing plays an important role in transmission of HBV to fresh users. Interventions directed at reducing the sharing of needles such as needle exchange programs and availability of bleach could play an important role in interrupting transmission. As transmission through sexual route could also be a contributory factor, encouraging safe sex practices would also help to limit transmission of hepatitis B. Finally immunizations with hepatitis B vaccine in infancy for long-term effect, or of adolescents provides an alternative approach for preventing HBV infection in the immediate future.

The fact that HIV prevention campaigns also have an effect on incidence of hepatitis B among drug users has been demonstrated in a study among drug users on a methadone maintenance treatment in Geneva. Over 700 IDUs in treatment between 1988 and 1995 were tested biannually for HIV, HBV, and HCV infection. The prevalence of these infections at entry into treatment declined dramatically over time for the three viruses. Comparing IDUs entering treatment after 1993, the prevalence of HIV was 38.2% versus 4.5%, of HBV 80.5% versus 20.1%, and of HCV 91.6% versus 29.8% respectively.[14] The data suggests that IDUs have changed risk-taking behaviour in response to HIV prevention campaigns.

In another case-control study conducted by the Seattle-king county Department of Public

Health, Washington, association between syringe exchange use and hepatitis B and C among IDUs was investigated. Non-exchange of syringe increased the risk of hepatitis B six-fold. (OR=5.5, 95% CI=1.5, 20.4). The results suggest that use of exchange can lead to a significant reduction in hepatitis B.[12,15]

While several programs aimed at harm reduction among IDUs specifically in relation to HIV/AIDS have been reported to be successful in the developed countries. Probably they are culturally and/or politically inapplicable. Nevertheless, success of some of interventions on small-scale have been encouraging and hold out hope for future. For example, the work of Lifesaving and Life-giving Society (LALS) in Kathmandu, Nepal;[16] Ikhlas, Kuala Lumpur, Malaysia.[17] Needle Syringe Exchange Programme, Mae Chan, Thailand[18] is commendable. In India, the Society for Serving the Urban poor, SHARAN, New Delhi[19] has successfully run a substitution program aimed at weaning off injecting drug users. In Manipur, the Society for HIV/AIDS and Lifeline Operations (SHALOM)[20] runs a program which includes syringe exchange, home and institutional detoxification and rehabilitation, use of bleach to clean needles, community education, recreational and vocational rehabilitation. So successful has been the program that the Manipur Government has included the harm reduction approach in the State AIDS policy.

As for HIV, coverage of interventions is critical to be effective. More than 80% coverage is desirable. Some of interventions work very well as pilot or demonstration projects, but suffer when they are scaled-up. For example in Nepal even after demonstration of successful impact (continued low prevalence under 2%) of early introduction of harm reduction measures in LALS' project,[16] recent report suggests that HIV and HCV sero-prevalence has started rising in a sample of drug users.[21] The lesson to learn is the need for rapid responses incorporating effective interventions and adequate coverage. Multi-level interventions and multi-sectoral involvement is key to success of such large-scale programs.

There is also a need to understand factors that facilitate injecting drug use. Some of the factors have been studied and include cost of heroin, the rate of police arrests, and social acceptance of drug injection. Certain geographical locations, settings and sub-populations have increased risk, there is a need to track changes in behavioural risk over time to contain the spread of HBV.[22,23] Many of the problems of HBV transmission among IDUs are linked to poverty, slum dwelling, unhygienic surroundings, non-availability of primary health care, clean water, sterile syringes, and high level of demoralization.[24-26] Without addressing these environment issues, it is doubtful whether full potential of interventions for IDUs will be realized.

REFERENCES

1. Narain JP, Jha A, Lal S, Salunke S. Risk factors for HIV transmission in India. *AIDS* 1994;8 (suppl 2):S77-82.
2. McLaughlin A. HIV/AIDS control in Manipur. *Asian Harm Reduction Newsletter* 1996(3).

3. Muddaliar S, Kumar SSM. Comparative analysis of HIV sexual and substance use risk behaviours among injecting heroin users and suprenorphine users in a drug treatment program. 58th Annual Scientific Meeting, College on Problems of Drug Dependence: Building International Research in Drug Abuse, opportunities and Challenges, India, 1996 (abstract).
4. Kumar MS, Muddaliar S, Thyagarajan SP, Kumar S, Selvanayagam A, Daniels D. Rapid assessment and response to injecting drug use in Madras. *South India Intt J Drug Policy* (in Press).
5. Panda S, Chatterjee A, Bhattacharjee S, Ray B, Saha MK, Bhattacharya SK. HIV, hepatitis B and sexual practices in the street-recruited injecting drug users of Calcutta: risk perception versus observed risks. *Intt J STD & AIDS*. 1998:9:214-8.
6. Saha MK, Chakrabarti S, Panda S, Naik TN, Manna B, Chatterjee A, Detels R, et al. Prevalence of HCV & HBV infection amongst HIV seropositive intravenous drug users & their non-injecting wives in Manipur, India. *Ind J Med Res* 2000,111:37-9.
7. Kaur U, Sahani SP, Bambery P, Kumar B, Chauhan A, Chawla VK, Dilawari JB. Sexual behaviour, drug use and hepatitis B infection in Chandigarh students. *Nat Med J India* 1996;9:156-9.
8. Levine OS, Vlahov D, Koehler J, Cohn S, Spronk AM, Nelson KE. Seroepidemiology of hepatitis B virus in a population of injecting drug users. *Am J Epidemiol* 1995;142:331-41.
9. Roy E, Haley N, Lemire N, Boivin JF, Leclerc P, Vincelette J. Hepatitis B virus infection among street youths in Montreal. *CMAJ* 1999;161:689-93.
10. Echevarria JE, Leon P, Lopex JA, Tenorio A, Domingo CJ, Echevarria JM. HBsAg subtype distribution among different populations of HBsAg carriers in Spain. *Eur J Epidemiol* 1995;11:39-45.
11. Lindh M, Horal P, Norkrans G. Acute hepatitis B in Western Sweden – genotypes and transmission routes. *Infection* 2000;28:161-3.
12. Hagan H, Jarlais DC, Friedman SR, Purchase D, Alter MJ. Reduced risk of hepatitis B and hepatitis C among injection drug users in the Tacome syringe exchange program. *Am J Public Health* 1995;85:1531-7.
13. Shreshtha SM, Shreshtha DM, Gafney TE, Maharajan KG, Tsuda F, Oka H. Hepatitis B and C infection among drug abusers in Nepal. *Trop Gastroenterol* 1996;17:212-3.
14. Brores B, Junet C, Bourquin M, Deglon JJ, Perrin L, Hirschel B. Prevalence and incidence rate of HIV, hepatitis B and C among drug users on methadone maintenance treatment in Geneva between 1988 and 1995. *AIDS* 1998;12:2059-66.
15. Osztrogonacz H, Gerevich J, Horvath G. Tolvaj G, David K. Prevalence of chronic viral hepatitis in drug abusers. *Orv Hetil* 2000;141:715-8.
16. Peak A, Rana S, Mahajan SH, Jolley D, Crofts N. Declining risk of HIV among injecting drug users in Kathmandu, Nepal: the impact of a harm reduction program. *AIDS* 1995;9:1067-70.
17. Narayanan P. Working with drug users in Kaula Lumpur. VIII Intl. Conference on Reduction of Drug Related Harm. Paris March 1997.
18. Gray J. Operating needle exchange programs in the hills of Thailand. *AIDS Care* 1995;7:489-99.
19. Dorabjee J, Samson L, Dyal Chand R. A community based intervention for injecting drug users in New Delhi Slums. Presented at VII International Conferences on the Reduction of Drug Related Harm. Hobart, March 1996.
20. Longkham B, Vanlalmuana P, Chinklolal T. An approach to reducing the impact of HIV/AIDS in Churachandpur. III International Conference on the Biopsychological Aspects of AIDS. Melbourne, June 1997 (abstract).
21. Karki BB, Upreti S. RAR Survey among drug users in Nepal, January 1999. Paper presented at the Inter-Country Technical Workshop for the prevention of Drug use and HIV/AIDS, organized by UNAIDS ESCAP, New Delhi 1999, June 1-4.

22. Lifson AR, Halcon LL. Substance abuse and high-risk needle-related behaviours among homeless youth in Minneapolis: implications for prevention. *J Urban Health* 2001;78:690-8.
23. Mcelrath K. Risk behaviours among injecting drug users in Northern Ireland. *Subst Use Misuse* 2001;36:2137-57.
24. Santolamazza M, Dell C, Monache M, Alvino A, Bacosi M, D'Jnnocenzo S, Gervo U, et al. Multiple viral infections in a group of intravenous drug users: hepatitis B virus exposure in the risk factor. *Eur J Gastroenterol Hepatol* 2001;13:1347-54.
25. Lemberg BD, Shaw-stiflel TA. Hepatic disease in injection drug users. *Infect Dis Clin North Am* 2002;16:667-79.
26. Panda S, Saha U, Pahari S, Mathan M, Poddar S, Meogi D, Sarkar M, et al. Drug use among the urban poor in Kolkata: behaviour and environment correlates of low HIV infection. *Natl Med J India* 2002;15:128-34.

Transfusion-associated hepatitis B after transfusion of blood negative for hepatitis B surface antigen

Shubhangi Saraswat, Vivek A Saraswat

After the discovery of the Australia antigen by Blumberg in 1969 and its identification as excess coat protein of hepatitis B virus (HBV), the putative agent responsible for serum hepatitis, tests for its routine detection were rapidly developed and introduced in clinical practice. Expectation of overcoming the problem of transfusion-associated hepatitis (TAH) were soon dashed when it was found that in most parts of the world only 20% or fewer cases of TAH were due to HBV, the remainder being due to the then unknown non-A non-B virus(es). Throughout the 1970's and 80's, tests for the detection of HBsAg were refined and improved, from agar-gel diffusion to reverse passive hemagglutination, enzyme-linked immunoassays and radio-immunoassays. Despite these newer tests, HBV could be implicated in the causation of only 20–25% of TAH. However, even as early as 1978,[1] it was suspected that TAH due to HBV was occurring despite transfusion of blood negative for HBsAg by the available tests. Accumulating data in the late 1980s and 90's has confirmed that this is indeed a clinical problem. Though this problem was first discovered and studied in the West, it is perhaps a much more pressing problem in Asia. Intermediate HBsAg prevalence areas of the world like India are especially vulnerable to this problem. In low prevalence areas, the risk of HBV infection being transmitted by HBsAg negative units is miniscule, given the very low prevalence of infection in the general population. On the other hand, in high prevalence areas like China, Taiwan and Hong Kong, though HBsAg rates are high and appreciable HBV transmission may be occurring through HBsAg negative units, the background prevalence of subclinical exposure and probable immunity to HBV is also high, with anti-HBc rates of 60–80%,[2] so that the proportion of HBV susceptible population and the risk of overt TAH-B may be low. Intermediate prevalence areas of the world like India seem to have the worst of both worlds, with high levels of HBV transmission, as suggested by high levels of HBV-DNA (4–24%)[3-5] among HBsAg negative voluntary donors and low frequency of anti-HBc

(~20%)[4,5] in the general population, so that risk of HBV sero-conversion or TAH-B due to HBsAg negative units is high.

MAGNITUDE OF THE PROBLEM

World Health Organization estimates suggest that 7 units of blood or components are transfused per hospital bed per annum. Based on this figure, it was estimated in 1997 that about 6 million units were needed every year in India to meet the needs of existing hospital beds. A national survey estimated that in India, annual blood collection was only one-third of this figure (1.9 million units), ~20% of which was being collected from voluntary, 30% from replacement and 50% from professional donors.[6] The incidence of TAH reported in small studies from India has been 15–17/1000 units transfused,[7,8] a figure much higher than in the West (1–2/1000)[9] or in Japan (0.038/1000). About 20% of these cases are due to HBV.[8,10] Using these figures, it can be estimated that at the present rate of blood transfusion, the annual incidence of TAH in India is approximately 30,000 cases, 6000 of which are due to HBV despite donor screening for HBsAg. In all probability, these figures are an underestimate. Although bleeding paid donors is now illegal, it is by no means certain that they have been completely eliminated from the donor pool. It is well documented that HBsAg positivity in this group (5–36%)[11] is much greater than in the general population (4.7%).[12] Apart from the morbidity and mortality of acute hepatitis B and its complications, 5–10% develop chronic liver disease, with ~30% ultimately likely to die of sequelae such as chronic hepatitis, liver cirrhosis and hepatocellular carcinoma. The financial burden incurred is enormous due to the following factors: (a) man-hours lost during the most productive phase of life, (b) repeated hospitalization, (c) antiviral therapy, (d) and the continued transmission of the virus within the general population.

TRENDS IN INCIDENCE OF TAH-B

Through the 1980s and 90's, even after the universal introduction of screening of all donated units with 3rd generation ELISA for HBsAg, the incidence of TAH varied from 1 to 16% in various parts of the world[7-10, 13-22] (Table 1). Though an overall reduction in the frequency of TAH has been noted after HBV screening, a process that has been markedly accelerated with the introduction of routine anti-HCV screening through the 1990s, it is worth noting that most countries have not succeeded in totally eliminating TAH-B. In the 1990s, 2.7–16.6% of TAH continues to be due to HBV even after 3rd generation ELISA screening for HBsAg. The wide variation in the frequency of TAH reported from various parts of the world and the differential impact of HBsAg screening on the occurrence of TAH-B may be due to differences in the prevalence of HBV markers in donors from different geographical areas as well as the wide variability in the protocol of the infectious disease marker tests being performed on donor blood. The Japanese Red Cross Non-A, Non-B Hepatitis Research Group[19] reported reduction in TAH from 7.7% before to 2.1% after anti-HCV screening

Table 1. Transfusion associated hepatitis: 1982-99

Author	Year	Country	N	TAH (%)	TAH-B (%)	TAH-C (%)	NANAB (%)
In the West							
Cossart	1982[9]	Australia	842	2	16.6	78	—
Collins	1983[13]	UK	248	2.4	—	—	3.2
Widell	1987[14]	Sweden	739	3.1	—	—	—
Feinman	1988[15]	Canada	576	9.2	—	—	—
Hoyos	1989[16]	Spain	112	11.6	7.7	—	92.3
Blajchman	1995[17]	Canada	—	2	—	—	—
In Asia							
Wang	1991[18]	China	296	12.5	2.7	64.8	32.4
JRC	1991[19]	Japan	—	7.7	0	—	—
Chung	1993[20]	Hong Kong	—	2.4	6.7	0.6	—
Huang	1994[21]	Taiwan	—	13.8	—	65	—
In India							
Patwari	1986[22]	Delhi	20	16	67	33	—
Dasarathy	1992[10]	Delhi	250	6.9	20	80	—
Saraswat	1996[7]	Lucknow	47	12.7	67	33	—
Saxena	1999[8]	Delhi	182	7.7	21	71	—

JRC – Japanese Red Cross

was introduced. They also found that TAH-B, which earlier accounted for 12% of TAH, was completely eliminated with no case of TAH-B reported since the policy of discarding all HBsAg positive and isolated anti-HBc positive units with hemagglutination inhibition (HAI) titers $\geq 2^6$ was implemented. This Japanese experience of identifying and discarding units positive for HBsAg and isolated, high-titer anti-HBc is unique and is the only instance of effective elimination of TAH-B from a population.

HBV-DNA in HBsAg negative blood

In Sardinia, where HBsAg positivity in the general population is 6.5%, Lai et al[3] found HBV-DNA by dot blot hybridization in 5% of 1411 HBsAg negative donors. In Taiwan, where chronic HBsAg positivity rate is 20%, Wang[18] failed to detect HBV-DNA by dot blot hybridization in 206 HBsAg negative voluntary blood donors with normal ALT but HBV-DNA was detected by PCR in 4%. From India, one center detected HBV-DNA in 9.8% of 500 HBsAg negative donor samples by dot blot hybridization,[4] while another center reported a figure of 24% by PCR in 126 voluntary units.[5] Reports from areas of low HBV prevalence have been mixed. In Germany,[23] HBV-DNA was detected after nested PCR in 10 HBsAg negative donors in plasma enriched with virus particles by ultracentrifugation; it was detected in only 30% without ultracentrifugation. Ninety percent of these samples also tested positive for anti-HBc. However, in USA, in a population with very low HBsAg (0.004%) and anti-HBc positivity (0.6%), HBV-DNA could not be amplified by PCR in any of 158 HBsAg negative, anti-HBc positive units.[24] Though the biologic role and significance of this hepatitis B viremia in areas with intermediate and high prevalence of HBV infection is uncertain, its implications for transfusion medicine are alarming. If these initial observations are substantiated in larger populations over a longer period of time, screening for HBV-DNA to identify this group of donors may become mandatory.

Some observations suggest that the presence of HBV-DNA in donor units does not necessarily result in transmission of TAH-B. Though HBV-DNA was detected by PCR in 9 of 206 HBsAg negative blood units, none of the recipients developed TAH-B, though developed non-A non-B TAH. The fact that all these units had tested negative for HBV-DNA by dot-blot hybridization suggests that only low level viremia was present and the dose of the virus transfused may have been too low to establish infection. Since it is known that while sensitive PCR assays can detect even a single viral particle,[25] 10^2 particles/ml is the minimum infectious dose in chimpanzees.[26] Alternatively, and more probably, it is likely that, in a hyperendemic country like Taiwan, many of the recipients may have had prior exposure to HBV and may already be immune to the virus, so that fresh exposure would not result in overt TAH. It was not studied whether any of the recipients seroconverted or not. These data also suggest that such units may transmit infection with other hepatitis viruses.

TAH-B AFTER TRANSFUSION OF HBsAg NEGATIVE BLOOD

Reports of TAH-B occurring after the transfusion of HBsAg negative blood first came in from USA[1] and Europe.[27,28] A female blood donor who had donated blood 25 times in 8 years and had repeatedly tested negative for HBsAg, was implicated in 3 clinical cases of TAH-B.[25] Thirteen of the 27 recipients of products prepared from these donations, who were alive and could be recalled for testing, were found to have acquired serologic markers of HBV infection. On subsequent testing, she was found to have high titers of anti-HBc and detectable HBV-DNA of subtype ayw.[29] DNA sequencing or quantitation were not reported. While most reports find detectable or high-titer anti-HBc[1,23,25] in HBsAg negative, HBV-DNA positive units, Thiers[26] reported DNA positivity in serum and liver of 3 patients in the absence of any detectable serologic markers of HBV infection and demonstrated that such units were infectious to chimpanzees.

At least 2 reports from India have documented clinical TAH-B after HBsAg negative transfusions.[7,8] TAH-B occurred in 4 of 47 (8.3%) recipients transfused 4 or more units of HBsAg negative blood during elective cardiac surgery.[7] Retesting stored donor sera demonstrated that each recipient had received 2 or more units negative for HBsAg but positive for HBV-DNA. Low level viremia was suspected in the implicated units, as, the units tested anti-HBc and HBV-DNA positive were persistently HBsAg negative with other EIAs while the HBV infection that developed in recipients was readily detected by standard HBsAg kits. Similarly, another study[8] reported TAH-B in 3/182 (1.6%) recipients, at least 1 of whom had received one HBsAg negative, HBV-DNA positive unit. TAH-B in the other 2 recipients appeared to have been caused by units in which HBsAg positivity was missed by the screening EIA used, but was picked up on subsequent testing with another HBsAg kit. These reports highlight the continuing transmission of HBV through HBsAg negative blood and emphasize the need for alternative tests to screen such donor units for HBV.

Recently, Jongerius[30] investigated HBV sero-conversion occurring in a multi-transfused patient who had received blood products from 200 donations screened for HBsAg. To trace the HBV-infectious unit, follow-up donor samples collected from all 200 voluntary, repeat donors 3 months or more after the implicated donation were tested for anti-HBc (172 from archived subsequent donations, 28 from called back donors). One of these tested positive for anti-HBc; platelets derived from the unit donated by this donor had been transfused to the recipient. On retesting stored serum from this donation, the unit was found to be HBsAg negative, anti-HBc negative but HBV-DNA positive. On looking back, products derived from this unit had caused transfusion associated HBV infection in 2 additional patients. This case highlights the problem of HBsAg negative units, probably donated in the window period of acute HBV infection, transmitting HBV infection that cannot be prevented by HBsAg or even anti-HBc screening; nothing short of screening for HBV-DNA would have prevented this infection.

Mechanisms

There is no single explanation for the phenomenon of TAH-B after transfusion of HBsAg negative blood. A false negative HBsAg test may result from (a) technical error in performance of the test, (b) presence of circulating HBsAg–anti-HBs immune complexes that may occur in persistent HBV infection[31] or (c) use of an insensitive HBsAg EIA. Retesting HBsAg negative samples implicated in transmitting TAH-B by a different kit, such as one using polyclonal anti-HBs, or in a different laboratory has resulted in positive tests for HBsAg.[8, 31]

Low level viremia

Currently available EIAs and RIA for HBsAg have a detection threshold of ~15–20 ng/ml, while most commercial and in-house PCR assays for HBV-DNA have detection threshold of 0.7 million genome equivalents or 2.5 pg/ml. The former two tests are quite adequate for routine clinical practice, since, in common or grden variety of chronic HBV infection, levels of viremia and antigenemia are far in excess of these thresholds. However, the minimum chimpanzee infective dose (MCID) is known to be 100 genomes/ml (0.36 fg/ml).[28] Thus, it is clear that the sensitivity of presently used tests is far below the level at which a blood unit may be infectious and that some blood units testing negative for HBsAg by currently available tests may be capable of transmitting HBV infection. This situation is perhaps the commonest mechanism by which apparently HBsAg negative units are found to transmit HBV infection. It should be suspected when units testing HBsAg negative during routine donor screening are implicated in transmitting wild type HBV infection detected by routinely used kits. On retesting, stored sera from implicated units may be found to be positive for HBsAg by a different EIA. Even if HBsAg is persistently negative in the original unit, it will invariably be found positive for anti-HBc and HBV-DNA.[7,8,31] This serologic profile (HBsAg negative, anti-HBc positive, HBV-DNA positive) suggests low level viremia in a donor unit capable of transmitting HBV infection. There are no reports quantifying level of HBV-DNA in such units. At least the Japanese experience suggests that these units are likely to be identified by testing for high-titer anti-HBc.[19]

Mutant virus infections

One of the foremost explanations for the phenomenon of TAH-B developing despite the transfusion of HBsAg negative blood has been the concern that false negative HBsAg tests may be due to S-gene HBV mutants in donor units. Given the facts that during persistent HBV infection ~25 mg of excess viral coat protein is produced daily and that random mutations occur at the rate of 2×10^{-4} base substitutions/site/year, the spontaneous emergence of a replication-competent variant not expressing immunologically detectable HBsAg was predicted in 1981.[32] The major envelope protein is encoded by the S gene of the HBV genome. Though over 10 serotypes of HBV have been described, the 4 major ones are *adw*, *ayw*, *adr* and *ayr*, based on the common 'a' determinant and the mutually exclusive d/y and w/r determinants. While domain 32–72 have T-cell epitopes, domain 110–160 contains the antigenic determinants that produce B-cell responses to HBsAg.[31] The 9 amino acid peptide analogue of the sequence 139–147 has been shown to produce anti-HBs that could be neutralized by all serotypes of HBsAg.[33] Additional epitopes have been mapped to HBsAg sequence 124–137. Thus, current data suggest that the composite sequence 124–147 appears to be the site for reactivity with various human anti-HBs/'a' and that mutations affecting this region are likely to produce virions that are not bound or poorly bound by anti-HBs, especially monoclonal anti-HBs directed at the 139–147 sequence. This would render the virus undetectable by many routinely used HBsAg EIAs that use such antibodies and may also result in HBV breakthrough infections despite vaccination with recombinant vaccines.[31]

Antibody escape mutant (AEM) in a vaccinated child was first reported from Italy.[34] A single mutation (G145A) in the 'a' determinant of the envelope protein was identified. Subsequent reports from Japan[35] and Singapore[36] have documented this AEM in vaccine recipients and in HBIg recipients for neonatal prophylaxis[37] and after liver transplantation.[38] It has been speculated that the AEM was mutant virus that had previously emerged spontaneously in the course of pre-existing chronic HBV infection and was selected under immune pressure of antibody induced by vaccination or infused as HBIg. At least in liver transplant recipients, the AEM reverted to wild type virus on cessation of immune pressure upon withdrawal of

HBIg. Though this AEM was capable of inducing infection in non-immune chimpanzees, it did not do so in immunized animals and fears of AEM epidemics sweeping through vaccinated and non-vaccinated populations have been discounted.[39] Thus, it appears highly unlikely that AEM virus is present in the general donor population to any significant extent or contributes at all to false negative HBsAg tests in donors. So far, there is no report of the AEM being implicated in any instance of HBV transmission by HBsAg negative blood. However, this may happen in the future if the proposed strategy of universal HBV vaccination of repeat donors is adopted.

Surface mutants that escape detection by several commonly used HBsAg screening tests and cause TAH-B have been reported.[40] A repeat blood donor tested HBsAg positive with Abbott EIA after having repeatedly tested negative with other EIAs on earlier donations. At this time, 4 other EIAs and 1 RIA for HBsAg routinely used for donor screening tested negative. The specificity of the positive Abbott EIA was confirmed by neutralizing serum with anti-HBs; additionally, HBeAg and anti-HBc were positive, anti-HBe and anti-HBs were negative while HBV-DNA was detectable by PCR in that unit. DNA sequencing revealed Q129R (Gln→Arg) and M133T (Met→Thr) substitutions in the 'a' determinant region of HBsAg. This report confirms the presence of surface mutants in the general population, raising the need for anti-HBc or HBV-DNA screening of donor blood. Limited data are available about the frequency of surface mutants in the general population, though a report from India[41] suggests that as much as 10% of HBV-related chronic liver disease may be due to surface mutants.

Precore mutants were implicated in a report of fulminant transfusion-associated hepatitis B in 8 recipients of HBsAg negative transfusions.[42] Two types of precore mutations were identified in the 124 HBV-DNA clones propagated from recipients: A G83A mutation converting codon 28 for Trp (TGG) to a stop codon (TAG) in 114 clones from these 8 patients and an insertion of 2 base pairs after codon 26 in 10 other clones from 1 patient. Anti-HBc testing identified some of the implicated donor units, suggesting that even this mutant may be identified by anti-HBc screening.

Blood units donated during the window period of acute HBV infection are likely to transmit infection. About 12–15% of transfusion associated HIV infections are thought to occur during the window period of HIV infection. In intermediate and high HBV prevalence regions of the world, appreciable inapparent, subclinical horizontal transmission may be occurring even in adult populations, as suggested by the high frequency (4–24%) of HBV-DNA in asymptomatic, HBsAg negative voluntary donors.[3-5, 19] Such transmission may contribute to window period infections, which are likely to be discovered only by meticulous investigation of TAH-B episodes or HBV sero-conversion in recipients.[30] The serologic profile (HBsAg negative, anti-HBc negative, HBV-DNA positive) of units from donors who may transmit HBV infection while in the window period of acute infection is such that these units are only likely to be identified if a policy of routine screening with HBV-DNA for all donor units were to be implemented. Few data are available to substantiate the occurrence and frequency of such window period infections and the contribution of this mechanism to the problem of HBsAg negative units transmitting HBV infection remains unknown.

Prevention strategies

A multi-pronged approach has to be adopted for preventing transfusion-associated hepatitis B infection transmitted by HBsAg negative units. Perhaps the ultimate solution to this problem will be elimination of HBV, a utopian ideal that can only be attained by a sustained, international effort to achieve universal immunization against HBV over the next few decades. The importance of adopting good blood banking practices in the interim period cannot be overemphasised. These include minimizing blood transfusion, moving over to autologous transfusions for elective surgery, making heterologous blood transfusion safer by improved donor selection, improved HBV screening of donor units, vaccination of repeat voluntary donors, and wider use of virus inactivation procedures.

Improving present procedures for screening for HBV in donor units is a daunting task. The challenges are mainly those of finding the logistically most feasible and cost-effective approach. Different approaches are needed for high and low prevalence regions of the world. For this purpose, strategies to be followed in the intermediate prevalence areas would have to be the same as for high prevalence areas. The options available in this regard are elimination of (a) all anti-HBc positive units; (b) units with isolated, high titer anti-HBc; and (c) HBV-DNA positive units from the donor pool.[43]

Anti-HBc screening

In West: Anti-HBc has long been a favorite surrogate marker in the West for a variety of transfusion associated infections such as NANB-TAH, HCV window period HIV infection and NANBNC infections. Following reports of TAH-B being transmitted by HBsAg negative, anti-HBc positive units, Hoofnagle[1] strongly advocated including anti-HBc along with HBsAg in the panel of donor screening tests. This was done by the American Association of Blood Banks (AABB) in the mid-1980s, since anti-HBc was also the best available surrogate marker for HCV and window period HIV infections at that time. Presently, AABB recommends discarding all units testing positive for anti-HBc. This is a strategy feasible in parts of the world, such as north America and northern Europe, with low rates of HBsAg and anti-HBc positivity. Here <1% units are likely to be discarded due to anti-HBc positivity. It is also clear, however, that most of the units so discarded will not be infectious for HBV. Isolated, low titer anti-HBc, especially in low prevalence areas, may represent nonspecific cross-reactivity. Persons with isolated anti-HBc identified during pre-vaccination testing of vaccine recipients in hepatitis B vaccination studies often mounted a primary rather than an anamnestic response to the vaccine, suggesting that they were HBV naïve.[2,44] Anti-HBc was present in

1.3% of 9238 East Anglian blood donors on screening but was confirmed only in 0.35%.[45] While 0.31% were positive for both anti-HBc and protective levels of anti-HBs, 0.04% had isolated anti-HBc positivity.[46] In none of the latter was HBV-DNA detectable on nested PCR. Finally, instances of anti-HBc negative units transmitting HBV have been reported[26, 30] suggesting that even discarding all anti-HBc positive units may not interdict the admittedly rare instances of window period acute HBV infections transmitting TAH-B. Nevertheless, discarding all anti-HBc positive units is the best available strategy for areas of the world where anti-HBc positivity is below 1%.

In Asia: A strong case may be made for adding anti-HBc screening to prevent TAH-B due to HBsAg negative units in high HBV prevalence areas of the world also. Anti-HBc is a reliable indicator of acute, persistent or past HBV infection. Most reports of TAH-B due to HBsAg negative blood report positive anti-HBc along with HBV-DNA in the incriminated units.[1, 7, 8, 25, 29-31, 40] Anti-HBc detects HBV infection in those with low level viremia and HBV mutant infection but not in possible window period donations. Exclusion of anti-HBc positive units from the donor pool is not practical in areas with intermediate HBsAg prevalence rates such as India where the anti-HBc positivity ranges from 17.6%[4] to 28%[5] in healthy donors. Discarding anti-HBc positive units would result in unacceptably high rates of donor rejection. In China, Taiwan, Hong Kong and Japan, due to even higher prevalence (60–80%) of anti-HBc in the general population, rejection of anti-HBc positive donors is even less practical. While the presence of both anti-HBs and anti-HBc is the feature of resolved infection, high-titer, isolated anti-HBc positivity is noted in persistent infection. Iizuka[43] tested for HBV-DNA in 294 blood units with anti-HBc positivity as the sole marker of HBV infection and found that 12/175 units with high hemagglutination inhibition anti-HBc titers ($>2^6$) tested positive for HBV-DNA compared to 0/119 units with HAI titers $<2^5$ ($p<0.01$). The Japanese experience[19] shows that blood supply can be preserved by discarding only units that are positive for anti-HBc in high-titres ($>2^6$ dilution by HAI) without sacrificing safety of blood. However, this encouraging experience has not been replicated elsewhere. Furthermore, this strategy involves added costs for testing all units for anti-HBs and anti-HBc as well as HBsAg and for quantitating levels of anti-HBc in all units positive for this marker.

Development of better tests for HBsAg

Third generation EIAs that use polyclonal rather than monoclonal anti-HBs for coating the wells in sandwich ELISA systems are more likely to bind surface mutant viruses since the avidity of the polyclonal antibody would be superior to that of the monoclonal in case of point mutations in the common 'a' determinant region of surface mutants. This may be particularly useful in regions where prevalence of surface mutants is high in the general population; so far, no such geographic regions have been identified worldwide, though an Indian report suggests that ~10% of HBV-related chronic liver disease in north India is due to HBsAg negative mutant virus infection.[41]

Simpler tests for HBV-DNA

It is intuitively more appealing to look directly for the presence of the virus by testing for HBV-DNA than looking for the virus indirectly using tests for antibodies. However, the elaborate, multi-step, time-consuming procedure used for DNA extraction, purification and PCR amplification has prevented the use of HBV-DNA testing for routine donor unit screening. Efforts have been made to simplify the PCR procedure by introducing automation and using only two thermal steps with a shift of 16°C, resulting in more efficient and reproducible amplification.[47] Another attempt at simplifying DNA extraction has been reported, in which HBV was isolated from plasma using polystyrene beads coated with monoclonal anti-Pre-S1, followed by proteinase K digestion of immunocaptured virions. Further modifications allowed flow cytometric analysis of HBV-specific PCR products. This technique has the potential for being adapted for simultaneous detection of multiple blood-borne viruses by an automated flow cytometric system.[48] It is also likely to identify the presence of different serotypes and mutant viruses since the anti-Pre-S1 used for virus capture is an epitope that is invariably highly conserved and all strains of HBV possibly have no mutations in the pre-S1 region involved in the virus receptor for host cells.[31]

Donor vaccination programs

Since voluntary blood donation programs are based on a bank of motivated, altruistic, repeat donors, a logical way to improve safety of donated blood is to implement a universal HBV vaccination program for this group. A cost–benefit analysis[39] comparing costs of hepatitis B vaccination for donors, including price of vaccine, duration of immunity, number of components transfused per donation with the costs incurred in the management of various courses that TAH-B may follow, found that universal immunization of blood donors is not only desirable but is also cost-effective for repeat donors in Germany.

Virus inactivation procedures

A variety of procedures have been tested for inactivating pathogens in the whole blood and components but few have found widespread application. Some procedures like β-propriolactone treatment and solvent–detergent treatment with the solvent tri-N-butyl phosphate (TNBP) and the detergent Tween 80 have been found promising for coagulation factor concentrates, achieving a >4.0 log reduction in levels of HBV, HCV, and HIV with a good safety record. Photo-inactivation procedures, using ultraviolet light after exposing whole blood or packed red cells to photosensitive compounds, such as psoralens or hematoporphyrin derivative (HPD) have been reported to inactivate most common RNA and DNA viruses. Illuminating single bags of plasma or cellular products to visible light after treating them with cationic dyes such as methylene blue, toluidine blue or neutral red has also been found to be effective against enveloped viruses.[49] However, none of these procedures have as yet been incorporated as routine practices in any centers and many await FDA approval. All these approaches help in reducing the incidence of TAH-B, although it has been emphasised that proper organization of the blood banks is crucial for achieving the goal.[50]

Over the last 25 years, routine screening of donated units with sensitive and specific tests for HBsAg has reduced but not eliminated the problem of transfusion associated hepatitis B (TAH-B). Even in the 21st century, 1–16% of TAH in different parts of the world continues to be due to HBV despite routine HBsAg screening. Numerous reports have documented the occurrence of TAH-B after the transfusion of units testing negative for HBsAg. A variety of explanations have emerged to explain this phenomenon: human error, insensitive HBsAg EIA kits, the use of monoclonal versus polyclonal anti-HBs for sandwich EIAs, low levels of viremia below the detection limit of routinely used EIA kits, the presence of surface mutants or antibody escape mutants (AEM) and the rare possibility of a unit being collected in the window period of an acute HBV infection. Except for the last situation, the presence of the virus is readily identified by the detection of high-titer anti-HBc ($\geq 2^6$ by HAI) and, in all cases, by the use of PCR amplification. Fears that TAH-B occurring despite screening for HBsAg maybe an increasing problem in intermediate and high HBV prevalence regions of the world have been fueled by reports that 4–24% of units collected from voluntary donors negative for HBsAg test positive for HBV-DNA in these areas. Until the dream of eliminating HBV from the world by universal immunization is achieved, the phenomenon of TAH-B occurring despite the use of HBsAg screened blood may be held in check by taking steps to improve the safety of heterologous blood transfusion. Besides using rigorous criteria for accepting voluntary donors, various measures proposed to eliminate this problem have included improved donor unit screening with better tests for HBsAg detection, routine anti-HBc screening, screening for isolated, high-titer anti-HBc, introduction of HBV-DNA screening, universal vaccination of repeat voluntary donors and routinely treating all donor units with virus inactivation procedures. The Japanese approach of rejecting all HBsAg positive and isolated, high-titer anti-HBc positive donor units has succeeded in eliminating TAH-B from Japan and is an example that warrants wider emulation in high prevalence areas of the world.

REFERENCES

1. Hoofnagle JH, Seeff LB, Bales ZB, Zimmermann HJ. Type B hepatitis after transfusion with blood containing antibody to hepatitis B core antigen. *N Engl J Med* 1978;298:1379-83.
2. Lok ASF, Lai CL, Wu PC. Prevalence of isolated antibody to hepatitis B core antigen in an area endemic for hepatitis B virus infection implications in hepatitis B vaccination programs. *Hepatology* 1988;8:766-70.
3. Lai ME, Farci P, Figus A, Balestrieri A, Arnone M, Vyas GN. Hepatitis B virus DNA in the serum of Sardinian donors negative for the hepatitis B surface antigen. *Blood* 1989;73:17-9.
4. Nagaraju K, Misra S, Saraswat S, Choudhary N, Masih B, Ramesh V, Naik S. High prevalence of HBV infectivity in blood donors detected by the dot-blot hybridization assay. *Vox Sang* 1994;67:183-6.
5. Nandi J, Banerjee K. Detection of hepatitis B virus DNA in donor blood by the polymerase chain reaction. *Natl Med J India* 1992;3:5-7.

6. Jolly JG. *Current status of blood transfusion program in India and the need for its reorganization.* In : Sarin SK, Hess G. Eds. Transfusion associated hepatitis: diagnosis, treatment and prevention. CBS Publishers & Distributors, New Delhi. 1997;pp. 49-56.
7. Saraswat S, Banerjee K, Chaudhary N, Mahant T, Khandekar P, Gupta RK, Naik S. Post-transfusion hepatitis type B following multiple transfusions of HBsAg-negative blood. *J Hepatol* 1996;25: 639-43.
8. Saxena R, Thakur V, Sood B, Guptan RC, Guruja S, Sarin SK. Transfusion associated hepatitis in a tertiary referral hospital in India. *Vox Sang* 1999;77:6-10.
9. Cossart YE, Kirsch S, Ismay SL. Post-transfusion hepatitis in Australia – report of the Australian Red Cross study. *Lancet* 1982;208-13.
10. Dasrathy S, Mishra SC, Acharya SK, Irshad M, Joshi YK, Venugopal P, Tandon BN. Prospective controlled study of PTH after cardiac surgery in a large referral hospital in India. *Liver* 1992;12: 116-20.
11. Sood B, Saxena R. *What is safe blood? In:* Sarin SK, Singal AK. Eds. Hepatitis B in India: Problems and Prevention. CBS Publishers & Distributors, New Delhi. 1996;pp.92-4.
12. Thyagarajan SP, Jayaraman S, Mohanvalli B. *Prevalence of HBV in general population of India. In:* Sarin SK, Singal AK. Eds. Hepatitis B in India: Problems and Prevention. CBS Publishers & Distributors, New Delhi. 1996;pp. 8-18.
13. Collins JD, Bassendine MF, Codd AA, Collins A, Ferner RE, James OFW. Prospective study of post-transfusion hepatitis after cardiac surgery in a British center. *Br Med J* 1983;18:122-46.
14. Widell A, Sundstrom G, Hansson BG, Fex G, Moestrup T, Nordenfelt E. Post-transfusion hepatitis type Non-A, Non-B in southern Sweden: occurrence and clinical significance. *Scand J Infect Dis* 1987; 19:603-10.
15. Feinman SV, Berris B, Bojarski S. Post-transfusion hepatitis in Toronto, Canada. *Gastroenterology* 1988;95:464-9.
16. Hoyos M, Sarrion JV, Perez-Castellanos T, Prieto M, Marty ML, Garrigues V, Berenguer J. Prospective assessment of donor blood screening for antibody to hepatitis B core antigen as a means of preventing post-transfusion non-A, non-B hepatitis. *Hepatology* 1989;9:449-51.
17. Blajchman MA, Bull SB, Feinmann SV. Post-transfusion hepatitis : impact of non-A, non-B hepatitis surrogate tests. *Lancet* 1995;3454:21-5.
18. Wang JT, Wang TH, Sheu JC, Shih LN, Lin JT, Chen DS. Detection of hepatitis B virus DNA by polymerase chain reaction in plasma of voluntary blood donors negative for hepatitis B surface antigen. *J Infect Dis* 1991;163:397-9.
19. Japanese Red Cross non-A, non-B Hepatitis Research Group. Effect of screening for hepatitis C virus antibody and hepatitis B core antibody on incidence of post-transfusion hepatitis. *Lancet* 1991; 338:1040-1.
20. Chung HT, Lee JSK, Lok ASF. Prevention of post-transfusion hepatitis B and C by screening for antibody to hepatitis C virus and antibody to HBcAg. *Hepatology* 1993;18:1045-9.
21. Huang YY, Yang SS, Wu CH, Shih WS, Huang CS, Chen PH, Lin YM, et al. Impact of screening blood donors for hepatitis C antibody on post-transfusion hepatitis: a prospective study with a second generation anti-hepatitis C virus assay. *Transfusion* 1994;34:661-5.
22. Patwari SI, Ershad M, Gandhi BM, Joshi YK, Nundy S, Tandon BN. Post-transfusion hepatitis: a prospective study. *Ind J Med Res* 1986;6:508-10.
23. Hennig H, Dennin RH, Hasse D, Kirchner H. HBV-DNA positive findings in HBsAg negative blood donors and patients. *Beitr Infusionsther Transfusionsmed* 1997;34:26-30.
24. Douglas DD, Taswell HF, Rakela J, Rabe D. Absence of hepatitis B virus DNA detected by polymerase chain reaction in blood donors who are hepatitis B surface antigen negative and antibody to

hepatitis B core antigen positive from a United States population with a low prevalence of hepatitis B serologic markers. *Transfusion* 1993;33:212-6.
25. Larzul D, Guigue F, Sninsky JJ, Mark DH, Brechot C, Guedson JL. Detection of hepatitis B virus sequences in serum by using in-vitro enzymatic amplification. *J Virol Methods* 1988;20:227-37.
26. Prince AM, Stephan W, Brotman B. β-propriolactone irradiation: a review of its effectiveness for inactivation of viruses in blood serivatives. *Rev Inf Dis* 1983;5:92-107.
27. Larsen J, Hetland G, Skaug K. Posttransfusion hepatitis B transmitted by blood from a hepatitis B surface antigen negative hepatitis B virus carrier. *Transfusion* 1990;30:431-2.
28. Thiers V, Nakajima E, Kremsdorf K, Mack D, Schellekens H, Driss F, Goudeau A, et al. Transmission of hepatitis B from hepatitis B seronegative subjects. *Lancet* 1988;2:1273-6.
29. Norder H, Hammas B, Larsen J, Skaug K, Magnius LO. Detection of HBV-DNA by PCR in serum from an HBsAg negative blood donor implicated in cases of post-transfusion hepatitis B. *Arch Virol Suppl* 1992;4:116-8.
30. Jongerius JM, van der Poel CL, van Leeuwen EF. A simple strategy to look back on post-transfusion hepatitis B in a multi-transfused patient. *Vox Sang* 1998;75:66-9.
31. Vyas GN. *Significance of HBV-DNA positivity in HBsAg negative donors. In :* Sarin SK, Hess G, Eds. Transfusion associated hepatitis: diagnosis, treatment and prevention: CBS Publishers & Distributors, New Delhi. 1997;49-56.
32. Lee HS, Ulrich PP, Vyas GN. Mutations in the S-gene affecting the immunologic determinants of the envelope protein of hepatitis B virus. *J Hepatol* 1991;13:S97-101.
33. Bhatnagar PK, Papas E, Blum HE, Milich DR, Nitecki D, Karels MJ, Vyas GN, et al. A synthetic analogue of hepatitis B surface antigen sequence 139-147 produces immune response specific for the common 'a' determinant. *Proc Natl Acad Sci USA* 1982;79:4400-4.
34. Zanetti AR, Tanzi E, Manzillo G, Maio G, Sbreglia C, Caporaso N, Thomas H, et al. Hepatitis B variants in Europe. *Lancet* 1988;2:1132-3.
35. Okamoto H, Yano K, Nozaki Y, Matsui A, Miyazaki H, Yamamoto K, Tsuda F, et al. Mutations within the S-gene of hepatitis B virus transmitted from mothers to babies immunized with hepatitis B immune globulin and vaccine. *Pediatr Res* 1992;32:264-8.
36. Oon CJ, Lim GK, Ye Z, Goh KT, Tan KL, Yo SL, Hopes E, et al. Molecular epidemiology of hepatitis B virus vaccine variants in Singapore. *Vaccine* 1995; 13:699-702.
37. Carman WF, Trautwein C, van Deursen FJ, Colman K, Dornan E, McIntyre G, Waters J, et al. Hepatitis B virus envelope variation after transplantation with and without hepatitis B immune globulin prophylaxis. *Hepatology* 1996;24:489-93.
38. McMahon G, Ehrlich PH, Mustafa ZA, McCarthy LA, Dottavio D, Tolpin MD, Nadler PI, et al. Genetic alterations in the gene encoding the major HBsAg: DNA and immunologic analysis of recurrent HBsAg derived from monoclonal antibody-treated liver transplant patients. *Hepatology* 1992;15:757-66.
39. Gesemann M, Gentner P, Scheiermann N. Hepatitis B vaccination of blood donors–a cost-benefit analysis. *Beitr Infusionther Transfusionsmed* 1994;32:110-2.
40. Jongerius JM, Wester M, Cuypers HT, van Oostendorp WR, Lelie PN, van der Poel, CL, van Leeuwen EF. New hepatitis B virus mutant form in a blood donor that is undetectable in several hepatitis B surface antigen screening assays. *Transfus Med* 1997;7:319-20.
41. Guptan RC, Thakur V, Sarin SK, Banerjee K, Khandekar P. Frequency and clinical profile of pre-core and surface hepatitis B mutants in Asian-Indian patients with chronic liver disease. *Am J Gastroenterol* 1996;91:1312-7.
42. Kojima M, Shimizu M, Tsuchimochi T, Koyasu M, Tanaka S, Iizuka H, Tanaka T, et al. Post-transfusion fulminant hepatitis B associated with precore-defective HBV mutants. *Vox Sang* 1991;60: 34-9.

43. Iizuka H, Ohmura K, Ishijima A, Satoh K, Tanaka T, Tsuda F, Okamoto H, et al. Correlation between anti-HBc titers and HBV-DNA in blood units without detectable HBsAg. *Vox Sang* 1992;63:107-11.
44. Draelos M, Morgen T, Shiffman RB, Sampliner RE. Significance of isolated antibody to hepatitis B core antigen determined by immune response to hepatitis B vaccination. *JAMA* 1987;258:1193-5.
45. Allain JP, Reeves I, Kitchen AD, Williamson LM. Feasibility and usefulness of an efficient anti-HBc screening program in blood donors. *Transfus Med* 1995;5:259-65.
46. Weber B, Melchior W, Gehrke R, Doerr HW, Berger A, Rabanau H. Hepatitis B virus markers in anti-HBc only positive individuals. *J Med Virol* 2001;64:312-9.
47. Larzul D, Chevrier D, Thiers V, Guedson JL. An automatic modified polymerase chain reaction procedure for hepatitis B virus detection. *J Virol Methods* 1990;27:49-60.
48. Yang G, Ulrich PP, Aiyer RA, Rawal BD, Vyas GN. Detection of hepatitis B virus in plasma using flow cytometric analyses of polymerase chain reaction-amplified DNA incorporating digoxigenin-11-dUTP. *Blood* 1993;81:1083-8.
49. Ray V, Kamath M. *Viral inactivation in blood products.* In: Sarin SK, Hess G, Eds. Transfusion associated hepatitis: diagnosis, treatment and prevention: CBS Publishers & Distributors, New Delhi. 1997; pp. 320-7.
50. Nanu A. Blood transfusion services: organization is integral to safety. *Natl Med J India* 2001;14:237-40.

8

Transmission of hepatitis B virus infection in patients with hematological disorders

Ved P Choudhry, Rajesh Kashyap

India has the second largest pool of subjects with hepatitis B virus infection in the world. There are a total of 43 million HBsAg positive subjects and of these 4.3 million are highly infectious (HBeAg positive).[1] Many of these HBV infected subjects are potential blood donors. A recent national survey on blood transfusion practices revealed that only 87% of the respondent blood banks screen blood for hepatitis B.[2] It is possible that a large number of blood banks may not be screening all the blood units for hepatitis B, even though it is mandatory by law. It has been observed that the positivity of HBsAg in multitransfused thalassemic children increased significantly over three years even when the children were being transfused HBsAg negative blood screened by ELISA at a tertiary centre.[3] Significant increase in HBsAg positivity in these children could be either due to poor quality control or not following the universal precautions strictly.

Patients with primary hematological disorders such as thalassemia, sickle cell anemia, hemophilia, aplastic anemia, or hematological malignancies receive multiple transfusions in the above scenario. Therefore, these patients are at a much higher risk of developing transfusion transmitted infections (TTI). Among various TTI, the risk of hepatitis B infection is much higher (9–30%) because of the higher prevalence of the HBV in the general population and its high infectivity.[4] Management of hematological disorders includes the treatment of underlying condition along with the supportive care to maintain hemoglobin, coagulation factors or platelets within the safe range. Inherited hematological disorders such as thalassemia, hemoglobinopathies, and coagulation disorders require blood products life-long while other states such as hematological malignancies, immune mediated hemolytic anemias, thrombocytopenia, etc. require blood components during the active stage of the disease. Prevalence of HBV in various hematological disorders is being reviewed along with the possible measures for prevention of TTI in patients with various hematological disorders.

THALASSEMIA

The main principle of management of thalassemia includes (a) maintaining hemoglobin level above 10 gm/dl by regular packed red cell transfusion, (b) chelation therapy to maintain the serum ferritin at a safe level, and (c) treatment of complications of the disease process.[5] Infants with thalassemia major or patients with other severe hemoglobinopathies need blood transfusion from early childhood. Prevalence of HBsAg positivity in our country varied from 0 to 59.6 percent of cases (Table 1). However, the evidence of recent or past hepatitis B infection varied between 43.7 and 80.0% of cases. HBsAg prevalence in multitransfused thalassemic children has declined. Over the last five years its prevalence has been observed between 0 and 21% as compared with 0 to 59.6% prior to 1995 among Indian subjects. The prevalence of HBV infection in thalassemic children from India is still higher as compared with the studies from the developed or other Asian countries (Table 2).

Table 1. Prevalence of hepatitis B in multi-transfused Indian thalassemic children

Authors	Place	Patients (n)	Per cent Positive			
			HBsAg	Anti-HBs	Anti-HBc	Overall
Mittal et al[6]	Delhi	27	14.8	48.1	51.9	74.1
Kapil[7]	Delhi	50	10.0	40.0	62.0	80.0
Gulati et al[8]	Chandigarh	100	6.0	73.0	49.0	76.0
Jolly et al[9]	Lucknow	251	15.5	–	–	–
William et al[10]	Delhi	54	7.4	–	59.2	66.6
Manglani et al[11]	Bombay	25	8.0	84.0	–	88
Chopra and Popli[12]	Delhi	37	59.6	–	–	–
Choudhry et al[13]	Delhi	102	29.4	1.0	–	65.7
Chopra et al[14]	Mumbai	50	21.0	–	–	–
Chaudhary[3]	Lucknow	39	17.9	17.9	–	43.7
Sharma and Sharma[15]	Jammu	58	0.0	–	–	–
Acharya et al[16]	Delhi	199	8.5	–	–	–

Table 2. Prevalence of hepatitis B in thalassemic children from other countries

Authors	Country	Number	Per cent Positive			
			HBsAg	Anti-HBs	Anti-HBc	Overall
Wonke et al[17]	UK	73	0	27.04	27.04	–
de-Montalembert[18]	Belgium	15	0.0	73.3	26.7	–
	France	172	5.9	76.2	23.3	–
	Italy	118	1.2	57.6	49.2	–
Cacopardo et al[19]	Italy	152	8	55.0	–	–
Dentico et al[20]	Italy	114	9.6	29.8	9.1	47.4
Al Fawaz and Ramia[21]	Arabia	20	0.0	26.7	0	26.7
Al Mahroos et al[22]	Bachanin	191	–	–	–	–
Jamal et al[23]	Malaysia	85	2.4	–	–	–

Prevalence of HBV infection in multitransfused thalassemic children in developed countries has declined as a result of universal hepatitis B vaccination program, stringent screening of donors, practice of repeat donors, practice of universal precautions, and improvement in hygienic and socio-economic standards. The prevalence of HBV infection even in some Asian countries is lower than our country. High prevalence of HBV infection in our country is possibly due to multiple factors, such as: (a) lack of awareness of blood transmitted infections in the general population and even in paramedical staff, (b) absence of national blood transfusion services, (c) poor quality control for screening of blood, (d) hepatitis B vaccine not being administered at diagnosis to a large number of thalassemic patients, and (e) lack of facilities at many centres for universal precautions and waste management.[24]

HEMOPHILIA

There are only a few studies regarding the prevalence of HBV infection in hemophiliacs from India. This could be attributed to lack of national hemophilia care program, poor availability of fresh frozen plasma, cryoprecipitate, and factor concentrates. Hemophilia Federation of India, a non-governmental organization (NGO), is primarily engaged in increasing the awareness of hemophilia, education of medical and paramedical staff, and providing the factor concentrates at an affordable price. Some small studies have revealed that HBsAg positivity varies between 5.6 and 24.3% against hemophiliacs (Table 3). Long-term follow-up studies from the developed countries have indicated that the prevalence of HBsAg positivity varied

Table 3. Prevalence of hepatitis B in hemophiliacs in India

Authors	Place	Number	HBsAg +ve (%)
Chandra et al[25]	Calcutta	47	22.5
		105	8.6
De et al[26]	Calcutta		9.0
Irshad and Singh[27]	Delhi	89	5.6
Sengupta et al[28]	Calcutta	37	24.3

between 4.5 and 57.3% of cases (Table 4). The incidence of HBV infection was significantly higher in patients who had received factor concentrates more than 10,000 units per year, older patients, and those hemophiliacs who were positive for HIV infection.[32,40] Over the last few years, prevalence of HBsAg positivity in developing countries has declined significantly as a result of hepatitis B vaccination during infancy, use of ultrapure factor concentrates which have been inactivated by at least two methods, use of DNA recombinant factors, besides strict adherence to universal precautions. Continuous education programs for hemophiliacs on preventive measures and to reduce the prevalence of infection and bleeding episodes have contributed significantly in reducing the prevalence of HBV infection among them.

Table 4. Prevalence of hepatitis B in hemophiliacs in Asian and developing countries

Authors	Place	Number	Per cent Positive HBsAg	Overall
Rollag et al[29]	Norway	324	28 44 (severe)	
Kacperska et al[30]	Warszaivie	100	*16.7 **4.5	
Chow et al[31]	Taiwan	11	9	82
Brenner et al[32]	Israel	117	–	90/62
Kumar et al[33]	USA	41	–	75.6
Kocabas et al[34]	Turkey	41	26.8	–
Akdeniz et al[35]	Turkey	73	57.3	–
Tradati et al[36]	Italy	385	7.6	–
Bentancor et al[37]	Uruguay	22		9.1
Shamri et al[38]	Karachi	27	7.4	–
Hill and Stein[39]	USA			< 1% under 10 yr

*   Patients on factor concentrates
** Patients getting only cryoprecipitate

LYMPHOPROLIFERATIVE DISORDERS

Patients with lymphoproliferative disorders are immunocompromized and are at a higher risk of developing transfusion transmitted infections. Prevalence of HBsAg positivity is higher at diagnosis in patients with AML than with ALL. Incidence of HBV infection increases proportionately with the duration of follow-up (Table 5).

Table 5. Prevalence of hepatitis B infection in lymphoproliferative disorders

Authors	Place	Number	Per cent Positive HBsAg	Overall
Kumar et al[41]	Lucknow	25	–	76
Dibenedetto et al[42]	Italy	90 (All)	0	–
Nag et al[43]	Mumbai	–	–	45
Kocabas et al[44]	Turkey	137	–	47.4
Dutta et al[45]	Delhi	51	–	37.5
Kebudi et al[46]	Turkey	50	0 (at diagnosis) 10 (at end of therapy)	4 (at diagnosis) 20 (at end of therapy)
Ramesh et al[47]	Chandigarh	35	16.3	24.3

Kumar et al[41] observed HBV infection in 76% of cases with lymphoproliferative disorders and HBsAg was persistently positive in 57.9% of cases indicating active viral replication. Chemotherapy suppresses the immune function and facilitates the viral replication and hepatic damage. Long-term impact of HBV infection in these patients needs to be evaluated in larger studies. The possibility that patients cured of lymphoproliferative disorders following chemotherapy may succumb to hepatitis or its sequelae cannot be excluded. Ehrmann et al[48] observed fulminant hepatitis with hepatic failure following withdrawal of chemotherapy. Fulminant hepatic failure was observed possibly as a result of reactivation of the infection.

Administration of the hepatitis B vaccine is an integral part of the management of these cases with hematological disorders. It is unethical to withhold chemotherapy for patients with lymphoproliferative disorders till immunization of these patients with hepatitis B vaccine. Therefore, patients with the lymphoproliferative disorder were being treated with chemotherapy along with hepatitis B vaccination. Results of these studies have been variable (Table 6). Protective levels of antibodies against surface antigen were achieved in less than 20% of cases in Indian patients which was much lower than Turkish study despite using five doses of vaccine and/or higher dose of vaccine. Poor sero-conversion in Indian patients could be secondary to poor nutritional status. Strategies to improve the sero-conversion have been recommended which include: (a) doubling the dose of the vaccine, (b) increasing the number of doses, and (c) using combination of passive along with active immunization schedule.[52] Combination of hepatitis B vaccine along with growth factors may improve the uptake. Large multicentric studies are essential to evolve an effective immunization schedule for these patients.

Table 6. Impact of hepatitis B immunization in lymphoproliferative disorders

Authors	Place	Vaccination schedule (months)	Anti-HBs (mIU/ml)	
			< 10	> 10
Goyal et al[49]	Mumbai	0, 1, 2, 12	19.7%	10.5%
Somjee et al[50]	Mumbai	0, 1, 2, 3, 4, 12	30.0%	19.0%
Meral et al[51]	Turkey	0, 1, 2, 12		Solid tumor 94% Leukemia 90% Lymphoma 74%
Ramesh et al[47]	Chandigarh	0, 1, 2, 6	–	18.8%

CONCLUSIONS

Prevalence of HBV infection in patients with various hematological disorders is high as a result of multiple transfusions of blood and blood products. These patients acquire HBV infection through blood or blood products even though the screening for blood products for HBV is mandatory. National survey on blood transfusion practices indicates that only 87% of blood donors were screened for HBV infection among 13% of blood banks who participated in the study.[2] The possibility that blood banks who were not following the strict screening of donors as per guidelines did not participate in the National survey cannot be excluded. Development of post-transfusion hepatitis in 6.9% of patients who received blood transfusion once during surgery suggests that screening of blood for HBsAg by ELISA alone was inadequate.[52] This hypothesis is being further supported as the positivity of HBsAg increased significantly over three years period at one center in multitransfused thalassemic patients who were being administered blood from voluntary donors which was negative for HBsAg by third generation ELISA.[3] It has been suggested by various studies[53, 54] that prevalence of HBV increased after the screening of blood for HBV was made mandatory. Thus, the current screening methods for HBV infection in our country are unsatisfactory. There is need to adopt more sensitive methods. It is suggested that the donors need to be tested for core antigen along with liver enzymes (alanine aminotransferase, aspartate aminotransferase), in addition to HBsAg to ensure that the blood and blood products are safe. In view of the shortage of blood, limited storage capacity, and lack of awareness, the practice of repeat donors may not be feasible for the present. However, efforts should be made to encourage voluntary blood donors.

Inclusion of the hepatitis B vaccine in the expanded universal immunization program needs to be implemented at the earliest. Prevalence of HBV infection among thalassemic and hemophiliac patients can be reduced significantly by the use of hepatitis B vaccine at the time of diagnosis. Thalassemic and hemophiliac patients and their families need to be educated regarding hepatitis B vaccination and the need for periodical booster doses. Immunocompromised patients and cases with lymphoproliferative disorders are at a higher risk of developing HBV infection and presence of HBV infection in them may adversely affect the long-term survival. The current hepatitis B vaccination schedule is not effective for patients with hematological disorders. Therefore, the strategies such as use of (a) higher dose, (b) 5–7 doses in place of 3 conventional doses, (c) passive and active immunization, and (d) hepatitis B vaccination along with growth factors, need to be evaluated in larger studies to determine the most effective mode of vaccination in patients with various hematological disorders.[55]

REFERENCES

1. Tandon BN. *Dimensions and issues of HBV control in India In:* Sarin SK, Singal AK, Eds. Hepatitis B in India: Problems and Prevention. CBS Publishers & Distributors, New Delhi 1996; pp. 1-4.
2. Kapoor D, Saxena R, Sood B, Sarin SK. Blood transfusion practices in India. Results of a national survey. *Indian J Gastroenterology* 2000;19:64-7.
3. Choudhury N, Saraswat S, Naveed M. Serological monitoring of thalassemia major patients for transfusion associated viral infections. *Ind J Med Res* 1998;107:263-8.
4. Guidelines for preventing HIV, HBV and other infections in the health care setting. *World Health Organization.* 1996; pp.1-5.

5. Choudhry VP, Desai N, Pati HP, Nanu A. Current management of homozygous beta thalassemia. *Indian Pediatr* 1991;28:1221-9.
6. Mittal MK, Vij JC, Talukdar B, Sachdev HPS, Saini L. Prevalence of hepatitis B virus markers in multitransfused thalassemic patients. *Indian Pediatr* 1988;25:161-5.
7. Kapil D. Growth and development, liver and cardiac status in thalassemia. Thesis submitted to All India Institute of Medical Sciences, New Delhi 1989.
8. Gulati S, Marwaha RK, Dilawari JB, Midhu V, Waler BN. Serological responses to hepatitis B virus infection in multitransfused thalassemic children. *Indian Pediatr* 1991;29:73-7.
9. Amarapukar DN, Kumar A, Vaidya S, Murti P, Bichile SK, Kalro RH, Desai HG. Frequency of hepatitis B, C and D and human immunodeficiency virus infection in multitransfused thalassemics. *Indian J Gastroenterol* 1992;11:80-1.
10. William TN, Wonke B, Donohue SM. A study of hepatitis B and C prevalence and liver function in multitransfused thalassemia and their parents. *Indian Pediatr* 1992;29:1119-24.
11. Manglani M, Kanabia S, Bhatia N, et al. Liver function tests hepatitis B markers and HIV in multiple transfused thalassemics. XXXII National Conference of Indian Academy of Pediatrics 1994;53-4 (abstract).
12. Chopra K, Popli V. Prevalence of hepatitis B and hepatitis C in multitransfused thalassemics. XXXII National Conference of Indian Academy of Pediatrics 1994;444-5 (abstract).
13. Choudhry VP, Acharya SK. Hepatitis B, C and D viral markers in multitransfused thalassemic children: long-term complications and present management. *Indian J Pediatr* 1995;62:655-68.
14. Chopra A, Nadkarni UB, Kshirsagar. Prevalence of hepatitis C virus infection and its comparison with HBV and HIV infections in multitransfused thalassemia major children in 35th National Conference IAP 1998;pp. 34 (abstract).
15. Sharma K, Sharma DB. HIV, hepatitis B, hepatitis C screening in multitransfused thalassemic children in V International Congress of Tropical Pediatrics Jaipur. *Hematology-Oncology* 1999;pp. 4.
16. Acharya SK, Choudhry VP, Panda SK, Dutta Gupta S, Bharati VV. Prevalence of hepatitis B & C virus infection among multitransfused thalassemic children: An Indian Scenario. *J Gastroenterol Hepatol* (submitted for publication).
17. Wonke B, Hoffbrand AV, Brown D, Dusheiko G, et al. Antibody to hepatitis C virus in multiple transfused patients with thalassemia major. *J Clin Pathol* 1990;43:638-40.
18. de Montalembert M, Costagliola DG, Lefrere JJ, Cornu G, Lombardo T, Cosentino S, Perrimond H, Guot R. Prevalence of markers for human immunodeficiency virus Types 1 and 2, human T-lymphotropic virus Type I, cytomegalovirus and hepatitis B and C virus in multiple transfused thalassemia patients. *Transfusion* 1992;32:509-12.
19. Cacopardo B, Russo R, Futuzzo F, Cosentino S, Lombardo T, La Rosa R, Celesia BM, et al. HCV and HBV infection among multitransfused thalassemics from eastern Sicily. *Infection* 1992;20:83-5.
20. Dentico P, Boungiorno R, Volpe A, Zavoianni A, DeMattra D, Sabato V. Long-term persistence of anti-HBs after hepatitis B immunization in thalassemic patients. *Infection* 1992;20:276-8.
21. al-Fawaz I, Ramia S. Decline in hepatitis B infection in sickle cell anemia and beta thalassemia major. *Arch Dis Child* 1993;69:594-6.
22. al Mahroos FT, Ebrahim A. Prevalence of hepatitis B, hepatitis C and human immune deficiency virus markers among patients with hereditary hemolytic anemia. *Ann Trop Pediatr* 1995;15:121-8.
23. Jamal R, Fadzillah G, Zulkiffi SZ, Yasmin M. Sero-prevalence of hepatitis B, hepatitis C, CMV and HIV in multiply transfused thalassemia patients. Results from a thalassemia day care centre in Malaysia. *Southeast Asian J Trop Med Publish Health* 1998;29:792-4.
24. Choudhry VP, Kashyap R, Acharya SK. Management of thalassemia. In: Gupta S. Ed. Recent Advances in Pediatrics. Jaypee Brothers, New Delhi, 2000;10:pp.179-94.
25. Chandra C, De M, Banerjee D, Bhattacharya DK. Emergence of seropositivity for HIV in multitransfused

hemophiliac of eastern India XXX Annual Conference of Indian Society of Hematology and Blood Transfusion 1989;pp.47.
26. De M, Banerjee D, Chandra S, Bhattacharya DK. HBV and HIV seropositivity in multitransfused hemophiliacs and thalassemia in eastern India. *Ind J Med Res* 1990;91:63-6.
27. Irshad M, Singh YN. Prevalence of HBV markers in hemophiliacs and eunuchs in India. *Indian J Gastroenterol* 1991;10:154.
28. Sengupta B, De M, Lahiri P, Bhattacharya DK. Sero surveillance of transmissible hepatitis B and C viruses in asymptomatic HIV infection in hemophiliacs. *Ind J Med Res* 1992;95:256-8.
29. Rollag H, Evensen SA, Froland SS, Glomstein A. Serological markers of hepatitis B virus and cytomegalovirus infections in Norwegians with coagulation factor defects. *Blut* 1990;60:93-6.
30. Kacperska E, Gloskowska – Moraczewska S, Seyfried H, Kalasinska – Kramer M, Cetnarowicz N, Lopaciuk S. Serological markers of hepatitis B virus and cytomegalovirus in patients with hemophilia. *Acta Hematol Pol* 1990;1:52-9.
31. Chow MP, Lin CK, Lin JJ, Chau WK, Ho CH, Chen SY, Lee SH et al. HIV, HBV and HCV seroposivitity in hemophiliac. *Zhorghua Min Guo Wei Sheng Wu Ji Mian Yi Xue Za Zhi* 1991;24: 339-44.
32. Brenner B, Schwartz S, Ben – Porath E, Taotaorsky I, Varon D, Martinowitz U. The prevalence and interaction of human immunodeficiency virus and hepatitis B virus infection in Israeli hemophiliacs. *Isr J Med Sci* 1991;10;557-61.
33. Kumar A, Kulkarni R, Murray DL, Gera R, Scott – Emuakpor AB, Bosma K, Penner JA. Serologic markers of viral hepatitis A, B, C and D in patients with hemophilia. *J Med Virol* 1993;41:205-9.
34. Kocabas E, Aksaray N, Alhan E, Yarkin F, Koksal F, Kilinc Y. Hepatitis B and C virus infection in Turkish children with hemophilia. *Acta Pediatr* 1997;86:1135-7.
35. Akdeniz C, Buyukpinarbasili Y, Zufilkar B. Hepatitis B seropositivity in patients with hemophilia. *Hemophilia* 1998;4:260 (abstract).
36. Tradati F, Colombo M, Mannucci PM, Rumi MG, De Fazio G, Gamba G, Ciavarella N, et al. A prospective multicenter study of hepatocellular carcinoma in Italian hemophiliacs with chronic hepatitis C. The study group of the association of Italian Hemophilia centers. *Blood* 1998;91:1173-7.
37. Bentancor N, Vila V, Zorrilia J, Meseia G, Parietti J, Gruells M, Zeballos E. Sero-prevalence of hepatitis in a cohort of hemophiliacs in Uruguay. *Hemophilia* 1998;4:260 (abstract).
38. Shamri T, Qureshi K, Ahmed S, Ahmed A. Prevalence of HBV, HCV and HIV in a group of hemophiliac patients. *Hemophilia* 1998;4:419 (abstract).
39. Hill HA, Stein SF. Viral infections among patients with hemophilia in a state of Georgia. *Am J Hematol* 1998;59:36-41.
40. Troisi CL, Hollinger FB, Hoots WK, Constant C, Gill J, Ragni M, Permley R, et al. A multicenter study of viral hepatitis in United States hemophiliac population. *Blood* 1993;81:412-8.
41. Kumar A, Mishra PK, Rana GS, Mehrotra R. Infection with hepatitis A, B, Delta and human immunodeficiency viruses in children receiving cycled cancer chemotherapy. *J Med Virology* 1992;37:83-6.
42. Dibenedetto Sp, Ragusa R, Sciacca A, DiCataldo DiA, Miraglia V, D Amico S, Lo Nigro L, et al. Incidence and morbidity of infection of hepatitis C virus in children with acute lymphoblastic leukemia. *Eur J Pediatr* 1994;153:271-5.
43. Nag S, Vaidya S, Pai S, Kelkar R, Advani SH. Hepatitis B viral infection in acute lymphoblastic leukemia. *Ind J Hemat Blood Transfusion* 1995;13:150.
44. Kocabas E, Aksaray N, Alhan E, Tanyeli P, Koksal F, Yarkin F. Hepatitis B and C Virus infection in turkish children with cancer. *Eur J Epidemiol* 1997;8:869-73.
45. Dutta U, Raina V, Garg PK, Gurbuxani S, Joshi YK, Bhargava M, Tandon RK. A prospective study

on the incidence of hepatitis B and C infection among patients with lymphoproliferative disorders. *Ind J Med Res* 1998;107:78-82.
46. Kabudi R, Ayan I, Yilmaz G, Akici F, Gorgun O, Badur S. Sero-prevalence of hepatitis B, hepatitis C and human immunodeficiency virus infection in children with cancer at diagnosis and following therapy in Turkey. *Med Ped Oncol* 2000;34:102-5.
47. Ramesh M, Marwaha RK, Chawla YK, Trehan A. Sero-conversion after hepatitis B vaccination in children receiving cancer chemotherapy. *Indian Pediatr* 2000;37:882-6.
48. Ehramann J Jr., Kucerova L, Jezdins ska V, Papajik T, Galuzskova D, Dusek J, Indark K, et al. Fulminant hepatitis caused by hepatitis B virus infection in the patients with hematological malignancies. Report of 5 cases. Acta Univ. *Palacki Olomic Fac Med* 1996;140:81-2.
49. Goyal S, Pai SK, Kelkar R, Advani SH. Hepatitis B vaccination in acute lymphoblastic leukemia. *Leuk Res* 1998;92:193-5.
50. Somjee S, Pai S, Kelkar R, Advani SH. Hepatitis B vaccination in acute lymphoblastic leukemia: results of an intensified immunization schedule. *Leuk Res* 1999;23:365-7.
51. Meral A, Sevinir B, Gunay U. Efficacy of immunization against hepatitis B virus infection in children with cancer. *Med Pediatr Oncol* 2000;35:47-51.
52. Dasarathy S, Misra SC, Acharya SK, Irshad M, Joshi YK, Venugopal P, Tandon BN. Prospective controlled study of post-transfusion hepatitis after cardiac surgery in a large referral hospital in India. *Liver* 1992;12:116-20.
53. Agarwal V, Prakash C, Yadav S, Chattopadhya D. Prevalence of transfusion transmitted infection in multitransfused children in relation to mandatory screening of HIV in donated blood. *Southeast Asian J Trop Med Public Health* 1997;4:699-703.
54. Ko WJ, Chow NK, Hsu RB, Chen YS, Wang SS, Chu SS, Lai MY. Hepatitis B virus infection in heart transplant recipients in a hepatitis B endemic area. *J Heart Lung Transplant* 2001;20:865-75.
55. Somjee S, Pai S, Parikh P, Banavali S, Kelkar R, Advamo S. Passive active prophylaxis against hepatitis B in children with acute lymphoblastic leukemia. *Leuk Res* 2002;26:989.

Section II

Pathogenesis, clinical presentation and diagnosis of hepatitis B

9

Immunopathogenesis and mechanisms of persistence of hepatitis B virus

Shobha Broor, Suma Ray

Approximately 5% of the world population is infected with the hepatitis B virus (HBV) causing liver disease of variable duration and severity. HBV infection in adults usually clears in majority with complete recovery. Some of the patients die due to fulminant hepatic failure. Five to ten percent of acutely infected adults develop chronic HBV infection which results in diverse clinical outcomes varying from asymptomatic chronic HBV infection to hepatocellular carcinoma.[1] Neonatally acquired HBV infection is, however, rarely cleared and over 90% of such children become chronically infected and develop chronic liver disease.[1]

HBV is a non-cytopathic DNA virus with a 3.2 kb circular genome that comprises many overlapping open reading frames coding for several structural and non-structural proteins like envelope (pre-S1, pre-S2, HBsAg), nucleocapsid (HBcAg, HBeAg), transactivating (X) and polymerase (pol) proteins. The pathogenic mechanism responsible for HBV related acute and chronic liver disease and the host determinants of hepato-carcinogenesis are only partially defined. The lack of *in vitro* culture system and narrow host range has hampered pathogenic studies. In order to establish a persistent infection in the host, HBV adopts a non-cytopathic mode of replication so as not to cause death of the host cell and avoid clearance by host antiviral immune response.[2] In general, T-cell mediated immune response to HBV-encoded antigens is responsible both for viral clearance and for disease pathogenesis during infection while humoral antibody response to viral envelope antigens contributes to the clearance of circulating virus particles. There are many host related and/or virus related factors that could be responsible for persistence of the HBV infection (Table 1).

HOST FACTORS

Immune Response to Hepatitis B Virus

Humoral Immune Responses

Antibody response to HBV envelope antigen (HBsAg) is a T-cell dependent process.[3] The

Table 1. Factors responsible for persistence of HBV infection

---
HOST FACTORS
  Immune response to hepatitis B virus
  - Humoral immune response
  - Cell-mediated immune response
  - Class II restricted T-lymphocyte response
  - Class I restricted T-lymphocyte response
  - Role of cytokines
  Tolerance
  - Neonatal tolerance
  - Adult onset tolerance
VIRAL FACTORS
  Infection of immunologically privileged sites
  Alteration of recognition molecules on the surface of infected cells
  Selective immune suppression
  Mutations in the virus leading to suppression of epitopes
---

anti-envelope antibodies are found in high titer in patients who clear the virus and recover from acute hepatitis, whereas in chronic HBV infection antibodies to envelope antigens are usually undetectable. Thus, these antibodies play a critical role in viral clearance by complexing with free viral particles and removing them from circulation or possibly by preventing the attachment and uptake of the virus by the cells. Antibodies to envelope antigen also contribute to the extrahepatic syndromes associated with HBV infection by forming antigen-antibody complexes.

On the other hand, the role of antibodies to nucleocapsid antigen (HBcAg and HBeAg) is not clear. These antibodies do not neutralize infectivity of the virus and they are present in high titers in both acute and chronic HBV infection. In experimental studies on chimpanzees, passively administered antibodies to HBeAg could provide protection.[4] The RNase H domain of viral polymerase also has an immunodominant epitope and antibodies to this epitope may reflect an ongoing viral replication.[5]

Cell-mediated immune response

The cellular immune responses to the envelope, nucleocapsid and polymerase antigens eliminate infected cells. The class I and class II restricted T-cell responses to the virus are vigorous, polyclonal and multispecific in acutely infected patients who successfully clear the virus and the responses are relatively weak and more narrowly focussed in chronically infected patients who do not clear the virus. The predominant cause of viral persistence during HBV infection is the development of a weak T-cell immune response to the viral antigens.

Class II restricted T-lymphocyte response

In acute hepatitis there is a vigorous HLA-II restricted CD4+ helper T-cell response to multiple epitopes on nucleocapsid antigen which is detectable in the peripheral blood. The CD4+ helper T-cell response to envelop antigen on the other hand is less vigorous. The reason for this absence of strong CD4+ T-cell response to envelop antigen is not clearly understood. It is speculated that envelope specific CD4+ T-cell response either becomes exhausted as a result of stimulation by high dose of the virus or paralyzed by high concentration of HBsAg.[1] In contrast, in vaccine recipient's envelope specific CD4+ T-cell response is good.[6] In chronic HBV infection, the HLA class II restricted T-cell response to all the viral antigens including HBcAg and HBeAg in the peripheral blood is weak as compared to acute hepatitis.[7,8] The nucleocapsid specific helper T-cell response is, however, accentuated during exacerbations of the disease. Preceding the exacerbation, the levels of HBV DNA and HBeAg go up and are followed by a sharp drop as the disease activity subsides.[9] The class II restricted nucleocapsid antigen specific T-cell response may thus be dependent upon critical levels of this antigen.[10] HBcAg specific helper T-cells also help HBV envelope specific B-cells to produce neutralizing antibodies by a process of "intermolecular" help.[11] Thus, nucleocapsid specific CD4+ T-cells play a key immunoregulatory role in the clearing or persistence of the virus.

Class I restricted T-lymphocyte (CTL) response

Antiviral CTL (HLA-I restricted) response is believed to play a major role in eradication of infection by killing of the virus infected cells. Patients with self-limiting acute hepatitis develop a vigorous polyclonal HLA-I restricted CTL response to epitopes in HBV envelope, nucleocapsid and polymerase proteins.[12,13] The CTL response to envelop antigen is very vigorous during acute infection as opposed to helper T-cell response. HBV persistence on the other hand is typically associated with a weak or undetectable virus specific CTL response. Weak CTL response is not only responsible for persistence of the virus but also leads to a slow and indolent necroinflammatory disease seen in chronic HBV infection. CTL response is also known to suppress HBV gene expression and replication which may also contribute to viral persistence. The basis for individual-to-individual variation in the generation of CTL response is not well understood and several possible mechanisms are suggested.

The CTL mediated immunopathology is a multistep process. In HBsAg transgenic mice, it has been shown that the earliest detectable pathological event following the entry of CTL into the liver is their attachment to HBsAg positive hepatocytes which they trigger to undergo apoptosis (Fig. 1).[14] This direct CTL-hepatocyte interaction results in the appearance of scattered acidophilic Councilman bodies (apoptotic hepatocytes) seen characteristically in

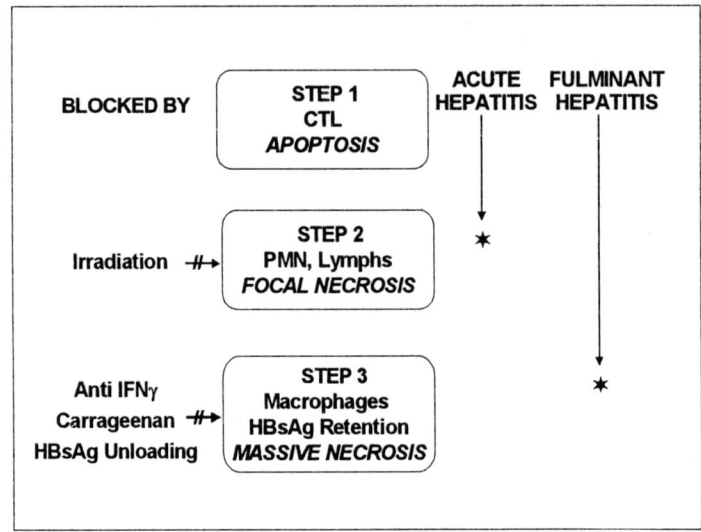

Fig. 1. CTL mediated immunopathogenesis of acute HBV infection

acute viral hepatitis in humans. The direct cytopathic effect is, however, limited to very few hepatocytes due to very low effector: target ratio. After about 4–12 hrs, the CTLs recruit many host derived antigen non-specific inflammatory cells into their vicinity. This results in the formation of necroinflammatory foci with hepatocellular necrosis extending to the periphery thus signifying that most of the hepatocytes are killed by cells other than the CTLs.[15] In most cases of acute viral hepatitis, not more than 5% of the hepatocytes are killed. However, in some cases the envelope antigen accumulates as non-secretable filamentous HBsAg particles in the endoplasmic reticulum of the hepatocytes giving them a ground glass appearance. These hepatocytes become very sensitive to destruction by gamma interferon secreted by the macrophages leading to fulminant hepatitis. This hypothesis suggests that fulminant hepatitis can be prevented by prior administration of neutralizing antibody to interferon gamma (IFN-γ) or by inactivation of macrophages by multiple injections of carrageenan.[15] CTLs, however, are not able to kill the virus infected cells in the extrahepatic sites due to the their microvascular anatomical barriers. Thus, the extrahepatic reservoirs of HBV might contribute to viral persistence.

Role of cytokines

The replication of HBV in the hepatocytes leads to the production of HBV virions and the release of HBsAg and HBeAg into the circulation, whereas HBcAg is trapped inside the liver cells. Both inside the liver and in the peripheral circulation the viral peptides are processed and expressed on antigen presenting cells (APC) along with major histocompatibility complex (MHC) II. The CD4 lymphocytes recognize the expressed antigens and get activated to produce Th-1 type of cytokines like IL-2 and IFN-γ, or Th-2 cytokines like IL-4, IL-5, IL-6,

IL-10. The Th-1 cytokines stimulate CD8+ T-lymphocytes, which recognize MHC-I linked viral peptides expressed on the hepatocytes and cause death of these infected cells through mediators like perforins.[16] Apart from antigen specific antigen non-specific killing of infected hepatocytes is carried out by inflammatory cells like macrophages and natural killer (NK) which are recruited to the site by Th-1 cytokines (Fig. 2). CD8+ cells also effect viral clearance by production of antiviral cytokines like TNF-α and IFN-γ. This cytokine-mediated non-cytolytic viral clearance is presently considered to be the most effective way of eradication of the HBV infection. The Th-1 cytokines like IFN-γ and TNF-α down regulate HBV gene expression and replication in the hepatocytes.[17] The Th-2 cytokines on the other hand act predominantly on B lymphocytes to produce humoral-mediated immunity, which clears the circulating virus particles and prevent re-infection of naïve hepatocytes. Hence, while a Th-1 type response eradicates the infected hepatocytes, the Th-2 type response takes care of the circulating virus. So, for clearance of HBV in a self-limiting infection, a pre-dominant Th-1 type response associated with a Th-2 type response is essential. If a predominant Th-2 response occurs instead of a Th-1 response, virus from the infected hepatocyte cannot be cleared and hence it persists. Interleukin-12 which is produced by APC regulates the balance between Th-1/Th-2 lymphocyte subsets.[18] IL-12 modulates macrophage response through the control of IFN-γ synthesis by Th-1 cells.[18] The balance between Th-1 and Th-2 cells specific for HBc/HBe is important in acute and chronic HBV infection. The factors which affect HBc/HBe specific Th-1/Th-2 cell balance include the concentration of HBc/HBe antigen, the host MHC and T-cell site recognition, T-cell tolerance and concentration of

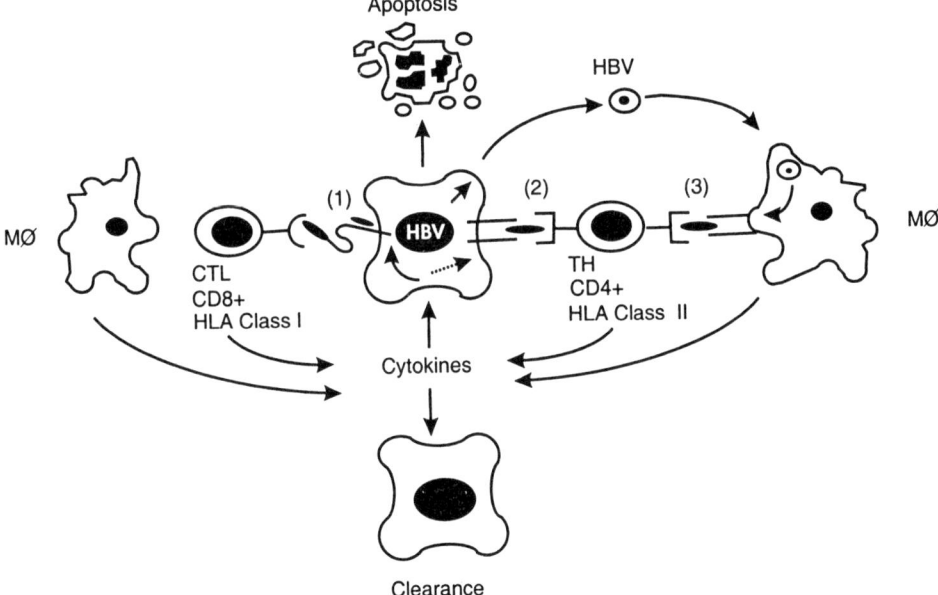

Fig. 2. Host-virus interaction and the mechanisms for clearence of the HBV

secreted HBe antigen in circulation which preferentially deletes Th-1 cells.[19] Deficiency of IL-12 production may cause a predominant Th-2 type response leading to persistence of HBV.

Tolerance

For a non-cytopathic virus to persist, it should be able to evade immune surveillance by either producing a weak immune response or by developing strategies to escape an efficient immune response. One of the ways to escape an immune response is by way of developing immune tolerance.

Neonatal tolerance

Clonal deletion of HBV specific T-cells due to transplacental infection of the fetus or transplacental passage of subviral antigens can play an important role in chronic infection seen in neonates. As neonates are able to respond well to hepatitis B virus vaccine during infancy, the immunological immaturity cannot be blamed.[20] Presumably there is a thymic deletion of MHC class II restricted HBV nucleocapsid specific helper T-cells due to transplacental exposure to HBeAg.[21] Tolerance occurs to other HBV antigens as well by negative selection of responding cells in thymus during development.

Adult onset tolerance

Immunological tolerance in adult onset infection may be caused by the exhaustion of CTLs by the high load of the virus[22] or by induction of apoptosis during extremely vigorous proliferative responses to an antigen, like superantigens.[23] During acute hepatitis B, patients mount a vigorous T-cell response to HBV nucleocapsid antigen.[8] Usually this response leads to clearance of the virus but it could result in overload exhaustion as is reported in lymphocytic choriomeningitis virus (LCMV) infection in mice.[20] This overload exhaustion causes tolerance leading to failure to eradicate the virus. While neonatal tolerance probably plays an important role in viral persistence in patients infected at birth, the basis for poor responsiveness in adult-onset infection is not well understood.

VIRAL FACTORS

Infection of immunologically privileged sites

Replication of HBV in a site not accessible to the immune system helps the virus to evade immune recognition. HBsAg-specific CTLs cannot reach HBsAg positive parenchymal cells in many organs due to the microvascular barriers that do not exist in the liver.[24] During naturally acquired HBV infection, HBV-specific CTLs are unable to recognize antigen expressed in the tissues like kidney, brain, testes, pancreas, etc., and thus allow it to persist in these extrahepatic sites.[25] The virions released from these immunologically protected sites can infect liver cells and stimulate memory T-cells, thereby contributing to viral persistence.

Alteration of recognition molecules on the surface of infected cells

Studies with adenovirus, cytomegalovirus and Epstein-Barr virus show that expression of HLA and other accessory molecules can be influenced by the virus themselves leading to inefficient recognition of infected cells by CTLs and the escape of the virus from immune clearance.[26] Although, there is no evidence that HBV exerts a direct negative influence on the expression of HLA or accessory molecules, recent findings suggest that HBcAg can suppress transcription of the β-interferon gene,[27] and the polymerase protein can inhibit the cellular response to IFNs-α and γ.[28] It may thus appear that HBV has the capacity to downregulate these immunoregulatory molecules and the accessory molecules they induce. It is also known that HBV integrates into the host genome during chronic infection, which interrupts at least one of the coding regions of the virus and is usually associated with extensive viral genomic rearrangement, thereby reducing its visibility to the host immune system.

Selective immune suppression

Viruses like HBV that infect lymphocytes and monocytes have the potential to cause selective or generalised immunosuppression of the host.[26] It has been shown for LCMV that infection in immunologically immature newborns selectively depletes the specific CTL response, whereas, persistent infection in an immunologically mature adult causes generalized immunosuppression of CTL response.[29] Similar immunosupression may also account for different patterns of chronicity observed in HBV infection. Class I envelope antigen-specific CTLs can also selectively kill HBsAg specific B-cells following uptake *via* the immunoglobulin receptor due to the ability of the exogenous soluble HBsAg to enter the class I processing pathway.[30] Thus, HBV-specific T-cells drawn to the site of antigen synthesis can take up viral envelope antigens, process and present them to the neighboring envelope-specific CTLs and clear the virus.

Mutations in the virus leading to suppression of epitopes

During acute HBV infection, most patients develop a strong CTL response against multiple epitopes in the viral envelope, nucleocapsid and polymerase proteins which is vigorous enough to be detected in the peripheral blood.[12,13] Mutations in both CD4+ and CD8+ T-cell epitopes have also been thought to be responsible for immune escape mechanism of HBV and may thereby be responsible for viral persistence.[31] The pre-core mutation could increase virus pathogenicity if truncated pre-core peptide is more efficiently processed with the generation of the high affinity class I restricted CTL epitope. It is likely that the viruses containing precore or any other mutation can display a positive growth advantage entirely independent of any immunological advantage that they may enjoy if they replicate more efficiently than their parental wild type virus. Besides rendering CTL epitopes invisible to T-cell recognition, substitution of T-cell receptor contact site can also influence the CTL response by creating analogue peptides that can still interact with the T-cell receptor but may not be able to deliver the stimulatory signal, thus acting as antagonists. T-cell receptor antagonists have recently been identified in two patients with chronic hepatitis.[32] If the major CTL response is directed towards such an epitope, it would give a selective survival advantage to the mutant viruses compared to the wild type virus. Since an individual HBV-infected cell generally contains many DNA copies of the virus, it may simultaneously express both variant as well as the wild type peptides on its surface. This would thus effectively protect the cell containing the mutant virus from the immune elimination by CTL specific for the wild type epitope. This mechanism might also lead to survival of the cells infected with both variant and wild type giving extra benefit for survival of variant viral population. Under such conditions this mechanism could contribute to persistence of HBV infection. Mutations in pre-S and/or S-region can also contribute to viral escape from immune surveillance by anti-HBs.[33-35] Single amino acid substitutions in the surface antigen have been shown to mediate escape from circulating anti-HBs.[36] Cirrhosis and HCC have been reported in patients with chronic HBV infection in the presence of anti-HBs.[37] Thus, the mutant virus has the potential to develop severe disease even in the presence of anti-HBs.

REFERENCES

1. Chisari FV. Hepatitis B virus immunopathogenesis. *Ann Rev Immunol* 1995;13:29-60.
2. Chisari FV, Fessari C, Mondelli MV. Hepatitis B virus structure and biology. *Micro Pathol* 1989;6:311-25.
3. Milich DR, McLachlan A. The nucleocapsid of hepatitis B virus is both a T-cell independent and a T-cell dependent antigen. *Science* 1986;234:1398-1401.
4. Stephan W, Prince AM, Brotman B. Modulation of hepatitis B infection by intravenous application of an immunoglobulin preparation that contains antibodies to hepatitis B e and core antigens but not to hepatitis B surface antigen. *J Virol* 1984;51:420-4.
5. Weimer T, Schodel F, Jung MC, Pape GR, Alberti A, Fattovich G, Beljaars H, et al. Antibodies to the RNase H domain of hepatitis B virus P protein are associated with ongoing viral replication. *J Virol* 1990;64:5665-8.
6. Celis E, Ou D, Otvos L. Recognition of hepatitis B surface antigen by human T-lymphocytes. Proliferative and cytotoxic responses to a major antigenic determinant defined by synthetic peptides. *J Immunol* 1988;140:1808-15.
7. Ferrari C, Penna A, Bertoletti A, Valli A, Antoni AD, Giuberti T, Cavalli A, et al. Cellular immune response to hepatitis B virus encoded antigens in acute and chronic hepatitis B virus infection. *J Immunol* 1990;145:3442-9.
8. Jung MC, Spengler U, Schraut W, Hoffman R, Zachoval R, Eisenburg J, Eichenlaub D, et al. Hepatitis B virus antigen-specific T-cell activation in patients with acute and chronic hepatitis B. *J Hepatol* 1991;13:310-7.
9. Tsai SL, Chen PJ, Lai MY, Yang PM, Sung JL, Huang JH, Hwang LH, et al. Acute exacerbations of chronic type B hepatitis are accompanied by increased T-cell responses to hepatitis B core and e antigens? Implications for hepatitis B e antigen sero-conversion. *J Clin Invest* 1992;89:87-96.
10. Maruyama T, Iino S, Koike K, Yasuda K, Milich DR. Serology of acute exacerbation in chronic hepatitis B. *Gastroenterology* 1993;105:1141-51.

11. Celis E, Kung PC, Chang TW. Hepatitis B virus-reactive human T-lymphocyte clones: antigen specificity and helper function for antibody synthesis. *J Immunol* 1984;132:1511-6.
12. Penna A, Chisari FV, Bertoletti A, Missale G, Fowler P, Giuberti T, Fiaccadori F, et al. Cytotoxic T-lymphocytes recognize an HLA-A2-restricted epitope within the hepatitis B virus nucleocapsid antigen. *J Exp Med* 1991;174:1565-70.
13. Nayersina R, Folwer P, Guilhot S, Missale G, Cerny A, Schlicht HJ, Vitiello A, et al. HLA-A2-restricted cytotoxic T-lymphocyte responses to multiple hepatitis B surface antigen epitopes during hepatitis B virus infection. *J Immunol* 1993;150:4659-71.
14. Ando K, Guidotti LG, Wirth S, Ishikawa T, Missale G, Moriyama T, Schreiber RD, et al. Class I restricted cytotoxic T-lymphocytes are directly cytopathic for their target cells in vivo. *J Immunol* 1994;152:3245-53.
15. Ando K, Moriyama T, Guidotti LG, Wirth S, Schreiber RD, Schlicht HJ, Huang SN, et al. Mechanisms of class I restricted immunopathology. A transgenic mouse model of fulminant hepatitis. *J Exp Med* 1993;178:1541-54.
16. Gilles PN, Guerrette DL, Ulevitch RJ, Schreiber RD, Chisari FV. Hepatitis B surface antigen retention sensitizes the hepatocyte to injury by physiologic concentrations of gamma interferon. *Hepatology* 1992;16:655-63.
17. Milich DR. Pathobiology of acute and chronic hepatitis B virus infection: an introduction. *J Viral Hepatitis* 1997;4 (suppl 2):25-30.
18. Gilles PN, Fey G, Chisari V. Tumor necrosis factor-alpha negatively regulates hepatitis B virus gene expression in transgenic mice. *J Virol* 1992;66:3955-60.
19. Milich DR. Influence of T-helper cell subsets and crossregulation in hepatitis B virus infection. *J Viral Hepatitis* 1997;4 (suppl 2):48-59.
20. Lee GC, Hwang LY, Beaseley RP, Chen SH, Lee TY. Immunogenicity of hepatitis B virus vaccine in healthy Chinese neonates. *J Infect Dis* 1983;148:526-9.
21. Milich DR, Jones JE, Hughes JL, Price J, Raney AK, McLachlan A. Is a function of the secreted hepatitis B e antigen to induce immunologic tolerance in utero? *Proc Natl Acad Sci USA* 1990;487:6599-6603.
22. Moskophidis D, Lechner F, Pircher H, Zinkernagel RM. Virus persistence in acutely infected immunocompetent mice by exhaustion of antiviral cytotoxic effector T-cells. *Nature* 1993;362:758-61.
23. Webb S, Morris C, Sprent J. Extrathymic tolerance of mature T-cells: clonal elimination as a consequence of immunity. *Cell* 1990;63:1249-56.
24. Ando K, Guidotti LG, Cerny A, Ishikawa T, Chisari FV. Access to antigen restricts cytotoxic T-lymphocyte function in vivo. *J Immunol* 1994;153:482-8.
25. Yoffe B, Burns DS, Bhatt HS, Combes B. Extrahepatic hepatitis B virus DNA sequences in patients with acute hepatitis B infection. *Hepatology* 1990;12:187-92.
26. Oldstone MB. Viral persistence. *Cell* 1989;56:517-20.
27. Whitten TM, Quets AT, Schloemer RH. Identification of the hepatitis B virus factor that inhibits expression of the beta interferon gene. *J Virol* 1991;65:4699-4704.
28. Foster GR, Ackrill AM, Goldin RD, Kerr IM, Thomas HC, Stark GR. Expression of the terminal protein region of hepatitis B virus inhibits cellular responses to interferons-alpha and gamma and double stranded RNA. *Proc Natl Acad Sci USA* 1991;88:2888-92.
29. Tishon A, Borrow P, Evans C, Oldstone MBA. Virus induced immunosupression: age at infection relates to a selective or a generalized defect. *Virology* 1993;195:397-405.
30. Barnaba V, Franco A, Alberti A, Benvenuto R, Balsano F. Selective killing of hepatitis B envelope antigen-specific B-cells by class I restricted, exogenous antigen specific T-lymphocytes. *Nature* 1990;345:258-60.

31. Sabao V, Tomiyama H, Sogi K, Tokunaga M, Ueno T, Saito S, Fujiyama S. The role of hepatitis B virus-specific memory CD8 T-cells in the control of viral replication. *J Hepatol* 2002;36:105-15.
32. Bertoletti A, Sette A, Scaccaglia P, Levrero M, Chisari FV, Fiaccadori F, et al. Natural variants of cytotoxic epitopes are T-cell receptor antagonists for antiviral cytotoxic T-cells. *Nature* 1994;369:407-10.
33. Kato J, Hasegawa K, Torii N, Yamaguchi K, Hayashi N. A molecular analysis of viral persistence in surface antigen-negative chronic hepatitis B. *Hepatology* 1996;23:389-95.
34. Jung MC, Pape GR. Immunology of hepatitis B infection. *Lancet Infect Dis* 2002;2:43-50.
35. Lok AS, McMohan BJ. Chronic hepatitis B. *Hepatology* 2001;34:1225-41.
36. Yamamoto K, Horikita M, Tsuda F, Itoh K, Akahane Y, Yotsumoto S, Okamoto H, et al. Naturally occurring escape mutants of hepatitis B virus with various mutations in the S-gene in carriers seropositive for antibody to hepatitis B surface antigen. *J Virol* 1994;68:2671-6.
37. Okoshi S, Igarashi M, Suda Ta, Iwamatsu H, Watanabe K. Ishihara K, Ogata N, et al. Remote development of hepato cellular carcinomain patients with liver cirrhosis type B serologically cured for HBs anti genemia with long-standing normalization of ALT values. *Dig Dis Sci* 2002;47;2002-6.

10

Incidentally detected asymptomatic HBsAg positive subjects

Amrinder S Puri, Sri R Agarwal

Widespread use of screening tests for hepatitis B surface antigen (HBsAg) in sixties and seventies in Europe and North America led to the detection of a large subset of asymptomatic individuals with circulating HBsAg. These were designated as "Hepatitis B Carriers". This term which is used widely comprises a "mixed bag" population. Thus, a patient with end stage renal disease who acquires HBsAg post-dialysis is lumped together with a healthy blood donor incidentally detected to have HBsAg. The natural history of the disease is likely to be very different in both the cases. For this and several other reasons, the term "Hepatitis B Carrier" has come under criticism.[1,2] Arguments have been made both for and against the change of this nomenclature but a clear consensus eludes the issue.[1-4]

Traditionally, studies on natural history of "carriers" were based mainly on voluntary blood donors incidentally detected to have HBsAg in their serum. These studies are likely to be skewed in their observations, as majority of the blood donors were male, belonged to a narrow age group (18-45 yr) and hence, not representative of the entire carrier pool.

An alternative term, "Incidentally Detected Asymptomatic Hepatitis B Subject (IDAHS)" has been suggested to overcome these shortcomings. To this bulky term, some workers have added another adjective "healthy".[2] IDAHS comprises individuals found positive for HBsAg during screening for varied reasons. Data on IDAHS are preliminary and only beginning to emerge.

DEFINITION AND NOMENCLATURE

The term IDAHS has not been clearly defined in the literature. Is it different from hepatitis B carrier? For the puritans, the answer is in the affirmative because of various reasons. First, the literature on carriers is based on voluntary blood donors from the West (low endemicity regions). There are inherent differences between this group and the large pool of carriers in Asia/Africa (high endemicity region) where a carrier pool is established early in childhood.

Second, a small group of IDAHS could theoretically be having anicteric hepatitis B. Third, the label carrier is given at the end of a gamut of investigations that may even include liver biopsy whereas IDAHS is usually the entry point of referral to a hepatologist. The key issue here is what proportion of IDAHS will have significant liver disease albeit asymptomatic whereas the remainder would then be labeled as true carriers. However, many workers would consider both the terms as synonyms. A pragmatic approach would be to consider IDAHS as the first step in algorithm of investigations for hepatitis B. Thus, the group of IDAHS would practically include those apparently healthy individuals testing positive for HBsAg during screening for varied reasons (Table 1). By definition, subjects with a co-existing morbid disease would be excluded.

Table 1. Reasons for HBsAg screening in healthy individuals

Voluntary blood donors
Health care professional
Household contacts of patients with HBV-related liver disease
Insurance policy requirement
Immigration formality
Executive health checkup
Organ donors
Hepatitis B screening camps

BASIC QUESTIONS ON IDAHS

In an attempt to describe this entity, five basic questions need to be addressed.

(a) What is the magnitude of the problem?
(b) What is the biochemical and serological profile of these patients?
(c) Is liver biopsy required in all subjects?
(d) What proportion of these patients has clinically silent chronic liver disease at presentation?
(e) What are the recommendations for work up and subsequent follow-up?

Magnitude of the problem

There are about 370 million chronic HBsAg positive subjects all over the world, out of which 45 million are in India alone.[5] This pool will continue to expand until universal vaccination programs reach the target population in Asia and Sub Saharan Africa. This pool may also increase as threshold of HBsAg testing becomes lower because of increasing awareness. Recently, Chandra et al[6] reported biochemical and serological profile of 370 IDAHS over a period of 4 years at a tertiary referral center in New Delhi.

Biochemical and serological profile of IDAHS

Analysis of data from different parts of the country shows little variation in serological profile. On the other hand, there is considerable variation in proportion of patients showing raised aminotransferases that have been reported in 0–72% of asymptomatic carriers.[3, 6-9] The main reasons for this variation are: (i) short follow up period, (ii) ingestion of alcohol or other hepatotoxic drugs, and (iii) the different reports taking different groups of patients. HBeAg positivity rate in the country lies in the narrow range between 9 and 33% with the exception of a single report by Tandon et al (9%).[3] Similarly, the entire country shows uniformly high positivity for anti-HBe (56–82%). HBV-DNA positivity is reported in 17–41% of subjects positive for anti-HBe (Table 2). Based on serological markers, Chandra et al[6] have suggested 3 subgroups: Group I-HBeAg positive and anti-HBe negative; Group II-HBeAg negative and anti-HBe positive; Group III-negative for both HBeAg and anti-HBe. Majority of patients in India belong to group II. Chandra et al[6] showed high percentage of HBV-DNA positivity in group II possibly because of the large number of precore mutants seen in their center. The positivity for anti-HBe is seen in 29–75% at a global level.[10-13]

Is liver biopsy necessary in all IDAHS?

Several large studies have shown that liver biopsies performed in incidentally detected individuals with normal transaminase levels show minimal evidence of liver disease. Koertz et al[14] compiled data from several studies to show that only 2% of these individuals showed ad-

Table 2. Biochemical and serological profile of IDAHS

Author	Elevated AST/ALT %	HBeAg positive %	Anti-HBe positive %	HBV-DNA positive %
Indian data				
Tandon[3]	0	0	NR	0
Arankalle et al[7]	NR	9	80	NR
Puri et al (UP)	19	37	56	NR
Chandra et al[6]	47-72	30	62	41 (eAb +ve)
Hari et al[8]	NR	1	82	17 (eAb +ve)
Singal[9]	10	5	5	5 (eAb +ve)
Global data				
Viola et al[10]	73	62	31	–
Stroffolini et al[11]	–	27	69	8.8
Alward et al[12]	–	69	29	–
Lindh et al[13]	60	22	75	–

UP–unpublished data
NR–not recorded

vanced liver disease in the form of cirrhosis/chronic active hepatitis. However, this figure increased by nearly ten-fold in a similar population with persistently elevated aminotransferase levels. Since antiviral therapy (interferon/lamivudine) is currently indicated only in patients with raised aminotransferase levels, liver biopsy, therefore, is recommended only when there is rise in aminotransferase levels.

What proportion of IDAHS has clinically silent/asymptomatic liver disease?

The answer to this question can be ascertained either by data on liver biopsies or by follow up studies showing progression from asymptomatic to symptomatic liver disease. Data from the West suggest that the vast majority of incidentally detected HBsAg positive subjects with normal liver enzymes do not show significant histological damage.[14] The commonest finding in this situation is the presence of ground glass hepatocytes with minimal portal tract inflammation. Available long-term follow-up studies from the West in healthy HBsAg positive subjects indicate an excellent prognosis and a low risk for development of cirrhosis and HCC.[15-17] In contrast to Caucasians, the outlook for the Asian HBsAg positive subjects is not so sanguine. In areas with high endemicity, like China and Taiwan, early acquisition of HBV leads to early liver damage perhaps before HBeAg seroconversion. Thus, of the 30 Hong Kong children who seroconverted at a mean age of 10 years, 15 had advanced liver disease, viz., fibrosis, cirrhosis or HCC. Indian experience is similar to the experience from China and Taiwan despite major difference in the HBsAg prevalence in these two regions. Chandra et al[18] showed Histological Activity Index (HAI) of >3 in 40% of IDAHS with normal enzymes and in 70% in subjects with raised enzymes. However, these authors have not elaborated what proportion of their patients had moderate or severe liver disease, i.e. HAI ≥ 9.

What are the recommendations for work up of IDAHS?

At an international conference held in New Delhi in 1998 on hepatitis B, it was suggested that the first step in the diagnostic algorithm of a person harboring HBsAg for > 6 months should be the determination of ALT.[19] HBeAg testing was recommended in all patients irrespective of ALT status. Anti-HBe test should be done if HBeAg is negative. In an HBeAg positive individual there is no need for routine testing of HBV-DNA except for prognostic or research purpose. In an anti-HBe positive individual, baseline HBV-DNA test should be done to determine the replicative status of the virus. Indications for liver biopsy in IDAHS have been discussed vide supra. Liver biopsy may also be performed as a part of study protocol in two other situations, where ALT is normal. First, in an anti-HBe positive individual with high HBV-DNA level and second, when HBeAg is persistently positive for ≥ 6 months (Fig. 1). The algorithm is to be used in connection with other tests and is not a substitute for history, physical examination, ultrasound examination or endoscopy that may establish the diagnosis of advanced liver disease.

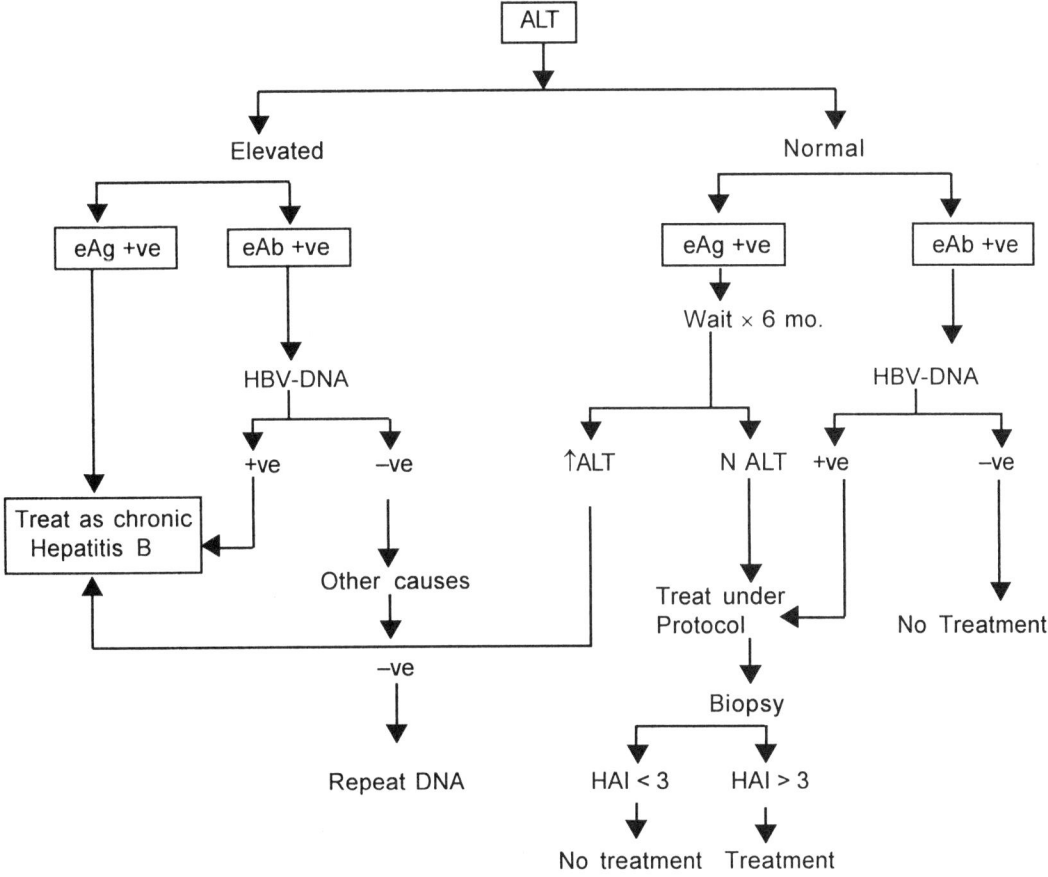

Fig. 1. Algorithm for diagnosis of an HBsAg positive subject

Chronic HBV infection is not a static disease. Constant interplay between host and viral factors may swing the pendulum temporarily towards either side. Unfortunately the liver can suffer in silence for long. By the time the disease becomes manifest, irreversible architectural damage may have been done. IDAHS are a subset, which provide the clinician a unique opportunity to arrest the disease at an early stage. However, not all IDAHS have chronic hepatitis and hence, there is a need for an algorithm which will separate healthy HBsAg positive subjects from those with liver disease. It remains to be seen if any of the existing antivirals or drugs of the future will ultimately reduce the HBV infected pool of the world and eradicate this virus that affects nearly 350 million people of the world.

REFERENCES

1. Hepatitis B and C – Asian perspectives: Preconference expert group deliberations. *Indian J Gastroenterol* 1999;18(suppl):S9-10.
2. Hoofnagle JH, Shafritz DA, Popper H. Chronic type B hepatitis and the healthy HBsAg carrier state. *Hepatology* 1987;7:758-63.
3. Tandon BN. Hepatitis B carrier, the correct nomenclature. *Natl Med J India* 1999;12:141-5.
4. Naik SR. Hepatitis B virus: infected or just carrying. *Indian J Gastroenterol* 2000;19:130-2.
5. Thyagarajan SP, Jayaram S, Mohanvalli B. *Prevalence of HBV in the general population of India.* In: Sarin SK, Singal AK, Eds. Hepatitis B in India – Problems and Prevention: CBS Publishers & Distributors, New Delhi 1996; pp.5-16.
6. Agarwal SR, Kapoor D, Chandra R, Thakur V, Sarin SK. Biochemical and serological profile of incidentally detected asymptomatic HBsAg positive subjects. *Indian J Gastroenterol* 1998;18(suppl 1):S29.
7. Arankalle VA, Chadha MS, Chobe LP. Five year follow-up of HBsAg carriers. *Indian J Gastroenterol* 1999;18(suppl):S27.
8. Hari R, Mohan KVK, Murugavel KG, Thyagarajan SP. Hepatitis B virus DNA in asymptomatic carriers: relationship with HBeAg/anti-HBe and titer status. *Indian J Gastroenterol* 1998;18(suppl):S25.
9. Singal AK. Follow-up of asymptonate HBsAg positive individuals detected during blood donation. *J Gastroenterol Hepatol* 2002 (abstract).
10. Viola LA, Barrison IG, Coleman JC, Paradinas FJ, Fluker JL, Evans BA. Natural history of liver disease in chronic hepatitis B surface antigen carriers. *Lancet* 1981;21:1156-9.
11. Stroffolini T, Sagnelli E, Rapicetta M, Felaco FM, Filippini P, Annella T, Petruzziello A. Hepatitis B virus DNA in chronic HBsAg carriers: correlation with HBeAg/anti-HBe status, anti-HD and liver histology. *Hepatogastroenterology* 1992;39:62-5.
12. Alward WL, McMahon BJ, Hall DB, Heyward WL, Francis DP, Bender TR. The long-term serological course of asymptomatic hepatitis B virus carriers and the development of hepatocellular carcinoma. *J Infect Dis* 1985;151:604-9.
13. Lindh M, Horal P, Dhillon AP, Norkrans G. Hepatitis B virus DNA levels, precore mutations, genotypes and histological activity in chronic hepatitis B. *J Viral Hep* 2000;7:258-67.
14. Koretz RL, Levin KH, Rebhun DJ, Gitnick GL. Hepatitis B surface antigen carriers – to biopsy or not to biopsy. *Gastroenterology* 1978:75:860-3.
15. de Franchis R, Meucci G, Vecchi M, Tatarella M, Colombo M, Del Nino E, Rumi MG, et al. The natural history of asymptomatic hepatitis B surface antigen carriers. *Ann Intern Med* 1993;118:191-4.
16. Villeneuve JP, Desrochers M, Infante Rivard C, Williams B, Raymond G, Bourcier M, Cote J. A long-term follow-up study of asymptomatic hepatitis B surface antigen positive carriers in Montreal. *Gastroenterology* 1994;106:1000-5.
17. Mcmahon BJ, Holck P, Bulkow Z, Snowball M. Serologic and Clinical Outcomes of 1536 Alarka natives chronically infected with hepatitis B virus. *Ann Intern Med* 2001;135:759-68.
18. Chandra R, Agarwal SR, Kapoor D, Sakhuja P, Malhotra V, Sarin SK. HBV carrier state – does it exist? *Indian J Gastroenterol* 1999;18(suppl):S29.
19. Hepatitis B and C–Asian perspectives. Consensus statement. *Indian J Gastroenterol* 1999;18(suppl):S16-20.

11

Clinical spectrum of hepatitis B virus infection in India

Anand Dotihal, Shiv K Sarin

Hepatitis B Virus (HBV) infection is a global health problem. Its protean clinical manifestations have been documented in great detail in the past three decades from almost all countries. However, wide geographic variations in the frequency and profile of acute and chronic infection exist. Moreover, the change in the profile of the disease due to the emergence of the mutant strains also merits attention. An updated information on the clinical spectrum of HBV would have a bearing on the approach to diagnosis, treatment and prevention strategies for hepatitis B in India.

Acute Viral Hepatitis

In India, hepatitis B virus is an important cause of sporadic acute viral hepatitis in adults, the incidence being 26% to 62% in various series.[1,2] In one study from Chandigarh involving 253 patients with sporadic acute viral hepatitis, 77 patients tested positive for HBsAg and on further analysis 64% had acute hepatitis B while 35% had exacerbation of chronic hepatitis B and 1% had co-infection with hepatitis B and E viruses.[3]

The occurrence of transfusion associated hepatitis (TAH) is reported to be 6.9% to 16%[4,5] in our country. Recent reviews estimate that 20% of TAH are due to HBV, i.e. 1.4% of all transfusion episodes. Anti-HBe positive blood (3.5%), HBV-DNA positive blood (0.7%), mutant HBV infection and low-level HBV viremia are some causes of TAH-B despite screening for HBsAg.

One study done in early 1990's found that 80% of TAH were due to non-A, non-B virus.[4] In a prospective study using current screening practices, Saxena et al[6] reported 7.7% occurrence of TAH among 182 patients who received blood, with 71.5% being due to hepatitis C. HBV was responsible for 1.6 % of cases even after donor blood was screened for HBsAg using monoclonal assay. As some (up to 10%) of the hepatitis B patients may harbor surface mutants[7] and about 9% of healthy adults have detectable HBV-DNA in their blood, further reduction in the incidence of TAH-B is only possible with additional and improved screening tests for hepatitis B. Similar view has been expressed by Saraswat et al.[8] The incidence of development of TAH also depends on the number of units of blood transfused. In multiply transfused patients, TAH may develop in more than 50% for hepatitis B and more than 30% for hepatitis C.[9]

An outbreak of hepatitis B has been reported by Singh et al from Gujarat related to the use of inadequately sterilized needles and syringes with a very high case fatality rate of 46.7%.[10]

Acute liver failure

Acute liver failure (ALF) complicates acute hepatitis B virus infection in less than 1% of patients. The same may occur if HBV co-infection or superinfection occurs with other viruses. In India, about 95% of ALF in whom etiology can be ascertained, are due to hepatotrophic viruses.[7] The reported causes of ALF in recent studies are shown in Table 1.

Table 1. Etiology of acute liver failure in India

Authors	Year	No. of Patients	HAV	HBV	HCV	HDV	HEV	Mixed	Non-A-E	Drugs
Acharya et al[10]	2000	458	4	11	4	0	23	6	47	5
Khuroo et al[12]	1997	119	3	15	3	3	38	–	39	1
Jaiswal et al[11]	1996	95	4	37	2	5	41	4	15	0

HBV alone was responsible for 2.4% of ALF in the series by Acharya et al and an additional 17 of 29 patients who had mixed viral infection had hepatitis B. However, the same group of investigators have elsewhere reported that 23.6% of their ALF patients were carriers for HBsAg and 19.1% had acute HBV infection defined by the presence of HBsAg and IgM anti-HBc. Jaiswal et al have reported ALF due to HBV in 27% of patients in central India. Mixed infection was infrequent in this series.[11] In Kashmir, HEV appears to be the commonest cause of ALF followed by HBV infection.[12]

It is reported that cryptic HBV infection, HCV infection, HEV infection can cause FHF without being detectable serologically especially in the early phase of the illness. One study evaluated 59 patients with ALF who had apparently non A-E infection, it was found that 39%, 3.3% and 1.6% of the patients had HBV-DNA, HCV RNA and HEV RNA in the serum respectively. The role of HBV mutants in ALF was also studied in the above patients by Acharya et al. None of the patients had mutation in the pre-core region and 5 of 59 patients with non A-E hepatitis had HBV-DNA in serum with the core region showing deletion and insertion of nucleotides. These changes might have been responsible for the absence of detectable IgM anti-HBc in the serum. The issue whether HBV causes ALF in the absence of standard serological markers for HBV, has to be evaluated further. It may be summarized that 10–37% patients of ALF in India are caused by HBV infection and mutations in the HBV genome are not uncommon.

The overall survival of the patients in ALF is around 33% with about 2/3rd of them dying within the first three days. Unlike the observations from the west, the etiology of ALF and the rapidity of onset of encephalopathy was not reported to influence the patient outcome in a large series.[13] The common causes of death in this series were cerebral edema and sepsis while renal failure and GI bleed rarely caused death.

Subacute Hepatic Failure

It is an ill-defined and controversial term. Subacute hepatic failure (SAHF) generally connotes the development of unequivocal ascites with or without encephalopathy in a patient four weeks after persistent or progressive jaundice. Presence of underlying chronic liver disease forms an exclusion criterion.

Initial studies found a prevalence rate of SAHF in 34% of all liver disease patients from the All India Institute of Medical Sciences. However, the reported incidence from all over the country has varied from 0 to 3%. More recently, Jaiswal et al report that 6.5% of their patients had SAHF. These figures suggest that a large majority of patients with CLD were included in the previous studies of SAHF. In fact, most people believe that the entity of subactue hepatic failure does not exist and patients presenting with these features have acute on chronic liver failure, a term widely used in the west.[14]

Viral hepatitis is the commonest cause of SAHF, especially HBV and HCV infection. HBV is implicated in 10% to 45% of patients of SAHF.

A mortality rate of 30-80% has been reported with renal failure, spontaneous bacterial peritonitis and GI bleed being the common causes of death. Chronic sequelae could develop in 60% of the survivors.[7]

CHRONIC HEPATITIS B

Chronic hepatitis B (CHB) continues to be an important cause of chronic liver disease (CLD) in India. The natural history in subjects who vertically acquire the infection includes an initial immunotolerent phase in childhood, characterized by high viral load and minimal ALT elevation followed by an immune clearance phase during which the e-antigen seroconversion occurs, usually in the second or the third decade and results in residual chronic HBV infection. In this state, the subject is HBsAg +ve, HBeAg –ve, anti-HBe+ve with low or undetectable HBV-DNA. The chance of developing progressive liver disease is higher in subjects with prolonged replicative phase. In some patients depending on the geographic area, a variable number develop raised ALT with high viral DNA in the face of e antibody positivity which potentially leads to progressive liver disease. Hepatocellular carcinoma, the sinister consequence of chronic HBV infection, can develop at any point during the course of infection with the risk being minimal in an incidentally detected HBsAg positive subject (IDAHS) vis-à-vis a cirrhotic and in a non-replicative versus a replicative infection.

There are only a few studies reported from India that have specifically addressed the issue of chronic hepatitis B (CHB). In one study,[15] 48 patients with chronic hepatitis were studied. Of them, 44 had chronic active hepatitis. Markers of HBV were positive in 50%, and 54% of these subjects had replicative phase of CHB. Hypoalbuminemia (< 3 gm%) was seen in more than 50% of patients suggesting that patients with CHB are detected at a late stage in India. Another study attempted to identify the frequency and determinants of chronicity following acute viral hepatitis. Marked hyperbilirubinemia at 4 weeks and bridging necrosis on histological examination were found to be important factors associated with delayed clearance of 's' antigen. The study concluded that 4.2% of patients with acute viral hepatitis developed chronic hepatitis.[16]

INCIDENTALLY DETECTED ASYMPTOMATIC HBsAg POSITIVE SUBJECTS (IDAHS)

This is a clinical situation that is frequently encountered with increasing awareness of HBV infection. These subjects are identified on routine screening for blood donation, health check-up or screening of family members of hepatitis B patients. These patients are potential candidates for transmission of HBV to others and at risk of developing long-term sequelae of chronic HBV infection. The profile of IDAHS has been studied by Chandra et al.[17] These investigators found that nearly one-third of the IDAHS have active viral replication i.e. HBeAg positive and the rest have anti-Hbe positivity. Those with raised ALT have significant histopathological lesions in both HBeAg positive or negative serological pattern.

CHRONIC LIVER DISEASE

Several studies have shown that infection with HBV is seen in more than 50% of patients with chronic liver disease in India. Two recent studies from Mumbai and Calcutta report that HBV was responsible for 16% and 35.4% of their patients with chronic liver disease. In a large series,[18] we have shown HBV positivity in 56% of patients with non-alcoholic cirrhosis (Table 2). HBV and HCV dual infection was seen in 13.5% of patients and the overall HBV

Table 2. Etiological spectrum of chronic liver disease in India

Author (yr.)	Patient (n)	HBV	HCV	HBV plus HCV Infection
Sundaram ('90)*	114	67.5%	–	–
Acharya ('90)	33	36.7%	15.2%	12.0%
Sarin ('95)	148	56%	10.8%	13.5%#

*Autopsy study #remaining 19.5% were diagnosed to have cryptogenic cirrhosis

positivity therefore reached around 70%. There was no difference in the frequency of HBV positivity in young adults and elderly patients with cirrhosis. A fair proportion of patients with chronic liver disease are HBV-DNA positive, suggesting HBV replication (Table 3). In one study it has been shown that eAg and HBV-DNA was detected in 26.5% and 52.9% of chronic active hepatitis, 45.5% and 81.8% of cirrhosis and 18.5% and 44.4% of asymptomatic chronic HBV infected subjects respectively. Thus, serum HBV-DNA is more sensitive than e-antigen in identifying the viral replication status.

Table 3. Profile of hepatitis B serology and HBV-DNA studies in HBV-related chronic liver disease

Group	Transfused (n=42)	Non-transfused (n=41)	Total n (%)
HBsAg + (eAg, Anti-HBc, DNA -)	21	7	28 (34%)
HBsAg+, eAg +, DNA +	3	12	15 (18%)
HBsAg+ eAg-, DNA +	7	4	11 (13%)
HBs+, Anti-HBc+, DNA+	7	11	18 (22%)
HBV-DNA + (HBsAg, Anti-HBc, eAg-)	4	7	11 (13%)
	42	41	83 (100%)

Could we clinically suspect the type of viral infection present in a patient with chronic liver disease? To investigate this, three groups of histologically proven chronic liver disease patients were studied: HCV related (n=30), HBV related (n=105) and dual infection with HBV and HCV (n=30). Patients with dual infection were younger, with a male dominance and a shorter duration of clinical illness compared to patients with HCV. Patients with chronic HCV more often presented in an indolent manner, with a prolonged history of low-grade fever (Table 4).

Table 4. Demographic and clinical profile of patients with HCV, HBV and dual infection

Parameter	Chronic HCV (n=30)	Chronic HBV (n=105)	Dual infection (n=30)
Mean age (yr.)	45.9±14.7	42.8±16.9	38.4±14.4*
Male:Female	20:10	85:20	26:4
Anorexia	7 (34.3%)	42 (40%)	12 (40%)
Bleeding	3 (10%)	49 (47%)	12 (40%)
Jaundice	12 (40%)	59 (56%)	16 (53%)
Fever	18 (60%)	39 (37%)	9 (30%)
Ascites	9 (30%)	57 (54%)	12 (40%)
Hepatomegaly	9 (30%)	46 (44%)	6 (20%)
Splenomegaly	9 (30%)	49 (47%)	6 (20%)
Mean Duration of illness (yr.)	6.9±1.2	3.2±1.4#	2.6±1.4*

* HCV Vs. dual infection $p<0.05$, # HCV Vs. HBV infection $p<0.05$

Serological Patterns of Chronic HBV Infection

Based on the virological profile, we can classify patients with chronic hepatitis and cirrhosis in the following manner:

i) HBsAg +ve, HBeAg +ve, HBV-DNA +ve

ii) HBsAg +ve, HBeAg –ve, HBV-DNA –ve

iii) HBsAg +ve, HBeAg –ve, anti-HBe +ve, HBV-DNA +ve

iv) HBsAg –ve, IgG anti-HBc +ve, HBV-DNA +ve

The first two category of patients have a "wild" type of HBV infection, while group three is likely to have a 'precore or core' mutant and group four, most likely is due to self limiting hepatitis B infection with persistent HBV-DNA. Rarely, such patients might have a 'surface mutant' form of HBV infection. There is limited data available on the natural history of 'wild' and 'mutant' forms of HBV in India.

HBV MUTANTS

Though HBV genome is compact and genetically efficient, a multitude of mutations have been described, some of which have clinical significance as shown in Table 5.

Table 5. Common hepatitis B mutant forms

Mutant form	Mutation	Biological significance
Pre-core	Single or multiple point mutations in the pre-C region, at codon 28 or 29, preventing HBeAg Secretion	Commonest mutation severe disease and fulminant hepatitis
Core	Clustering mutations in core gene often associated with pre-core mutations	Progressive liver disease
Envelope :		
Vaccine escape mutant	G145R mutation in 'a' region	Vaccine failure, rarely chronic liver disease
Non-Vaccine induced	Spontaneous mutation of nucleotide encoding a sequence 139-147	Chronic liver disease, post-transfusion hepatitis due to HBsAg negative, DNA +ve blood, HCC
Polymerase gene mutation	M552V/I mutation involving YMDD locus of domain C or L528M in domain B	Occur during lamivudine treatment
Other Mutations		
X gene		
Pre-S gene		

The clinically significant mutations occur in the following genes: (i) Pre-core (ii) Polymerase, and, (iii) Surface gene

Pre-core mutation

These mutations result from one of the several point mutations in the precore region, resulting in the loss of signal peptide, which is involved in the secretion of e antigen. The virological profile of chronic hepatitis due to pre-core variant is HBsAg +ve, HBeAg –ve, anti-HBe +ve, HBV-DNA >10^5 copies/ml and can be confirmed by either direct genomic sequencing, Restricted Fragment Length Polymorphism (RFLP), Line Probe Assay or ligase chain reaction. Pre-core mutation imposes difficult problems in the treatment with antivirals and also for monitoring the efficacy of the therapy.

Infection with pre-core mutant virus can occur *de-novo* or develop during the course of typical HBV infection. In the former case, acute and fulminant hepatitis can occur but chronic HBV infection does not develop as a result of aggressive immune response elicited.[19]

The prevalence of e minus CHB is linked often to non-A genotype of HBV especially genotype D. Data regarding viral genotype and its significance has been recently published from India. The occurrence of HBV genotype A is as frequently noted as genotype D (46% and 48% respectively) and the latter was more prevalent in young (below 40 years) patients with hepato-cellular carcinoma HCC and in those with severe liver disease.[20]

Pre-core mutants have been described in apparently healthy subjects with chronic HBV infection as well as in patients with chronic hepatitis B. Studies from Pune report that 21.5% of HBsAg positive subjects have pre-core mutation and an additional 17.6% have mixture of wild and mutant forms.[19] In another study, all patients with acute hepatitis or fulminant hepatic failure due to HBV had both wild and precore variants.[21] In patients with chronic liver disease, the prevalence is reported to be 15.5% in Delhi[22] and 9.5%-14% in Calcutta and 33.3% from Hyderabad.[23] In a recent study, Amarapurkar et al have shown that 61% of their chronic hepatitis B infection were due to e minus virus. In these patients, normal ALT was noted in 54%, HBV-DNA (b DNA assay) in 40%. Majority of those with HBV-DNA had elevated ALT. Hepatitis and cirrhosis was noted in 20% and 26% respectively.[24] Histological appearance of wild and e minus CHB were studied by Sakuja et al[25] who found similar activity scores but higher stage of fibrosis in the latter group. Studies from west on the natural history of this virus suggest frequent flares, a more rapid course and a higher incidence of hepatocellular carcinoma compared to wild type of HBV infection. In a prospective short term follow up study of 51 patients with e minus CHB for 28.8 mo, Sharma et al report that nearly 75% of the patients were decompensated at presentation. These patients suffered frequent ALT flares with an average interval of 10.2 mo between the flares. An increase in ALT>2 ULN was associated with florid decompensation.[26] Further studies with a more precise definition of a flare and long-term follow-up are needed.

S-gene mutation

Mutations are described in the pre-S and S-gene regions, which contain HLA-1 restricted cytotoxic T-cell epitopes resulting in immune, escape mutants. In addition, secretion of small s protein may also be affected. These mutations are important as they are involved in the diagnosis and prevention of HBV infection. S-gene mutations usually arise under immune pressure either following vaccination/immunoprophylaxis in a newborn or in post-liver transplant setting receiving HBIg. A report from Taiwan has noted increased prevalence of 's' mutants of HBV in children from 7.8% to 25% following implementation of vaccination which was accompanied by a decrease in chronic HBV infection rate. The significance of this mutation is unclear but continued monitoring is necessary. However, acute and chronic hepatitis and fuliminant hepatic failure have been reported. The prevalence of surface mutants in India has varied from none[27] to 10%.[22] Joshi et al found a prevalence rate of 6.2% and 3.2% in CHB and subjects with chronic HBV infection respectively.[23]

In a comparative study on the clinical profile of HBeAg negative and HBsAg negative mutants versus wild type chronic hepatitis B, Guptan et al[22] found that patients with HBsAg negative, HBV-DNA positive chronic liver disease were younger, and more often presented with quiescent cirrhosis with a higher frequency of development of HCC. (Table 6).

Table 6. Demographic and clinical profile of chronic liver disease due to the wild and the mutant HBV forms

Parameter	HBeAg-ve (n=18)	HBsAg-ve HBV-DVA+ (n=13)	Wild Type (n=41)
Mean age (yr.)	36.7 (11.9)	30.1 (12.4)#	39.9 (14)
Male: Female	14:4	8:5	28:13
Anorexia	11 (61%)	5 (38%)	17 (41.4%)
Fever	10 (55.5%)	3 (23%)#	25 (61%)
Jaundice	10 (55.5%)	3 (23%)#	25 (61%)
Ascites	13 (67%)	3 (23%)*	17 (41%)
GI bleed	4 (22%)	5 (38%)	19 (46%)
Mean duration of illness (yr.)	2.4±2.14	5.0±1.6**	3.2±1.4#

\# $P<0.05$ between HBsAg –ve and the wild type
* $p<0.05$, ** $p<0.01$, between the HBeAg –ve and the HBsAg –ve infection

Polymerase gene mutations

The polymerase gene has four distinct regions. YMDD locus in the C domain of reverse transcriptase/HBV-DNA polymerase region is highly conserved and naturally occurring mutations are rare in this region. Mutations in the DNA polymerase gene confer genotypic resistance to nucleoside analogue lamivudine or famiclovir in patients if the drugs are given for more than 6 months. Several mutations have been described in this gene either alone or in combination (Table 5). *In vitro* studies have shown that YMDD variant has reduced replication competence though recent studies have identified emergence of concomitant mutations that restore its replication potential. It is important to note that development of YMDD variant does not preclude HBeAg seroconversion. Kazim et al have reported the prevalence of lamivudine induced mutations in the P-gene. Two groups of patients with chronic hepatitis B were treated with lamivudine. In first group (9 patients) that received lamivudine for nine months, none developed YMDD mutation while, 5 of the 17 (29%) patients in the second group developed YM5521/VDD mutation after a mean period of 16.4 months. and three of these patients had in addition L528M and two novel double mutations, Q563S and L577G in between B and C domains of the P-gene. The significance of these mutations remains to be seen. Concomitant mutations in the 'a' determinant region of the S-gene, that structurally overlaps the P-gene were not observed despite lamivudine induced mutations in the P gene. In this study, pre-treatment viral load, ALT levels and the presence of e-antibody did not influence the selection of lamivudine resistant strains.[28]

The contribution of HBV infection in HBsAg negative CLD has been evaluated in atleast two studies. Sujata et al[29] reported that of the 62 patients with CLD who were HBsAg negative, only two had HBV-DNA in their serum by PCR. Both the patients had cirrhosis and were positive for total core antibody. The authors concluded that silent HBV infection is rare in patients with CLD in India. In contrast to this, the results of a study from Lucknow suggest that HBV infection is the commonest cause of cryptogenic liver disease.[30] In this study, HBV-DNA was detected in 57% of the 35 patients diagnosed as cryptogenic CLD. In both these studies, no sequencing studies were undertaken for the S-gene region.

HEPATOCELLULAR CARCINOMA

Viral hepatitis and cirrhosis constitute an important risk factor for the development of HCC. The estimated incidence of new HCC in India was about 12,750 in 2001, accounting for 1.6% of all cancers.[31] Prevalence of HCC is lower in Indians than in most parts of the world despite some pockets of contamination of food with aflatoxin and moderately high prevalence of hepatitis B and hepatitis C. Throughout the country. HBV is the single most important etiological association (80%) while HCV plays a lesser role in the development of HCC in India.[31] An autopsy study from south India which studied the prevalence of surface antigen in the liver tissue of HCC patients reported a prevalence rate of 80% in those who had cirrhosis and 75% in those without cirrhosis. Tandon et al had observed HBV infection in nearly 60% patients with HCC. In a recent study from Delhi,[32] etiological associations were carefully studied in patients with HCC (Table 7). In this study, cirrhosis was common (76%) and was seen more often in CLD due to viral etiology than other causes. Nearly half of the patients with HCC presented with decompensated liver disease. It is important to observe that 26 (49%) patients with hepatitis B related CLD had mutated virus. Of them, twelve

Table 7. Possible etiologic associations in hepatocellular carcinoma patients in India

Group	Patients	Cirrhotic	Non-cirrhotic
Total patients	74	56	18
HBV-related	53	46 (87)*	7 (13)
HBV alone	47	36 (77)	11 (23)
HCV alone	3	3 (100)	0
Alcohol alone	3	1 (33)	2 (67)
HBV + alcohol	11	11 (100)	0
HBV + HCV + alcohol	2	2 (100)	0
HBV + HCV	6	6 (100)	0
Unknown	15	6 (40)	9 (60)

Figures in parentheses are percentage.
*Includes all patients of hepatocellular carcinoma in whom infection with HBV was detected.

patients had serology suggestive of precore / core mutation and 14 patients had an HBsAg negative status. About 39% patients had more than one pre-disposing factor and aflatoxin B was not a significant etiological agent. It is possible that testing liver tissue for aflatoxin B could be more representative than serological testing. In the only study from India that evaluated the presence of HBV-DNA by PCR in the biopsy specimen obtained from the tumor, 90% positivity was reported, while seropositivity for HBsAg and HBeAg by ELISA were noted in 71% and 40% respectively thereby suggesting possible mutations in the S-gene and C / Pre-C gene. Use of primers that encompass more than one region of the viral genome has been suggested to pick-up HCC cells bearing incomplete HBV genomes.[33] In the same study, p53 tumor suppressor gene mutation was observed in only 3 of 21 liver biopsy specimens from patients with HCC thereby implying that this mutation may not be the crucial event in the molecular oncogenesis of HCC in India.[33,34]

Important Issues pertaining to HBV infection in India that need to be addressed in future:

1. Incidence and profile of liver disease among family contacts. Our own experience is that among the relatives of the index patient with HBV-related CLD, 23% of e antigen positive versus 38% of e negative contacts have histologically proven chronic liver disease with their virological profile being similar to the index patient.[35]
2. Coinfection with other viruses. Clinical experience with HBV infection in association with hepatitis C or HIV is limited. We have observed 14% and 8% incidence of HBV and HCV among our patients with CLD and HCC respectively. Others have noted a lower (3%) incidence, and a high rate of occurrence of HCC in this group of patients.[36] The concurrence of HBV and HIV infection is reported as high as 33% from Chandigarh with most of them being acquired heterosexually. Definitely, more data is required to reveal the natural history of coinfections in our country.

3. Perinatal versus horizontally acquired infection. The natural history of perinatally acquired HBV infection seen in hyperendemic areas is well studied unlike the horizontally transmitted disease that is more prevalent in low endemic areas like India.

In summary, several new aspects of the HBV related liver diseases are being recognized and much more needs to be known. The spectrum of mutant virus related liver disease needs serious attention in India and calls for better diagnostic and therapeutic approach.

REFERENCES

1. Tandon BN, Nayak NC, Tandon HD, Bijlani L, Joshi YK, Gandhi BM. Madanagopalan N, et al. Acute viral hepatitis with bridging necrosis. Collaborative study on chronic hepatitis. *Liver* 1983;3:140-6.
2. Tandon BN, Gandhi BM, Joshi YK. Etiological spectrum of viral hepatitis and prevalence of hepatitis A and B virus infection in north India. *Bull WHO* 1984;62:67-73.
3. Khandelwal I, Prasad SR, Sreshta J, Pal SR, et al. Etiological spectrum of acute sporadic viral hepatitis amongst adults in chandigarh. *Ind J Med Res* 1990;91:91-3.
4. Dasarathy S, Misra SC, Acharya SK, Irshad M, Joshi YK, Venugopal P, Tandon BN. Prospective controlled study of post transfusion hepatitis after cardiac surgery in a large referal hospital in India. *Liver* 1992;12:116-20.
5. Patwari SI, Irshad M, Gandhi BM, Joshi YK, Nundy S, Tandon BN. Post transfusion hepatitis—A prospective study. *Ind J Med Res* 1986;84:508-10.
6. Saxena R, Thakur V, Sood B, Guptan RC, Gururaja S, Sarin SK. Transfusion-associated hepatitis in a tertiary referral hospital in India: A prospective study. *Vox Sang* 1999;77:6-10.
7. Acharya SK, Panda SK, Saxena A, Gupta SD. Acute hepatic failure in India: A perspective from the East. *J Gastroenterol Hepatol* 2000;15:473-9.
8. Saraswat S, Banerjee K, Chowdhury N, Mahant T, Khandekar P, Gupta, RK, Naik S. Post-transfusion hepatitis B following multiple transfusions of HBsAg negative blood. *J Hepatol* 1996; 25:639-43.
9. Nanu A. Blood Transfusion services: Organisation is integral to safety. *Natl Med J Ind* 2001;14: 237-40.
10. Singh J, Bhatia R, Gandhi JC, Kaswekar AP, Khare S, Patel SB, Oza VB, et al. Outbreak of viral hepatitis B in rural community of India linked to inadequately sterilized needles and syringes. *Bull WHO* 1998;76:93-8.
11. Jaiswal SB, Chitnis DS, Asolkar MV, Naik G, Artwani KK. Etiology and prognostic factors in hepatic failure in central India. *Trop Gastroenterol* 1996;17:217-20.
12. Khuroo MS. Acute liver failure in India. *Hepatology* 1997;26:244-6.
13. Acharya SK, Dasarathy S, Kumar TL, Sushma S, Prasanna KS, Tandon A, Sreenivas V, et al. Fulminant hepatitis in a tropical population: Clinical course, cause, and early predictors of outcome. *Hepatology* 1996;23:1448-55.
14. Heemann U, Treichel U, Loock J, Phillipp T, Gerken G, Malago M, Klammt S, et al. Albumin dialysis in cirrhosis with superimposed acute liver injury: a prospective controlled study. *Hepatology* 2002; 36:949-58.
15. Acharya SK, Panda SK, Duphare H, Dasarathy S, Ramesh R, Jameel S, Nijhawan S, et al. Chronic hepatitis in large Indian hospital. *Natl Med J Ind* 1993;6:202-6.
16. Krishnamurthy L, Singh DS, Tandon HD, Tandon BN, et al. Chronic active hepatitis. *Ind J Med Res* 1976;64:1376-84.

17. Chandra R, Kapoor D, Aggarwal SR, et al. Profile of asymptomatic chronic HBV infection in India–End of the carrier saga? *Indian J Gastroenterol* 2001;20:A6.
18. Sarin SK, Chari S, Sundaram KR, Ahuja RK, Anand BS, Broor SL, et al. Young *vs.* adult cirrhotics: a prospective comparative analysis of clinical profile, natural course and survival. *Gut* 1988;29:101-7.
19. Hadziyannis SJ, Vassilopoulos D. Hepatitis B e antigen negative chronic hepatitis B. *Hepatology* 2001;34:617-24.
20. Thakur V, Guptan RC, Kazim SN, Malhotra V, Sarin SK, et al. Profile, spectrum and significance of HBV genotypes in chronic liver disease patients in the Indian subcontinent. *J Gastroenterol Hepatol* 2002;17:165-70.
21. Rana SS, Kailash U, Das BC, et al. Detection of pre-core mutant of hepatitis B in patients of acute viral hepatitis and fulminant hepatic failure using ligase chain reaction and its clinical implications. *Indian J Gastroenterol* 2001;20:A5.
22. Guptan RC, Thakur V, Sarin SK, Banerjee K, Khandekar P. Frequency and clinical profile of precore and surface hepatitis B mutants in Asian-Indian patients with chronic liver disease. *Am J Gastroenterol* 1996;91:1312-7.
23. Joshi N, Kumar A, Kumar N, et al. Frequency of precore and surface mutants in HBV related chronic liver diseases and in incidentally detected asymptomatic HBsAg positive subjects. *Indian J Gastroenterol* 2001;20:A89.
24. Amarapurkar DN, Baijal R, Kulsrestha PP, Agal S, Chakraborty MR, Pramanik SS, et al. Profile of hepatitis B e negative chronic hepatitis B. *Indian J Gastroenterol* 2002;21:99-101.
25. Puja S, Vena M, Gondal R, et al. Histological spectrum of chronic hepatitis B in precore mutants and wild type HBV infection. *Indian J Gastroenterol* 2001;20:A77.
26. Sharma J, Ramchandani M, Aggarwal SR, et al. Natural history of anti-HBe positive chronic hepatitis B–a prospective study. *Indian J Gastroenterol* 2001;20:A11.
27. Tandon BN, Acharya SK, Tandon A. Epidemiology of hepatitis B virus infection in India. *Gut* 1996;38 (suppl) 2:S56-9.
28. Wakil SM, Kazim SN, Khan SA, Raisuddin S, Parvez MK, Guptan RC, Thakur V, et al. Prevalence and profile of mutations associated with lamivudine therapy in Indian patients with chronic hepatitis B in the surface and polymerase genes of hepatitis B virus. *J Med Virol* 2002;68:311-8.
29. Radhakrishnan S, Abraham P, Raghuraman S, Kabrawala M, Eapen CE, Sridharan G, Chandy G. Infrequent occurrence of silent HBV infection among Indian patients with chronic liver disease. *Indian J Gastroenterol* 2001;20:87-9.
30. Aggarwal N, Naik S, Kini D, et al. Hepatitis B infection is seen in majority of cases of cryptogenic and alcoholic liver cirrhosis. *Indian J Gastroenterol* 2001;20(suppl 1):C5
31. Dhir V, Mohandas KM. Epidemiology of digestive tract cancers in India. III. Liver. *Indian J Gastroenterol* 1998;17:100-3.
32. Sarin SK, Thakur V, Guptan RC, Saigal S, Malhotra V, Thyagarajan SP, Das BC. Profile of hepatocellular carcinoma in India: an insight into the possible etiologic associations. *J Gastroenterol Hepatol* 2001;16:666-73.
33. Jayasree RS, Shreedhar H. p53 tumor suppressor genes in hepatocellular carcinoma in India. *Cancer* 2000;89:2322.
34. Katiyar S, Dash BC, Thakur V, Guptan RC, Sarin SK, Das BC. p53 tumor suppressor gene mutations in hepatocellular carcinoma patients in India. *Cancer* 2000;88:1565-73.
35. Thakur V, Guptan RC, Malhotra V, Basir SF, Sarin SK, et al. Prevalence of hepatitis B infection within family contacts of chronic liver disease patients: Does HBeAg positivity really matter? *J Assoc Physicians India* 2002;50:1386-94.
36. Xes SA, Kumar M, Minz S, Sharma HP, Shahi SK, et al. Prevalence hepatitis B and hepatitis C virus coinfection in chronic liver disease. *Ind J Pathol Microbiol* 2001;44:253-5.

12

Extrahepatic manifestations of hepatitis B

Mahesh P Sharma, Govind K Makharia

Hepatitis B virus (HBV) has tissue tropism for the liver and liver is the primary site for HBV replication.[1,2] An important step in tissue tropism is the binding of HBV envelope proteins to specific receptors on the hepatocytes, but the exact mechanisms for attachment and penetration of the virus in the hepatocytes have not been elucidated.[3,4] Despite strong tissue tropism of HBV for the liver, viral particles (HBV-DNA, replicative intermediates and/or viral transcripts) have been detected in other tissues, including peripheral blood mononuclear cells, bile duct epithelium, endothelium, pancreatic acinar cells, emulsified corneal tissue, and cultured lymphoblastoid cells.[1,5-7] They have also been found in lymphnodes, spleen, gonads, thyroid gland, kidneys, adrenals and cultured bone marrow cells during the acute phase of HBV infection.[1,5-7] Thus, the manifestations of hepatitis B virus infection are not limited only to the liver, but it also produces a number of systemic manifestations.[1,2,5-11]

Extrahepatic manifestations have been described both in patients with either acute or chronic viral hepatitis and occur in about 10–20% of the patients.[6-9] Extrahepatic manifestations associated with acute viral hepatitis are self-limiting and transient but the syndromes associated with chronic viral hepatitis may add significantly to the morbidity and mortality.

The two main mechanisms responsible for extrahepatic manifestations associated with HBV are either direct involvement of the target tissue by the HBV or immune complex mediated. Despite presence of HBV in the extrahepatic tissues, direct cytopathological alterations have not been demonstrated. Thus, virus specific immune complex injury remains the most plausible explanation for a number of syndromes associated with HBV, including serum sickness, polyarteritis nodosa (PAN), glomerulonephritis, neuropathies and pancreatitis.[1-2,6-11] Conversely, hematopoietic stem cell suppression may be mediated directly by HBV infection which blocks the maturational development of bone-marrow progenitor cells.

The various systemic manifestations of chronic HBV infection are listed in Table 1.

Table 1. Systemic manifestations of hepatitis B virus

Systemic manifestations associated with HBV infection	
Cardiovascular	EKG abnormalities
	Hypotension
	Cardiomegaly
Pulmonary	Pleural effusion
Neuropsychiatric	Higher mental function abnormalities
	Polyneuropathy
	Guillain-Barré syndrome
Hematologic	Aplastic anemia
	Agranulocytosis
	Hemolysis
Pancreatic	Acute pancreatitis
Diseases associated with HBV infection	
Serum sickness like syndrome	
Polyarteritis nodosa	
Glomerulonephritis	
Cryglobulinemia	
Papular acrodermatitis	

EXTRAHEPATIC MANIFESTATIONS OF HBV INFECTION

Cardiopulmonary manifestations

There is lack of well designed prospective studies evaluating the occurrence of cardiac manifestations in patients with both complicated and uncomplicated hepatitis B. Based on the available literature, it appears that patients with uncomplicated hepatitis rarely manifest with significant cardiac disease; however, in fulminant hepatic failure, cardiac disease may contribute to the cause of death.[7, 12-14]

The clinical findings in affected patients mostly include asymptomatic electrocardiographic abnormalities (low voltage complexes, left axis deviation, T-wave changes, prolongation of PR and QT intervals), various arrhythmias (sinus bradycardia, tachycardia, atrial flutter, atrial fibrillation and ventricular premature complexes). However, in some patients hypotension and sudden death may occur.[12, 13] The original belief that sinus bradycardia results from depression of sinus node by high levels of circulating bilirubin is not well established. In fact bradycardia is found when jaundice is not present, and most jaundiced patients do not have bradycardia.[20] We also observed bradycardia in a patient who was recovering from fulminant hepatic failure and when his serum bilirubin was decreasing. Bradycardia, when present, may reflect inflammation of the myocardial conduction system.[6, 13] Pericardial effusion, often hemorrhagic, has also been reported and HBsAg has occasionally been demonstrated in the pericardial fluid.[6]

Pleural effusion can rarely occur during the course of acute viral hepatitis B. The fluid when present is inflammatory (exudative). In addition, HBsAg, antibody to HBcAg, HBeAg and Dane particles have been identified in the pleural fluid. The effusion disappears spontaneously with the improvement of the hepatic disease.[6, 15]

Hematological manifestations

Viral hepatitis may be associated with two forms of hematological alterations. The first form, which includes mild lymphocytosis and a minor decrease in hematocrit, is common in the course of acute viral hepatitis and always reverts to normal as hepatic disease subsides.[1, 6-7, 14] Acute viral hepatitis in addition may precipitate hemolytic anemia, especially in patients with glucose-6-phosphate dehydrogenase deficiency.

The more serious hematological disorders associated with acute viral hepatitis include aplastic anemia, agranulocytosis, pure red cell aplasia and thrombocytopenia.[16-18] Pancytopenia develops more frequently in males than in females and the average age at onset is approximately 20 years. The interval between the onset of jaundice and the appearance of pancytopenia is 2 to 12 weeks. Usually this complication develops within a year of acute viral hepatitis, however, it has been reported to occur later. The associated hepatic disease usually is mild and the patient frequently is in the recovery phase when aplasia develops.[7, 14] Liver biopsies, when done, have shown the features of resolving hepatitis. Bone marrow examination shows hypoplasia or aplasia. Treatment of this condition with corticosteroids, androgenic steroids and splenectomy have not been successful.[7, 14] Bone marrow transplantation has been shown to have promise. Prognosis of this condition is poor and only 15% of the patients survive. The pathogenesis of bone marrow suppression has been postulated to be direct infiltration of bone marrow by HBV and inhibition of erythrogenesis.

Isolated agranulocytosis is an uncommon hematological complication where total leucocyte count may be normal, but neutrophilic cells usually are less than 5%. Bone marrow is hypercellular. Maturation arrest in the myelocytic series is the cause of agranulocytosis.[8]

Neurological manifestations

Neurological manifestations in the course of uncomplicated acute viral hepatitis are uncommon and include apathy, irritability, difficulty in concentration, headache and photophobia. The course of acute viral hepatitis has also been complicated by more serious neurological diseases, such as aseptic meningitis, encephalitis, myelitis, seizures, and even status epilepticus.[6, 14, 19] Guillain-Barré syndrome has been noted to be a complication of acute viral hepatitis. HBsAg has been shown to be present in cerebrospinal fluid in patients with such complications.[20]

Occurrence of polyneuropathy (peripheral and cranial) is somewhat more common. Even among patients with viral hepatitis who do not have overt neurological symptoms, impairment of nerve conduction velocities have been demonstrated.[21] Loss of appetite and alteration in food preferences are important features of acute viral hepatitis and this has been attributed to impairment of gustatory and olfactory acuity.[22, 23] A suggested mechanism for the disturbed olfaction derives from the finding that retinol binding protein, the specific transport protein for vitamin A is decreased during acute viral hepatitis.

Pancreatic diseases

Acute pancreatitis is a frequent complication of fulminant hepatic failure.[24, 25] Elevation in serum amylase activity is found in 20% to 30% of the patients and morphological evidence of pancreatitis may be present in upto 50% of the cases.

DISEASES/SYNDROMES ETIOLOGICALLY ASSOCIATED WITH HBV INFECTION

Serum sickness like syndrome

Acute viral hepatitis is sometimes heralded by a serum sickness like syndrome consisting of fever, arthralgia, arthritis, skin rashes, angioneurotic edema and occasionally hematuria and proteinuria.[26-28] This syndrome usually precedes the onset of jaundice by a few days to 4 weeks and may be the primary or only manifestation of anicteric hepatitis B infection.[6-7, 14, 26-28] Fever is generally more than 100°F and may exceed 102°F. The average duration of joint symptoms is estimated to be approximately 20 days. Symptoms mostly disappear with the onset of jaundice, however, they may sometimes persist. Joint involvement may be localized or generalized. It is usually symmetrical with swelling, tenderness, and inflammation. The areas most frequently involved in decreasing order of frequency are the proximal interphalangeal joints, knees, ankles, shoulders, wrists, small joints of the feet, elbows, cervical spine and lumbar spine.[26-28] Occasionally subcutaneous nodules have also been seen on the extensor surfaces. Morning stiffness is common. Synovial fluid is usually positive for HBsAg. Skin rashes commonly accompany joint manifestations. These may take any of these forms such as urticarial, maculopapular, petechial, scarlantiniform, annular erythematous plaques, and nodular.[6, 14, 28]

Polyarteritis nodosa

Polyarteritis nodosa (PAN) is a serious extrahepatic manifestation associated with multiple viral infections, including hepatitis B, hepatitis C, human immunodeficiency virus, cytomegalovirus, herpes zoster virus, herpes simplex virus and Elstein-Barr virus, but the strongest relationship has been observed with the hepatitis B virus.[1, 2, 6, 7, 9, 14, 29, 30] Although vasculitis associated with viral hepatitis was identified as early as 1940s, the association between viral infection and vasculitis could be established only after the discovery of hepatitis B virus.[14, 29] Hepatitis B surface antigen (HBsAg) has been reported to be found in about 10–50% of the patients with established PAN.[6, 7, 9, 14, 29, 30] The immunopathogenetic mechanisms responsible for vascular injury in PAN are incompletely understood and based on both experimental and clinical studies is thought to be immune complex mediated.[6-7, 30-31] In HBV-related PAN, immune complexes consisting of HBsAg, anti-HBs, immunoglobulins (IgG and IgM), and complement have been demonstrated by immunoflorescence in fibrinoid lesions in the walls of the blood vessels.[30] However, the presence of circulating immune complexes in the serum has been variable.[5, 31] According to these models, immune complexes activate the complement cascade, and the activated products of complement in turn attract and activate neutrophils.

Pathology

The characteristic lesion of PAN is focal segmental necrotizing vasculitis involving medium and small-sized muscular arteries, less commonly arterioles and only rarely venules.[32] The lesions may involve most organs, however, involvement of pulmonary and splenic arteries is less commonly seen. The inflammation is characterized by fibrinoid necrosis and pleomorphic cellular infiltration consisting predominantly of polymorphonuclear leucocytes. Arterial aneurysms and thrombosis can occur at the site of the lesion. Healing of these lesions can lead to vessel occlusion or regression of aneurysms. Another histologic feature characteristic of PAN is co-existence of active vasculitis, healing lesion or a normal artery in different tissues or in different parts of the same tissue.[6, 10, 32]

Clinical features

There is no age or sex predilection. Majority of the patients present with constitutional symptoms (malaise, fever and weight loss) which are associated with more classical symptoms such as arthralgia, mononeuritis multiplex, hypertension, renal disease, skin rashes, livido reticularis and gastrointestinal manifestations.[2, 10, 33-35] Fever has no specific character. The spectrum of the clinical presentation may vary from an apparently limited disease to fulminant polyvisceral failure. Therefore, management of such patients requires a comprehensive multi-disciplinary approach.

Digestive tract involvement is one of the most severe manifestations of PAN. Abdominal pain has been noted in 34% of the patients and to establish always the exact cause of abdominal pain has been difficult. Abdominal pain may be the first manifestation of gastrointestinal vasculitis. Gastrointestinal bleeding and bowel perforation can occur. Patients with malabsorption, pancreatitis, vasculitis of gallbladder and appendix have also been described.[10, 33, 35] Liver involvement, such as infarction and hematomas can exist. Among the diagnostic criteria led down by the American College of Rheumatology for the diagnosis of polyarteritis nodosa, presence of HBsAg is an important component (Table 2).[36]

HBV and PAN-special characteristics

The immunological process responsible for development of PAN occurs early in the course

Table 2. Criteria for the diagnosis of polyarteritis nodosa

Weight loss > 4 kg
Livido reticularis (mottled reticular pattern over the skin)
Testicular pain or tenderness
Mononeuritis multiplex, mononeuropathy or polyneuropathy
Hypertension (diastolic BP > 90 mm Hg)
Elevated blood urea nitrogen or creatinine
Hepatitis B virus infection
Angiographic abnormalities (aneurysms, occlusions)
Biopsy of small or medium sized arteries containing polymorphonuclear cells

---

Note : A patient with vasculitis is diagnosed to have polyarteritis nodosa if at least three of these 10 criteria are present.[36] The presence of any three or more criteria yield a sensitivity of 82.2% and specificity of 86.6%.

of HBV infection. In a French study, Guillevin et al[37] could date the onset of infection by HBV. They observed that if PAN developed in them, it developed in less than 6 months after HBV infection. During the course of vasculitis, hepatic disease is moderate clinically and even at histology, liver shows only moderate inflammation. There is no apparent relationship between the severity of vasculitis and the severity of the hepatic disease. Actually hepatic disease often remains quiescent. Thus, PAN may be the first and the only presentation of HBV infection.[37-39a]

The clinical features of HBV-related PAN are more or less same as those without HBV infection, however, according to a large study, malignant hypertension, renal infarction and epididymo-orchitis are seen more commonly in the former.[37-39] HBV-related PAN is mostly acute and initially severe, but the outcome is usually excellent for both PAN and hepatitis if adequate treatment is prescribed.[10, 37-39]

Treatment

The decision regarding treatment of PAN depends upon the extent, severity of involvement of organs, and the rate of progression of disease.[10, 37, 40-42] Approach to a patient with PAN with and without HBV infection is different. The conventional treatment of PAN includes corticosteroids and cyclophosphamide.[10, 40-43] However, when associated with HBV, treatment of PAN with corticosteroids and cyclophosphamide have shown to enhance the viral replication,[10, 40-43] in the long run they perpetuate chronic hepatitis B infection and facilitate progression towards cirrhosis which may be complicated further by hepatocellular carcinoma.[10, 37, 44] Although, the natural history of PAN is not marked by remissions and relapses, a PAN patient with concomitant HBV infection may suffer relapses and complications despite combinations of high doses of corticosteroids and cyclophosphamide. The high level of HBV replication with immunosuppressive treatment may be one of the reasons for treatment failure.

Treatment of PAN associated with HBV include antiviral drugs (vidarabine[37], famciclovir[45, 46] or lamivudine[47, 48a]) and interferon-α–2b in combination with either plasmapharesis or immunosuppressive drugs.[37, 49-52] Efficacy of IFN-α and antiviral drugs have been well established in the treatment of chronic hepatitis B infection. Based on the efficacy of antiviral drugs in chronic hepatitis B and plasmapharesis in PAN, combination of these two have been used sequentially.[37, 53, 54] In this form of therapy, short-term (2 weeks) corticosteroids are administered initially to control rapidly the life-threatening manifestations of PAN, and subsequently steroids are withdrawn abruptly to enhance immune-mediated clearance of HBV-infected hepatocytes. This is followed by plasma exchanges to control the course of PAN without adding corticosteroids or cyclophosphamide.[53, 54]

Combination of antiviral drugs and plasmapharesis : In HBV-related PAN, a combination of antiviral drugs (vidarabine[37] and IFN-α–2b[52]) and plasma exchanges have been used with impressive overall therapeutic results. In a large prospective study[37, 41] patients with HBV-related PAN were treated with vidarabine (35 patients) or IFN-α–2b (6 patients) in combination with plasmapharesis. Treatment protocol was as follows: initially every patient was given prednisolone at a dose of 1 mg/kg/day during the first week of treatment and then its dose was tapered rapidly and subsequently stopped at the end of the second week. Every patient underwent plasma exchanges beginning just after the patient's inclusion in the study. During the first two weeks, 6 sessions of plasma exchange were given, followed by 4 sessions in next 3 weeks, 3 sessions in next 3 weeks, 3 sessions per week and subsequently 2 sessions per week. After stopping prednisolone, each patient was given vidarabine for 3 weeks, administered by continuous intravenous infusion at a dose of 15mg/kg/day during the second and third weeks. Vidarabine was stopped immediately before and reintroduced after each plasma exchange session. When HBeAg/anti-HBe seroconversion was not obtained within 4 months, a second cycle of vidarabine without plasma exchange was offered.[56] In another 6 patients, IFN-α2b was used in doses of 3 million units 3 times a week in place of vidarabine. Rest of the protocol remained the same. With above combination of treatment, sero-conversion from HBeAg to anti-HBe was obtained in 21 of 41 (51.2%) patients and total viral clearance (seroconversion from HBsAg to anti-HBs and HBeAg to anti-HBe) was documented in 10 (24.4%) patients. Ten-year survival rate was 83%.[37] These results were much better than those obtained by corticosteroid with or without cyclophosphamide and plasma exchanges with which sero-conversion had been rare.

Combination of famciclovir and IFN-α-2b : In an isolated case report,[46] a 56 years old man with HBV-related PAN who failed to respond to combination of prednisolone and IFN-α-2b, was treated with a combination of IFN-α-2b (5 million units 3 times per week) and famciclovir (500 mg three times a day orally) and 5 mg of prednisolone daily. Under this regime HBV-DNA rapidly declined which was accompanied by a significant improvement in clinical symptoms. After 1 year of famciclovir treatment, HBeAg sero-conversion was also noted. Famciclovir at lower doses (125 mg three times per day) have been continued on a long-term basis in this index patient.

Combination of IFN-α or lamivudine and immunosuppressive drugs : Furthermore, in isolated case reports, patients with HBV-related PAN have been treated successfully with a combination of immunosuppressive therapy (to control manifestations of PAN) and lamivudine (to control HBV replication).[47,48]

A final protocol of treatment of HBV-related PAN has still not been devised. However, since evidence of efficacy of newer and potent anti-viral drugs in hepatitis B viral infection are accumulating, a simpler and more effective regimen to treat HBV-related PAN is on the horizon.

Glomerulonephritis

Although, the association of renal disease and acute viral hepatitis has been recognized long before the discovery of HBV, the first human case demonstrating presence of HBV immune-complexes in the kidney of a person with glomerulonephritis was reported by Combes et al[55] in 1971. This patient, with known chronic hepatitis B, developed severe proteinuria, hypo-albuminemia, and peripheral edema. Renal histology revealed membranous glomerulonephritis, whereas immunoflorescence deposits of IgG, C3 and HBsAg were seen throughout the glomerular capillary loops.[55]

Pathogenesis

It is thought that the pathogenesis of HBV-related glomerulonephritis is most likely due to deposition of circulating immune complexes containing HBV-antigens. It is also speculated that when a viral infection becomes persistent, the heightened immune response by the patient favour circulating immune complex formation, with their deposition ultimately in various organs.[2,7,56-60] The factors that influence the formation, clearance, and deposition of immune complexes are not clearly understood. Current evidence suggests that the size and composition (antigen/antibody ratio) are important determinants of immune complex induced tissue injury.

Appearance of immune complexes in patients with HBV infection is not an uncommon phenomenon as a number of investigators have demonstrated such immune complexes during the course of acute viral hepatitis even in the absence of clinically evident renal disease. Thus, it may be possible that many patients with acute viral hepatitis develop an immune complex mediated renal lesions although transient.[61] Indeed, an autopsy study of patients who died with acute or chronic HBV infection, indicated that kidney lesions (membranous GN, membranoproliferative GN) were found in 15–20% of the patients, however, these patients had no clinical evidence for renal disease.[62]

Extrahepatic manifestations of hepatitis B   119

The association of HBV and GN is based on certain facts which are as follows.

(a) demonstration of deposition of immune complexes containing HBsAg-anti-HBs and HBeAg-anti-HBe in the glomeruli,
(b) demonstration of HBV-DNA in the kidney biopsy, and
(c) reversal of glomerulonephritis both clinically and histologically by eradication of the HBV.

Pathology

Several histological findings have been reported in renal biopsies in patients with glomerulonephritis associated with chronic HBV infection. These include, membranous GN, membranoproliferative GN, mesangiocapillary GN, mesangioproliferative GN and focal glomerulosclerosis.[11, 58, 59, 63, 64] Overall, membranous GN is the most common type of HBV-related GN. Whereas in children, the most common type of HBV-related GN has been membranous, in adults membranoproliferative has been the commonest and more severe lesion.[58, 59] Histologically, membranous GN is usually associated with capillary wall deposits of HBsAg.[65, 66] Occasionally, a spectrum of glomerular lesions are seen on a single kidney biopsy.

Clinical manifestations

HBV-related GN occurs mainly in children, predominantly males, in areas of world where HBV infection is endemic, such as Asia, Africa and Eastern Europe.[2, 6, 11] The most frequent presentation of HBV-related GN is nephrotic syndrome. At presentation in childhood, significant renal failure is infrequent, and if present should prompt investigations for causes other than HBV-related GN.[2, 63] The diagnosis of HBV-related GN is usually established by[2, 6, 14] (a) serological evidence of HBV infection, (b) the presence of an immune complex GN on the kidney biopsy, and (c) by demonstrating glomerular deposits containing one or more HBV-related antigens (HBsAg, HBeAg, HBcAg) by immunochemical staining.

In addition, most patients have evidence of activation of classical complement cascade, with low serum levels of C_3 and C_4. Most patients with HBV-related GN have active viral replication, as shown by presence of HBV-DNA, DNA polymerase, and HBeAg in serum and HBcAg or replicative intermediates of HBV-DNA in the liver. There is no correlation between the severity of renal disease and the severity of underlying chronic hepatitis. In fact in many of such patients, the liver disease may not be clinically manifest.[11, 58, 59, 63] Remissions in chronic hepatitis B are usually accompanied by improvement in the renal disease.[66, 67]

Natural history

The course of HBV-related glomerulonephritis is different in children and adults. In those who acquire disease in childhood, progression to renal failure is uncommon. Eighty-five percent of them achieve remission spontaneously by two years and 95% by 5–7 years.[2, 5, 63]

The course in adults is not that benign and in many of them, the glomerular disease progresses relentlessly to renal failure.[2, 60]

Treatment

Corticosteroids and immunosuppressive drugs are important components of treatment for glomerulonephritis. However, these drugs are not suitable for treatment of HBV-related GN. Most of the patients with HBV-related GN who received corticosteroids have either had no beneficial effects or have only transient or incomplete remissions. Because most of the young patients with the disease achieve spontaneous remission by 2–3 years, and there is a risk of steroid induced worsening of the liver disease, corticosteroids are not recommended for young patients with HBV-related GN.[2, 68]

As sero-conversion of HBV infection leads to remission of HBV-related GN, the most logical way to treat HBV-related GN is to treat HBV by antiviral drugs.[11, 63-64, 69-73] Quite convincing evidence based data have been accumulated supporting this form of therapy.[63-64, 69-74] Conjeevaran et al[11] have reported a small series of 15 patients with chronic hepatitis B and glomerulonephritis (membranous 10, and membranoproliferative 5) treated with IFN-α-2b (5 million units subcutaneously daily for 16 weeks), and have shown a long term serological response with sustained loss of HBeAg and HBV-DNA in 8 (53%) patients. Seven of eight responders also had gradual but marked improvement in proteinuria. All eight responders had membranous GN, whereas four of seven non-responders had membranoproliferative GN.

Lin[63] has reported the effect of IFN treatment in 40 children who failed to respond to corticosteroids. Of the 40 children with membranous GN, 20 patients were treated with IFN-α and 20 patients received supportive treatment only. All 20 children who received IFN were free of proteinuria after 1 year of follow up, and 40% of them had HBeAg sero-conversion. By contrast, in the group receiving only supportive treatment, none of them seroconverted and only 50% had improvement in proteinuria while the remainder persisted with heavy proteinuria.

In adults, the results of IFN treatment for HBV-related GN are not always encouraging. In a report of 5 adult patients with HBV-related GN, only 1 achieved complete remission with sero-conversion. According to the limited experience of IFN in HBV-related GN, it has been observed that patients with GN have higher response rate in the liver disease than in patients without glomerulonephritis (53% vs. an average of 30–40%).[11, 75] This may be because of the fact that patients with extrahepatic manifestations have an enhanced immunologic response, i.e. they appear to produce high levels of immune complexes. This greater degree of immunologic reactivity could also predispose them to a better response to IFN therapy.

The good predictors of response to IFN therapy in the treatment of HBV-related GN have been identified to be shorter duration of the disease, higher level of liver transaminases, lower viral load (HBV-DNA) and younger age.[75] The results of IFN treatment also depend upon the histological type of GN, the best results being reported to be with membranous GN and poorer with membranoproliferative GN.[2, 11] There are also reports of successful treatment of other varieties of GN (mesangiocapillary, mesangioproliferative) with IFN.[64, 76]

Cryoglobulinemia

Cryoglobulinemia connotes the presence in the serum of immunoglobulins that precipitate reversibly with cooling. The type of cryoglobulinemia depends on the composition of the immunoglobulins. Cryoglobulinemia type I (monoclonal) consists of monoclonal immunoglobulins (IgM, IgG), type II (mixed) consists of monoclonal IgM and polyclonal IgG, whereas type III (polyclonal) consists of both polyclonal IgM and IgG. In most of the type II and type III cryoglobulinemia, no etiological factors are identified and are thus classified as essential mixed cryoglobulinemia (ECM). In those patients with type II and type III cryoglobulinemia where a cause is identified (secondary cryoglobulinemia), the causes include infections, autoimmune diseases, and chronic liver disease.[2]

Although, the association of mixed cryoglobulinemia with chronic liver disease has been recognized for many years, its clinical significance, however, is not clear. Controversy arose over whether the cryoglobulinemia was the cause, or the consequence, of underlying chronic liver disease. Recently, the association of chronic liver disease and mixed cryoglobulinemia to a certain extent has been clarified.[77] In a prospective study of patients with chronic liver disease of varied etiology, prevalence of mixed cryoglobulinemia was found to be high (41.5%). However, it was higher in patients with chronic HCV infection (54.3%) than in patients with chronic HBV infection (15%) and in patients with other causes of the liver disease (32%). Although, biochemical evidence for mixed cryoglobulinemia was found commonly in chronic liver disease, the presence of clinical syndrome was infrequent.[77, 78] These observations support the concept that a persistent viremia can continuously stimulate production of monoclonal and polyclonal immunoglobulins. Synovitis, vasculitis, purpura, peripheral neuropathy, renal failure, and Raynaud's phenomenon are the usual clinical features of cryoglobulinemia.[2, 6] Reports on the therapy of HBV-related mixed cryoglobulinemia are limited. More experience is necessary before antiviral therapy can be routinely prescribed for an uncommonly observed HBV-related mixed cryoglobulinemia.

Papular acrodermatitis of childhood (Gianotti's Crosti Syndrome)

A distinctive disease of childhood, papular acrodermatitis is characterized by skin eruptions, lymphadenopathy and mild, usually anicteric acute hepatitis due to hepatitis B virus.[79] In an epidemic of the disease in Matsuyama City, Japan, 153 cases occurred in a period of two and half years and 91.7% of the patients were younger than 4 years.[80]

The disease begins with the onset of skin eruptions which are usually flat, erythematopapular and non-pruritic. They appear symmetrically on the face, buttocks and limbs. Mucous membrane is mostly spared. The eruptions takes several weeks to evolve and lasts approximately 15 to 20 days. Lymphnodes enlargement involves mainly the inguinal and axillary areas, and may last for 2 to 3 months. Evidence of acute hepatitis may conicide with the onset of the skin lesions or more commonly begins as the dermatitis starts to wane. Aminotransferases levels are often high, whereas serum bilirubin levels are almost always normal in the affected children, but those adults who acquire the disease from children are likely to become icteric.[2, 79, 80]

REFERENCES

1. Hollinger FB. *Hepatitis B virus. In:* Fields BN, Knipe DM, Howley PM, Chanock RM, Monath TP, Melnick JL, Roizman B. Eds. Fields virology, 3rd ed. Philadelphia, Lippincott-Raven, 1996;2739-2807.
2. Wilson RA. Extrahepatic manifestations of chronic viral hepatitis. *Am J Gastroenterol* 1997;92:4-17.
3. Leenders WP, Hertogs K, Moshage H, Yap SH. Host and tissue tropism of hepatitis B virus. *Liver* 1992;12:51-5.
4. Hertogs K, Leenders WPJ, Depla E, De Bruin WCC, Meheus L, Raymackers J, Moshage H, et al. Endonexin II, present on human liver plasma membranes, Is a specific binding protein of small hepatitis B virus (HBV) envelope protein. *Virology* 1993;197:549-57.
5. Chan HL, Ghany MG, Lok ASF. *Hepatitis B. In:* Schiff ER, Sorrell M, Maddrey WL, Eds, Schiff's Diseases of the Liver, 8th ed. Philadelphia: Lippincott-Raven, 1999;pp.757-92.
6. Seeff LB. *Diagnosis, therapy and prognosis of viral hepatitis. In:* Zakim D, Boyer TD, Eds. Hepatology: A Textbook of Liver Diseases, 3rd ed. Philadelphia: WB Saunders Company 1996;pp.1067-1145.
7. Czaja AJ, Carpenter HA, Santrach PJ, Moore B. Immunologic features and HLA associations in chronic viral hepatitis. *Gastroenterology* 1995;108:157-64.
8. Shusterman N, London WT. Hepatitis B and immune complex disease. *N Engl J Med* 1984; 310:43-6.
9. Czaja AJ. Extra hepatitis immunologic features of chronic viral hepatitis. *Dig Dis* 1997;15:125-44.
10. Lhote F, Guillevin L. Polyarteritis nodosa, microscopic polyangiitis and Churg-Strauss Syndrome – clinical aspects and treatment. *Rheum Dis Clin North Am* 1995;21:911-47.
11. Conjeevaran HS, Hoofnagle JH, Austin HA, Park Y, Fried MW, Di Bisieglic AM. Long-term outcome of hepatitis B virus-related glomerulonephritis after therapy with interferon-alpha. *Gastroenterology* 1995;109:540-6.
12. Bell H. Cardiac manifestations of viral hepatitis. *JAMA* 1971;218:387-91.
13. Arnon R, Ehrlich R. Hepatitis, bradycardia, and the use of a cardiac pacemaker. *JAMA* 1974; 228:1024-5.
14. Dusheiko G. *Hepatitis B. In:* Bircher J, Benhamou J-P, McIntyre N, Rizzetto M, Rodes J, Eds. Oxford Textbook of Hepatology. Oxford: Oxford University Press 1999:pp. 876-95.
15. Tabor E, Russell P, Gerety RJ, Barker LF, Hillis WD, Jockson DR. Hepatitis B surface antigen and e antigen in pleural effusion. A case report. *Gastroenterology* 1977;73:1157-9.
16. Camitta BM, Nathan DG, Forman EN, Parkman R, Rappeport JM, Orellana TD. Post-hepatitic severe aplastic anemia—an indication for early bone marrow transplantation. *Blood* 1974;43:473-83.
17. Casciato DA, Klein CA, Kaplowitz N, Scott JL. Aplastic anemia associated with type B viral hepatitis. *Arch Intern Med* 1978;138:1557-8.
18. Nagaraju M, Weitzman S, Baumann G. Viral hepatitis and agranulocytosis. *Am J Dig Dis* 1973;18:247.
19. Apstein MD, Koff E, Koff RS. Neuropsychological dysfunction in acute viral hepatitis. *Digestion* 1979;19:349.

20. Tabor E. Guillain-Barre syndrome and other neurologic syndromes in hepatitis A, B, and non-A non-B. *J Med Virol* 1987;21:207-16.
21. Tsukada N, Koh CS, Owa M, Nubuo Y. Chronic neuropathy associated with immune complexes of hepatitis B virus. *J Neurol Sci* 1983;61:193-210.
22. Smith FR, Henkin RK, Dell RB. Disorders gustatory acuity in liver disease. *Gastroenterology* 1976; 70:568-71.
23. Henkin RI, Smith FR. Hyposmia in acute viral hepatitis. *Lancet* 1971;1:823-6.
24. Parbhoo SP, Welch J, Sherlock A. Acute pancreatitis in patients with fulminant hepatic failure. *Gut* 1973;14:428.
25. Shimoda T, Shikata T, Karasawa T, Tsukagoshi S, Yoshimura M, Sakurai I. Light microscopic localization of hepatitis B virus antigens in the human pancreas: possibility of multiplication of hepatitis B virus antigens in the human pancreas. *Gastroenterology* 1981;81:998-1005.
26. Alarcon GS, Townes AS. Arthritis in viral hepatitis. Report of two cases and review of the literature. *Johns Hopkins Med J* 1973;132:1-15.
27. Wands JR, Mann E, Alpert E, Isselbacher KJ. The pathogenesis of arthritis with acute-B surface antigen-positive hepatitis. Complement activation and characterization of circulating immune complexes. *J Clin Invest* 1975;55:930-6.
28. Steigman AJ. Rashes and arthropathy in viral hepatitis. *Mt Sinai J Med* 1973;40:752.
29. Gocke DJ, Hsu K, Morgan C, Bombardieri S, Lockshin M, Christian CL. Association between polyarteritis nodosa and Australia antigen. *Lancet* 1970;2:1149-53.
30. Guillevin L, Ronco P, Verroust P. Circulating immune complexes in systemic necrotizing vasculitis of the polyarteritis nodosa group. Comparison of HBV-related polyarteritis nodosa and Churg-Strauss angiitis. *J Autoimmun* 1990;3:789-92.
31. Trepo CG, Zuckerman AJ, Bird RC, Prince AM. The role of circulating hepatitis B antigen-antibody immune complexes in the pathogenesis of vascular and hepatic manifestations in polyarteritis nodosa. *J Clin Pathol* 1974;27:863-8.
32. Lie JT. Diagnostic histopathology of major systemic and pulmonary vasculitic syndromes. *Rheum Dis Clin North Am* 1990;16:269-92.
33. Frohnert PP, Sheps SG. Long-term follow-up study of periarteritis nodosa. *Am J Med* 1967;43:8-14.
34. Cohen RD, Conn DL, Astrup DM. Clinical features, prognosis and response to treatment in polyarteritis. *Mayo Clin Proc* 1980;55:146-55.
35. Guillevin L, Le Thi Huong D, Godeau P, Jais P, Wechsler B. Clinical findings and prognosis of polyarteritis nodosa and Churg-Strauss angiitis: A study in 165 patients. *Br J Rheumatol* 1988;27:258-64.
36. Lightfoot RW Jr., Michel BA, Bloch DA, Hunder GG, Zvaifler NJ, McShane DJ, Arend WP, et al. The American College of Rheumatology 1990 criteria for the classification of polyarteritis nodosa. *Arthritis Rheum* 1990;33:1088-93.
37. Guillevin L, Lhote F, Gayraud M, Cohen P, Jarrousse B, Lortholary O, Thibult N. Prognostic factors in polyarteritis nodosa and churg-Strauss syndrome. A perspective study in 342 patients. *Medicine* 1996;75:17-28.
38. Guillevin L, Lhote F, Jarrousse B, Bironne P, Barrier J, Deny P, Trepo C, et al. Polyarteritis nodosa related to hepatitis B virus. A retrospective study of 66 patients. *Ann Med Intern* 1992;143 (suppl 1):63-74.
39. Lhote F, Cohen P, Guillevin L. Polyarteritis nodosa, microscopic polyangitis and Churg-Strauss syndrome. *Lupus* 1998;7:238-58.
39a. Trepo C, Guillvin C. Polyarteritis nodosa and extrahepatic manifestations of HBV infection: the case against autoimmune intervention in pathogenesis. *J Autoimmun* 2001;16:269-74.

40. Guillevin L. Treatment of classic polyarteritis nodosa in 1999. *Nephrol Dial Transplant* 1999; 14:1077-9.
41. Conn DL. Polyarteritis. *Rheum Dis Clin North Am* 1990;16:341-62.
42. Guillevin L, Lhote F, Gherardi R. The spectrum and treatment of virus-associated vasculitides. *Curr Opin Rheumatol* 1997;9:31-6.
43. Guillevin L, Jarrousse B, Lok C, Lhote F, Jais JP, Le Thi Huong DU D, Bussel A. Long-term follow-up after treatment of periarteritis nodosa and Churg-Strauss angiitis with comparison of steroids, plasma exchange and cyclophosphamide to steroids, plasma exchange. A prospective randomized trial of 71 patients. *J Rheumatol* 1991;18:567-74.
44. Lam KC, Lai CL, Trepo C, Wu PC. Deleterious effect of prednisolone in HBsAg-positive chronic active hepatitis. *N Engl J Med* 1981;304:380-6.
45. Kruger M, Boker KH, Zeidler H, Manns MP. Treatment of hepatitis B related polyarteritis nodosa with famciclovir and interferon-alpha-2b. *J Hepatol* 1997;26:935-9.
46. Molloy PJ, Friendlander L, Van-Thiel DH, Kania RJ. Combined interferon, famciclovir and GM-CSF treatment of HBV infection in an individual with polyarteritis nodosa. *Hepatogastroenterology* 1999;46:2529-31.
47. Wicki J, Olivieri J, Pizzolato G, Guillevin L, Dayer JM, Chizzolini C. Successful treatment of polyarteritis nodosa related to hepatitis B virus with a combination of lamivudine and interferon alpha. *Rheumatology-Oxford* 1999;38:183-5.
48. Maclachlan D, Battegay M, Jacob AL. Successful treatment of hepatitis B associated polyarteritis nodosa with a combination of lamivudine and conventional immunosuppressive therapy: a case report. *Rheumatology-Oxford* 2000;39:106-8.
48a. Filer A, Hughes A, Kane K, Mutimer D, Jobanputra P. Successful treatment of hepatitis B-associated vasculitis using lamivudine as the sole therapeutic agent. *Rheumatology-Oxford* 2001; 40:1064-5.
49. Simsek H, Telatar H. Successful treatment of hepatitis B virus associated polyarteritis nodosa by interferon-alpha alone. *J Clin Gastroenterol* 1995;20:263-5.
50. Sonnatag KC, Schwarz-Eywill M, Hunstein W. Is interferon alpha a therapy for hepatitis B associated polyarteritis nodosa. *Br J Rheumatol* 1995;34:86-7.
51. Avsar E, Savas B, Tozun N, Ulusoy NB, Kalayci C. Successful treatment of polyarteritis nodosa related to hepatitis B virus with interferon-alpha as first line therapy. *J Hepatol* 1998;28:525-6.
52. Guillevin L, Lhote F, Sauvaget F, Deblois P, Rossi F, Levallois D, Pourrat J, et al. Treatment of polyarteritis nodosa related to hepatitis B virus with interferon-alpha and plasma exchanges. *Ann Rheum Dis* 1994;53:334-7.
52a. Duzova A, Bakkaloglu A, Yuce A, Ozen S, Kocak N. Successful treatment of polyarteritis nodosa with interferon-alpha in a nine month old girl. *Eur J Pediatr* 2001;16:269-74.
53. Guillevin L, Le Clerc P, Cohen P, Lhote F, Jarrousse B, Gayraud M, Leon A, et al. Treatment of severe polyarteritis nodosa without HBV infection and Churg-Strauss syndrome: A prospective tiral in 57 patients comparing prednisone, pulse cyclophosphamide with or without plasma exchanges. *Arthritis Rheum* 1993;35(suppl 9):S96 (abstract).
54. Guillevin L, Lhote F, Leon A, Fauvelle F, Vivitski L, Trepo C. Treatment of polyarteritis nodosa related to hepatitis B virus with short-term steroid therapy associated with antiviral agents and plasma exchanges. A prospective trial in 33 patients. *J Rheumatol* 1993;20:289-98.
55. Combes B, Shorey J, Barrera A, Stastny P, Eigenbrodt EH, Hull AR, Carter NW. Glomerulonephritis with deposition of Australia antigen-antibody complexes in glomerular basement membrane. *Lancet* 1971;2:234-7.
56. Brzosko WJ, Krawczynski K, Nazarewicz T, Morzycka M, Nowoslawski A. Glomerulonephritis

associated with hepatitis B surface antigen immune complexes in children. *Lancet* 1974;2:477-81.
57. Takekoshi Y, Tanaka M, Shida N, Satake Y, Saheki Y, Matsumoto S. Strong association between membranous nephropathy and hepatitis B surface antigenemia in Japanese children. *Lancet* 1987;2:1065-8.
58. Johnson RJ, Goluser WG. Hepatitis B infection and renal disease: clinical immunopathogenetic and therapeutic considerations. *Kidney Int* 1990;37:663-76.
59. Venkataseshan VS, Lieberman K, Kim DU, Thung SN, Dikman S, D' Agati V, Susin M. Hepatitis B-associated glomerulonephritis: Pathology, pathogenesis, and clinical course. *Medicine (Baltimore)* 1990;69:200-16.
60. Lai KN, Li PK, Lui SF, Au TC, Tam JS, Tong KL, Lai FM. Membranous nephropathy related to hepatitis B virus in adults. *N Engl J Med* 1991;324:1457-63.
61. Eknoyan G, Gyorkey F, Dichoso C, Martinez Maldonado M, Suki WN, Gyorkey P. Renal morphological and immunological changes associated with acute viral hepatitis. *Kidney Int* 1972;1:413-9.
62. Morzycka M, Slusarczyk J. Kidney glomerular pathology in various forms of acute and chronic hepatitis. *Arch Pathol Lab Med* 1979;103:38-41.
63. Lin CY. Treatment of hepatitis B virus-associated membranous nephropathy with recombinant alpha-interferon. *Kidney Int* 1995;47:225-30.
64. Dhiman RK, Kohli HS, Das G, Joshi K, Chawla Y, Sakhuja V. Remission of HBV-related mesangioproliferative glomerulonephritis after interferon therapy. *Nephrol Dial Transplant* 1999; 14:176-8.
65. Ohba S, Kimura K, Mise N, Konno Y, Suzuki N, Miyashita K, Tojo A, et al. Differential localization of s and e antigens in hepatitis B virus-related glomerulonephritis. *Clin Nephrol* 1997;48:44-7.
66. Altiparmak MR, Pamlk ON, Pamuk GE, Mert A, Ataman R, Sardengecti K. Prevalence of serum antibodies to hepatitis B and C viruses in patients with primary glomerulonephritis. *J Nephrol* 2001;14:388-91.
67. Knecht GL, Chisari FV. Reversibility of hepatitis B virus-induced glomerulonephritis and chronic active glomerulonephritis and chronic active hepatitis after spontaneous clearance of serum hepatitis B surface antigens. *Gastroenterology* 1978;75:1152-6.
68. Lai KN, Tam JS, Kin HJ, Lai FM. The therapeutic dilemma of the usage of corticosteroid in patients with membranous nephropathy and persistent hepatitis B virus surface antigenemia. *Nephron* 1990;54:12-7.
69. Garcia G, Scullard G, Smith C, Weissberg J, Alexander S, Robinson WS, Gregory P, et al. Preliminary observation of hepatitis B-associated membranous glomerulonephritis treated with leukocyte interferon. *Hepatology* 1985;5:317-20.
70. Mizushima N, Kanai K, Matsuda H, Matsumoto M, Tamakoshi K, Ishii H, Nakajima T, et al. Improvement of proteinuria in a case of hepatitis B-associated glomerulonephritis after treatment with interferon. *Gastroenterology* 1987;92:524-6.
71. de Man RA, Schalm SW, Van der Heijden AJ, ten Kate FW, Wolff ED, Heijtink RA. Improvement of hepatitis B-associated glomerulonephritis after antiviral combination therapy. *J Hepatol* 1989;8: 367-72.
72. Lok ASF. Antiviral therapy of the Asian patient with chronic hepatitis B. *Semin Liver Dis* 1993; 13:360-6.
73. Gonzalo A, Mampaso F, Barcena R, Gallego N, Ortuno J. Membranous nephropathy associated with hepatitis B virus infection: long-term clinical and histological outcome. *Nephrol Dial Transplant* 1999;14: 416-8.
74. Al-wakeel J, Mitwalli A, Tarif N, Al Mohaya S, Malik G, Khalil M. Role of interferon-alpha in the treatment of primary glomerulonephritis. *Am J Kidney Dis* 1999;33:1142-6.

75. Hoofnagle JH. Therapy of acute and chronic viral hepatitis. *Adv Intern Med* 1994;39:241-75.
76. Abbas NA, Pitt MA, Green AT, Solomon LR. Successful treatment of hepatitis B virus (HBV)-associated membranopoliferative glomerulonephritis (MPGN) with alpha-interferon. *Nephrol Dial Transplant* 1999;14:1272-5.
77. Lunel F, Musset L, Cacoub P, Franguel L, Cresta P, Perrin M, Grippon P, et al. Cryoglobulinemia in chronic liver disease: Role of hepatitis C virus and liver damage. *Gastroenterology* 1994;106:1291-1300.
78. McMahon BJ, Alberts SR, Wainwright RB, Bulkow L, Lanier AP. Hepatitis B-related sequalae: Prospective study in 1400 hepatitis B surface antigen-positive Alaska native carriers. *Arch Intern Med* 1990;150:1051-4.
79. Gianotti F. Papular acrodermatitis of childhood—an Australia antigen disease. *Arch Dis Child* 1973; 48:794-9.
80. Ishimaru Y, Ishimaru H, Toda G, Baba K, Mayumi M. An epidemic of infantile papular acrodermatitis (Gianotti's disease) in Japan associated with hepatitis-B surface, subtype ayw. *Lancet* 1976;1:707-9.

13

Hepatitis B virus mutants: clinical presentation, diagnosis and management

Stephen Locarnini, Angeline Bartholomeusz

Almost 400 million people will be infected with hepatitis B virus (HBV) by the end of the year 2000.[1-3] This is equivalent to about 5% of the world's population and more than ten times the number infected with the human immunodeficiency virus (HIV). Up to half of these hepatitis B surface antigen (HBsAg) positive individuals will succumb to the clinical sequelae as a consequence of the persistent HBV carriage, i.e., development of liver failure and/or hepatocellular carcinoma.[4]

Hepatitis B virus can cause both acute and chronic liver disease. The outcome depends on the interplay between the virus, the hepatocyte and the host's immune response.[5] Under most circumstances, HBV is not cytopathic and it is the infected host's immune response that is responsible for the liver damage during infection.[6] In specialized circumstances, such as orthotopic liver transplantation (OLT), with its extensive use of immunosuppressive agents, HBV can be directly cytopathic for hepatocytes causing unique histopathological conditions such as fibrosing cholestatic hepatitis (FCH),[7] which before the advent of specific antiviral therapy,[8] was invariably fatal.

Over the past decade, increasing attention has been focused on the contribution of HBV mutants to the clinical course of acute or chronic infection.[9,10] Mutants of HBV including those in the precore,[9] core[11] and pre-S2 regions[12], can display enhanced virulence with increased levels of viral replication.[11] In addition, viral mutations may influence response to treatment: precore or core mutations may modulate response to interferon-alpha and drug-selected polymerase mutations can result in reduced or absent sensitivity of viral replication to antiviral nucleoside analogues, while envelope protein mutants can escape antibody-mediated neutralization reducing efficacy of hepatitis B immune globulin (HBIg) and the prophylactic vaccine.[12]

Thus, antiviral chemotherapy remains the major treatment option for controlling chronic HBV infection, with the immune modulating agent interferon-alpha and the antiviral compound lamivudine (LMV) being the only two FDA–approved treatments. The registration of LMV was only a recent event and a number of new deoxynucleoside analogues and derivatives are also approaching final stages of clinical development. These include Entecavir, Famciclovir, Clevudine, Emtricitabine and Adefovir Dipivoxil. These new anti-HBV drugs are capable of reducing viral loads very rapidly, but the initial response is invariably followed by a very much slower elimination of residual virus.[13] The long-term treatment which is required to eliminate residual virus carries with it increased risks for cumulative toxicity and drug resistance. Fortunately, experience to date indicates that toxicity is not a major problem with these newer nucleoside analogues, so emergence of drug resistance during the slower phase of HBV elimination appears most likely to become the single significant obstacle blocking progress towards the eventual control of chronic infection.[14]

MOLECULAR VIROLOGY OF HBV

HBV is a small, DNA-containing virus with four overlapping open reading frames (Fig. 1). The 4 genes are core (precore and core proteins), surface (Pre-S and S proteins), X and polymerase. The core gene encodes the core nucleocapsid protein and the secreted, soluble hepatitis B 'e' antigen (HBeAg) protein. The surface gene encodes pre-S1, pre-S2 and S protein, yielding the large, middle and small surface proteins, respectively. The X-gene encodes the X protein, which has transactivating properties and may be important in hepatic carcinogenesis. The polymerase gene encodes a large protein with functions critical for packaging and DNA replication (including priming, RNA- and DNA-dependent DNA polymerase, and RNaseH activities).[10-12]

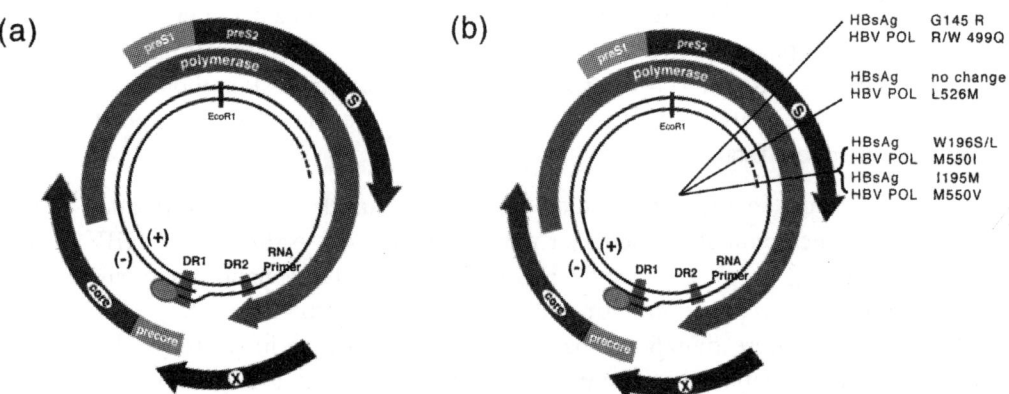

Fig. 1. The organization of the HBV genome modified from Hunt et al [11] (a). The (+) and (-) DNA strands are represented by the inner circle. The DNA polymerase is attached to the 5' terminus of the (-) DNA strand. Also indicated are the EcoR1 site, the direct repeat sequences DR1 and DR2 and the RNA primer. The four open reading frames are shown by the arrows. (b) The important antiviral resistant and vaccine escape mutations which alter codons in the overlapping polymerase and S-genes are noted.

Although HBV is a DNA virus, replication is through an RNA-replicative intermediate requiring an active viral reverse transcriptase/polymerase enzyme (Fig. 2).[10] The reverse transcriptase (for both HBV and HIV) is believed to lack a conventional proofreading function

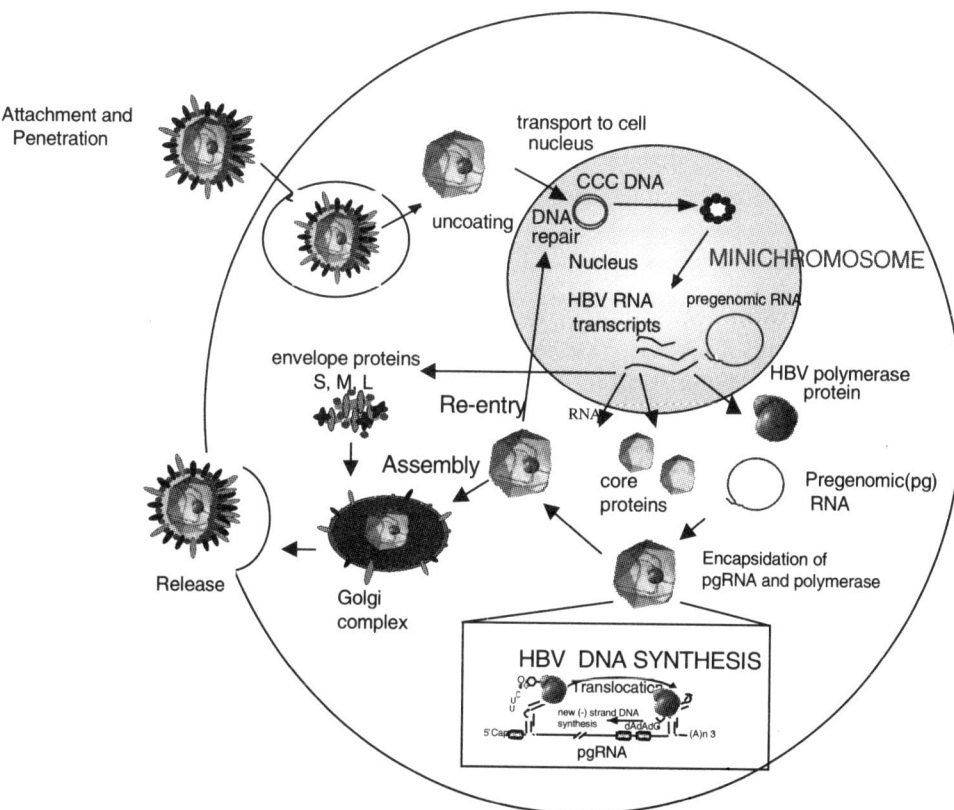

Fig. 2. Hepatitis B virus replication cycle. The virus in the serum adheres to the surface of the hepatocytes through a receptor. Through the process of endocytosis the virus enters the cell and is uncoated to remove the envelope proteins. The viral core particles bind to the nuclear pore and the HBV genome enters the nucleus. In the nucleus the HBV-DNA is repaired and chromatinized to form a minichromosome. The minichromosome is used as the transcriptional template for RNA synthesis by RNA Polymerase II. The HBV RNA is transported into the cytoplasm where the viral proteins are made. The pre-genomic RNA is encapsidated. In the viral RNA cores DNA synthesis occurs through a process of reverse transcription and also DNA synthesis. The viral cores can be either transported back into the nucleus for further genomic amplification or are enveloped and secreted into the blood.

which is found in other polymerases. Therefore, HBV exhibits a mutation rate more than 10-fold higher than other DNA viruses,[11] which has been estimated at approximately 1 nucleotide/10,000 bases/infection year.[15] The rates for nucleotide substitutions vary in chronic HBV compared to those determined in the liver transplant setting after HBV recurrence. The natural evolutionary rate for the HBV genome is approximately 1.4 to 3.2×10^{-5} substitutions/site/year.[15, 16] In the liver transplant setting, it is almost 100-fold higher in the range of 1.1×10^{-2} to 5.9×10^{-3} substitutions/site/year[17] The much higher substitution rate in the liver transplant setting may be due to a number of factors including possible reinfection of the liver allograft by a different subpopulation of the virus which may have been present in extra hepatic sites pre-transplantation. Reinfection of the new liver also occurs at a very rapid rate, which may promote an increased mutation rate for the virus. The high substitution rate may also be a result of the immunosuppression regime associated with transplantation, or by the treatment with HBIg. Finally, fidelity of replication by HBV polymerase may be affected by the concentration of the intracellular deoxynucleotide triphosphate pools.[18]

PRE-C/C-GENE MUTANTS

The HBV C-gene contains two in-frame start codons (Fig. 3a). The region between the first (pre-C ATG) and second (C ATG) start codons is designated the "pre-C" region. The basal core promoter [BCP] (nucleotides 1744 to 1804), residing in the overlapping X open reading frame region (X-ORF), controls transcription of both precore and core regions and directs the synthesis of two mRNAs, the pre-core mRNA and the pregenomic/C mRNA (Fig. 3b). The pre-core mRNA encodes HBeAg. The pregenomic/C mRNA encodes the core protein, the DNA polymerase and itself acts as the pregenomic RNA, the template for reverse transcription.[10]

A variety of precore/core mutants have been described.[18, 19] The two major groups of mutations which affect HBeAg synthesis are precore protein mutations and mutations in the basal core promoter (BCP) at nt 1762 and nt 1764, all resulting in diminished production of HBeAg and a resultant increased host immune response. Precore mutations frequently occur temporally related to core gene mutations/deletions (see below). Mutations in the BCP are likely to increase viral replication and enhance disease activity.[19]

Precore protein mutations

There are three major types of mutations which block HBeAg protein production. The first reported precore mutant viruses contained a mutation at nt 1896 [G1896A] that caused a stop codon (TGG changed to TAG) in the precore ORF thus abolishing HBeAg production[20-22] (Fig. 3a). The second type of mutation inactivates the pre-C ATG initiation codon (position 1814) whilst the third type comprises insertions or deletions in the pre-C region that lead to a frameshift in the protein. All three types of mutations prevent translation of the precore protein from the pre-C mRNA, whereas the translation of the core protein from the pregenomic/C mRNA remains unaffected.[23]

Marked geographical differences in the prevalence of the precore stop mutant viruses have been noted.[12] Only 10% of HBV isolates from USA in patients with fulminant hepatitis[24] and 12% to 27% of isolates from USA and Europe in patients with chronic active hepatitis exhibit these precore stop mutations[24,25] whereas 47% to 60% of isolates from patients with chronic active hepatitis in Asia, Africa, Southern Europe, and the Middle East exhibit these stop mutations.[25]

Lok et al[26] demonstrated the important link between the precore stop mutation and HBV genotype. Nucleotide (nt) 1896 is a guanosine (G) and is found within the RNA structural element, involved in encapsidation, epsilon. This is base paired with nt 1858 and mutations at nt 1858, in conjunction with the precore stop mutation at nt 1896 can enhance viral base pairing within the stem-loop region of epsilon. In patients with genotype A HBV infections (the predominant genotype in North America and parts of Europe), nt 1858 is a C. In this genotype, both a mutation at nt 1896 (G to A) and nt 1858 (C to T) would be required to stabilize the stem-loop structure. Without a compensatory mutation at nt 1858 in genotype A HBV, impaired base pairing results when C-1858 tries to pair with a A-1896, which destabilizes the stem-loop structure of the packaging signal. Without a stable epsilon for packaging, decreased encapsidation and consequently decreased replication may occur. Thus, precore stop codon mutations may be less frequent in genotype A because of the requirement for two mutational events.[12] Stability of epsilon is critical for replication because binding of the polymerase to epsilon is important for the pregenomic RNA to be packaged and for priming of genomic replication. In contrast, HBV sequences in more than 50% of subjects with chronic HBV infection from Asia, Africa, or the Middle East already contain a T at nt 1858 and, therefore, only require a single mutation at nt 1896 to yield a precore mutant with stable stem-loop pairing. Therefore, the higher frequency of precore stop mutant HBV in patients harbouring these other genotypes (genotypes B, C, D and E) where nt 1858 is a T, is simply a reflection of the requirement of only a single mutation (G1896A) needed to cause a stop codon and a stable stem-loop structure for epsilon.[25]

Basal core promoter mutations

Mutations in the BCP especially at nt 1762 and nt 1764, resulting in T-1762 and/or A1764, have been detected in patients with persistent infection[27], fulminant hepatitis,[28] as well as in immunosuppressed patients[29] (Fig. 3b, c). The double mutation at T-1762 and A1764 together is associated with a decrease in HBeAg and an increase in viral load.[30] Li et al (30) have demonstrated diminished binding of liver-specific transcription factors, resulting in a decrease in precore mRNA transcription and thus HBeAg, but unchanged amounts of HBV pregenomic/C mRNA. This mutation does not appear to affect the transcription of the pregenomic/C mRNA as the translation of the core protein and subsequent viral genomic can proceed via an alternative initiation site downstream from the precore mRNA initiation site. Since the relative proportion of precore/core RNA is altered by this mutation, viral replication efficiency may be affected.[12, 27]

Interestingly, the detection of the single A to T-1762 change in HBV isolates from patients was found to correlate with HBeAg sero-conversion and histological inflammation.[31] Thus, it has been suggested that this single mutation may be a useful marker to identify those patients who may be primed for subsequent sero-conversion.[31]

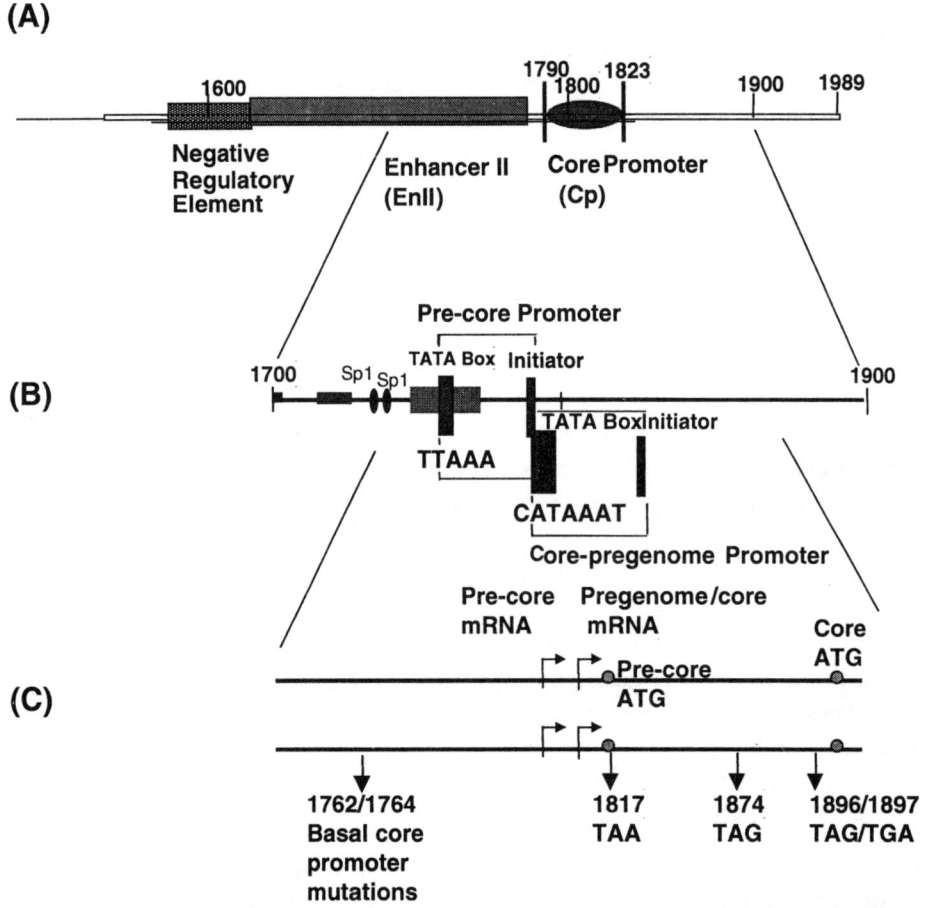

Fig. 3. The precore/core promoter region and the precore and basal core promoter mutants. (a) The negative regulatory element and the enhancer II region precede the core promoter. (b) The region encompassing the precore promoter and the core promoter including regions which are important for transcription such as the Sp1 binding sites and the TATA box are indicated. (c) The sites for initiation of the precore and core mRNA and protein and the location of important basal core mutations and precore mutations are indicated.

Baumert et al[32] have examined cultured cells transfected with HBV BCP mutants in order to determine a potential mechanism to account for the increased HBV virulence. The precore stop mutants do not usually increase the level of viral replication in similar *in vitro* cell culture models.[33] In contrast, BCP mutations of HBV were found to cause increased core protein expression and viral replication,[28] suggesting that BCP mutations may increase HBV virulence by up-regulating viral replication. More recent studies from this group[30] using cells transfected with BCP mutants, have found that associated and corresponding X protein mutations suppressed precore RNA transcription, but, due to the "creation" of a hepatocyte nuclear factor 1 (HNF-1) binding site, there was increased core RNA expression resulting in an overall enhancement of viral replication.

Core protein mutations

The core protein can be divided into two major domains, the N-terminal assembly domain up to amino acid position 144 and the functionally important, arginine-rich C-terminal domain. The C-terminal domain is required for binding of the pregenomic RNA and genome replication, as well as being involved in nuclear transportation.[10]

The prevalence of HBc/e amino acid changes is very similar to that of pre-C defects seen during particular stages of chronic infection. Core protein sequences of HBV from patients in the HBeAg-positive immune tolerant phase contain none or very few amino acid changes. However, once patients enter the immune clearance phase, the mean rate of HBc/e amino acid changes increases by more than five-fold, clustering onto 36 hot-spot positions.[10] These hot-spot positions have been linked to major cytotoxic T-lymphocyte (CTL) [amino-acid 18-30] and T-helper (T_H) cell [amino-acid 50-70] regions, and two B-cell [HBc/e1 and HBc/e2] epitopes at amino-acid residues 75-90 and 120-140 respectively. A burst of amino acid changes emerges together with the pre-C defect, usually concomitant with sero-conversion to anti-HBe, consistent with the T and B-cell immune selection pressures directed against these epitopes.[10]

Deletions to the core protein have been detected in many patients. Such core gene deletions may alter core protein, thereby decreasing immune recognition by cytotoxic T-cells, which is essential in viral clearance. It would be predicted that HBV with extensive core gene deletion mutants which result in the absence of core nucleocapsid protein would be replication incompetent as they could not produce viable virus and would require rescue by wild-type virus, i.e. these viruses could only replicate in the presence of low levels of wild-type HBV. Patients with core deletion mutants of HBV demonstrate low serum HBV-DNA levels indicating restricted replicative capacity.[34] These patients often mount a more vigorous immune response due to the loss of immunologic tolerance, with a resultant increase in HBeAg seroconversion and higher HAI scores.

Ehata et al[35] have examined the appearance of precore and core mutations in three groups:

fulminant hepatitis ($n=5$), severe exacerbation of hepatitis ($n=10$), and self-limited acute hepatitis ($n=9$). All patients with fulminant or severe hepatitis exhibited core mutations, but not all exhibited precore mutations, suggesting that core mutations may be more virulent than precore mutations. In 15 patients followed-up pre- and post-OLT, precore, core gene, and core promoter mutations were evaluated in HBV isolates.[36] Patients harbouring HBV with precore mutations exhibited significantly greater number of mutations (11.7 vs. 2.7) than those without precore mutations. Severe HBV recurrence post-transplantation was not associated with mutations in the BCP. The cytotoxic T-lymphocyte epitope in amino acid (aa) 18 to 30 was well-conserved, with mutations detected in only 2 of 15 patients. The greatest genomic variation was found in the central region of the core gene, as noted previously by Ehata et al.[33] Patients exhibiting severe post-transplantation HBV recurrence exhibited significantly more precore/core mutations and had a greater likelihood of being genotype D pre-transplantation. The number of patients in each of the two studies was small, and larger patient number investigations are required to resolve the potential significance and relevance of these mutations.

Precore/core protein mutations and interferon alpha therapy

Both HBV core and HBeAg are known to be important in the generation of the host's immune response to acute and chronic HBV infection,[5] with the core antigen epitopes 18 to 30 involved in the HLA-A2-restricted cytotoxic T lymphocyte response. Schepis et al[37] examined precore and core gene variability pre- and post-interferon-alpha therapy in HBV isolates from 25 Italian children with chronic HBV infection with a median age of 6 years. HBeAg sero-conversion occurred in 16 of 25 children and HBsAg sero-conversion occurred in 3 of 25 patients. Viral genomes were highly conserved pre- and post-therapy although up to 14 silent mutations were found in the sequenced isolates. Only one of the children exhibited HBV isolates with a precore stop mutation pre-interferon therapy and 2 of 25 children developed HBeAg-defective viruses post-therapy.[12] Zhang et al[38] examined interferon response in adults from the Mediterranean area as a function of precore sequence variability in HBV isolates. Seventeen of 35 patients exhibited a response to treatment (HBeAg sero-conversion) although 5 patients subsequently relapsed. Successful response to interferon-alpha was not related to the pre-treatment HBV-DNA level or dose of interferon-alpha, but did vary by precore sequence of HBV isolates. A significantly greater proportion ($PL<0.02$) of treatment responders contained HBV isolates with wild-type precore sequences in contrast to the precore stop mutation seen in non-responders[38] suggesting that precore mutants are associated with decreased interferon-alpha responsiveness.

In one of the largest European based studies, Brunetto and colleagues[39] studied spontaneous and interferon-alpha-associated HBV clearance in 115 patients who were then monitored for up to 30 months post-treatment. Fifty-nine patients received interferon-alpha and 56 remained untreated.[39] Pre-therapy, approximately half of the patients were found to be infected with wild-type HBV whilst half carried precore stop mutants. Spontaneous HBV clearance occurred in 28% of patients infected with HBV with wild-type precore regions whilst no patients spontaneously cleared HBV if they were infected with precore stop mutants. Similarly, interferon-alpha–associated HBV clearance was noted in 47% of patients carrying HBV with wild-type precore regions whilst only 19% of those patients with precore stop mutations were found to clear viraemia.[39] A significant diminution in both spontaneous and interferon-alpha-associated HBV clearance was attributed to the presence of precore stop mutations. These results support the use of interferon-alpha therapy early in chronic HBV before the acquisition of precore mutants.[12]

Naoumov et al[40] examined the development of hepatitis B precore-core gene mutations in isolates obtained from 12 USA patients before, during, and after interferon-alpha therapy. Interferon-alpha responders exhibited HBV isolates with significantly ($P<0.001$) fewer precore or core missense mutations (24 mutations noted in 23 serum samples) in comparison to the non-responders (141 mutations noted in 23 samples). No changes were detected in the precore or core region after interferon-alpha-associated sero-conversion in these isolates. The most notable changes were substitutions resulting in alterations in the CTL epitope at amino acids 18 to 30 of the core protein in all non-responders, suggesting that this region may influence interferon-alpha response.[12]

Fattovich et al[41] examined HBV isolates obtained over time from 55 Italian patients and found that core, but not precore mutations, were more predictive of the response to interferon therapy. Major core mutations which resulted in protein substitutions in B and T-cell epitopes were more frequently seen in non-responders. As with previous studies, the development of precore mutations during interferon-alpha therapy was usually associated with non-response. To summarise then, the pivotal mutations influencing interferon-alpha response in hepatitis B remain unclear but alterations in both precore and core sequences have been shown to influence response to therapy.[12]

X-GENE MUTANTS

The X protein is a non-structural protein encoded by the X-gene which can transactivate a variety of promoters *in vitro*[42] by activating signalling pathways.[43] X has been reported to interact with a number of nuclear proteins involved in cell cycle regulation, DNA repair and transcription. Due to the overlap of the basal core promoter (BCP) with the X-gene, the core promoter mutations often affect the structure and possibly the function of the X protein (see above). Nearly all deletions/insertions in the BCP shift the X-gene frame and lead to the production of truncated X proteins. These X proteins lack a domain in the C-terminus (around amino-acid 130–140) which is essential for transactivation activity.[44] The amino acid changes that are introduced in the X protein by the 1762-T/1764-A BCP mutations do not affect the transcriptional function of X.

PRE S/S-GENE MUTANTS

The S-gene encodes the three surface proteins of HBV. It is divided into the pre-S1 region the pre-S2 region and the S region. Three corresponding mRNAs serve for the synthesis of these proteins. The pre-S1 promoter is located upstream of the S gene, whereas transcription of the pre-S2 and S mRNAs is directed by the S promoter, which is located within the pre-S1 region. The pre-S region overlaps with the spacer domain of the P protein, which is dispensable for P protein function, while the S region overlaps with the essential reverse transcriptase domain[45] (Figs. 1 and 4).

Surface mutations have obvious clinical relevance in the prevention of HBV due to impact on prophylactic vaccination as well as laboratory-based diagnosis. Several large HBV vaccination programs in endemic regions have revealed a 2% to 3% incidence of vaccine escape mutants resulting from alterations in the HBsAg protein.[12] Generally, the amino-acid (aa) substitution of glycine for arginine at aa 145 of the S protein makes this epitope unlikely to bind to antibodies generated to wild-type HBsAg. The 'a' determinant of the HBsAg is a peptide sequence located between aa 116–160 which represents the major immune target of polyclonal antibody to the HBsAg. This antibody reactivity is directed mainly against the second loop of this determinant, located in aa 139–147.[46] In patients infected with HBV exhibiting surface mutations affecting the 'a' determinant, the mutant HBsAg may not be detectable by commonly used HBsAg assays, especially if based on monoclonal antibody "capture" reagents. As a result, these mutants do represent a potential public health issue since patients harbouring HBV with these surface mutants remain infectious but do not exhibit readily detectable HBsAg.[12]

Trautwein and colleagues[47] followed the natural history of disease in 20 patients with HBV infection pre- and post-OLT. Ninety percent (18/20) of patients exhibited mutations in the pre-S region both pre- and post-OLT. In one particular patient, who developed fatal FCH post-OLT, a mutation in the CCAAT-box of the S promoter was found. This change spanned the pre-S2 start codon. A wild-type CCAAT-box directs the normal transcription of the S-promoter and suppresses the level of the pre-S transcript, resulting in greater production of small surface protein (S) and a lesser amount of large surface protein (L). The mutant carrying the altered CCAAT-box was found to have reduced binding of transcription factors which caused enhanced transcription of the 2.4 kb mRNA transcript relative to the 2.1 kb mRNA. The increased expression of large surface protein (L) almost certainly contributed to a cytopathic effect in hepatocytes due to intracellular retention of the envelope protein, precipitating FCH.[47, 48]

The incidence of surface gene mutations in isolates from 20 patients with HBV reinfection after liver transplantation despite hepatitis B immune globulin (HBIg) administration was examined.[49] Pre-transplantation, only 5% (1/20) of patients were found to exhibit mutations in HBV isolates affecting the 'a' determinant of HBsAg. However, post-OLT, 50% of patients exhibited significant surface gene mutations in isolates affecting the 'a' determinant. The development of these surface gene mutations correlated with the duration of HBIg therapy. In contrast, a case series examining the outcome of liver transplantation in 55 HBV-infected patients revealed only an 8.3% incidence of surface mutations in HBV isolates at 2 years post-OLT.[50] Regimes of HBIg differ amongst transplantation centres almost certainly affecting the outcome and severity of HBV recurrence post-OLT.[9, 17, 29, 36, 46, 47, 49, 50]

Several reports have characterized the clinical course of nonimmunosuppressed patients infected with HBV expressing surface gene mutations. Santantonio et al[51] identified a number of subjects with chronic HBV infection in Italy who were infected with HBV genomes that contained almost complete pre-S2 deletions. These patients tended to have more aggressive or advanced liver disease indicating that pre-S2 deletion mutants prevail with the evolution of chronic HBV infection.[51] In the livers of these patients, intrahepatic accumulation of envelope proteins was observed. This mutation prevents translation of the middle surface protein. Mutations in the pre-S2 region have also been carefully examined in HBV isolates prepared four patients, who experienced fulminant hepatitis with a mutant expressing a pre-S2 start codon mutation.[52]

Such mutations could diminish immune recognition and clearance of the protein or alternatively cause intracellular accumulation of the large surface protein due to the imbalance in L and S levels as outlined by Trautwein et al.[47, 48] The role of the pre-S2 region has been examined in cellular transfection models using HBV deletion mutants.[48, 53] These models have suggested that the C-terminal region of the pre-S1 protein and the N-terminal region of the pre-S2 protein may alter binding affinities of the surface protein to the nucleocapsid[53] and conclusively demonstrated the importance of the molar ratio of the S and L protein translation required for normal assembly and release.[48]

P-GENE MUTATIONS

The HBV P protein mediates encapsidation of the pregenomic RNA into the core particle and synthesizes the HBV-DNA genome therein.[54] It has three enzymatic activities: DNA synthesis priming activity, RNA-dependent (RT) and DNA-dependent DNA polymerase activity, and RNaseH activity. These activities of the P protein are located in different domains[45] with primase encoded N-terminally, followed by the non-essential spacer region; thereafter follows the polymerase activity domain after which is located the RNaseH domain at the C-terminal end of the protein. The HBV RT contains several regions that are conserved in other RNA-dependent polymerases. These regions have been designated domains A to F, where domain F is located upstream of domain A (Fig. 4).[55, 56] The "YMDD" motif of HBV is located in the C domain. The polymerase protein of HBV has not been crystallized, however, there is amino acid similarity with HIV in the conserved domains and these comparable regions may be involved in NTP binding and substrate recognition. In the analysis of the X-ray crystal structure of HIV it was proposed that domains A, C, D and F may participate

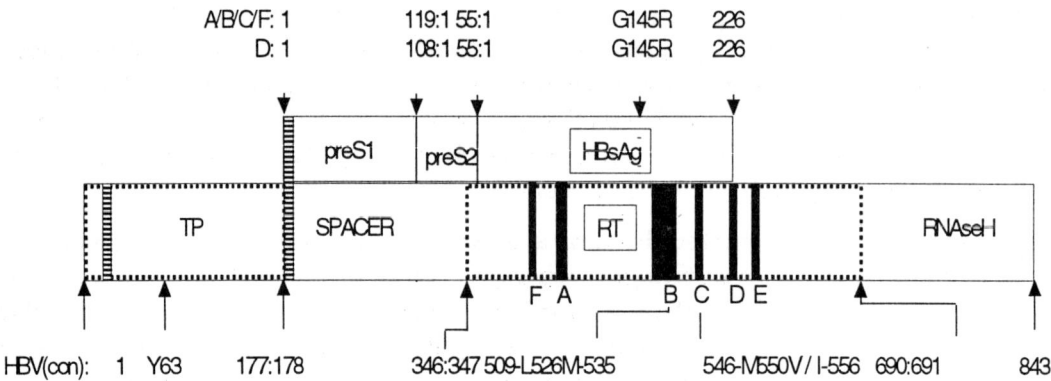

Fig. 4. Organisation of the HBV polymerase. The different domains the terminal protein (TP), spacer region, reverse transcriptase (RT) and RNAse H domain of the HBV polymerase are indicated with a dotted line. The conserved domains within the reverse transcriptase are indicated by shaded boxes. The numbering for HBV consensus sequence in which the methionine in the "YMDD" motif is designated 550 is shown and this corresponds to the numbering for genotypes B, C and F. The overlapping reading frame encoding pre-S1, pre-S2, and HBsAg is also shown. This figure was modified from Stuyver et al 2000.[73]

directly in nucleotide triphosphate (NTP) binding and catalysis.[57, 58] Domains B and E may be involved in the positioning of the template-primer relative to the active site, in which domain B forms part of the "template grip" and domain E forms the "primer grip".[59]

Hepatitis B virus quasi-species with mutations in the polymerase gene have been detected in patients undergoing antiviral therapy (Table 1). On exposure to lamivudine therapy, discrete polymerase nt polymorphisms result in amino acid changes in codon L526M (the template binding site of the polymerase or domain B) or codon M550I/V of the YMDD motif (the catalytic site of the polymerase or domain C), or both. These mutations significantly decrease the *in vitro* sensitivity of the polymerase to lamivudine-associated chain termination.[60, 61] Similarly, after famciclovir therapy, polymerase mutations in codon L526M markedly decrease famciclovir efficacy.[62]

The development of genotypic resistance to nucleoside analogue therapy has been closely followed up in patients undergoing OLT. In an early trial of lamivudine therapy in liver transplant patients in Europe,[63] 1 of 10 exhibited HBV isolates with LMV resistant HBV at 24 weeks post-transplantation. One year post-transplantation, the patient's liver histology revealed moderate chronic hepatitis with immunostaining strongly positive for HBcAg.

In immunocompetent patients receiving lamivudine for 52 weeks in the treatment of chronic hepatitis B, 14% to 32% developed LMV resistant HBV mutants.[64] As in liver transplantation patients, these mutants usually appear in the second 6 months of treatment. Despite the development of HBV expressing the resistant polymerase (L526M plus M550V or M550I

Table 1. Mutations in HBV polymerase protein associated with drug resistance to LMV and FCV with the corresponding change in HBsAg

FCV Mutations		HBsAg Mutations
H436N/Y	A Domain	no change
V519L	B Domain	E164D
P523L	B Domain	no change
L526M/V	B Domain	no change
T530S		not published
V553I	C Domain	W199 Stop/no change
N/S/H584K	D Domain	After end HBsAg
R588K	D Domain	After end HBsAg
LMV Mutations		HBsAg Mutations
I399S		not published
F512L	B Domain	A157D
V519L	B Domain	E164D
L526M/V	B Domain	no change
T530S		not published
A546V		not published
M550I	C Domain	W196S, W196L
V533I	C Domain	M198I/W199S
S559T		not published
S565P		S565R
L575V		not published
M550V	C Domain	I195M
ADV Mutations		
None to date		

alone), these patients largely exhibited continued suppression of HBV-DNA, significantly improved serum ALT values, and continued histological response when compared with untreated control patients.[64] However, longer follow-up is clearly required. In comparison to untreated control patients, lamivudine-treated patients harbouring drug-resistant HBV mutants had somewhat higher incidence of ALT elevations during treatment (24% vs 14%). No increased incidence of hepatic insufficiency or adverse events was noted in patients harbouring HBV LMV resistant mutants. Careful clinical and virological monitoring of these mutants is essential in order to define their significance in the natural history of drug-treated HBV infections.

CLINICAL PRESENTATION OF HBV MUTANTS

In an infected individual, at any point in time, HBV exists as a quasispecies and there is good scientific evidence that the major single mutations of HBV, such as the G1896A precore mutation, the G145R envelope mutation and even the M550V polymerase mutation occur spontaneously in the absence of any selection pressure, i.e., they pre-exist. The majority of infections caused by HBV generate a typical and usually predictable course of HBeAg-positive "wild-type" HBV infection, the clinical outcome of which depends on the age, gender and immune competence of the particular individual.[4] However, in uncommon circumstances, transmission of a particular mutant can occur. For example, mother to baby transmission of the G145R vaccine escape mutation, but this becomes significant usually in the setting of the selection pressure of active immunization. Similarly, transmission of the HBeAg-negative precore HBV mutant, either horizontally or perinatally, has been documented with various clinical outcomes ranging from mild disease to fulminant hepatic failure. The exact virological or clinical basis for virulence of HBV has not been conclusively identified. However, over the course of the 20–30 year span of persistent HBV infection and as the patient sequentially "passes" through the immune tolerant phase, the immune elimination phase and finally the "latent" phase,[65] the HBV quasispecies profile in that individual changes enormously. This is primarily driven by significant immune based selection pressures, which can account for the appearance of such bizarre mutants as the pre-S2 deletion mutations and other multiply mutated forms of HBV.[10]

In the case of severe or fulminant hepatitis B, Carman[66] has proposed a pathogenesis model that particular motifs from various parts of the HBV genome and its ORFs, if they occur together on the one genome, are more likely to be linked to the development of severe infection. For example, "fulminant motifs" have been identified in the BCP, X-gene, precore region, and the negative regulating element (NRE) of the BCP. Thus any combinations of any of these "fulminant motifs" are more likely to be associated with potentially virulent HBV. For example, an HBV genome exhibiting the combination of G1896A plus aberrant X-gene mutant or a BCP change plus aberrant X-gene mutant. This hypothesis requires *in vitro* and/or *in vivo* confirmation.

DETECTION OF HBV MUTANTS

The largest number of published reports on HBV mutants is based on sequence analysis of polymerase chain reaction (PCR)-amplified genome fragments from serum, liver and peripheral blood mononuclear cell (PBMC) specimens of patients with different clinical courses of HBV infection. The technique most commonly used for characterization of the sequence variability of amplified DNA is direct sequencing or sequencing of an appropriate number of cloned fragments. These methods detect variants if they make up around 10% of the virus population. For identification of minor subpopulations of specific mutants (0.1–0.01% of the virus population), methods for selective amplification of mutated HBV-DNA by PCR or ligase chain reaction[67, 68] have been established. Analysis of DNA single-strand conformation polymorphism is particularly useful for tracking transmission routes on the basis of sequence heterogeneity.[69]

Real time PCR is a useful improvement in quantitative assessment of viral load measurements.[70] For this technique, amplification can be monitored by incorporation of a fluorescent dye (SYBR Green I) which binds to double-stranded DNA or, alternatively, with hybridization probes using fluorescence resonance energy transfer (FRET). To set up FRET, two probes are used that will bind adjacent to the site of mutation juxtaposed to internal sites of the PCR product. The 3'-end of one probe contains a donor fluoreophore and the 5'-end of the adjacent probe contains an acceptor fluorephore. During FRET, the donor fluor is excited by a light source and emits a signal which is absorbed by the adjacent acceptor fluor; this in turn also emits a light signal but of a different wavelength. By measuring the different wavelengths, the specificity of the target can be determined and quantitated. This has been successfully applied to HBV and in particular, the detection of lamivudine resistant mutants in clinical samples.[70]

Molecular beacon technology is a further refinement of the recent success of molecular technology as applied to infectious diseases and is ideally suited to detect HBV mutations. The beacons, each labelled with a different fluorophore, can be designed to discriminate and accurately identify the mutant nucleotide sequence.[71, 72] Finally a line probe assay (LiPa) has been developed for monitoring drug resistance in HBV-infected patients during antiviral therapy[73] which can successfully detect and discriminate the complex quasispecies nature of HBV. It is much more sensitive than PCR-direct sequencing and can detect particular quasispecies at around 1–3% of the virus population.

The use of complete HBV genomic sequencing, also using PCR amplification, has greatly expanded the number of mutations identified, many of which are silent or do not alter the amino acid sequence in a particular open reading frame.[74] However, some of the silent mutations identified may cause an amino acid change in an overlapping reading frame. This has focused attention on the interdependency of multiple mutations, with each potentially having effects on more than one viral protein, for example the catalytic domain of the polymerase and the neutralization region of the envelope directly overlap (Fig. 1).

MANAGEMENT OF HBV MUTANTS

From the preceding discussion, only lamivudine and interferon alpha are licensed for the treatment of chronic hepatitis B. For patients with HBeAg-positive chronic hepatitis B who have normal or near normal serum alanine amino transferase (ALT) levels, treatment does not appear to be indicated. However, for those patients with a serum ALT greater than five times the upper limit of normal (ULN) and who are viraemic, lamivudine treatment should be considered; whilst for patients with a serum ALT of greater than 2, but less than 5 times ULN, treatment with either lamivudine or interferon are reasonable options following the appropriate counselling of the patient.[75-79] The recommended duration of interferon-alpha therapy is usually 4–6 months. The precore/core mutants which can be selected during interferon-alpha treatment have been discussed above. In the case of lamivudine, drug-resistant mutants appear in the second 6 month period of treatment and continue to emerge with duration of therapy. Certainly, once a patient has undergone HBeAg sero-conversion with HBV-DNA loss then treatment can be stopped, typically after one month. The optimal duration of therapy still needs to be resolved against the increasing frequency of drug resistance versus HBeAg sero-conversion. Most physicians treat for 12 months in the first instance and then carefully assess the clinical situation and virological status.

For patients with HBeAg-negative chronic hepatitis B, the position is a little more complex. Patients with normal serum ALT do not require conventional antiviral therapy, whilst patients with raised serum ALT, greater than twice the ULN, do warrant therapeutic intervention. In most cases, treatment with either interferon-alpha or lamivudine is only chemosuppressive and when treatment is discontinued, clinical and virological relapse is usually observed. Furthermore, drug-resistant mutations appear to be selected at a higher frequency in this group.[80] Thus, there is a significant number of patients where current therapy is of little or no long term benefit.

In those patients whose HBV contains lamivudine resistant mutants or they are interferon-alpha non-responsive, there are newer antiviral agents such as adefovir dipivoxil and entecavir which are in phase III clinical development, which may become available in future as part of the antiviral treatment. It is known that adefovir dipivoxil is highly active against lamivudine resistant HBV[81-83] and entecavir appears to have some activity against these viruses as well.[84] The patterns of resistance of the HBV polymerase observed during famciclovir and lamivudine long-term therapy are becoming complex (Table 1). Furthermore, the pattern of antiviral cross-resistance has only been established based on clinical (Table 2) and some limited virological parameters. However, there are now *in vitro* systems for measuring antiviral cross-

Table 2. Antiviral cross resistance: clinical studies

- *Lamivudine resistance*
  - Group 1: L526M plus M550V   (B plus C Domain)
  - Group 2: M550I   (C domain)
  - Group 3: F512L + L526M +/- M550V (B and/or C Domain)
  - Group 4: L426V/I + M550I   (A plus C Domain)
  - Group 5: L526M + M550I   (B plus C Domain)

  - Groups 1–5 resistant to famciclovir
  - All groups sensitive to adefovir dipivoxil

- *Famciclovir resistance*
  - A, B and C domain, typically L526M
    - Isolates sensitive to lamivudine, but lamivudine resistance emerges more quickly.
    - Isolates sensitive to adefovir dipivoxil

- *Adefovir Dipivoxil resistance*
  - None to date

resistance including an HBV-DNA polymerase assay[81, 82] and the recombinant-HBV baculovirus[85] as well as transient transfection cell culture systems.[86] Thus the development of new agents effective against HBV can be implemented into treatment strategies that include combination antiviral therapy based on maximal antiviral efficacy against a background of maximising the barriers to the development of drug-resistance.[87]

SUMMARY AND CONCLUSIONS

From the preceding discussion, infection with the HBV can result in a diverse clinical spectrum and eventual patient outcome. Attempts to control HBV prophylactically with vaccination and therapeutically with antiviral agents has met with great success. However, this success needs to be tempered against the recognition of selected mutants which have the ability to escape control and establish their own particular "niche". Future challenges will be based on our ability to detect and characterize these HBV mutants and find new therapeutic approaches to reduce their significance as well.

REFERENCES

1. Hollinger F, Ed. Hepatitis B Virus. Third ed. Philadelphia: Lippincott-Raven Publishers, 1996; pp.996.
2. Mast EE, Alter MJ, Margolis HS. Strategies to prevent and control hepatitis B and C virus infections: a global perspective. *Vaccine* 1999;17:1730-3.
3. Mahoney FJ. Update on diagnosis, management, and prevention of hepatitis B virus infection. *Clin Microbiol Rev* 1999;12:351-66.
4. Lee W. Hepatitis B virus infection. *N Engl J Med* 1997;337:1733-45.
5. Chisari F, Ferrari C. Hepatitis B virus immunopathogenesis. *Ann Rev Immunol* 1995;13:29-60.
6. Guidotti LG, Rochford R, Chung J, Shapiro M, Purcell R, Chisari FV. Viral clearance without destruction of infected cells during acute HBV infection. *Science* 1999;284:825-9.
7. Lau JY, Bain VG, Davies SE, O'Grady JG, Alberti A, Alexander GJ, William R. High-level expression of hepatitis B viral antigens in fibrosing cholestatic hepatitis. *Gastroenterology* 1992;102:956-62.
8. Angus P, Richards M, Bowden S, Ireton J, Sinclair R, Jones B, Locarnini S. Combination chemotherapy controls severe post-liver transplant recurrence of hepatitis B virus infection. *J Gastroenterol Hepatol* 1993;8:353-7.
9. Angus PW, Locarnini SA, McCaughan G, Jones RM, McMillan J, Bowden S. Hepatitis B virus precore mutant infection is associated with severe recurrent disease following liver transplantation. *Hepatology* 1995;21:14-8.
10. Gunther S, Fischer L, Pult I, Sterneck M, Will H. Naturally occurring variants of hepatitis B virus. *Adv Virus Res* 1999;52:25-137.
11. Hunt CM, McGill JM, Allen MI, Condreay LD. Clinical relevance of hepatitis B viral mutations. *Hepatology* 2000;31:1037-44.
12. Blum HE. Variants of hepatitis B, C and D viruses: molecular biology and clinical significance. *Digestion* 1995;56:85-95.
13. Tsiang M, Rooney JF, Toole JJ, Gibbs CS. Biphasic clearance kinetics of hepatitis B virus from patients during adefovir dipivoxil therapy. *Hepatology* 1999;29:1863-9.

14. Shaw T, Locarnini S. Combination chemotherapy for hepatitis B virus: the final solution? *Hepatology* 2000;32:430-2.
15. Okamoto H, Imai M, Kametani M, Nakamura T, Mayumi M. Genomic heterogeneity of hepatitis B virus in a 54-year-old woman who contracted the infection through materno-fetal transmission. *Jpn J Exp Med* 1987;57:231-6.
16. Orito E, Mizokami M, Ina Y, Moriyama EN, Kameshima N, Yamamoto M, Gojobori T. Host-independent evolution and a genetic classification of the hepadnavirus family based on nucleotide sequences. *Proc Natl Acad Sci USA* 1989;86:7059-62.
17. Sterneck M, Gunther S, Gerlach J, Naoumov NV, Santantonio T, Fischer L, Rogiers X, et al. Hepatitis B virus sequence changes evolving in liver transplant recipients with fulminant hepatitis. *J Hepatol* 1997;26:754-64.
18. Gunther S, Sommer G, Pilkat U, Iwanska A, Wain-Hobson S, Will H, Meyerhans A. Naturally occurring hepatitis B virus genomes bearing the hallmarks of retroviral G–A hypermutation. *Virology* 1997;235:104-8.
19. Miyakawa Y, Okamoto H, Mayumi M. The molecular basis of hepatitis B 'e' antigen (HBeAg) negative infections. *J Viral Hepat* 1997;4:1-8.
20. Hadziyannis S. Hepatitis B e antigen negative chronic hepatitis B: from clinical recognition to pathogenesis and treatment. *Viral Hepatitis Reviews* 1995;1:7-36.
21. Brunetto M, Stemler M, Schodel F, Will H, Ottobrelli A, Rizzetto M. Identification of HBV variants which cannot produce precore derived HBeAg and may be responsible for severe hepatitis. *J Gastroenterol Hepatol* 1989;21:151-4.
22. Carman WF, Jacyna MR, Hadziyannis S, Karayiannis P, McGarvey MJ, Makris A, Thomas HC. Mutation preventing formation of hepatitis B 'e' antigen in patients with chronic hepatitis B infection. *Lancet* 1989;2:588-91.
23. Tong SP, Brotman B, Li JS, Vitvitski L, Pascal D, Prince AM, Trepo C. *In vitro* and *in vivo* replication capacity of the precore region defective hepatitis B virus variants. *J Hepatol* 1991;13:S68-73.
24. Laskus T, Rakela J, Nowicki MJ, Persing DH. Hepatitis B virus core promoter sequence analysis in fulminant and chronic hepatitis B. *Gastroenterology* 1995;109:1618-23.
25. Lindh M, Horal P, Dhillon AP, Furuta Y, Norkrans G. Hepatitis B virus carriers without precore mutations in hepatitis B e antigen-negative stage show more severe liver damage. *Hepatology* 1996;24:494-501.
26. Lok AS, Akarca U, Greene S. Mutations in the precore region of hepatitis B virus serve to enhance the stability of the secondary structure of the pre-genome encapsidation signal. *Proc Natl Acad Sci USA* 1994;91:4077-81.
27. Buckwold VE, Xu Z, Chen M, Yen TS, Ou JH. Effects of a naturally occurring mutation in the hepatitis B virus basal core promoter on precore gene expression and viral replication. *J Virol* 1996;70:5845-51.
28. Baumert T, Rogers S, Hawegawa J, Liang T. Two core promoter mutations identified in a hepatitis B virus strain associated with fulminant hepatitis result in enhanced viral replication. *J Clin Invest* 1996;98:2268-76.
29. Gunther S, Piwon N, Iwanska A, Schilling R, Meisel H, Will H. Type, prevalence, and significance of core promoter/enhancer II mutations in hepatitis B viruses from immunosuppressed patients with severe liver disease. *J Virol* 1996;70:8318-31.
30. Li J, Buckwold V, Hon M, Ou J. Mechanism of suppression of hepatitis B virus precore RNA transcription by a frequent double mutation. *J Virol* 1999;73:1239-44.
31. Lindh M, Gustavson C, Mardberg K, Norkrans G, Dhillon AP, Horal P. Mutation of nucleotide 1,762 in the core promoter region during hepatitis B e sero-conversion and its relation to liver damage in hepatitis B e antigen carriers. *J Med Virol* 1998;55:185-90.

32. Baumert TF, Marrone A, Vergalla J, Liang TJ. Naturally occurring mutations define a novel function of the hepatitis B virus core promoter in core protein expression. *J Virol* 1998;72:6785-95.
33. Hasegawa K, Huang J, Rogers SA, Blum HE, Liang TJ. Enhanced replication of a hepatitis B virus mutant associated with an epidemic of fulminant hepatitis. *J Virol* 1994;68:1651-9.
34. Marinos G, Torre F, Gunther S, Thomas MG, Will H, Williams R, Naoumov NV. Hepatitis B virus variants with core gene deletions in the evolution of chronic hepatitis B infection. *Gastroenterology* 1996;111:183-92.
35. Ehata T, Omata M, Chuang WL, Yokosuka O, Ito Y, Hosoda K, Ohto M. Mutations in core nucleotide sequence of hepatitis B virus correlate with fulminant and severe hepatitis. *J Clin Invest* 1993;91:1206-13.
36. McMillan JS, Bowden DS, Angus PW, McCaughan GW, Locarnini SA. Mutations in the hepatitis B virus precore/core gene promoter in patients with severe recurrent disease following liver transplantation. *Hepatology* 1996;24:1371-8.
37. Schepis F, Verucchi G, Pollicino T, Attard L, Brancatelli S, Longo G, Raimondo G. Outcome of liver disease and response to interferon treatment are not influenced by hepatitis B virus core gene variability in children with chronic type B hepatitis. *J Hepatol* 1997;26:765-70.
38. Zhang X, Zoulim F, Habersetzer F, Xiong S, Trepo C. Analysis of hepatitis B virus genotypes and precore region variability during interferon treatment of HBe antigen negative chronic hepatitis B. *J Med Virol* 1996;48:8-16.
39. Brunetto MR, Giarin M, Saracco G, Oliveri F, Calvo P, Capra G, Randone A, et al. Hepatitis B virus unable to secrete e antigen and response to interferon in chronic hepatitis B. *Gastroenterology* 1993;105:845-50.
40. Naoumov NV, Thomas MG, Mason AL, Chokshi S, Bodicky CJ, Farzaneh F, William R, et al. Genomic variations in the hepatitis B core gene: a possible factor influencing response to interferon-alpha treatment. *Gastroenterology* 1995;108:505-14.
41. Fattovich G, McIntyre G, Thursz M, Colman K, Giuliano G, Alberti A, Thomas HC, et al. Hepatitis B virus precore/core variation and interferon therapy. *Hepatology* 1995;22:1355-62.
42. Rossner MT. Review: hepatitis B virus X-gene product: a promiscuous transcriptional activator. *J Med Virol* 1992;36:101-17.
43. Benn J, Schneider RJ. Hepatitis B virus HBx protein activates Ras-GTP complex formation and establishes a Ras, Raf, MAP kinase signaling cascade. *Proc Natl Acad Sci USA* 1994;91:10350-4.
44. Arii M, Takada S, Koike K. Identification of three essential regions of hepatitis B virus X protein for trans-activation function. *Oncogene* 1992;7:397-403.
45. Radziwill G, Tucker W, Schaller H. Mutational analysis of the hepatitis B virus P gene product: domain structure and RNase H activity. *J Virol* 1990;64:613-20.
46. Carman WF, Trautwein C, van Deursen FJ, Colman K, Dornan E, McIntyre G, Waters J, et al. Hepatitis B virus envelope variation after transplantation with and without hepatitis B immune globulin prophylaxis. *Hepatology* 1996;24:489-93.
47. Trautwein C, Schrem H, Tillmann HL, Kubicka S, Walker D, Boker KH, Maschek HJ, et al. Hepatitis B virus mutations in the pre-S genome before and after liver transplantation. *Hepatology* 1996;24:482-8.
48. Bock CT, Tillmann HL, Maschek HJ, Manns MP, Trautwein C. A preS mutation isolated from a patient with chronic hepatitis B infection leads to virus retention and misassembly. *Gastroenterology* 1997;113:1976-82.
49. Ghany MG, Ayola B, Villamil FG, Gish RG, Rojter S, Vierling JM, Lok AS. Hepatitis B virus S mutants in liver transplant recipients who were reinfected despite hepatitis B immune globulin prophylaxis. *Hepatology* 1998;27:213-22.

50. Terrault NA, Zhou S, McCory RW, Pruett TL, Lake JR, Roberts JP, Ascher NL, et al. Incidence and clinical consequences of surface and polymerase gene mutations in liver transplant recipients on hepatitis B immunoglobulin. *Hepatology* 1998;28:555-61.
51. Santantonio T, Jung MC, Schneider R, Fernholz D, Milella M, Monno L, Pastore G, et al. Hepatitis B virus genomes that cannot synthesize pre-S2 proteins occur frequently and as dominant virus populations in chronic carriers in Italy. *Virology* 1992;188:948-52.
52. Pollicino T, Zanetti AR, Cacciola I, Petit MA, Smedile A, Campo S, Sagliocca L, et al. Pre-S2 defective hepatitis B virus infection in patients with fulminant hepatitis. *Hepatology* 1997;26:495-9.
53. Le Seyec J, Chouteau P, Cannie I, Guguen-Guillouzo C, Gripon P. Role of the pre-S2 domain of the large envelope protein in hepatitis B virus assembly and infectivity. *J Virol* 1998;72:5573-8.
54. Bartenschlager R, Schaller H. Hepadnaviral assembly is initiated by polymerase binding to the encapsidation signal in the viral RNA genome. *Embo J* 1992;11:3413-20.
55. Poch O, Sauvaget I, Delarue M, Tordo N. Identification of four conserved motifs among the RNA-dependent polymerase encoding elements. *European Molecular Biology Organisation* 1989;8:3867-74.
56. Lesburg CA, Cable MB, Ferrari E, Hong Z, Mannaino F, Weber PC. Crystal structure of the RNA-dependent RNA polymerase from hepatitis C virus reveals a fully encircled active site. *Nat Structure Biol* 1999;6:937-43.
57. Huang H, Chopra R, Verdine GL, Harrison SC. Structure of a covalently trapped catalytic complex of HIV-1 reverse transcriptase: implications for drug resistance [see comments]. *Science* 1998; 282:1669-75.
58. Jacobo-Molina A, Ding J, Nanni RG, Clark AD, Lu X, Tantillo C, Williams RL, et al. Crystal structure of human immunodeficiency virus type 1 reverse transcriptase complexed with double-stranded DNA at 3.0 A resolution shows bent DNA. *Proc Natl Acad of Sci USA* 1993;90:6320-4.
59. Nanni R, Ding J, Jocobo-Molina A, Hughes S, Arnold E. Review of HIV-1 reverse transcriptase three dimensional structure: Implications for drug design. *Perspectives Drug Discovery Design* 1993;1:129-50.
60. Allen MI, Deslauriers M, Andrews CW, Tipples GA, Walters KA, Tyrrell DL, Brown N, et al. Identification and characterisation of mutations in hepatitis B virus resistant to lamivudine. Lamivudine Clinical Investigation Group. *Hepatology* 1998;27:1670-7.
61. Bartholomew MM, Jansen RW, Jeffers LJ, Reddy KR, Johnson LC, Bunzendahl H, Condreay LD, et al. Hepatitis B virus resistance to lamivudine given for recurrent infection after orthotopic liver transplantation. *Lancet* 1997;349:20-2.
62. Aye T, Bartholomeusz A, Shaw T, Breschkin A, Gronen L, Bowden D. Hepatitis B virus polymerase mutations during famciclovir therapy in patients following liver transplantation. *Hepatology* 1996;24(suppl):285A (abstract).
63. Grellier L, Mutimer D, Ahmed M, Brown D, Burroughs AK, Rolles K, McMaster P, et al. Lamivudine prophylaxis against reinfection in liver transplantation for hepatitis B cirrhosis. *Lancet* 1996;348:1212-5.
64. Atkins M, Hunt C, Brown N, Gray F, Sanathanan L, Woessner M. Clinical significance of YMDD mutant hepatitis B virus (HBV) in a large cohort of lamivudine-treated hepatitis B patients. *Hepatology* 1998;28:398A.
65. Lok AS. Treatment of chronic hepatitis B. *J Viral Hepat* 1994;1:105-24.
66. Carman WF. Personal communication. 1997.
67. Protzer-Knolle U, Knolle P, Schiedhelm E, Meyer zum Buschenfelde KH, Gerken G. Semiquantitative assessment of precore stop-codon mutant and wildtype hepatitis B virus during the course of chronic hepatitis B using a new PCR-based assay. *Arch Virol* 1996;141:2091-2101.
68. Minamitani S, Nishiguchi S, Kuroki T, Otani S, Monna T. Detection by ligase chain reaction of precore mutant of hepatitis B virus. *Hepatology* 1997;25:223-5.

69. Hardie DR, Kannemeyer J, Stannard LM. DNA single strand conformation polymorphism identifies five defined strains of hepatitis B virus (HBV) during an outbreak of HBV infection in an oncology unit. *J Med Virol* 1996;49:49-54.
70. Cane PA, Cook P, Ratcliffe D, Mutimer D, Pillay D. Use of real-time PCR and fluorimetry to detect lamivudine resistance-associated mutations in hepatitis B virus. *Antimicrob Agents Chemother* 1999;43: 1600-8.
71. Tyagi S, Kramer FR. Molecular beacons: probes that fluoresce upon hybridization. *Nat Biotechnol* 1996;14:303-8.
72. Marras S, Kramer F, Tyagi S. Multiplex detection of single-nucleotide variations using molecular beacons. *Genetics Analysis* 1999;14:151-6.
73. Stuyver L, Van Geyt C, De Gendt S, Van Reybroeck G, Zoulim F, Leroux-Roels G, Rossau R. Line probe assay for monitoring drug resistance in hepatitis B virus-infected patients during antiviral therapy. *J Clin Microbiol* 2000;38:702-7.
74. Gunther S, Li BC, Miska S, Kruger DH, Meisel H, Will H. A novel method for efficient amplification of whole hepatitis B virus genomes permits rapid functional analysis and reveals deletion mutants in immunosuppressed patients. *J Virol* 1995;69:5437-44.
75. Rizzetto M. Efficacy of lamivudine in HBeAg–negative chronic hepatitis B. *J Med Virol* 2002;66: 435-51.
76. Hadziyannis SH. Interferon-alpha therapy in HBeAg–negative chronic hepatitis B: new data in support of long-term efficacy. *J Hepatol* 2002;36:280-2.
77. Brunetto MR, Oliveri R, Coco B, Leandro G, Colombatto P, Gorinj M, Bonino F. Outcome of anti-HBe positive chronic hepatitis B in alpha-interferon treated and untreated patients: a long-term cohort study. *J Hepatol* 2002;36:263-70.
78. Lin CC, Wu JC, Chang TT, Huang YH, Wang YJ, Tsay SH, Chow NH, et al. Long-term evaluation of recombinant interferon-alpha-2b in the treatment of patients with hepatitis B 'e' antigen-negative chronic hepatitis B in Taiwan. *J Viral Hepat* 2001;8:438-46.
79. Papatheocloridis GV, Hadziyannis SJ. Diagnosis and management of precore mutant hepatitis B. *J Viral Hepat* 2001;8:311-21.
80. Tassopoulos NC, Volpes R, Pastore G, Heathcote J, Buti M, Goldin RD, Hawley S, et al. Efficacy of lamivudine in patients with hepatitis Be antigen-negative/hepatitis B virus DNA-positive (precore mutant) chronic hepatitis B. Lamivudine Precore Mutant Study Group. *Hepatology* 1999;29:889-96.
81. Xiong X, Flores C, Yang H, Toole JJ, Gibbs CS. Mutations in hepatitis B DNA polymerase associated with resistance to lamivudine do not confer resistance to adefovir in vitro. *Hepatology* 1998;28:1669-73.
82. Xiong X, Yang H, Westland C, Zou R, Gibbs C. In vitro evaluation of hepatitis B virus polymerase mutations associated with famciclovir resistance. *Hepatology* 2000;31:219-24.
83. Perrillo R, Schiff E, Yoshida E, Statler A, Hirsch K, Wright T, Gutfreund K, et al. Adefovir dipivoxil for the treatment of lamivudine-resistant hepatitis B mutants. *Hepatology* 2000;32:129-34.
84. Colonno R. Personal communication. 2000.
85. Delaney WEt, Isom HC. Hepatitis B virus replication in human HepG2 cells mediated by hepatitis B virus recombinant baculovirus. *Hepatology* 1998;28:1134-46.
86. Chin R, Shaw T, Torresi J, Sozzi V, Trautwein C, Bock T, Manns M, et al. In vitro susceptibilities of wild-type or drug-resistant hepatitis B virus to (-) - beta - D - 2, 6-diaminopurine dioxolane and 2'-fluoro-5 methyl - beta - L - arabino furanosyluracil. *Antimicrob Agents Chemother* 2001;45:2495-501.
87. Locarnini S, Birch C. Antiviral chemotherapy for chronic hepatitis B infection: Lessons learned from treating HIV infected patients. *J Hepatology* 1999;30:536-50.

14

Acute-on-chronic liver disease in reference to hepatitis B

Saroj K Sinha, Kartar Singh

Hepatitis B virus (HBV) is an important cause of acute hepatitis, chronic hepatitis, and hepatocellular carcinoma. The clinical manifestations and outcome of HBV infection depend on the age at which the infection is acquired, the level of HBV replication, and the immune status of the host. Perinatal and childhood infection is usually associated with few or no symptoms but there is a high-risk of chronicity. In contrast, HBV infection in adults usually leads to symptomatic acute hepatitis, however, the risk of chronicity is low. The acute and chronic forms of hepatitis related to HBV are well recognised entities. Sometimes, patients with chronic HBV infection present with acute deterioration in hepatocellular function which can be labelled as acute on chronic hepatitis. Similarly, patients with chronic hepatitis of other etiologies may deteriorate acutely due to HBV infection. With wider availability of various serological markers for different hepatitis viruses, this entity is more commonly recognised now. Acute on chronic hepatitis can be part of natural history of chronic HBV infection or can result from unrelated causes of hepatitis.

ETIOLOGY

The different causes of acute on chronic hepatitis in patients with chronic HBV infection are listed in Table 1.

Spontaneous exacerbations in hepatocellular damage are common in the natural history of chronic HBV infection.[1,2] Some of these exacerbations may be associated with HBeAg sero-conversion (i.e. conversion from HBeAg positive status to anti-HBe positive status). Such acute exacerbations of hepatocellular injury are believed to be caused by sudden increase in immune mediated lysis of hepatocytes. Some of the studies have found that these exacerbations are often preceded by an increase in serum HBV-DNA level and change in distribution of HBcAg from nuclear to cytoplasmic location in the hepatocytes. Not all such exacerbations lead to HBeAg sero-conversion. Some patients have suboptimal immune response and

Table 1. Causes of acute-on-chronic hepatitis in patients with HBV infection

---
Reactivation or change in replication status of HBV
Sero-conversion from HBeAg to anti-HBe
Superinfection with hepatitis D virus (HDV)
Infection with other hepatitis viruses
- Hepatitis A virus (HAV)
- Hepatitis C virus (HCV)
- Hepatitis E virus (HEV)
- Epstein Barr virus (EBV)
- Cytomegalo virus (CMV)

Withdrawal of immuno-suppressive drugs, e.g. steroids, cytotoxic chemotherapy, etc.
Alcoholic liver disease
Acute HBV infection in patients with chronic hepatitis of other etiology
Treatment with interferon
Miscellaneous causes
- Systemic sepsis
- Ischemic hepatitis
- Congestive hepatitis
- Portal or hepatic vein thrombosis
- Massive gastrointestinal bleeding
---

abortive immune clearance of the virus. These patients may develop recurrent exacerbations of chronic hepatitis with or without transient loss of HBeAg. Rarely IgM anti-HBc response may occur with such an exacerbation confusing the picture with acute hepatitis B. Recently high frequency of mutations at codon 130 in HBV core region have been reported to occur during such acute exacerbations.[3] Reports on the use of lamivudine for treatment of episodes of spontaneous acute exacerbations in patients with chronic hepatitis B have appeared recently.[4]

Hepatitis D virus (HDV) is a negative stranded RNA virus which depends on HBV (a DNA virus) for its propagation. HDV can be acquired as coinfection with HBV or as superinfection on chronic HBV infection. After superinfection, the risk of chronicity of HDV infection is very high. It has been estimated that about 5% of the HBsAg positive subjects globally are also infected with HDV. Prevalence of HDV infection among HBsAg positive subjects in the Asian countries has been reported to be high. The figures for India vary from 7.3% to 15.5% in patient with fulminant hepatic failure and 6.1% to 19% in patients with chronic liver disease.[1, 5-9]

Incidence and prevalence of HDV infection appears to be decreasing in most parts of the world. In a study from Spain, prevalence of HDV infection among patients with HBV related chronic liver disease was 15.1% during the period 1979-1985 which decreased to 7.1% during the period 1985-1992.[10] The incidence of new HDV infection in the same study was only 1.4% during 44.6±31.9 months of follow-up. In a study from Taiwan which included patients with fulminant hepatic failure (FHF) or subacute hepatic failure (SAHF), 14 out of 32 patients with evidence of chronic HBV infection were found to have HDV superinfection.[11] In another study from New Delhi which included 48 patients of chronic hepatitis, 34 patients had evidence of chronic HBV infection and 10 were positive for antibodies to HDV.[12]

HDV superinfection may manifest with acute hepatitis like or fulminant hepatic failure like picture. HDV superinfection of a subject with chronic HBV infection can be mistaken for flare up of chronic hepatitis B unless serological test is done to demonstrate the HDV infection. Detection of hepatitis delta antigen (HDAg) and/or IgM anti-HDAg confirms acute HDV infection. HDV RNA can be detected in the liver or serum by hybridization or RT-PCR.[11] HDV infection alters the course of chronic hepatitis B. Although the severity of underlying chronic hepatitis increases, titers of HBsAg, HBeAg and HBV-DNA in serum tend to fall and may even become undetectable. HDV infection may inhibit replication of HBV in some patients.

Mode of transmission of hepatitis C virus (HCV) is similar to HBV. The course of chronic hepatitis B may be altered by acquisition of HCV infection.[13] Acute HCV infection upon chronic HBV infection can manifest either as FHF or acute hepatitis (actually acute on chronic hepatitis).[14-24] In a study from Taiwan, 23% of patients with acute hepatitis C superimposed on chronic HBV infection had fulminant hepatic failure.[19] Similar results have been reported from other countries also.[19,20] The risk of FHF in HBsAg positive subjects with acute hepatitis C did not correlate with age and gender of patients, HCV genotype, concurrent hepatitis G virus infection, serum titre of HBV-DNA and serum titre of HCV RNA on admission.[19] It remains unknown whether severity of hepatocellular damage in such a setting correlates with the pre-existent HBV replication status or histological changes in the liver.[19,20]

It has been shown that acute hepatitis C virus infection in patients with chronic HBV infection can suppress some of the markers of HBV infection and can even replace HBV as a cause of continuing hepatitis.[14,15,21-24] Hence, in some instances of HCV superinfection of subjects with chronic HBV infection or concomitant dual infection, some of the markers of HBV infection may not be detectable in serum and severe liver damage may be erroneously attributed to HCV alone.[15,21,24-30] In most of such instances, HBV-DNA can be detected in the liver tissue.[27,28]

Hepatitis A virus (HAV) infection in a patient with chronic HBV infection may manifest either as acute hepatitis like or fulminant hepatic failure like clinical picture. It is widely believed that acute hepatitis A is more severe and carries higher mortality in patients with chronic hepatitis B virus infection.[31-36] In an epidemic in Shanghai city, out of 310,746 cases of acute hepatitis A, HBsAg was detected in 8.8% of cases.[31] Risk of mortality (mostly related to fulminant hepatic failure) in HBsAg positive patients was 5.6 fold higher than HBsAg negative subjects. Data from the United States of America also strongly support the finding that hepatitis A is more severe in patients with chronic HBV infection.[31] However, a Japanese study concluded that severe hepatitis A occurred primarily in patients with chronic hepatitis B whereas HAV infection in healthy HBsAg positive subjects was probably not different from infection in patients without HBV infection.[31] In contrast, a prospective study from Greece concluded that acute hepatitis A on current or even past HBV infection is associated with higher peak aminotransferases suggesting increased severity.[31] However, some case series have suggested that course and outcome of hepatitis A is not different in patients with chronic HBV infection.[31, 36]

Acute hepatitis A can be confirmed by detection of IgM anti-HAV in serum. Acute hepatitis A can alter the serum markers of HBV. Transient decrease in HBsAg titres, transient suppression of HBV replication, sero-conversion from HBeAg to anti-HBe and transient disappearance of HBV-DNA from serum have been reported with acute hepatitis A on underlying chronic HBV infection. These facts should be kept in mind when one is evaluating a patient for acute on chronic hepatitis.

Like hepatitis A, acute hepatitis E virus (HEV) infection can also occur in patients with chronic HBV infection. Severity and mortality with acute hepatitis E may be higher in patients with chronic hepatitis B than in previously normal subjects.[22, 37] Clinically, it may manifest as acute hepatitis like or fulminant hepatic failure like clinical picture. Acute hepatitis E can be confirmed by detection of IgM anti-HEV in serum. HEV RNA may be detectable in liver, bile, stool and serum during acute stage of the disease. The summary of global and the Indian data on the occurrence of acute hepatitis on underlying chronic liver disease can be seen in Tables 2 and 3.

Chronic alcohol abusers and patients with alcoholic liver disease are at higher risk for acquisition of HBV and HCV than general population. Several studies have documented higher prevalence of HBV and HCV in alcoholic patients.[38-45] Prevalence of these viral infections increases with severity of underlying liver disease. In a study from Korea which included 162 alcoholic patients, 29% were HBsAg positive and 10.5% had positive serology for HCV.[45] But none of the patients had both HBsAg and anti-HCV positivity. Acquisition of HBV in a patient with underlying alcoholic liver disease may result in decompensation (acute on chronic hepatitis). Conversely, deterioration in liver function in a patient with chronic HBV infection may occur due to continued alcohol consumption. In such cases where two or more etiological factors can be responsible for liver disease, histology of the liver may identify the dominant offending agent.[41] Whenever unexplained deterioration occurs in a patient with alcoholic liver disease, evidence for superadded viral hepatitis should be sought. Prognosis of both

Table 2. Acute-on-chronic hepatitis—selected global data

Country (Year) Ref. no.	Japan 1991 (23)	Spain 1995 (10)	Taiwan 1994 (11)	Taiwan 1990 (14)	Taiwan 1998 (16)	Taiwan 1994 (18)	France 1993 (17)	USA 1985 (42)	Italy 1998 (36)	Italy 1998 (36)	Japan 1999 (21)	Korea 2000 (45)	USA 2001 (46)	Italy 2000 (47)
Sample population	FHF	Chronic HBV	FHF SAHF	AH	AH sporadic	FHF	FHF	Alcoholic + AH	CHB	CHC	CHC	Alcoholic	CHC	CHB
	%	%	%	%	%	%	%	%	%	%	%	%	%	%
Number of patients (n)	21	696	32	532	273	62	40	20	163	432	2014	162	1092	834
Anti-HAV (IgG)													38	
Anti-HAV (IgM)				2.1	2.9				6.1	3.9				
HBsAg +			84.3	61.3	63.0	74.2	42.5	10			49.9	29	67	
Anti-HBc (total)														
Anti-HBc (IgM)	26.2		21.8	12.8	13.2	8.1	12.5							
Anti-HDV		9.6	37.5			17.7								8.3
Anti-HCV	29		9.3									10.5		
HCV-RNA	33		18.6				20					11.7		
Anti-HEV (IgM)			3.1											
Mixed infection	42.3			61.3	63									
HAV+HBV									6.1					
HBV+HDV		9.6	44		21	17.7								
HBV+HCV	14.1		9.3			9.6	20					0		
HAV+HCV	4.7									3.9				

FHF–Fulminant hepatic failure, SAHF–Subacute hepatic failure, AH–Acute hepatitis, CHB–Chronic hepatitis B, CHC–Chronic hepatitis C.

Table 3. Acute-on-chronic hepatitis—Indian data (selected)

City (Year) Ref. no.	Ludhiana 1995 (5)	Indore 1998 (6)	Indore 1998 (6)	Chandigarh 1994 (48)	Indore 1996 (7)	Delhi 1993 (8)	Delhi 1991 (49)	Delhi 1989 (50)	Delhi 1993 (12)
Sample population	AH Children %	AH Adults %	AH Children %	AH Epidemic %	Hepatic failure %	CHB %	AH %	AH %	CH %
Number of patients	52	140	167	1273	122	40	405	496	48
Anti-HAV (IgG)									
Anti-HAV (IgM)	10	6.4	46.1	8.2	3.2		5.9	55.8	
HBsAg +ve	24			4.4		100	26		71
Anti-HBc (total)				29.4					
Anti-HBc (IgM)		18.6	15.0	8.4	27.8		8.4	20.2	
HDV	7.7	0.6			4.1	10			21
Anti-HCV	2	1.4	0.5		8.1				15
Anti-HEV (IgM)		44.3	7.2	90	31.9				
Mixed infection					25.4		17.6	15.8	
HAV+HBV	6							0.8	
HBV+HDV	12				4.1	10			21
HBV+HCV					1.6				
HAV+HCV									
Undiagnosed	42	29.3	31.1		1.6			23.2	

AH – Acute hepatitis, CHB – Chronic hepatitis B, CH – Chronic hepatitis

acute and chronic viral hepatitis is worse in alcoholic patients. Additionally, HBV and HCV infections increase the risk of hepatocellular carcinoma in patients with alcoholic liver disease.[43, 45] In one study, rate of development of hepatocellular carcinoma was 6.1% among alcoholics who were negative for HBsAg and anti-HCV, 23.5% when they were positive for HBsAg and 34% if they were positive for HCV antibody.[45]

Drug-induced liver disease in patients with chronic HBV infection may present with acute on chronic hepatitis. Patients with chronic HBV[46-50] infection constitute high-risk group for hepatotoxicity related to anti-tubercular drugs. The same may be true for several other potentially hepatotoxic drugs. Thus, these patients should be monitored clinically as well as biochemically whenever a potentially hepatotoxic drug is administered.[51] Outcome of the drug-induced liver disease in patients with chronic hepatitis B may be worse than that in previously healthy subjects.

Administration of steroids, cancer chemotherapy and other immunosuppressive drugs increase the replication of HBV in the liver. Sudden withdrawal of these drugs results in augmented immune mediated destruction of hepatocytes, rise in transaminases and deterioration in hepatocellular function. Similar phenomenon may occur if lamivudine treatment is withdrawn before HBeAg sero-conversion. In chronic hepatitis B patients with poor hepatic reserve, this may manifest as decompensated liver disease.

In patients with chronic hepatitis B, acute deterioration in liver function may occur in a variety of conditions, e.g. systemic infection (viral, bacterial or fungal), gastrointestinal bleeding, hypotension from any cause, hepatic congestion from any cause, portal vein thrombosis, hepatic vein thrombosis, etc.

MODES OF PRESENTATION

The different modes of presentation of acute on chronic hepatitis are enlisted in Table 4.

Table 4. Modes of presentation of acute on chronic hepatitis

Acute hepatitis like picture
Sudden worsening of course of chronic hepatitis
Fulminant hepatic failure like picture
Subacute hepatic failure like picture
Hepatic decompensation in a patient with chronic liver disease
• Hepatic encephalopathy
• Ascites
• Coagulopathy
• Hemorrage
Only biochemical deterioration of chronic hepatitis

Presentation of acute on chronic hepatitis is extremely varied and ranges from mere biochemical abnormalities in almost asymptomatic patient to fulminant hepatic failure like picture. The clinical presentation depends upon the severity of acute liver injury, severity of chronic hepatitis and hepatic reserve at the time of acute insult.

If chronic hepatitis is recognised already, the diagnosis of acute on chronic hepatitis may be easy. However, in patients with unrecognised chronic HBV infection, the clinical presentation may closely mimic acute hepatitis. In areas with high prevalence of HBV, most of the cases of apparently acute hepatitis may be actually acute hepatitis superimposed on chronic HBV infection.[14,16]

Acute hepatitis A or E superimposed on chronic HBV infection may present like fulminant hepatic failure (Fig. 1). Acute hepatitis C occurring in otherwise healthy adults rarely presents with fulminant hepatic failure. But acute HCV infection in patients with chronic HBV infection may present like fulminant hepatic failure in as much as 23% of cases.[19]

Another mode of presentation of acute on chronic hepatitis is sudden occurrence of hepatic decompensation in a patient with compensated chronic liver disease. The typical examples are acute hepatitis B in a patient with chronic alcoholic liver disease and HDV superinfection in chronic hepatitis B patients.

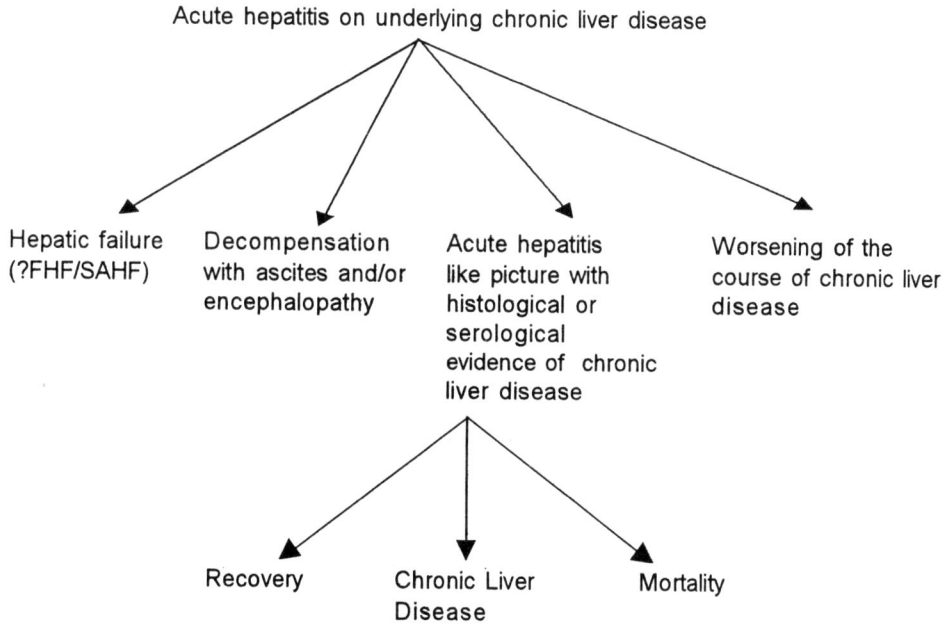

Fig. 1. Possible clinical manifestations and outcomes of acute hepatitis in a patient with nic liver disease

DIAGNOSIS

Complete diagnosis of acute on chronic hepatitis in addition to an attentive experienced hepatologist requiring facilities for various serological markers for different hepatitis viruses, qualitative and quantitative tests for viral RNA and DNA (preferably RT-PCR and PCR) and experienced histopathologist. Availability of facilities for immunocytochemical staining of tissue sections is desirable.

In a previously diagnosed case of chronic hepatitis, acute deterioration in hepatocellular function may be easily diagnosed as acute on chronic hepatitis. However, chronic hepatitis may go unrecognised for long periods of time. Thus, evidence for underlying chronic liver disease should be sought in patients presenting with apparent acute hepatitis or fulminant hepatic failure. The algorithm for diagnosis of patients with acuate-on-chronic liver disease is depicted in Fig. 2.

HBsAg is the most commonly used serological marker for HBV infection. However, HBsAg negativity does not completely rule out HBV as a cause of liver disease. When suspicion of

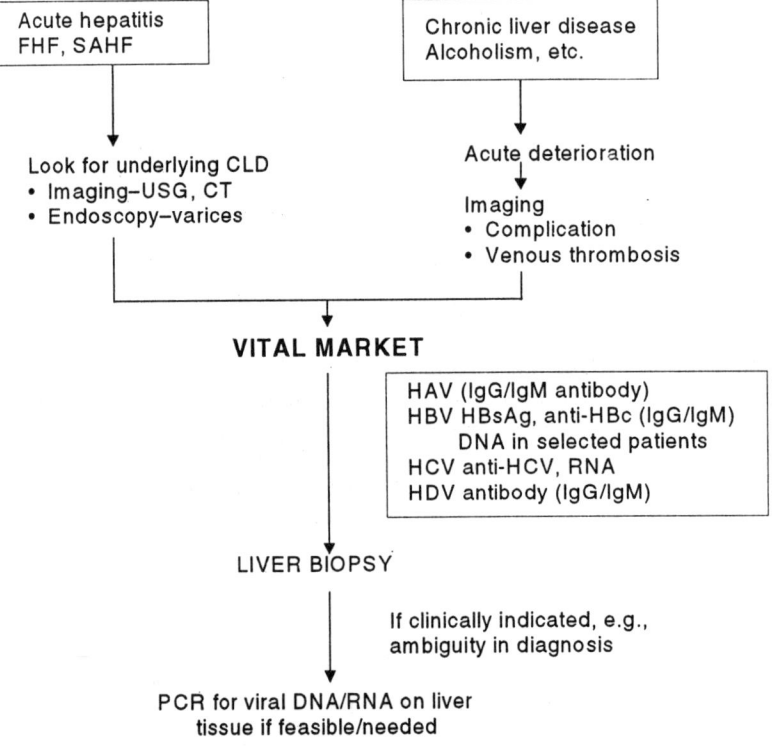

Fig. 2. Suggested algorithm for the diagnosis of acute-on-chronic liver disease

HBV infection is high but HBsAg is found to be negative, serum HBV-DNA and anti-HBc (total) should be tested. Rarely HBV-DNA may not be detectable in the serum but can be detected in the liver tissue.[28] As acute infection with HAV, HCV, or HDV in a patient with chronic HBV infection may decrease the titers of HBsAg and HBV-DNA in serum transiently, repeated testing for more than one marker may be useful. For diagnosis of acute HBV infection, IgM anti-HBc is an excellent test, but can rarely be falsely positive during phase of HBeAg sero-conversion, i.e. acute on chronic hepatitis. If a patient presents with acute hepatitis-like picture and is found to be HBsAg positive but IgM anti-HBc negative, he should be tested for other hepatitis viruses. Liver biopsy in such patients may reveal evidence of chronic hepatitis in addition to changes of acute hepatocellular injury. Immunocytochemical staining of the liver section may also be helpful. IgG anti-HBc suggests past HBV infection whereas high titres of anti-HBs generally rules out HBV as etiology of liver disease. HBeAg positivity in the serum signifies replicative stage of HBV infection but its negativity does not rule out replication. Sero-conversion from HBeAg to anti-HBe can lead to flare up of hepatitis but it is generally considered a good sign suggesting conversion to non-replicative phase of HBV infection.

Antibodies to HCV can be detected in the serum by ELISA or RIBA but they may take weeks to months to be detectable after acute infection. Sensitivity and specificity of third and fourth generation antibody assays are better than older assays. Serum HCV RNA test by RT-PCR is much more reliable test for diagnosis of acute or chronic HCV infection. Single test for HCV RNA may be negative as viremia may be intermittent. Acute hepatitis C occurring in a patient with chronic HBV infection may be diagnosed by HCV RNA positivity, HBsAg positivity and anti-HBc (IgM) negativity.

Acute HDV infection may be diagnosed by testing for IgM anti-HDAg and HDAg in serum. Sensitivity of a single test is not very high. Test for HDV RNA by RT-PCR is more sensitive and more reliable. In HDV/HBV co-infection, IgM anti-HBc will be positive whereas in case of HDV superinfection IgM anti-HBc is negative.

Reliable antibody test for hepatitis E virus (IgM anti-HEV for recent infection, IgG anti-HEV for past infection) is now widely available. HEV RNA can be detected in bile, blood, serum, and liver in acute stage. Similarly reliable tests for CMV and EBV are available now.

Drug-induced liver disease may be difficult to diagnose as no serological test will clinch the diagnosis and rechallenge may be unethical and risky. Liver biopsy may be helpful at times. Changes of chronic hepatitis may be reliably detected on liver biopsy. Similarly, when both alcohol and viral etiology are likely on the basis of history and serological findings, liver biopsy may identify the chief culprit.[41, 51-53] Immune staining of the tissue sections for various viral antigens may also help.

Thus, acute on chronic hepatitis may be a more common entity than generally recognised, particularly in developing countries like India where extensive serological testing for various hepatitis viruses and liver biopsy are not routinely done in clinical practice. Diagnosis of acute on chronic hepatitis requires an attentive hepatologist, good laboratory support, and at times invasive procedures like liver biopsy. This exercise of making complete diagnosis may be time and money consuming but results may have very significant bearing on the final treatment plan and outcome of the patients.

REFERENCES

1. Sarin SK. *Clinical spectrum of hepatitis B in India.* In: Sarin SK, Singal AK, Eds. Hepatitis B in India: Problems and Prevention. CBS Publishers & Distributors, New Delhi, 1996;pp. 51-3.
2. Perrillo RP. Acute flares in chronic hepatitis B: Natural and unnatural history of an immunologically mediated liver disease. *Gastroenterology* 2001;120:1009-22.
3. Okumura A, Ishikawa T Yoshioka K, Yuasa R, Fukuzawa Y, Kakumu S. Mutations at codon 130 in hepatitis B virus (HBV) core region increases remarkably during acute exacerbation of hepatitis in chronic HBV carriers. *J Gastroenterol* 2001;36:103-10.
4. Tsubota A, Arase Y, Saitoh S, Kobayashi M, Suzuki Y, Suzuki F, Chayama K, et al. Lamivudine therapy for spontaneously occurring severe acute exacerbation in chronic hepatitis B virus infection: a preliminary study. *Am J Gastroenterol* 2001;96:557-62.
5. Ghuman HK, Kaur S. Delta – hepatitis. *Ind J Paediatr* 1995;62:691-3.
6. Jaiswal SP, Chitnis DS, Jain AK, Inamdar S, Jain KS, Jain SC, Naik GD. Etiologic spectrum among acute viral hepatitis cases in Central India. *Indian J Gastroenterol* 1998;17:113.
7. Jaiswal SB, Chitnis DS, Asolkar MV, Naik G, Artwani KK. Aetiology and prognostic factors in hepatic failure in Central India. *Trop Gastroenterol* 1996;17:217-20.
8. Gupta P, Kar P, Chakravarty A, Jain A. Delta virus infection in cirrhotics in a north Indian hospital. *JAPI* 1993;41:503-4.
9. Tandon BN, Gandhi BM, Joshi YK. Etiological spectrum of viral hepatitis and prevalence of markers of hepatitis A and B virus infection in north India. *Bull WHO* 1984;62:67-73.
10. Navascues CA, Rodriguez M, Sotorrio NG, Sala P, Linares A, Suarez A, Rodrigo L, et al. Epidemiology of hepatitis D virus infection: changes in last 14 years. *Am J Gastroenterol* 1995;90:1981-4.
11. Wu JC, Chen CL, Hou MC, Chen TZ, Lee SD, Lo KJ. Multiple viral infection as the most common cause of fulminant and subfulminant viral hepatitis in an area endemic for hepatitis B: application and limitations of the polymerase chain reaction. *Hepatology* 1994;19:836-40.
12. Acharya SK, Panda SK, Duphare H, Dasarathy S, Ramash R, Jameel S, Nijhawan S, et al. Chronic hepatitis in a large Indian hospital. *Nat Med J Ind* 1993;6:202-6.
13. Sato S, Fujiyama S, Tanaka M, Yamasaki K, Kuramoto I, Kawano S, Sato T, et al. Coinfection of hepatitis C virus in patients with chronic hepatitis B infection. *J Hepatol* 1994;21:159-66.
14. Chu CM, Liaw YF. The incidence of fulminant hepatic failure in acute viral hepatitis in Taiwan: increased risk in patients with pre-existing HBsAg carrier state. *Infection* 1990;18:200-3.
15. Lau GK, Wu PC, Lo CK, Lau V, Lam SK. Histological changes of concurrent hepatitis C virus infection in asymptomatic hepatitis B virus patients. *J Gastroenterol Hepatol* 1998;13:52-6.
16. Chu CM, Sheen IS, Liaw YF. The aetiology of acute hepatitis in Taiwan: acute hepatitis superimposed on HBsAg carrier state as the main aetiology of acute hepatitis in areas with high HBsAg carrier rate. *Infection* 1988;16:233-7.
17. Feray C, Gigou M, Samuel D, Reyes G, Bemuan J, Reynes M, Bismuth H, et al. Hepatitis C virus RNA and hepatitis B virus DNA in serum and liver of patients with fulminant hepatitis. *Gastroenterology* 1993;104:549-55.

18. Chu CM, Sheen IS, Liaw YF. Role of hepatitis C virus in fulminant viral hepatitis in area with endemic hepatitis A and B. *Gastroenterology* 1994;107:189-95.
19. Chu CM, Yeh CT, Liaw YF. Fulminant hepatic failure in acute hepatitis C: increased risk in chronic carriers of hepatitis B virus. *Gut* 1999;45:613-7.
20. Lau GKK, Williams R. HCV in hepatic failure: West and East do not meet. *Gut* 1999;45:481-2.
21. Marusawa H, Osaki Y, Kimura T, Ito K, Yamashita Y, Egnchi T, Kudi M, et al. High prevalence of anti-hepatitis B virus serological markers in patients with hepatitis C virus related chronic liver disease in Japan. *Gut* 1999;45:284-8.
22. Liang TJ, Jeffers L, Reddy RK, Silva MO, Cheinquer H, Findor A, De Medina M, et al. Fulminant or subfulminant non-A, non-B viral hepatitis: the role of hepatitis C and E viruses. *Gastroenterology* 1993;104:556-62.
23. Yanagi M, Kaneko S, Unoura M, Murakami S, Kobayashi K, Susihara J, Ohnishi H, et al. Hepatitis C virus in fulminant hepatic failure. *New Engl J Med* 1991;324:1895-6.
24. Liaw YF, Tsai SL, Chang JJ, Sheen IS, Chien RN, Lin DY, Chu CM, et al. Displacement of hepatitis B virus by hepatitis C virus as cause of continuing chronic hepatitis. *Gastroenterology* 1994;106:1048-53.
25. Sheen IS, Liaw YF, Chu CM, Pao CC. Role of hepatitis C virus infection in spontaneous hepatitis B surface antigen clearance during chronic hepatitis B virus infection. *J Infect Dis* 1992;165:831-4.
26. Zarski JP, Bohn B, Bastie A, Pawlotsky JM, Baud M, Bost-Bozeau F, Tran Van Nhieu J, et al. Characteristics of patients with dual infection by hepatitis B and C viruses. *J Hepatol* 1998;28:27-33.
27. Villa E, Grottola A, Buttafoc P, Trande P, Merighi A, Fratti N, Seium Y, et al. Evidence for hepatitis B virus infection in patients with chronic hepatitis C with and without serological markers of hepatitis B. *Dig Dis Sci* 1995;40:8-13.
28. Brechot C, Degos F, Lugassy C, Thiers V, Zafrani S, Franco D, Bismuth H, et al. Hepatitis B virus DNA in patients with chronic liver disease and negative tests for hepatitis B surface antigen. *N Engl J Med* 1985;312:270-6.
29. Pontisso P, Ruvoletto MG, Fattovich G, Chemello L, Gallorini A, Ruol A, Alberti A. Clinical and virological profiles in patients with multiple hepatitis virus infection. *Gastroenterology* 1993;105:1529-33.
30. Cramp ME. HBV + HCV = HCC ? *Gut* 1999;45:168-9.
31. Keeffe EB. Is hepatitis A more severe in patients with chronic hepatitis B and other chronic liver diseases? *Am J Gastroenterol* 1995;90:201-5.
32. Zaachoval R, Roggendorf M, Deinhardt F. Hepatitis A infection in chronic carriers of hepatitis B virus. *Hepatology* 1983;3:528-31.
33. Viola LA, Barrison IG, Coleman JC, Murray-Lyon IM. The clinical course of acute type A hepatitis in chronic HBsAg carriers—a report of 3 cases. *Postgrad Med J* 1982;58:80-1.
34. Conteas C, Kao H, Rakela J, Weliky B. Acute type A hepatitis in three patients with chronic HBV infection. *Dig Dis Sci* 1983;28:684-6.
35. Zachoval R, Roggendort M, Deinhardt F. Hepatitis A infection in chronic carriers of hepatitis B virus. *Hepatology* 1983;3:528-31.
36. Vento S, Garofano T, Renzini C, Cainelli F, Casali F, Ghironzi G, Ferraro T, et al. Fulminant hepatitis associated with hepatitis A virus superinfection in patient with chronic hepatitis C. *N Engl J Med* 1998;338:286-90.
37. Wright TL, Mamish D, Combs C, Kim M, Donegan E, Ferrell L, Lake J, et al. Hepatitis B virus and apparent fulminant non-A, non-B hepatitis. *Lancet* 1992;339:952-5.
38. Mendenhall CL, Seeff L, Diehl AM, Ghosn SJ, French SW, Gartside PS, Ronster SD, et al. Antibodies to hepatitis B virus and hepatitis C virus in alcoholic hepatitis and cirrhosis: their prevalence and clinical relevance. The VA Coperative Study Group *Hepatology* 1991;14:581-9.

39. Shiomi S, Kuroki T, Minamitani S, Ueda T, Nishiguchi S, Nakajima S, Seki S, et al. Effect of drinking on outcome of cirrhosis in patients with hepatitis B or C. *J Gastroenterol Hepatol* 1992;7:274-86.
40. Fong TL, Kanel GC, Conrad A, Valinluck B, Charboneau F, Adkins RH. Clinical significance of concomitant hepatitis C infection in patients with alcoholic liver disease. *Hepatology* 1994;19:554-7.
41. Brillanti S, Masci C, Siringo S, Di Febo G, Miglioli M, Barbara L. Serological and histological aspects of hepatitis C virus infection in alcoholic patients. *J Hepatol* 1991;13:347-50.
42. Fellar A, Uchida T, Rakela J. Acute viral hepatitis superimposed on alcoholic liver cirrhosis: clinical and histopathologic features. *Liver* 1985;5:239-46.
43. Ohnishi K, Iida S, Iwama S, Goto N, Nomura F, Takashi M, Mishima A, et al. The effect of chronic habitual alcohol intake on development of liver cirrhosis and hepatocellular carcinoma: relation to hepatitis B surface antigen carriage. *Cancer* 1982;49:672-7.
44. Tasake S, Takada A. Alcohol abuse and liver disease: True, true, but not necessarily related. *Gastroenterology* 1991;101:1744-51.
45. Kwon SY, Ahm MS, Chang HJ. Clinical significance of hepatitis C virus infection to alcoholics with cirrhosis in Korea. *J Gastroenterol Hepatol* 2000;15:1282-6.
46. Siddiqui F, Mutchnick M, Kinzie J, Peleman R, Naylor P, Ehrinpreis M. Prevalence of hepatitis A virus and hepatitis B virus immunity in patients with polymerase chain reaction – confirmed hepatitis C: implication for vaccination strategy. *Am J Gastroenterol* 2001;96:858-63.
47. Gaeta GB, Stroffolini T, Chiaramonte M, Ascione T, Stomainolo G, Lobello S, Sagnell E, et al. Chronic hepatitis D: a vanishing disease? An Italian multicentre study. *Hepatology* 2000;32:824-7.
48. Dilawari JB, Singh K, Chawla YK, Ramesh GN, Chauhan A, Bhusnurmath SR, Sharma TR, et al. Hepatitis E virus: Epidemiological clinical and serological studies of a north Indian epidemic. *Indian J Gastroenterol* 1994;13:44-8.
49. Ichhpujani RL, Riley LW, Duggal L, Kumari S, Gupta PS, Sehgal S. Demographic features of sporadic acute hepatitis as determined by viral hepatitis markers. *J Commun Dis* 1991;23:138-43.
50. Panda SK, Datta R, Gupta A, Kamat RS, Madangopalan N, Bhan MK, Rath B, et al. Etiologic spectrum of acute sporadic viral hepatitis in children in India. *Trop Gastroenterol* 1989;10:106-10.
51. Ormerod LP. Hepatotoxicity of anti-tuberculosis drugs. *Thorax* 1996;51:111-3.
52. Yamanaka T, Shiraki K, Nakazaawa S, Okano H, Ito T, Deguchi M, Takare K, et al. Impact of hepatitis B and C viruses infection on the clinical prognosis of alcoholic liver cirrhosis. *Anti Cancer Res* 2001;21: 2937-40.
53. Saigal S, Kapoor D, Tandon N, Thakur V, Guptan RC, Agarwal SR, Sarin SK. High seroprevalence and clinical significance of hepatitis B and C infection in hospitalized patients with alcoholic cirrhosis. *J Assoc Phys India* 2002;50:1002-6.

15

Reactivation of hepatitis B virus infection

George K Lau, Xunrong Luo

Hepatitis due to reactivation of hepatitis B virus (HBV) is a well recognized complication in patients with chronic HBV infection receiving cytotoxic or immunosuppressive therapy.[1-4] It has been reported in HBsAg positive subjects receiving organ transplant or cytotoxic chemotherapy.[2,4,5] Even in HBsAg negative patients who had past HBV infection (hepatitis B core antibody; anti-HBc positive), HBV reactivation has been reported after immunosuppression.[1]

PATHOGENESIS OF HBV REACTIVATION AFTER IMMUNOSUPPRESSION

Careful prospective serological testing of subjects with chronic HBV infection who had HBV reactivation after chemotherapy showed that immunosuppression enhances HBV replication. This is reflected by increase in serum levels of hepatitis B 'e' antigen (HBeAg) and HBV-DNA polymerase, and naïve hepatocyte infection with HBV.[2] Withdrawal of cytotoxic or immunosuppressive drugs may lead to restoration of immune function, resulting in rapid destruction of infected hepatocytes. This can lead to hepatitis, hepatic failure, and even death.[1,6] The occurrence and severity of HBV reactivation after chemotherapy is unpredictable.

IN VITRO AND *IN VIVO* EFFECT OF IMMUNOSUPPRESSIVE AGENTS ON HEPATITIS B VIRUS

Most current clinical protocols for post-transplantation immunosuppression include a combination of corticosteroids, azathioprine, and cyclosporin A. There are at least 2 mechanisms by which immunosuppressive agents may increase HBV expression. As the host immune response to the virus plays a pivotal role in determining the outcome of HBV infection, suppression of the immune response is likely to increase the replication of HBV. However, the immunosuppressive agents may have a direct effect on the viral replication. *In vitro*, corticosteroids have been shown to increase HBV-DNA and RNA production by stimulating HBV transcription,[7-9] by binding to the glucocorticoid responsive element (GRE) and augmenting the HBV enhancer I. However, it is controversial whether corticosteroids increase the secretion of HBsAg and HBeAg.[7, 8, 10] At higher concentrations, azathioprine increases the total intracellular levels of HBV-DNA and RNA, as well as secreted virus. The main change in the intracellular replicative forms was an increase in HBVcccDNA. However, the levels of HBsAg and HBeAg secreted from the cells were not increased.[11]

Cyclosporin A had no apparent effect on the replication of HBV and did not alter intracellular or secreted HBsAg and nucleocapsid antigen levels. The effects of 'cyclosporin A' on viral replication have not been studied clinically in patients with chronic HBV infection. In woodchuck hepatitis virus (WHV)–infected animals, short-term 'cyclosporin A' treatment had no effect on the viral replication.[12, 13] However, long-term 'cyclosporin A' treatment was associated with decreased acute-phase liver injury and increased viremia.[13] In addition, cyclosporin A-treated woodchucks developed chronic infections at a higher rate compared with immunocompetent woodchucks.[12, 13] Hence, 'cyclosporin A' probably enhanced WHV replication indirectly by selectively inhibiting the T-cells. Combinations of all three immunosuppressive agents caused an eightfold increase in levels of intracellular HBV-DNA when cells were exposed to concentrations of each drug typically found in the clinical situation.[11] From a virological standpoint, cyclosoporin A appears to be the agent that least enhances HBV replication. However, at lower concentrations, azathioprine and prednisolone did not appear to stimulate HBV replication. Thus, the doses of these compounds should be kept as low as possible in the clinical practice.

DIAGNOSIS OF HBV REACTIVATION

HBV reactivation is best defined as an increase in the replication of HBV in patients with chronic/past HBV infection. In a patient with acute hepatitis, evidence of HBV reactivation needs to be confirmed to make the diagnosis of reactivation of hepatitis B (Fig. 1). In the setting of bone marrow transplantation, other causes of liver derangement, such as veno-occlusive disease (VOD), graft vs. host disease/rejection or superinfection with cytomegalovirus or herpes simplex virus, should be excluded.[14, 15] Diagnosis of hepatitis due to HBV reactivation in patients with chronic/past HBV infection depends mainly on serial determinations of hepatitis markers in the serum.[16] The key issue is the demonstration of increased HBV replication in patients with serological evidence of chronic/past HBV infection. First, serological evidence of HBV reactivation, such as anti-HBe positive or HBeAg negative to HBeAg positive, anti-HBs positive to HBsAg positive, should be obtained. However, HBsAg positive patients could suffer from reactivation even if they remain HBeAg negative. Sequence analysis of the HBV, isolated from these patients had demonstrated the presence of point mutation in the pre-core region that inhibited the synthesis of HBeAg.[17-21] Therefore, it would be better to demonstrate the presence of HBV reactivation by showing an increase of serum HBV-DNA by quantitation. Second, the patient should have serological evidence of chronic HBV infection. In other words, they should at least be HBsAg positive, preferably for

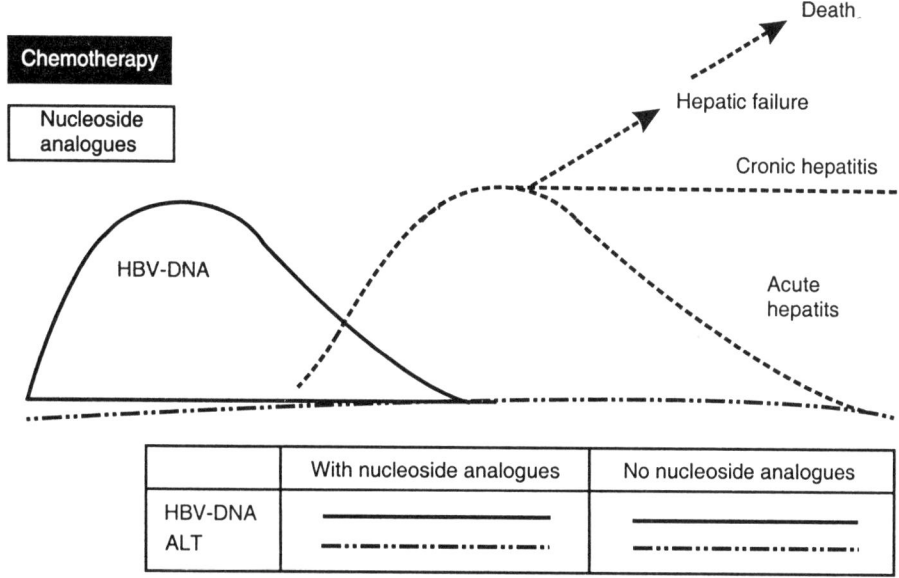

Fig. 1. Hepatitis due to HBV reactivation is characterised by the initial phase of enhanced viral replication followed by an immune attack on HBV-laden hepatocytes, resulting in hepatitis. The use of nucleoside analogues in the initial phase could theoretically reduce viral replication and the occurrence of hepatitis and its subsequent sequalae

at least 6 months, before HBV reactivation. In practice, this might be difficult if testing of HBV markers is not done routinely before the institution of cytotoxic chemotherapy. This is particularly the case if the patient is taking herbal drugs, which might contain immunosuppressive elements such as, steroids. HBV reactivation had also been reported in HBsAg negative patients with serological evidence of past infection (anti-HBc positive) after immunosuppressive therapy. In "HBsAg negative" patients, who are strongly suspected to have HBV reactivation, testing of HBsAg just by monoclonal antibody-based ELISA might not be adequate as mutation in the major neutralising epitope cluster might render a false negative result with these assays.[22] In these instances, polyclonal assay and testing of HBV-DNA should be performed.[23, 24] Other serological markers like anti-HBc IgM can differentiate between acute HBV infection and HBV reactivation in patients with chronic HBV infection.[25-27]

MANAGEMENT OF HBV REACTIVATION

Treatment of hepatitis due to HBV reactivation involves the use of either antiviral agents; such as ganciclovir,[28] lamivudine,[29, 32-35] famciclovir[30, 31] or foscarnet,[28, 36] immunosuppressive agents; such as steroids or liver protective agents; such as prostaglandin E2.[44] Results on the use of these agents have been generally disappointing. It is either because of their late administration or their ineffectiveness (Table 1). Another approach involves the pre-emptive use of nucleo-

Table 1. Summary of clinical trials on the use of nucleoside analogues in patients with reactivation of hepatitis B

Ref. No.	No. of patients	Baseline HBV serology	Underlying medical diseases	Treatment preceding HBV reactivation	Treatment of reactivation	Outcome
29	5	HBeAg+	Solid tumors or NHL	Chemotherapy	Lamivudine	Acute hepatitis; 4/5 recovered; 1/5 died of progression of disease
30	1	HBeAg unclear	CLL*	Fludarabine	FCV, then LMV after FCV failure	Resolved
32	1	HBeAg+	Invasive breast Carcinoma	Chemotherapy	Lamivudine	Acute hepatitis resolved with early treatment
33	1	HBeAg+	Non-Hodgkin lymphoma, stage IVb	Steroid based chemotherapy, radiotherapy	Lamivudine failure	Recovered from liver
44	1	HBeAg+	AML	T-cell depleted marrow allogeneic HSCT	Orthotopic liver transplant	Fatal hepatic failure
39	1	HBeAg+	ITP	Steroid	Reinstitution of steroid therapy	Acute hepatitis progressed to chronic hepatitis with severe compensated fibrosis
45	1	HBeAg+	Erosive rheumatoid arthritis	Methotrexate	Orthotopic liver transplant	Fulminant hepatic failure requiring OLT; maintained HBsAg+ post transplant
46	1	HBeAg+	Idiopathic nephritic syndrome	Steroid		Rapid steroid taper and concomitant ciclosporin; acute hepatitis resolved
40	1	HBeAg+	CML	Allogeneic Bone marrow transplant	CsA discontinued; Prednisone started	Fatal hepatic failure

Contd.

Contd.

Ref. No.	No. of patients	Baseline HBV serology	Underlying medical diseases	Treatment preceding HBV reactivation	Treatment of reactivation	Outcome
17	5	Precore ; BCP variants	Solid tumors (breast, germ cell, SCLC)	Cytotoxic agents (with dexamethasone as antiaemetic)	3/5 treated with Lamivudine 2/5 no treatment	Treated: 2 died (1 from progression of disease), 1 recovered; untreated: 1 died of hepatic failure, 1 recovered
37	1	Core-gene mutation	Non-Hodgkin lymphoma	Chemotherapy	IFN	Acute hepatitis
42	1	Precore mutation in signal sequence	CML	Allogeneic BMT	Prostaglandin E2	Fatal hepatic failure
28	1	Precore variants	AML	Allogeneic BMT	Gancyclovir and foscarnet	Died of fibrosing cholestatic hepatitis
38	3	Precore variants	Non-Hodgkin lymphoma	Steroid based chemotherapy	IFN-beta + CsA+ ALS	2/3 severe hepatitis, resolved with treatment; 1/3 fatal hepatic failure
34	1	anti-HBs+, anti-HBc+	Follicular small cell lymphoma	Chemotherapy	Lamivudine	Recovered from acute hepatitis and cleared HBsAg
36	1	anti-HBs+, anti-HBc+	ESRD and cadeveric renal transplant	12 weeks post-transplant; on immunosuppressants and steroid pulses for acute graft rejection	Withdrawal of steroid and azathiaprine; foscarnet started	Liver failure resolved with treatment
41	1	anti-HBs+, anti-HBc+	Lymphoma	Steroid taper	Corticosteroid	Fatal hepatic failur

Abbreviations : NHL–non-Hodgkin lymphoma; AML–acute myeloid lymphoma; CML–chronic myeloid leukemia; CLL–chronic lymphcytic leukaemia; SCLC–small-cell lung cancer; APUD–neuroendocrine tumour; CsA–cyclosporin A; FCV–famciclovir; ESRD–end-staged renal diseases; ITP–idiopathic thrombocytopenic purpura; IFN–Interferon

side analogues, such as lamivudine or famciclovir (Fig. 2). As the hepatitis due to HBV reactivation is preceded by HBV reactivation, suppression of HBV replication with nucleoside analogues is likely to decrease the liver injury and in turn the hepatitis due to HBV reactivation. In our center, eight HBsAg positive patients who received allogeneic bone marrow transplantations (BMT) were given oral famciclovir 250 mg three times daily, starting at least one week prior to BMT and continuing for 24 weeks after transplantation. During the treatment period after BMT, if patients had an elevation of serum HBV-DNA > 10 times the previous level or turned from negative to positive, then the dose of famciclovir was increased to 500 mg three times daily. Clinical and serological outcomes of these patients were compared with 24 HBsAg positive recipients of allogeneic BMT who did not receive famciclovir

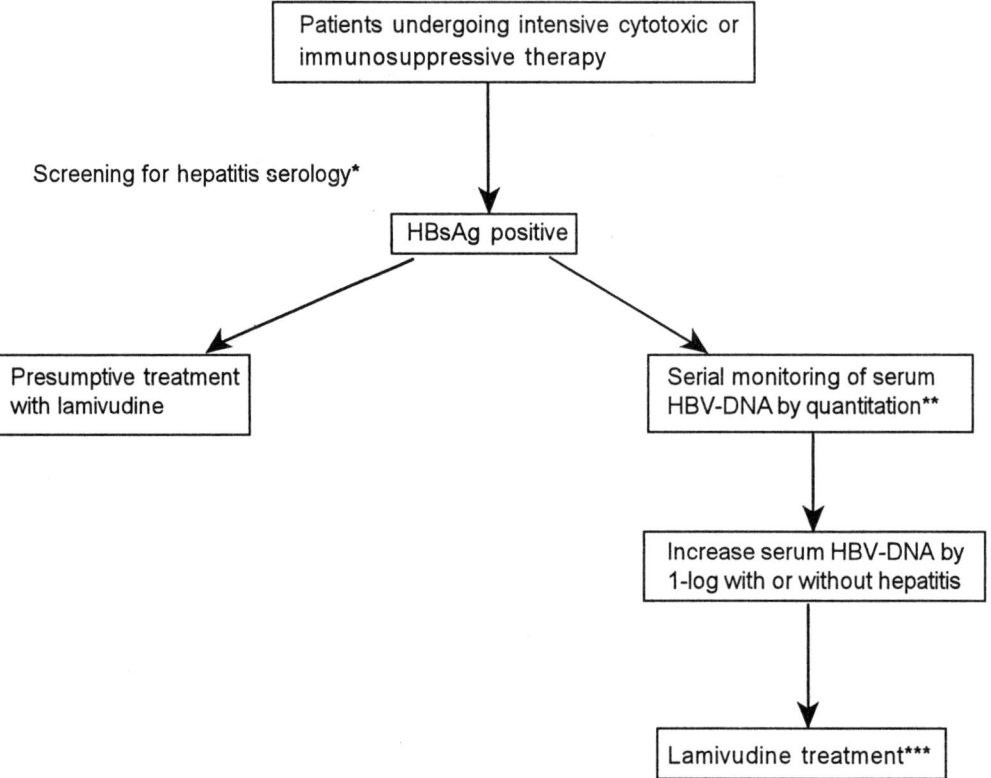

* HBsAg, HBeAg, anti-HBe
** Digene Hydrid-Capture™ II (Murex Diagnostics Ltd, Dartford, UK)
*** at the dose of 100 mg daily

Fig. 2. Management of chronic HBV infection in Chinese patients being treated with cytotoxic or immunosuppressive therapy

(historical controls). After BMT, hepatitis due to HBV reactivation was significantly reduced in those HBsAg positive patients who receive famciclovir prophylaxis.[43] Currently, higher dose of 500 mg three time a day is being evaluated at Queen Mary Hospital, Hong Kong.

REFERENCES

1. Nagington J, Cossart YE, Cohen BJ. Reactivation of hepatitis B after transplantation operations. *Lancet* 1977;68:105-12.
2. Locasciulli A, Bacigalupo A, Van-Lint MT, Chemello L, Pontisso P, Occhini D, Uderzo C, et al. Hepatitis B virus (HBV) infection and liver disease after allogeneic bone marrow transplantation: a report of 30 cases. *Bone Marrow Transplant* 1990;6:25-9.
3. Hoofnagle JH, Dusheiko GM, Schafer DF, Jones EA, Micetich KC, Young RC, Costa J. Reactivation of chronic hepatitis B virus infection by cancer chemotherapy. *Ann Intern Med* 1982;96(4):447-9.
4. Pariente EA, Goudeau A, Dubois F, Degott C, Gluckman E, Devergie A, Brechot C, et al. Fulminant hepatitis due to reactivation of chronic hepatitis B virus infection after allogeneic bone marrow transplantation. *Dig Dis Sci* 1988;33:1185-91.
5. Reed EC, Myerson D, Corey HT, Meyers JD. Allogeneic marrow transplantation in patients positive for hepatitis B surface antigen. *Blood* 1991;77:195-200.
6. Wands JR, Chura CM, Roll FJ, Maddrey WC. Serial studies of hepatitis-associated antigen and antibody in patients receiving antitumor chemotherapy for myeloproliferative and lymphoproliferative disorders. *Gastroenterology* 1975;68:105-12.
7. Tur-Kaspa R, Burk RD, Shaul Y, Shafritz DA. Hepatitis B virus DNA contains a glucocorticoid-responsive element. *Proc Natl Acad Sci USA* 1986;83(6):1627-31.
8. Chou CK, Wang LH, Lin HM, Chi CW. Glucocorticoid stimulates hepatitis B viral gene expression in cultured hepatoma cells. *Hepatology* 1992;16:13-8.
9. Gripon P, Diot C, Corlu A, Guguen-Guillouzo C. Regulation by dimethylsulfoxide, insulin, and corticosteroids of hepatitis B virus replication in a transfected human hepatoma cell line. *J Med Virol* 1989;28:193-9.
10. Doong SL, Tsai CH, Schinazi RF, Liotta DC, Cheng YC. Inhibition of the replication of hepatitis B virus in vitro by 2'-3'-didieoxy-3'-thiacytidine and related analogues. *Proc Nat Acad Sci USA* 1991;88:8495-9.
11. McMillan JS, Shaw T, Angus PW, Locarnini SA. Effect of immunosuppressive and antiviral agents on hepatitis B virus replication in vitro. *Hepatology* 1995; 22:36-43.
12. Cote PJ, Korba BE, Steinberg H, Ramirez-Mejia C, Baldwin B, Hornbuckle WE, Tennant BC, et al. Cyclosporin A modulates the course of woodchuck hepatitis virus infection and induces chronicity. *J Immunol* 1991;146:3138-44.
13. Cote PJ, Korba BE, Baldwin B, Hornbuckle WE, Tennant BC, Gerin JL. Immunosuppression with cyclosporine during the incubation period of experimental woodchuck hepatitis virus infection increases the frequency of chronic infection in adult woodchucks. *J Infect Dis* 1992;166:628-31.
14. Jones RJ, Lee KS, Beschorner WE, Vogel VG, Grochow LB, Braine-HG, Vogelsang GB, et al. Venoocclusive disease of the liver following bone marrow transplantation. *Transplantation* 1987;44:778-83.
15. Glucksberg H, Storb R, Fefer A, Buckner CD, Neiman PE, Clift RA, Lerner KG, et al. Clinical manifestations of graft-versus-host disease in human recipients of marrow from HL-A-matched sibling donors. *Transplantation* 1974;18;295-304.
16. Davis GL, Hoofnagle JH. Reactivation of chronic hepatitis B virus infection. *Gastroenterology* 1987;92:2028-31.

17. Steinberg JL, Yeo W, Zhong S, Chan JY, Tam JS, Chan PK, Leung NW, et al. Hepatitis B virus reactivation in patients undergoing cytotoxic chemotherapy for solid tumors: precore/core mutations may play an important role. *J Med Virol* 60:249-55.
18. Cooksley WG, McIvor CA. Fibrosing cholestatic hepatitis and HBV after bone marrow transplantation. *Biomed Pharmacother* 1995;49:117-24.
19. McIvor C, Morton J, Bryant A, Cooksley WG, Durrant S, Walker N. Fatal reactivation of pre-core mutant hepatitis B virus associated with fibrosing cholestatic hepatitis after bone marrow transplantation. *Ann Intern Med* 1994;121:274-5.
20. Mason WS, Taylor J, Hull R. Retroid virus genome replication. *Adv Virus Res* 1987;32:35-96.
21. Talbodec N, Loriot MA, Gigou M, Guigonis V, Boyer N, Bezeaud A, Erlinger S, et al. Hepatitis B virus pre-core mutations and HBeAg negative reactivation of chronic hepatitis B after interferon therapy. *Liver* 1995;15:93-8.
22. Carman WF, Korula J, Wallace L, MacPhee R, Mimms L, Decker R. Fulminant reactivation of hepatitis B due to envelope protein mutant that escaped detection by monoclonal HBsAg ELISA. *Lancet* 1995;345:1406-7.
23. Niederau C, Heintges T, Lange S, Goldmann G, Niederau CM, Mohr L, Haussinger D. Long-term follow-up of HBeAg-positive patients treated with interferon alfa for chronic hepatitis B. *N Engl J Med* 1996;334:1422-7.
24. Grellier L, Mutimer D, Ahmed M, Brown D, Burroughs AK, Rolles K, McMaster P, et al. Lamivudine prophylaxis against reinfection in liver transplantation for hepatitis B cirrhosis. *Lancet* 1996;348:1212-5.
25. Kryger P. Significance of anti-HBc IgM in the differential diagnosis of viral hepatitis. *J Virol Methods* 1985;10:283-9.
26. Chau KH, Hargie MP, Decker RH, Mushahwar IK, Overby LR. Serodiagnosis of recent hepatitis B infection by IgM class anti-HBc. *Hepatology* 1983;3:142-9.
27. Colloredo Mels G, Bellati G, Leandro G, Brunetto MR, Vicari O, Piantino P, Borzio M, et al. Role of IgM antibody to hepatitis B core antigen in the diagnosis of hepatitis B exacerbations. *Arch Virol Suppl* 1993;8:203-11.
28. McIvor C, Morton J, Bryant A, Cooksley WG, Durrant S, Walker N. Fatal reactivation of pre-core mutant hepatitis B virus associated with fibrosing cholestatic hepatitis after bone marrow transplantation. *Ann Intern Med* 1994;121:274-5.
29. Yeo W, Steinberg JL, Tam JS, Chan PK, Leung NW, Lam KC, Mok TS, et al. Lamivudine in the treatment of hepatitis B virus reactivation during cytotoxic chemotherapy. *J Med Virol* 1999;59:263-9.
30. Yagci M, Sucak GT, Haznedar R. Fludarabine and risk of hepatitis B virus reactivation in chronic lymphocytic leukemia. *Am J Hematol* 2000;64:233-4.
31. Manns MP, Nevhaus P, Atkinson GK, Griffin KE, Yeang Y, Young CL, Vollmas J, et al. Famciclovir treatment of hepatitis B infection following liver transplantation: a long-term, multi-centre study. *Transpl Infect Dis* 2001;3:16-23.
32. Maguire CM, Crawford DH, Hourigan LF, Clouston AD, Walpole ET, Powell EE. Case report: lamivudine therapy for submassive hepatic necrosis due to reactivation of hepatitis B following chemotherapy. *J Gastroenterol Hepatol* 1999;14:801-3.
33. Clark FL, Drummond MW, Chambers S, Chapman BA, Patton WN. Successful treatment with lamivudine for fulminant reactivated hepatitis B infection following intensive therapy for high-grade non-Hodgkin's lymphoma. *Ann Oncol* 1998;9:385-7.
34. Ahmed A, Keeffe EB. Lamivudine therapy for chemotherapy-induced reactivation of hepatitis B virus infection. *Am J Gastroenterol* 1999;94:249-51.
35. Rossi G, Pelizzari A, Motta M, Puoti M. Primary prophylaxis with lamivudine of hepatitis B virus reactivation in chronic HBsAg carriers with lymphoid malignancies treated with chemotherapy. *Br J Haematol* 2001;115:58-62.

36. Grotz W, Rasenack J, Benzing T, Berthold H, Peters T, Walter E, Schollmeyer P, et al. Occurrence and management of hepatitis B virus reactivation following kidney transplantation. *Clin Nephrol* 1998; 49:385-8.
37. Sato T, Kato J, Kawanishi J, Kogawa K, Ohya M, Sakamaki S, Niitsu Y. Acute exacerbation of hepatitis due to reactivation of hepatitis B virus with mutations in the core region after chemotherapy for malignant lymphoma. *J Gastroenterol* 1997;32:668-71.
38. Yoshiba M, Sekiyama K, Sugata F, Okamoto H, Yamamoto K, Yotsumoto S. Reactivation of precore mutant hepatitis B virus leading to fulminant hepatic failure following cytotoxic treatment. *Dig Dis Sci* 1992;37:1253-9.
39. Lau JY, Bird GL, Gimson AE, Alexander GJ, Williams R. Treatment of HBV reactivation after withdrawal of immunosuppression. *Lancet* 1991;337:802.
40. Pariente EA, Goudeau A, Dubois F, Degott C, Gluckman E, Devergie A, Brechot C, et al. Fulminant hepatitis due to reactivation of chronic hepatitis B virus infection after allogeneic bone marrow transplantation. *Dig Dis Sci* 1988;33:1185-91.
41. Hammond A, Ramersdorfer C, Palitzsch KD, Scholmerich J, Lock G. Fatal liver failure after corticosteroid treatment of a hepatitis B virus carrier. *Dtsch Med Wochenschr* 1999;124:687-90.
42. Caselitz M, Link H, Hein R, Maschek H, Boker K, Poliwoda H, Manns MP. Hepatitis B associated liver failure following bone marrow transplantation. *J Hepatol* 1997;27:572-7.
43. Lau GKK, Liang R, Wu PC, Lee CK, Lim WL, Au WY. Use of famciclovir to prevent HBV reactivation in HBsAg–positive recipients after allogeneic bone marrow transplantation. *J Hepatol* 1998; 28: 359-68.
44. Mertens T, Kock J, Hampl W, Schlicht HJ, Tillmann HL, Oldhafer KJ, Manns MP, et al. Reactivated fulminant hepatitis B virus replication after bone marrow transplantation: clinical course and possible treatment with ganciclovir. *J Hepatol* 1996;25:968-71.
45. Flowers MA, Heathcote J, Wanless IR, Sherman M, Reynolds WJ, Cameron RG, Levy GA, et al. Fulminant hepatitis as a consequence of reactivation of hepatitis B virus infection after discontinuation of low-dose methotrexate therapy. *Ann Intern Med* 1990;112:381-2.
46. Rostoker G, Rosenbaum J, Maadi A, Nedelec G, Deforge L, Vidaud M, Lang P, et al. Reactivation of hepatitis B virus by corticosteroids in a case of idiopathic nephrotic syndrome. *Nephron* 1990;56:224.

16

Kinetics of hepatitis B virus and its relevance to the clinician

Mark Thursz

In patients with chronic hepatitis B virus infection, prior to the HBeAg sero-conversion, plasma levels of the virus are fairly steady over short periods of time (weeks to months). However, underlying this steady level is a highly dynamic situation with fairly rapid rates of new virus production and viral elimination. Furthermore, the infected cells from which new viruses arise are also in a dynamic state. Immunological responses from cytotoxic T-lymphocytes eliminate infected cells and at the same time viral particles are constantly infecting susceptible cells. A number of recent advances in biological sciences have facilitated the dissection of these processes revealing novel insights into the biology of this important viral infection.

The measurement of viral kinetics is the study of changes in virus levels over periods of time, particularly after significant biological events such as the introduction of anti-viral therapy. Three important developments have contributed to the emergence of viral kinetic studies: (a) over the last few years we have attained the ability to measure viral DNA levels for HBV in serum with acceptable levels of accuracy and sensitivity; (b) potent inhibitors of HBV replication, suitable for use in humans, have been developed and licensed; and (c) mathematicians have recently started to apply their expertise to the study of fundamental biological problems.

MATHEMATICAL MODELS

The kinetics of HBV infection have been described by Nowak et al[1] in mathematical terms as a series of differential equations. Like most clinicians, with a rusty memory of calculus, I had some initial difficulty in understanding these equations. I hope that the explanation below may help other clinicians to understand the mathematics but a thorough understanding of the equations is by no means essential for understanding the general principals and the clinical implications.

The first of these equations describes the changes in the number of uninfected hepatocytes (x) over time. It assumes that new uninfected, but susceptible, hepatocytes are produced at a rate λ and die at a rate d. Uninfected hepatocytes become infected at a rate which is proportional to the amount of free virus v, the number of uninfected hepatocytes x and is expressed by the term bvx where b is a rate constant. Therefore the first equation is written as:

$$dx/dt = \lambda - dx - bvx \qquad [1]$$

The changes in the number of infected cells over time (y) incorporates terms for the rate at which unifected hepatocytes become infected (bvx as above) and the rate at which infected hepatocytes die, ay, where a is a rate constant. Therefore, the second equation is written as:

$$dy/dt = bvx - ay \qquad [2]$$

The changes in the amount of free virus load over time depend on the rate of production from infected cells (ky, where k is a rate constant for the production rate in individual hepatocytes) and the rate at which free virus is removed (uv, where u is the decay rate, i.e. a rate constant for the removal rate of viral particles). Therefore, the third equation is written as:

$$dv/dt = ky - uv \qquad [3]$$

When lamivudine is introduced, assuming that it is 100% efficient, then k (the rate of new virus production) becomes 0 and $dv/dt = -uv$. If v_t is the amount of free virus at time t then v_0 is the amount of virus at the beginning of treatment ($t = 0$) it can be deduced that

$$v_t = v_0 e^{-ut} \qquad [4]$$

In the steady state situation which is found in chronic hepatitis the amount of free virus is constant and therefore $dv/dt = 0$ and $ky = -uv$. A value for u has already been estimated and v_0, the amount of free virus has can be directly measured, hence a value for ky_0 can be estimated. The decay rate for virus producing cells was estimated by comparing ky_0 and ky_1: $a = ky_1 / ky_0$.

The rate of virus growth once therapy is withdrawn is described by the equation

$$v(t) = v_1 e^{-ut} + (ky_1 / u)(1 - e^{-ut}) \qquad [5]$$

or

$$ky_1 = u(v(t) - v_1 e^{-ut}) / (1 - e^{-ut}) v_1 \qquad [6]$$

The amount of free virus at the end of treatment can be measured directly and a value for u was already estimated therefore an estimate for ky_1 could be made.

Two modifications to the basic equations have subsequently been proposed; the first modification introduced a term for the efficacy of inhibition of viral production[1] and the second modification was made to explain the effect of removing infected hepatocytes which were still producing viral particles.[2]

A simple mathematical term was applied to the rate of virus production from infected hepatocytes (ky) to allow a drug efficacy of less than 100%. Therefore if p is the efficacy of a drug ($p = 1$ is 100% efficient) then the rate of virus production during therapy could be described by the term $(1-p)\, ky$ and equation 3 becomes:

$$dv/dt = (1-p)\, ky - uv. \qquad [7]$$

or

$$v(t) = (1-p)\, v_0 + p v_0 e^{-ut} \qquad [8]$$

The initial mathematical model proposed by Nowak described the changes in free virus during the initial period of treatment and therefore made the assumption that the number of infected and virus producing hepatocytes did not change significantly during this period. However, a more complex solution was provided by Tsiang et al[2] to describe the changes which occur after the first 20 days of treatment. This solution incorporates terms for the decay of infected and virus producing hepatocytes:

$$v(t) = v_0 e^{-ut} + \frac{(1-p)\, u v_0\, (e^{-at} - e^{-ut})}{u - a} \qquad [9]$$

Although equation 9 appears fairly complex it can be seen that the initial term is the same as equation 4 and describes the exponential decay in free virus at the beginning of treatment and the second term describes a slower second phase decline in free virus.

Measurement of kinetics and estimation of parameters

Using clinical data from patients treated with lamivudine Nowak estimated the decay rate of free viral particles (u) to be 0.67 corresponding to a $T_{1/2}$ for viral particles of 1 day. Furthermore the total virus production per day was estimated to be 10^{10}–10^{12} viral particles per day.

When a term for the efficiency of inhibition of viral production was incorporated and compared with clinical data (equation 6), the level of viral inhibition produced by different doses of lamivudine was calculated. Thus 20 mg inhibits 87% of viral replication, 100 mg inhibits 96% of viral replication and 600 mg inhibits 99% of viral replication.

Nowak et al[1], estimate the decay rate of virus producing cells by comparing the rate of virus production from infected hepatocytes before treatment (ky_0) and after treatment (ky_1) where the decay rate $a = ky_1 / ky_0$. These estimates gave a mean decay rate of 0.04 per day and infected cells were calculated to have a $T_{1/2}$ of between 10 and 100 days.

The mathematical models can only be of use if they accurately predict the real life data.

Tsiang et al[2] compared the models to data from 10 patients treated with adefovir dipivoxil.[2] Although Nowak's equation 4 predicts the initial phase of viral decay fairly well it is clear that the decline in free virus is not entirely exponential during this phase and the curves fit the data more accurately when the term for drug efficacy is introduced (equation 6). However, neither of these equations fits the data for the second phase of viral decay which is much slower than the initial phase. The modifications made by Tsiang, which incorporated a complex term for the removal of productively infected hepatocytes, accurately predicts the second phase decline in viral load.

Correlation with clinical findings

HBV is not cytopathic and therefore release of ALT is thought to arise from the lysis of infected hepatocytes by the immune system. High ALT levels imply that the immune response to the virus is greater and there is a higher turnover of infected cells. It would, therefore, be predicted that pretreatment ALT levels should correlate with the decay rate of the virus infected hepatocytes as calculated by using the mathematical models and the measurements of viral load. Nowak confirmed that this correlation is indeed present.

Data are now available which reveal the clinical significance of these predictions in that the rate of viral elimination (HBeAg sero-conversion) occurs more frequently and earlier in patients with high pretreatment ALT levels.[3, 4]

The mathematical models may prove to be useful in predicting another parameter of treatment–the duration of therapy. In patients with an infected hepatocyte half-life of 10 days and a drug efficiency of 100% treatment for 1 year should be sufficient to eliminate the virus. However, in patients with an infected hepatocyte half-life of 100 days treatment for one year would still leave a significant number of infected hepatocytes and complete elimination would require up to 100 years of therapy. Theoretically, therefore the duration of treatment necessary to completely eliminate the virus could be predicted from the estimation of infected cell half-life. This value could be calculated from the slope of the viral decay curve during the second phase of free virus decline after measuring plasma viral loads at timepoints between 20 and 40 days after the start of treatment. In patients with raised ALT values and HBeAg detectable at the start of treatment, these predictions may not be relevant as patients are likely to be treated until HBeAg sero-conversion occurs. In patients with low ALT levels at the beginning of treatment a prediction of the duration of therapy required to completely eliminate the virus may assist in determining whether treatment with reverse transcriptase inhibitors as monotherapy is a realistic option. In particular the emergence of resistant mutants is likely to occur during the course of therapy. Alternative options such as abandoning treatment or adding immunomodulatory drugs such as interferon may be considered. In patients infected with the HBeAg negative variant of HBV there is no sero-conversion event to guide when treatment may be discontinued. In theory, the required duration of therapy could be predicted from the slope of the second phase viral decay profile.

The end stage complications of HBV infection such as cirrhosis and hepatocellular carcinoma are thought to arise from the cycles of cell lysis and proliferation. Using the mathematical models, this rate of cell turnover can be estimated and where cell turnover rates are low it would be predicted that the risk of complications is low and the need for treatment is reduced. Thus measuring the rate of cell turnover during a relatively short period of reverse transcriptase inhibitor therapy may predict which patients need and will respond to treatment and those patients who will not respond and who are unlikely to need treatment. Clearly this hypothesis needs to be tested in clinical practice before it can be applied.

REFERENCES

1. Nowak MA, Bonhoeffer S, Hill AM, Boehme R, Thomas HC, McDade H. Viral dynamics in hepatitis B virus infection. *Proc Natl Acad Sci USA* 1996;93:4398-4402.
2. Tsiang M, Rooney JF, Toole JJ, Gibbs CS. Biphasic clearance kinetics of hepatitis B virus from patients during adefovir dipivoxil therapy. *Hepatology* 1999;29:1863-9.
3. Chien RN, Liaw YF, Atkins M. Pretherapy alanine transaminase level as a determinant for hepatitis B e antigen sero-conversion during lamivudine therapy in patients with chronic hepatitis B. Asian Hepatitis Lamivudine Trial Group. *Hepatology* 1999;30:770-4.
4. Murray JM, Whalley SA, Brown D, Webster GJ, Emery VC, Dnsheiko GM, Perelson AS. Kinetics of acute hepatitis B virus infection in humans. *J Exp Med* 2001;193:847-54.

17

Hepatitis B virus genotypes: an overview

Varsha Thakur, Shiv K Sarin

HBV GENOME STRUCTURE

Hepatitis B virus belongs to the genus orthohepadenavirus of family hepadnavirus. Having been found in various animals like duck, heron, woodchuk, ground squirrel, and primates hepadnavirus have undergone a long history of evolution. HBV is the prototype member of hepadnavirus family and is the only human representative of this family. It has a circular, partially double stranded DNA genome of 3.2 Kb containing 4 overlapping open reading frames.[1] Relative to other double stranded DNA viruses, HBV is capable of independent replication. HBV utilizes genetic material economically because proteins are encoded from overlapping translation frames, and all regulatory signal sequences reside within protein encoding sequences. The 4 open reading frames (ORFs) of HBV represent the gene sequence that encode the virus nucleocapsid (core), envelop (surface), virus replicase (polymerase) and virus gene expression protein (X-protein). Three major unspliced messenger RNA (mRNA) transcripts are synthesized by a cell derived RNA polymerase.[2] The longest 3.5 kilobase terminally redundant transcript is used both as a template for genome replication by reverse transcription as the mRNA for expression of the core and polymerase proteins. The other two transcripts direct the synthesis of the virus envelop proteins. A 2.4 Kb transcript contains RNA sequences specifying the pre-surface 1, pre-surface 2 and surface protein gene sequences, whereas a 2.1 Kb transcript contains RNA sequences specifying the pre-surface 2 and surface protein gene sequence. Another 0.9 Kb transcript contains RNA sequence which codes for X protein. The largest ORF is the polymerase which overlaps more than 63% of other ORF's. The surface ORF is contained completely within the polymerase ORF whereas the core and X gene ORF's overlap the polymerase over 23 and 39% of their sequence length respectively.

HBV has a rare genetic arrangement because all the *cis*-acting regulatory elements i.e., nucleotide sequence used as binding sites for protein involved in the gene regulation or genome replication, reside within gene sequences. The sequences involved in the replication of HBV genome are: (i) the short direct repeats DR_1 and DR_2 and the (ii) the U_5 like sequence. DR_1, DR_2 and U_5 like regions are located within the pre-core ORF, polymerase/X-ORF and the terminal repeats of the linear HBV-RNA pre-genome. The four types of signal sequences that appear to be involved in the HBV gene expression are: (i) the promoter, (ii) the enhancer, (iii) the poly-A addition signal, and (iv) the glucocorticoid responsive element (GRE).

A promoter is a nucleotide sequence that acts as a binding site for RNA polymerase, a host cell derived enzyme that synthesizes RNA from a DNA template. Most eukaryotic cell and viral proteins are expressed from poly-A^+ mRNA transcripts synthesized by RNA polymerase II. Since there are three major HBV mRNA transcripts, there are at least 3 RNA polymerase II promoters located near the 5' end of each of the virus transcripts. The promoter for the 3.5 kb mRNA is located within the X gene sequence, whereas that for the 2.4 kb transcript is within the polymerase gene sequence, 5' to the pre-surface initiation codon. The promoter for the 2.1 kb transcript is located within a region that encodes both polymerase and pre-surface protein in overlapping translation frames.

The HBV enhancer element involved in increasing the level of viral transcription has been found to be located within the polymerase ORF with no overlapping gene sequence.

Poly-A addition signal sequences are nucleotide sequences that are essential for the termination of the transcription. This signal sequence is located in the region of core ORF. This region is well conserved as all the HBV transcripts use this single poly-A additional sequence and thus all virus transcripts share a common 3' terminus. A GRE is a segment of DNA that binds a hormone receptor which in turn acts to increase the level of transcription of a given gene. This sequence has been localized to a region where the polymerase and surface ORFs overlap (Fig. 1).

GEOGRAPHIC DISTRIBUTION OF HBV GENOTYPE

HBV replicates by the reverse transcription of an RNA intermediate.[3] This process involves errors, because it is not controlled by the proof reading enzymes.[4,5] The rate of nucleotide substitution for the HBV is estimated to be 10^4 fold higher than the human genome.[6] Assuming the rate of nucleotide substitution of $1.4–3.2 \times 10^5$/site/year,[7] the evolution of HBV probably started approximately 3000 years ago. On the basis of surface gene analysis, 9 subtypes of HBV have been described.[8,9] However, genetic differences are not limited to S-gene as they are found all over the HBV genome with the highest variation within the Pre-S region. Depending upon the inter-group divergence of 8% or more in the complete genome nucleotide sequence or 4.1% divergence or more of the surface gene,[9,10] HBV can be divided into seven genotypes, A to H.[9,11-16] Additionally, 5 HBV genotypes have been isolated from gibbons, chimpanzees, gorillas and orangutans.[17-22]

HBV genotypes have a characteristic distribution.[23] The genomic group of HBV generally

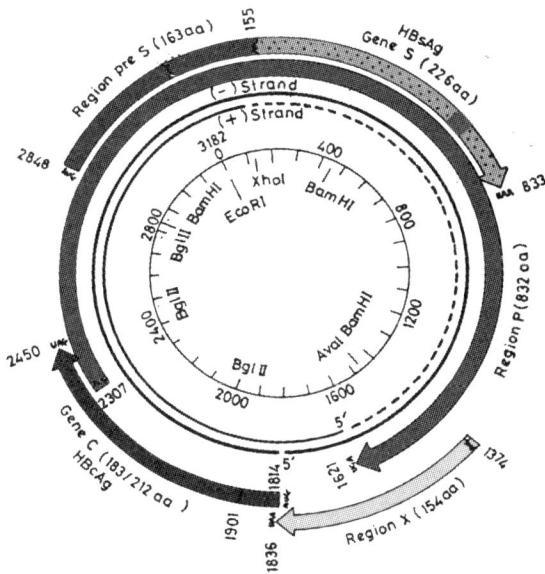

Fig. 1. Structure of circular, partially double-stranded genome of hepatitis B virus

gives an idea about the geographical area of origin. The HBV isolates belonging to the same subtype/genotype are believed to have an evolutionary relationship, and have been used for tracing the routes of HBV transmission and geographical migration of subjects with chronic HBV infection.[23,24] Genotypes A and D were originally widely distributed in the Old World (areas having old history of origin) and genotype F is confined to the new world. In general, genotype A is prevalent in two geographical groups, one western Europe and the other east and south Africa, separated by the D strain in Mediterranean area. The A strain might therefore represent a more ancient genomic group, which has been replaced in the Mediterranean region by the subsequently evolved strain D. Genotypes B and C were confined to the original population of the Far east.

Limited geographical distribution of strains B and C suggests that they have evolved there more recently. In fact, genotypes B, C and D seem to be prevalent in the regions of the world that are densely populated. Genotype D was found to be the most widespread one, predominating in Mediterranean area and the near east as far as India. This genotype was also found in aboriginal population in Asia, from Indonesia and Papua to Alaska. Genotype E has so far only been found in West Africa,[25] genotype F belongs to the New World like Polynesia, central America.[26,27] Genotype G is found in United States and Europe.[28,29] Recently there is an addition in the list of HBV genotypes, designated as Genotype H. The complete genomes were sequenced for ten hepatitis B virus (HBV) strains. Two of them, from Spain and Sweden, were most similar to genotype D. Five of them were from Central America and belonged to genotype F. Two strains from Nicaragua and one from Los Angeles, USA, showed divergences of 3.1–4.1% within the small S-gene from genotype F strains and were recognized previously as a divergent clade within genotype F. The complete genomes of the two genotype D strains were found to differ from published genotype D strains by 2.8–4.6%. Their S-genes encoded Lys(122), Thr(127) and Lys(160), corresponding to the putative new subtype adw3 within this genotype, previously known to specify ayw2, ayw3 or, rarely, ayw4. The complete genomes of the three divergent strains diverged by 0.8 to 2.5% from each other, 7.2 to 10.2% from genotype F strains and 13.2 to 15.7% from other HBV strains. Since pairwise comparisons of 82 complete HBV genomes of intratypic and intertypic divergences ranged from 0.1 to 7.4% and 6.8 to 17.1%, respectively, the three sequenced strains should represent a new HBV genotype, for which the designation H is proposed.[16] In the polymerase region, the three strains had 16 unique conserved amino acid residues not present in genotype F strains. So far, genotype H has been encountered in Nicaragua, Mexico and California. Phylogenetic analysis of the complete genomes and subgenomes of the three strains showed them clustering with genotype F but forming a separate branch supported by 100% bootstrap. Being most similar to genotype F, known to be an Amerindian genotype, genotype H has most likely split off from genotype F within the New World (Table 1, Fig. 2).

Table 1. Geographic distribution of HBV genotypes: Global/Asia

Genotype	Global	Asia
A	NW Europe, North America, Central America, Argentina	India
B	——	SE Asia, China, Japan
C	Australia	SE Asia, China, Japan
D	Europe, Argentina, Mongolia	Middle East, India
E	Africa	——
F	American Natives, Polynesia, Central and South America	——
G	United States, France	——
H	Nicaragua, Mexico and California	——

MOLECULAR BASIS OF HBV GENOTYPES

Hepatitis B virus has 4 overlapping open reading frames. The core gene of the HBV is divided into pre-core and core region, and it encodes both the hepatitis core protein (HBcAg) and the "e" antigen (HBeAg). It is well documented that there is a correlation between hepatitis B viral genotypes and mutation in the pre-core and core promoter region, which results in the cessation of HBeAg production.[30-33]

In HBV genome, positions 1847 to 1917 are part of a pregenomic RNA encapsidation signal,

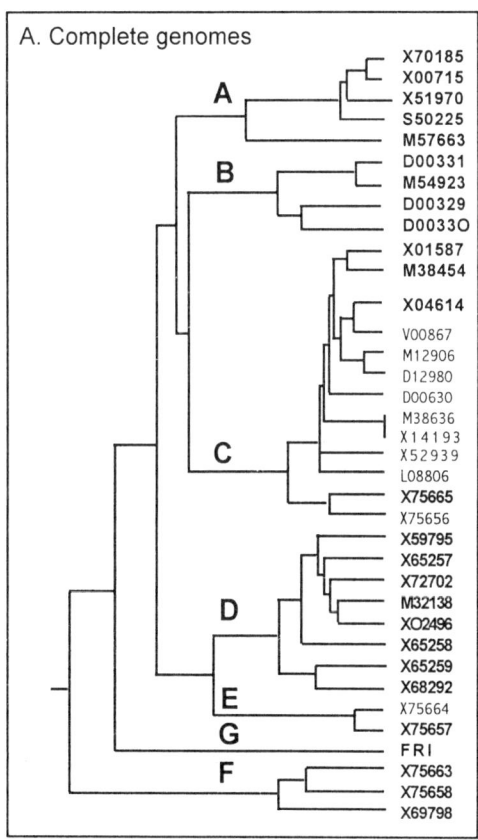

Fig. 2. Phylogenetic tree of HBV isolate of different genotype constructed with sequences of complete genome. Virus isolates are indicated by their gene bank accession number (Stuyver, et al)[11]

consisting of a hairpin RNA structure. This has two functions: encapsidation of HBV genome together with the viral polymerase and activation of the viral polymerase.[34-36] The commonest mutation in the pre-core region is a G to A substitution at nucleotide 1896, which creates a premature stop codon (M_1) consequently leading to cessation of HBeAg production. The basis for the genotype dependent selection of the M1 mutation is associated with the need to maintain base pairing of the stem loop structure of the pre-genomic encapsulation sequence epsilon (ε).[37, 38] HBV genotypes B, C and D generally have a 'T' at nucleotide 1858, which is directly opposite to the nucleotide 1896 in the stem of epsilon. However, in genotype A, frequently 'C' is present at nucleotide 1858 which forms a more stable bond in the wild type HBV strain with "G" at 1896 rather than a variant sequence with "A" at 1896 (M1 mutation).[39] The mutation M2 with G to A transition at nucleotide 1899 (GGC-GAC) also produces the best base pairing with an additional A to T change at nucleotide 1850. These additional mutations which result in the same encapsidation structure found in other genotypes except A, permit the best base pairing in the hair pin structure.[38, 40] The presence of M1 or M1+M2 mutation in genotype A without additional changes, would be thermodynamically unfavourable. The structural alterations mainly in the bulge lead to the high positivity of stabilization energy, which is essential for the reverse transcription of viral RNA[36] (Fig. 3).

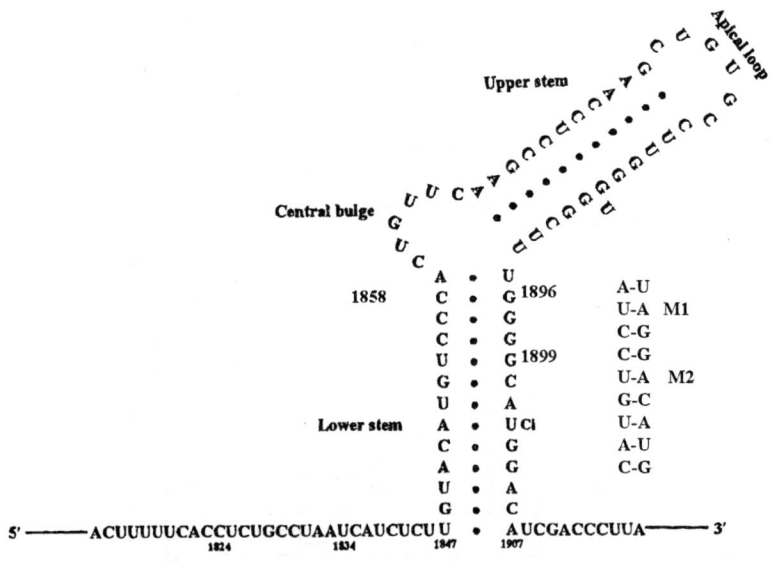

Fig. 3. Predicted secondary structure of pre genomic HBV RNA encapsidation signal showing: (A) base pairing in genotype A. (B) The effect of precore mutation (M1 and M2) in the base pairing in genotype D. The substitution C to U at 1858 permits correct base pairing with M1 variant in genotype D.

Recently, the mechanism which maintains HBeAg production has been explored in HBV genotype G in spite of the presence of 2 loop codons in the pre-core region.[41] Based on the partial sequencing of few clones, they found that all 4 patients with genotype G, who were HBeAg positive, were co-infected with genotype A. In patients who seroconverted to 'e' antibody, a shift from predominant genotype A to predominant genotype G took place.

Correlation of HBV genotype and subtype

The geographical distribution of different subtypes of HBV is well documented. These are ayw1, ayw2, ayw3, ayw4, ayr, adw2, adw4, adrq+, adrq-.[24] To some extent there is correlation between subtypes and genotypes of HBV.[27] Although some subtypes are genetically heterogenous, which encode more than one genotype. The genetic variability of HBV strain to some degree is influenced by their antigenic expression.

In general, strain adw2 shows a considerable heterogeneity and is found to be associated with genotypes A, B, C and G. African and Vietnamese genomes encoding ayw1, and ayr were found in genotypes A and B respectively.[28] However, genotype C was also found associated with serotypes ayr, adrq+ and adrq−. The strain ayw2 and ayw3 were found in genotype D. It has been shown that the strain ayw4 and ayw4q− belonged to genotype E and F respectively (Table 2).

Table 2. Correlation of HBV genotypes and serotypes

Genotype	Serotype
A	adw2, ayw1
B	adw2, ayw1
C	ayr, adrq+, adrq−, adw2
D	ayw2, ayw3
E	ayw4
F	adw4q−
G	adw2

Diagnostic tools

HBV genotypes reflect the genetic relatedness between viral strains more reliably than the serotypes. As genotypes of HBV are classified based upon the 4 to 8% of genomic variability of the whole genomes, several methods have been used for HBV genotyping which include direct sequencing/phylogenetic analysis,[42] restriction fragment length polymorphism (RFLP),[43,44] multiplex polymerase chain reaction,[45] differential hybridization techniques[46] and enzyme linked immunoassay.

Full genomic sequences are ideal for genotype assignment, but sequence determination is very expensive and time consuming. However, sequencing of small fragments of S, pre-S and core gene have been used in many studies for genotype determination using phylogenetic tree construction. It has been shown that phylogenetic analysis of S-gene and full length HBV genome by the N-J method generates trees which clearly separate genetic clusters. They were identical with 82–100% boot strap values.[43] Upon these analysis it has been concluded that genotypes can be determined by S-gene sequencing. However, sequencing is not the method of choice for large number of specimens. Therefore a less complicated and less cumbersome method; RFLP was developed to genotype HBV in large number of samples. This method is based on the identification of genomic positions that not only reflect reliably the genotype difference but also harbor restriction sites that allow the identification of these differences. HBV genotype determination using RFLP included amplification of S-gene[43] or pre-S gene.[44] The sequence of the S-gene is more conserved than the pre-S region because S-gene overlaps reverse transcriptase active site in the P-gene which is encoded in a different frame.[47] Therefore, S-gene is more suitable for genotyping. However, pre-S region is the most variable part of the HBV genome. Lindh et al[44] have shown that pre-S analysis yields the same genotype grouping as the S-gene with the exception of NCBI sequence of subtype ayw carrying a 33 base pair deletion, typical of genotype D. This sequence was classified as genotype A by S-region analysis and genotype D by pre-S analysis. Thus, genotyping by RFLP of the pre-S region is useful, specifically for genotype D.

A method using multiplex PCR,[45] 6 primer sets were designed for each of the six genotypes according to the specific sequence and used separately for PCR. The genotypes were identified according to the positive PCR results.

HBV GENOTYPES AND LIVER DISEASE

In different parts of the world different HBV genotypes contribute widely to the severity of liver disease as a result of differences in the replication rates and the capability to escape immune clearance. Genotypic classification of other hepatotropic viruses such as hepatitis C virus (HCV) and hepatitis D virus (HDV) is also well documented.[48,49] The relationship between HCV or HDV genotypes with the severity of liver disease remains controversial, although HCV genotype 1b and HDV genotype 1 were found to be more pathogenic than others.[49,50] Recently, clinical relevance of HBV genotypes has been described from several parts of the world. A number of HBV strains have been found to display alteration of epitopes, resulting in escape from the host immune recognition, enhanced replication, resistance to antiviral therapy or facilitated cell attachment and or penetration.[51] HBV strain with an adenine (A) to thymine (T) transversion at nucleotide 1762 and a G to A transition at nucleotide 1764 in the basal core promoter region are generally found to be present in chronic hepatitis, fulminant hepatitis and HCC and less often in asymptomatic subjects with chronic HBV infection and immune suppressed patients.[52] It has been suggested that changes in the secondary structure of the pre genome creates T1762/A1764 mutation which may increase viral replication through increase in core protein synthesis and creation of a binding site for transcription factor HNF1 (hepatoyte nuclear factor).[53]

Severity of liver disease

East A correlation between HBV genotype and liver disease has been described in several studies from east Asia.[54] A high prevalence of genotype B and C is found in eastern part of Asia including Japan, China, Taiwan, etc. Most of the studies from this region of Asia have found higher prevalence of HBeAg in patients with genotype C than genotype B, suggesting higher HBeAg clearance rate among patients with genotype B.[31,32,55,56] A Japanese study including 466 patients found presence of HBeAg in 53% of genotype C versus 16% of genotype B.[32] A recent study of 269 Chinese patients showed that spontaneous HBeAg seroconversion occurred nearly one decade earlier among patients with genotype B.[57] In a study from Japan, deranged serum ALT level was uncommon with serotype adw, mainly genotype B as compared with serotype adr, mainly genotype C.[58] Another study found that HBsAg positive subjects with genotype B had lower histological activity score.[31] A recent study from Hong Kong has correlated severe icteric flare-up in chronic HBV infection with viral genotype. Ninety one percent patients with IF had genotype B which was significantly higher than the asymptomatic HBsAg positive subjects, early cirrhosis and decompensated cirrhosis patients. On the other hand, genotype C was the predominant strain at different stages of chronic liver disease.[59] A study involving 490 Chinese patients found that genotype C was more prevalent in patients with cirrhosis.[55] Possibly longer duration of high level of HBV replication may contribute to more active liver disease and higher progression to cirrhosis in genotype C.

West Unlike Asia excluding India, genotypes A, D and F are prevalent in the western part of the world. A study from Switzerland involving only 65 patients have shown that genotype A was more common in patients with chronic HBV infection whereas genotype D was more frequent with resolving acute infection.[60] Acute liver failure and association of HBV genotype was studied in the United states. Hepatitis B virus infection was found in 9 of the 139 patients studied with acute liver failure. HBV genotypes A, B, C, and F were present in 4, 3, 1, and 1 patients respectively. Seven of the nine patients had pre-core and core promoter variants.[61]

Indian experience

Limited information is available on the prevalence, profile and significance of HBV genotypes in chronic HBV infection in the Indian subcontinent. A couple of isolated studies from India have studied the prevalence of HBV genotypes, their correlation to severity of liver disease and the outcome of interferon therapy.[62,63] Two available studies reveal that genotypes A and D are predominant in HBV related chronic liver disease patients of Indian origin (Fig. 4). Of the 130 patients studied at our center, 60 (46%) belonged to genotype A and 63 (48%) revealed the presence of genotype D. In the remaining seven (6%), patients, mixed genotype A and D were found. Patients infected with mixed genotype were younger.[62]

Genotypes A and D were originally widely distributed in the old world. The prevalence of genotype A in Indian population indicates a possible similar source of infection as in the European population. This observation has an important epidemiological implication which could be due to migration between India and UK over the past 300 years. Genotypes of HBV are subtype specific. In the Indian population the most prevalent sub types of HBV are adw and ayw, although a few reports document the presence of subtype adr in the southern part of India.[64] Presence of genotypes A and D in Indian population is well correlated to the prevalence of subtype adw and ayw. Genotype A in India and Europe is again subtype related as subtype adw encoded by genotype A is prevalent in the Western world. Other prevalent genotype of HBV in India is D, encoded by the strain ayw2 and ayw3, which are prevalent in the Indian population.

↑ Nt418 (S-gene)

Patient1	CCTGCTGCTA	TGCCTCATCT	TCTTGTTGGT	TCTTCTGGAC	TATCAAGGTA
Patient2	CCTGCTGCTA	TGCCTCATCT	TCTTGTTGGT	TCTTCTGGAC	TATCAAGGTA
Patient3	CCTGCTGCTA	TGCCTCATCT	TCTTGTTGGT	TCTTCTGGAC	TATCAAGGTA
Patient4	CCTGCTGCTA	GGCCTCATCT	TCTTATTGGT	TCTTCTGGAT	TATCAAGGTA
Patient5	CCTGCTGCTA	TGCCTCATCT	TCTTGTTGGT	TCTTCTGGAC	TATCAAGGTA
Patient6	CCTGCTGCTA	TGCCTCATCT	TCTTGTTGGT	TCTTCTGGAC	TATCAAGGTA
Patient7	CCTGCTGCTA	TGCCTCATCT	TCTTATTGGT	TCTTCTGGAT	TATCAAGGTA
Patient8	CCTGCTGCTA	TGCCTCATCT	TCTTGTTGGT	TCTTCTGGAC	TATCAAGGTA
Patient9	CCTGAGCTA	TGCCTCATCT	TCTTGTTGGT	TCTTCTGGAC	TATCAAGGTA
Patient10	CCTGCTGCTA	TGCCTCATCT	TCTTGTTGGT	TCTTCTGGAC	TATCAAGGTA
Patient11	CCTGCTGCTA	TGCCTCATCT	TCTTGTTGGT	TCTTCTGGAC	TATCAAGGTA
Patient12	CCTGCTGCTA	TGCCACATCT	TCTTGTTGGT	TCTTCTGGAC	TATCAAGGTA
Patient13	CCTGCTGCTA	TGCCACATCT	TCTTGTTGGT	TCTTCTGGAC	TATCAAGGTA
Patient14	CCTGCTGCTA	TGCCTCATCT	TCTTGTTGGT	TCTTCTGGAC	TATCAAGGTA
Patient15	CCTGCTGCTA	TGCCTCATCT	TCTTGTTGGT	TCTTCTGGAC	TATCAAGGTA
Patient16	CCTGCTGCTA	TGCCTCATCT	TCTTGTTGGT	TCTTCTGGAC	TATCAAGGTA
Patient17	CCTGCTGCTA	TGCCTCATCT	TCTTGTTGGT	TCTTCTGGAC	TATCAAGGTA
Patient1	TGTTGCCCGT	TTGTCCTCTA	ATTCCAGGAT	CTTCAACCAC	CAGCGTGGGA
Patient2	TGTTGCCCGT	TTGTCCTCTA	ATTCCAGGAT	CTTCAACCAC	CAGCGTGGGA
Patient3	TGTTGCCCGT	TTGTCCTCTA	ATTCCAGGAT	CTTCAACCAC	CAGCACGGGA
Patient4	TGTTGCCCGT	TTGTCCTCTA	ATTCCAGGAT	CAACAACAAC	CAGTACGGGA
Patient5	TGTTGCCCGT	TTGTCCTCTA	ATTCCAGGAT	CTTCAACCAC	CAGCGTGGGA
Patient6	TGTTGCCCGT	TTGTCCTCTA	ATTCCAGGAT	CTTCAACCAC	CAGCGTGGGA
Patient7	TGTTGCCCGT	TTGTCCTCTA	ATTCCAGGAT	CATCGACAAC	CAGTACGGGA
Patient8	TGTTGCCCGT	TTGTCCTCTA	ATTCCAGGAT	CTTCAACCAC	CAGCACGGGA
Patient9	TGTTGCCCGT	TTGTCCTCTA	ATTCCAGGAT	CTTCAACCAC	CAGCACGGGA
Patient10	TGTTGCCCGT	TTGTCCTCTA	ATTCCAGGAT	CTTCAACCAC	CAGCGTGGGA
Patient11	TGTTGCCCGT	TTGTCCTCTA	ATTCCAGGAT	CTTCAACCAC	CAGCGTGGGA
Patient12	TGTTGCCCGT	TTGTCCTCTA	ATTCCAGGAT	CTTCAACCAC	CAGCACGGGA
Patient13	TGTTGCCCGT	TTGTCCTCTA	ATTCCAGGAT	CTTCAACCAC	CAGCACGGGA
Patient14	TGTTGCCCGT	TTGTCCTCTA	ATTCCAGGAT	CTTCAACCAC	CAGTACGGGA
Patient15	TGTTGCCCGT	TTGTCCTCTA	ATTCCAGGAT	CTTCAACCAC	CAGTACGGGA
Patient16	TGTTGCCCGT	TTGTCCTCTA	ATTCCAGGAT	CTTCAACCAC	CAGCGTGGGA
Patient17	TGTTGCCCGT	TTGTCCTCTA	ATTCCAGGAT	CTTCAACCAC	CAGCGTGGGA
Patient1	CCATGCAGAA	CCTGCACGAC	TACTGTTCAA	GGAACCTCTA	TGTATCCCTC
Patient2	CCATGCAGAA	CCTGCACGAC	TACTGTTCAA	GGAACCTCTA	TGTATCCCTC
Patient3	CCATGCAGAA	CCTGCACGAC	TCCTGCTCAA	GGAACCTCTA	TGTATCCCTC
Patient4	CCCTGCAAAA	CCTGCACGAC	TCCTGCTCAA	GGCAACTCTA	TGTTTCCCTC
Patient5	CCATGCAGAA	CCTGCACGAC	TACTGTTCAA	GGAACCTCTA	TGTATCCCTC
Patient6	CCATGCAGAA	CCTGCACGAC	TACTGTTCAA	GGAACCTCTA	TGTATCCCTC
Patient7	CCCTGCAAAA	CCTGCACGAC	TCCTGCTAAG	GCCAATCTTA	TGTTTCCCTC
Patient8	CCATGCAGAA	CCTGCACGAC	TCCTGCTCAA	GGAACCTCTA	TGTATCCCTC
Patient9	CCATGCAGAA	CCTGCACGAC	TACTGTTCAA	GGAACCTCTA	TGTATCCCTC
Patient10	CCATGCAGAA	CCTGCACGAC	TACTGTTCAA	GGAACCTCTA	TGTATCCCTC
Patient11	CCATGCAGAA	CCTGCACGAG	TACTGTTCAA	GGAACCTCTA	TGTATCCCTC
Patient12	CCACTGAGAA	CCTGCACGAC	TCCTGCTCAA	GGAACCTCTA	TGTATCCCTC
Patient13	CCATGCAGAA	CCTGCACGAC	TCCTGCTCAA	GGAACCTCTA	TGTATCCCTC
Patient14	CCATGCAGAA	CCTGCACGAC	TCCTGCTCAA	GGAACCTCTA	TGTATCCCTC
Patient15	CCATGCAGAA	CCTGCACGAC	TCCTGCTCAA	GGAACCTCTA	TGTATCCCTC
Patient16	CCATGCAGAA	CCTGCACGAC	TACTGTTCAA	GGAACCTCTA	TGTATCCCTC
Patient17	CCATGCAGAA	CCTGCACGAC	TACTGTTCAA	GGAACCTCTA	TGTATCCCTC

nt618 (S-gene)

Patient1	CTGTTGCTGTA	CCAAACCTTC	GGACGGAAAT	TGCACCTGTA	TTCCCATCCC
Patient2	CTGTTCCTGTA	CCAAACCTTC	GGACGGAAAT	TGCACCTGTA	TTCCCATCCC
Patient3	CTGTTGCTGTA	CCAAACCTTC	GGACGGAAAT	TGCACCTGTA	TTCCCATCCC
Patient4	ATGCTGCTGTA	CAAAACCTAC	GGATGGAAAT	TGCACCTGTA	TTCCCATCCC
Patient5	CTGTTGCTGTA	CCAAACCTTC	GGACGGAAAT	TGCACCTGTA	TTCCCATCCC
Patient6	CTGTTGCTGTA	CCAAACCTTC	GGACGGAAAT	TGCACCTGTA	TTCCCATCCC
Patient7	ATGTTGCTGTA	CAAAACCTAC	GGATGGAAAT	TGCACCTGTA	TTCCCATCCC
Patient8	CTGTTGCTGTA	CCAAACCTTC	GGACGGAAAT	TGCACCTGTA	TTCCCATCCC
Patient9	CTGTTGCTGTA	CCAAACCTTC	GGACGGAAAT	TGCACCTGTA	TTCCCATCCC
Patient10	CTGTTGCTGTA	CCAAACCTTC	GGACGGAAAT	TGCACCTGTA	TTCCCATCCC
Patient11	CTGTTGCTGT-	CCAAACCTTC	GGACGGAAAT	TGCACCTGTA	TTCCCATCCC
Patient12	CTGTTGCTGTA	CCAAACCTTC	GGACGGAAAT	TGCACCTGTA	TTCCCATCCC
Patient13	CTGTTGCTGTA	CCAAACCTTC	GGACGGAAAT	TGCACCTGTA	TTCCCATCCC
Patient14	CTGTTCCTGTA	CCCCCCCTTC	GGACGGAAAT	TGCACCTGTA	TTCCCATCCC
Patient15	CTGTTCCTGTA	CCCCCCCTTC	GGACGGAAAT	TGCACCTGTA	TTCCCATCCC
Patient16	CTGTTGCTGTA	CCAAACCTTC	GGACGGAAAT	TGCACCTGTA	TTCCCATCCC
Patient17	CTGTTGCTGTA	CCAAACCTTC	GGACGGAAAT	TGCACCTGTA	TTCCCATCCC

Fig. 4. Variability of S-gene sequence (nt 418-618) of 17 Indian patients showing differences between genotypes A and D. Patients 4 and 7 show clustering with the sequence of genotype A[62]

The relationship of genotype with severity of liver disease may also depend on the inherent biological difference in the genotype. It has been shown in the Indian population that genotype A was more common in patients with milder disease. In one study from New Delhi, 130 chronic HBV infected patients were studied. Of them 52 were incidentally detected asymptomatic hepatitis B surface antigen positive subjects (IDAHS), 48 were cirrhotic and 30 had hepatocellular carcinoma. Genotype distribution in relation to severity of liver disease in the IDAHS group was assessed on the basis of histological activity index (HAI), Child's score and age of the patient. In the IDAHS group, subjects were divided into (i) HAI < 4 and (ii) HAI > 4. The presence of genotype D was significantly higher in IDAHS with HAI >4 (53 vs. 32%, p<0.05). In IDAHS subjects infected with genotype D, none had HAI of <4.

On the other hand, genotype A was more common in patients with a milder disease (HAI <4). In patients with severe disease, the percentage of genotype D was significantly higher as compared to genotype A (61 vs. 39%, p<0.05).

Development of hepatocellular carcinoma (HCC)

Hepatitis B virus X gene of HBV genome encodes two proteins that have potent transactivation properties on viral as well as cellular gene.[65] Thus X gene plays the role of a candidate gene in the development of HCC. The coding sequence overlaps the enhancer and core promoter region which are important for HBV replication. Mutations in this region alter amino acid in X protein and thus HBV gene expression. Precisely basal core promoter could be a candidate molecular marker for the pathogenic differences among the HBV genotypes.

East Studies from Taiwan and Japan have shown that genotype C is associated with the development of HCC and has lower response rate to interferon therapy as compared to genotype B.[54-56] The data related to the association of HBV genotypes and development of HCC is contradictory. One study found that genotype B is associated with the development of HCC at an earlier stage,[31] however, it was not confirmed by other studies.[32, 55, 56] Development of HCC was also found to be associated with core promoter mutation in patients of Chinese origin. This study revealed that genotype C causes more severe disease.[66] This hypothesis was supported by the Japanese investigators. They found that development of HCC occurred in 21% vs. 71% in patients infected with HBV genotypes B and C respectively. They also found that patients with genotype C showed poor response to embolization therapy.[67]

West In western countries, HCC associated with HBV or HCV infection usually occurs in cirrhotic liver. In Caucasian patients with compensated cirrhosis, HCC was found to be associated with 2% HBV and 2.5% HCV infection respectively.[68]

India The only available study from Indian sub-continent, compared the association of HBV genotypes in patients with HCC and IDAHS. The study revealed that genotype D was more prevalent in HCC patients of < 40 years of age as compared to IDAHS (63% vs. 49%, $p < 0.06$).[62]

HEPATITIS B VIRUS GENOTYPES AND ANTIVIRAL THERAPIES

Interferon A pathogenic difference among various HBV genotypes is well established. In addition pre-core stop codon mutant (G1896A) and core promoter mutants (A1762T and G1764A) have been reported to influence the therapeutic response to interferon.[69-72] These results prompted investigators to hypothesize an association between interferon response and HBV genotypes.

East From eastern Asia, Kao et al studied 68 patients and found that the rate of HBeAg loss was significantly higher in patients with genotype B compared to those with genotype C (41% vs. 15%).[54] Japanese investigators studied correlation of HBV genotype to Interferon response in patients with acute HBV infection. Interferon was given to the seven patients with acute prolonged HBV infection, and four of them responded by clearing hepatitis B e antigen (HBeAg) and surface antigen (HBsAg) from the serum. Of the four responders, one was infected with HBV genotype B and three with genotype C. HBsAg persisted in the remaining three patients all of whom were infected with HBV genotype A, and HBeAg stayed positive in one of them. These results indicate that HBV genotype A prevails in Japanese patients with acute hepatitis B, and suggest a high efficacy of interferon in the adult patients with acute prolonged HBV infection, except in those infected with HBV genotype A.[73]

West In a German study including 64 patients, the rate of interferon induced HBeAg seroconversion was higher among patients with genotype A than those with genotype D (37% vs. 6%).[70] In another study from the west, consisting of 35 HBeAg negative patients, those with genotype A responded better than genotype D/E (70% vs. 40%).[72] Little is known about co-infection among several hepatitis B virus (HBV) genotypes. In a recent study from Sweden, genotypic coinfection were found in 20 (67%) of 30 hepatitis B e antigen-positive patients treated with interferon (IFN). In 8 of these patients, coinfection or genotype shifts were detectable by direct sequencing or standard pre-S genotyping. In most of these cases, genotypic changes were detected after a >2-log decrease or increase of the HBV-DNA level. The presence of genotype mixtures did not significantly influence IFN response. Because quasi-species selection may occur at or shortly after transmission, patients might acquire HBV infection from subjects who appear to be infected with different genotypes.[74]

India In a small study on 24 HBeAg positive patients, a better response to interferon therapy was seen in patients with genotype D than genotype A.[63]

Lamivudine

Correlation between HBV genotype and response to lamuvidine therapy is being evaluated. Lamuvidine, nucleoside analogue, is a potent inhibitor of a HBV reverse transcriptase.[75] It has been shown that lamivudine rapidly suppresses HBV replication, improves liver histology in both HBeAg +ve and anti-HBe positive patients with chronic hepatitis B virus infection.[76-80] However, the use of lamivudine is hampered due to the selection of drug resistant HBV variants. Strains of HBV with lamivudine resistance associated mutation have been detected in 14-32% of patients after 1 year of treatment,[76-78, 81] the frequency increasing to 38%, 57% and 66% after 2, 3 and 4 years of treatment respectively.[82-84] The heterogeneity in disease manifestation and response to antiviral treatment in different parts of the world could be influenced by the varied geographic distribution of HBV strains.

East The natural history of hepatitis B virus infection in patients with Asian ethnicity is different as the onset of infection in these people occurs perinatally or at early childhood. A number of clinical trials to assess the efficacy of lamivudine in the treatment of chronic HBV infection have been carried out in China, Korea, Taiwan, and Japan. However, only a few studies have correlated the lamivudine response with HBV genotype. A study from a Taiwan compared HBV genotypes between 42 patients with sustained response and 43 patients who relapsed. All the patients received lamivudine for a mean period of 16 months. The follow-up period was 12–60 months. Stepwise logistic regression analysis showed that genotype B was the only predictor (odds ratio 7.793, 95% confidence interval, p=0.002) for sustained response.[85] Another study from Japan studied only five patients with chronic hepatitis B who showed HBV breakthrough after taking lamivudine for 1 year.[86] HBV genotype and lamivudine resistant mutations of the polymerase gene were determined. All the five patients were genotype C. Four patients had substitution of valine or isoleucine in place of leucine at residue 426 in P-gene together with M550I. In the remaining patient, change from leucine to methionine at residue 428 was found with M550V in the P-gene. Based on these observations, the investigators concluded that the occurrence of HBV polymerase mutation at residue 426 in combination with M550I is common in Japanese HBV genotype C infected patients who develop resistance to lamivudine.

West In a study by Buti et al,[87] of the 27 patients, 16 had genotype A and 11 genotype D. After one year of therapy, virological and biochemical response was similar in genotype A (62.5%) and genotype D (64%) patients. After two years of therapy, it was 53% vs. 55% for genotype A and D respectively. Thus, they concluded that HBV genotype does not play an important role in the response to lamivudine therapy. There is limited data on a small number of patients on the association of HBV genotype and response to lamivudine therapy.[78, 79] On the other hand, there are a few studies available in the literature correlating the HBV subtype with lamivudine response.[79, 80] In a series of 43 patients, 22 had subtype adw and 21 had subtype ayw. Response to lamivudine therapy determined at 12 months showed that subtype ayw responds significantly better than subtype adw.

India The predominant HBV genotypes in India are A and D. Limited information is available regarding the association of response of lamivudine therapy with genotype from the Indian subcontinent. Seventy-six consecutive liver biopsy proven HBV related chronic liver disease patients were studied by our group;[88] 26 (34%) were responders and 50 (66%) non-responders. There was no difference in the profile and pre-therapy viral load among the responders and non-responders. In group I, of the 26 responders, 8 (31%) had genotype A and 18 (69%) had genotype D. Similarly in group II, of the 50 non-responders, 20 (40%) had genotype A and 30 (60%) had genotype D. Patients with genotype D achieved higher SVR than genotype A. Long term follow-up of these patients is awaited.

The available literature from all over the world suggests, that HBV genotypes would become a useful tool for studying the natural history of HBV, tracing the route of HBV infection and most importantly, for predicting the response to antiviral therapies. Since genotypes are associated with different viral mutations, larger studies should be carried out to determine their relevance to therapeutic outcomes. Additional studies from different geographical regions are needed for complete understanding of the utility of HBV genotype in predicting the response to lamivudine therapy. Such an information would be of help in better patient selection for lamivudine therapy and possibly even the choice of antiviral drugs.

REFERENCES

1. Tiollais P, Pource C, Dejean A. The hepatitis B virus. *Nature* 1985;317:489-95.
2. Will H, Reiser W, Weimer T, Pfaff E, Buschar M, Sprengel R, Cattaneo R, et al. Replication strategy of hepatitis B virus. *J Virol* 1987;61:904-11.
3. Summers J and Mason WS. Replication of the genome of a hepatitis B-like virus by reverse transcription of an RNA intermediate. *Cell* 1982;29:408-15.
4. Holland J, Spindler K, Horodyzki F, Grabou E, Nechol S, Vandepol S. Rapid evolution of RNA genomes. *Science* 1982;215:1577-85.
5. Steinhauer DA, Holland JJ. Direct method for quantitation of extreme polymerase error frequencies at selected single base sites in viral RNA. *J Virol* 1986;57:219-28.
6. Orito E, Mizokami M, Ina Y, Moriyama N, Kameshima N, Yamamoto M, Gojobori T, et al. Host independent evolution and antigenic classification of the hepadnavirus family based on nucleotide sequences. *Proc Natl Acad Sci USA* 1989;86:7059-62.
7. Okamoto H, Imai M, Kametani M, Nakamura T, Mayumi M. Genomic heterogeneity of hepatitis B virus in a 54 year old woman who contracted the infection through materno-fetal transmission. *Jpn J Exp Med* 1987;57:231-6.
8. Yotsumoto S, Okamoto H, Tsuda F, Miyakawa Y, Mayumi M. Sub typing hepatitis B virus DNA in free or integrated forms by amplification of the S-gene sequence by the polymerase chain reaction and single track sequencing for adenine. *J Virol Methods* 1990;28:107-16.
9. Norder H, Courouce AM, Magnius LO. Complete genome, phylogenetic relatedness and structural proteins of six strains of the hepatitis B virus, four of which represent two new genotypes. *Virology* 1994;198:489-503.
10. Okamoto H, Tsuda F, Sakagawa H, Sastrosoewignjo RI, Imai M, Miyakawa Y, Mayumi M. Typing hepatitis B virus by homology in nucleotide sequence comparison of surface antigen subtypes. *J Gen Virol* 1988;69:2575-83.
11. Stuyver L, De Gendt S, Van Geyt C, Zoulim F, Fried M, Schinazi RF, Rossau R. A new genotype of hepatitis B virus. Complete genome and phylogenetic relatedness. *J Gen Virol* 2000;81:67-74.

12. Fuiyama A, Miyanohara A, Nozaki C, Yoneyama T, Ohtomo N, Matsubara K. Cloning and structural analysis of hepatitis B virus DNA, sub type adr. *Nucleic acids Res* 1983;11:4601-46.
13. Galibert F, Mandart E, Fitousri F, Tiollais P, Charnay P. Nucleotide sequence of the hepatitis B virus genome (subtype ayw) cloned in E. coli. *Nature* 1979;28:1:646-50.
14. Okamoto H, Imai M, Shimozaki M, Hoshi Y, Lizuka H, Gotanda T, Tsuda F, et al. Nucleotide sequence of a cloned hepatitis B virus genome, subtype ayr; comparison with genomes of the other three subtypes. *J Gen Virol* 1986;67:2305-14.
15. Valenzuel P, Quiroga M, Zavidar J, Gray H, Rutler WJ. The nucleotide sequence of the hepatitis B viral genome and the identification of the major viral genes. New York Academic Press, 1980.
16. Arauz-Ruiz P, Norder H, Robertson BH, Magnius LO. Genotype H: a new Ameri-indian genotype of hepatitis B virus revealed in Central America. *J Gen Virol* 2002;83:2059-73.
17. Mimms LT, Solomon LR, Ebert JW, Fields H. Unique Pre-S sequence in a gibbon derived hepatitis B virus variant. *Biochem Biophys Res Commun* 1993;195:186-91.
18. Norder H, Ebert JW, Fields HA, Mushashwar IK, Magnius LO. Complete sequencing of a gibbon hepatitis B virus genome reveals a unique genotype distantly related to the chimpanzees hepatitis B virus. *Virology* 1996;218:214-23.
19. Vaudin M, Wolstenholem AJ, Tsiuaye KN, Zuckerman AJ, Harrison TJ. The complete nucleotide sequence of the genome of a hepatitis B virus isolated from a naturally infected chimpanzee. *J Gen Virol* 1988;69:1388-9.
20. Zuckerman AJ, Thorrnton A, Howard CR, Tsiquaye KN, Jones DM, Brambell MR. Hepatitis B outbreak among chimpanzees at the London Zoo. *Lancet* 1978;8091:652-4.
21. Grethe S, Hecked JO, Riets Chel W, Hufwert F. Molecular epidemiology of hepatitis B virus variants in non-human Primates. *J Virol* 2000;74:5377-82.
22. Warren KS, Heeney JL, Swan RA, Heriyanto Verschor EJ. A new group of hepadnaviruses naturally infected organgutans. *Virology* 1999;73:7860-5.
23. Norder H, Hammas B, Lee SD, Bele C. Courouce AM, Mushawar IK, Magnius LO. Genetic relatedness of hepatitis B viral strains of diverse geographical origin and natural variation in the primary structure of the surface gene. *J Gen Virol* 1993;74:1341-8.
24. Courouce-Pauty AM, Plancon A, Soulier JP. Distribution of HBsAg subtype in the world. *Vox Sang* 1983;44:197-211.
25. Morozou V, Pisorava M, Groudenin M. Homologues recombination between different genotypes of hepatitis B. *Virus gene* 2000;60:55-65.
26. Nakano T, Lu L, Hu X, Mizokami M, Orito E, Shapiro C, Hadler S, et al. Characterization of hepatitis B virus genotypes among Yucpa Indians in Venezuela. *J Gen Virol* 2001;82:359-65.
27. Aranz RP, Norder H, Visona KA, Magnius LO. Genotype F Prevalence in HBV infected patients of Hispanic origin in central America and may carry the Pre-core stop mutant. *J Med Virol* 1997;51:305-12.
28. Norder H, Courouce AM, Magnius LO. Comparison of the amino acid sequence of nine different serotype of hepatitis B surface antigen and genomic classification of the corresponding hepatitis B virus strains. *J Gen Virol* 1992a;73:1201-8.
29. Norder H, Courouce AM, Magnius LO. Molecular basis of hepatitis B virus serotype variation within the four major subtypes. *J Gen Virol* 1992b;73:3141-5.
30. Frias FR, Buti M, Jardi R, Cotrina M, Viladomiu L, Estaban R, Guarbia J. Hepatitis B virus infection: Pre-core mutants and its relation to viral genotype and core mutations. *Hepatology* 1995;22:1641-7,
31. Rodrighez-Frias F, Buti M, Jardi R, Cotrina M, Viladomiu L, Esteban R, Guardia J. Hepatitis B virus infection: pre-core mutants and its relation to viral genotypes and core mutations. *Hepatology* 1995;22:1641-7.

32. Lindh M, Hannoun C, Dhillon AP, Norkrans G, Horal P. Core promoter mutations and genotypes in relation to viral replication and liver damage in East Asian hepatitis B virus carriers. *J Infect Dis* 1999;179:775-82.
33. Orito E, Mizokami M, Sakugawa H, Michitaka K, Ishikawa K, Ichida T, Okanoue T, et al. A case control study for clinical and molecular biological differences between hepatitis B virus of genotypes B and C. Japan HBV genotype research group. *Hepatology*. 2001;33:218-23.
34. Junkee-Niepmann M, Bartens chlager R, Schaller H. A short cis acting sequence is required for hepatitis B virus pre genome encapsidation and sufficient of foreign RNA. *EMBO J* 1990;9:3389-96.
35. Pollack JR, Ganem D. An RNA stem loop structure directs hepatitis B virus genomic RNA encapsidation. *J Virol* 1993;67:3254-63.
36. Wang GH, Zoulium F, Leper EH, Kilson J, Seeger C. Role of RNA in enzymatic activity of the reverse transcriptase of hepatitis B viruses. *J Virol* 1994;68:8437-42.
37. Li JS, Tong SP, Wen YM, Vitvitsky L. Zang Q, Trepo C. Hepatitis B virus genotype A rarely circulates as an HBe minus mutant; possible contribution of single nucleotide in the pre-core region. *J Virol* 1993;67:5402-10.
38. Lok AS, Akarca U, Greene S. Mutations in the pre-core region of hepatitis B virus serve to enhance the stability of the secondary structure of the pregenome encapsidation signal. *Proc Natl Acad Sci USA* 1994;91:4077-81.
39. Lindh M, Andersson AS, Gusdal A. Genotypes, nt 1858 variants, and geographic origin of hepatitis B virus large sclare analysis using a new genotyping method. *J Infect Dis* 1997;175:1285-93.
40. Laskus T, Rakela J, Persing DH. The stem loop structure of the cis-encapsidation signal is highly conserved in naturally occurring hepatitis B virus variants. *Virology* 1994;20:809-12.
41. Kato M, Orito E, Gish RG, Bzowej N, Newsom M, Sagauchi F, Suzuki S, et al. Hepatitis B 'e' antigen in sera from individuals infected with hepatitis B virus of genotype G. *Hepatology* 2002;35:922-9.
42. Ohba K, Mizokami M, Ohuo T, Suzuki K, Orito E, Lau JV, Ina U, et al, Relationship between serotype and genotype of hepatitis B virus: genetic classification of HBV by use of surface gene. *Virus Res* 1995;39:25-34.
43. Mizokami M, Nakano T, Orito OE, Tanaka Y, Sakugawa H, Mukaide M, Robertson BH. Hepatitis B virus genotype assignment using restriction fragment length polymorphism. *FEBS Lett* 1999;450:66-71.
44. Lindh M, Gongalez JE, Norkrans G, Horal P. Genotyping of hepatitis B virus by restriction pattern analysis of a Pre-S amplicon. *J Virol methods* 1998;72:163-74.
45. Yang J, Luo K, Guo Y, Dai L, Yan L, Hou J. Classification of genotyping hepatitis B virus with multiplex PCR. *Zhonghua, Gan Zang Bing Za Zhi* 2002;10:55-7.
46. Vangeyt C, DeGendt S, rombant A, Wyseur A, Maertens G, Rossau R, Stuyver L. *A line probe assay for hepatitis B virus genotypes*. In: Schinazi RF, Somma dossi JP, Thomas H, eds. Therapies for viral hepatitis. London. *International Medical Press* 1998;1399-1450.
47. Mizokami M, Orito E, Ohba K, Ikeo K, Lau JYN, Gojobori T. *J Mol Evol* 1997;44(suppl 1):S83-90.
48. Simmonds P, Alberti A, Bonino F, Bradley DW, Brechot C, Brouwer JT, et al. A proposed system for nomenclature for genotypes of hepatitis C virus. *Hepatology* 1994;19:1321-4.
49. Wu JC, Choo KB, Chen CM, Chen TZ, Huo T1, Lee SD. Genotyping of hepatitis D virus by restriction fragment length polymorphism and relation to outcome of hepatitis D. *Lancet* 1995;346:939-41.
50. Kao JH, Chen DJ, Lai MY, Yang PM, Sheu JC, Wang TH, Chen DS, et al. Genotypes of hepatitis C virus in Taiwan and the progression of liver disease. *J Clin Gastroenterol* 1995;21:233-7.
51. Gunther S, Fischer L, Pult I, Sterneck M, Will H. Naturally occurring variants of hepatitis B virus. *Adv Virus Res* 1999;52:125-37.

52. Hunt CM, Mc Gill JM, Allen MI, Condreay LD. Clinical relevance of hepatitis B viral mutations. *Hepatology* 2000;31:1037-44.
53. Kramvis A, Kew MC. The core promoter of hepatitis B virus. *J Viral Hepatitis* 1999;6:415-27.
54. Kao JH, Chen PJ, Lai MY, Chen DS. Hepatitis B genotypes correlate with clinical outcomes in patients with chronic hepatitis B. *Gastroenterology* 2000;118:554-9.
55. Ding X, Mizokami M, Yao G, Xu B, Orito E, Ueda R, Nakanishi M, et al. Hepatitis B virus genotype distribution among chronic hepatitis B virus carrier in Shanghai, China. *Intervirology* 2001;44:43-7.
56. Fujie H, Moriya J, Shintani Y, Yotsuyanagi H, lind S, Koike K, et al. Hepatitis B virus genotypes and hepatocellular carcinoma in Japan. *Gastroenterology* 2001;120:1564-5.
57. Chu CJ, Hussain M, Lok AS. Hepatitis B virus genotype B is associated with earlier HBeAg seroconversion compared to hepatitits B virus genotype C. *Gastroenterology* 2002;122:1756-62.
58. Shiina S, Fujino H, Uta V, Tagawa K, Unuma T, Yoneyama M, Ohmori T, et al. Relationship of HBsAg subtypes with HBeAg/anti-HBc status and chronic liver disease part I: analysis of 1744 HBsAg carriers. *Am J Gastroenterol* 1991;86:866-71.
59. Chan HL, Tsang SW, Wong ML, Tse CH, Leung NW, Chan FK, Sung JJ. Genotype B hepatitis B virus is associated with severe icteric flare-up of chronic hepatitis B virus infection in Hong Kong. *Am J Gastroenterol* 2002; 97:2629-33.
60. Mayerat C, Mantegani A, Frei PC. Does hepatitis B virus (HBV) genotype in influence the clinical outcome of HBV infection? *J Viral hepatitis* 1999;6:299-304.
61. Teo EK, Ostapowicz G, Hussain M, Lee WM, Fontana RJ, Lok AS. The US ALF study group (Acute Liver Failure). Hepatitis B infection in patients with acute liver failure in the United States. *Hepatology* 2001;33:972-6.
62. Thakur V, Guptan RC, Kazim SN, Malhotra V, Sarin SK. Profile, Spectrum and Significance of HBV genotype in chronic liver disease patients in the Indian subcontinent. *J Gastroenterol Hepatol* 2002;17: 165-70.
63. Thakur V, Maerten G, Guptan RC, Kazim SN, Sarin SK. Hepatitis B virus genotype variability and its influence on anti-viral therapy in HBeAg positive chronic hepatitis B in India. *Hepatology* 1998;28:216A.
64. Thyagarajan SP, Jayaram S, Mohanavalli B. *Prevalence of HBV in the general population of India. In:* Sarin SK, Singal AK, eds. Hepatitis B in India: Problems and Prevention. CBS Publishers & Distributors, New Delhi 1996;5-16.
65. Koike K. Hepatitis B virus HBx gene and hepato carcinogenesis. *Intervirology* 1995;38:134-42.
66. Fang ZL, Yang J, Ge X, Zhuang H, Gong J, Li R, Ling R, Harrison TJ. Core promoter mutations (A1762T and G1764A) and viral genotype in chronic hepatitis B and hepatocellular carcinoma in Guangxi, China. *J Med Virol* 2002;68:33-40.
67. Tsubota A, Arase Y, Ren F, Tanaka H, Ikeda K, Kumada H. Genotype may correlate with liver carcinogenesis and tumor characteristics in cirrhotic patients infected with hepatitis B virus subtype adw. *J Med Virol* 2001;65:257-65.
68. Fattovich G. Progression of hepatitis B and C to hepatocellular carcinoma in Western countries. *Hepatogastroenterology* 1998;45:1206-13.
69. Fattovich G, McIntyre G, Thursz M, Cotman K, Guiliano G, Alberti A, Thomas HC, et al. Hepatitis B virus precore/core variation and interferon therapy. *Hepatology* 1995;22:955-62.
70. Erhardt A, Reineke U, Blondin D, Gerlich WH, Adams O, Heintges T, Neiderau C, et al. Mutation of the core promoter and response to interferon treatment in chronic replicative hepatitis B. *Hepatology* 2000;31:716-25.
71. Hunt CM, McGill JM, Allen MI, Condreay LD, Clinical relevance of hepatitis B viral mutations. *Hepatology* 2000;31:1037-44.
72. Zhang Z, Zoulium F, Habersetzer F, Xiong S, Trepo C. Analysis of hepatitis B virus genotype and pre-

core region variability during interferon treatment of HBeAg negative chronic hepatitis *Br J Med Virol* 1996;48: 8-16.
73. Kobayashi M, Arare Y, Ikeda K, Tsubota A, Suzuki Y, Saitoh S, Kobayashi M, et al. Viral genotypes and response to interferon in patients with acute prolonged HBV infection of adulthood in Japan. *J Med Virol* 2002;68:522-8.
74. Hannoun C, Krogsgaard K, Horal P, Lindh M. Genotype mixture of hepatitis B virus in patients treated with interferon. *J Infect Dis* 2002;186:752-9.
75. Jarvis B, Faulds D. Lamivudine: A review of its therapeutic potential in chronic hepatitis B. *Drugs* 1999;58:101-41.
76. Lai CL, Chien RN, Leung NW, Chang TT, Guan R, Tai DI, Ng KY, et al. A one-year trial of lamivudine for chronic hepatitis B. Asia Hepatitis Lamivudine Study Group. *N Engl J Med* 1998;339: 61-8.
77. Dienstag JL, Schiff ER, Wright TL, Perrillo RP, Hann HWL, Goodman Z, Crowther L, et al. Lamivudine as initial treatment for chronic hepatitis B in the United States. *N Engl J Med* 1999;341: 1256-63.
78. Lau DT, Khokhar MF, Doo E, Ghany MG, Herion D, Park Y, Kleiner DE, et al. Long-term therapy of chronic hepatitis B with lamivudine. *Hepatology* 2000;32:828-34.
79. Santantonio T, Mazzola M, Iacovazzi T, Miglieta A, Guastadisegni A, Postore G. Long-term follow-up of patients with anti-HBe/HBV-DNA – positive chronic hepatitis B treated for 12 months with lamivudine. *J Hepatol* 2000;32:300-6.
80. Tasopoulos NC, Volpes R, Pastore G, Heathcote J, Buti M, Goldin R, Hawlet S, et al. Efficacy of lamivudine in patients with hepatitis B e antigen negative/hepatitis B virus DNA positive (precore mutant) chronic hepatitis B. *Hepatology* 1999;29:889-96.
81. Schalm SW, Heathcote J, Cianciara J, Farrell G, Sherman M, William B, Dhillon A, et al. Lamivudine and alpha-interferon combination treatment of patients with chronic hepatitis B infection: a randomized trial. *Gut* 2000;46:562-8.
82. Liaw YF, Leung NWY, Chang TT, Guan R, Tai DI, Ng KY, Chien RN, et al. Effects of extended lamivudine therapy in Asian patients with chronic hepatitis B. *Gastroenterology* 2000;119:172-80.
83. Leung NW, Lai CL, Chang TT, Guan R, Lee CM, Ng KY, Lim SG, et al. Extended lamivudine treatment in patients with chronic hepatitis B enhances hepatitis B e antigen seroconversion ratio, results after 3 years of therapy. *Hepatology* 2001;33:1527-32.
84. Chang TT, Lai CL, Liaw YF, et al. Incremental increase in HBeAg sero-conversion and continued ALT normalization in Asian chronic HBV patients treated with lamivudine for four years. *Antiviral therapy* 2000;5(suppl 1);B44 (abstract).
85. Chien RN, Liaw YF, Tsai SL, Yeh CT, Chu CM. HBV genotype is the major factor for durability of HBeAg responses to Lamivudine therapy. *Gastroenterological J Taiwan* 2002; 19:65.
86. Ogata N, Fujii K, Takigawa S, Nomoto M, Ichida T, Asakura H. Novel patterns of amino acid mutations in the hepatitis B virus polymerase in association with resistance to Lamivudine therapy in Japanese patients with chronic hepatitis B. *J Med Virol* 1999;59:270-6.
87. Buti M, Cotrina M, Valdes A, Jardi R, Frias FR, Esteban R. Is hepatitis B virus subtype testing useful in predicting virological response and resistance to Lamivudine? *J Hepatol* 2002;36:445-6.
88. Thakur V, Rehman S, Guptan RC, Kazim SN, Kumar S, Malhotra V, Sarin SK. Clinical utility of HBV genotype to predict outcome of lamivudine therapy in patients with chronic hepatitis B. *Indian J Gastroenterol* 2002;21:A103 (abstract).

18

Diagnosis of hepatitis B virus infection

Ashwani K Singal

The diagnosis of HBV infection is a little complex because of the presence of different viral antigens and antibodies and the ability of HBV to produce chronic hepatic inflammation leading to intricate serological profiles. The diagnosis was revolutionized by the discovery of Australia antigen, now called HBsAg, by Blumberg et al in 1965.[1] Later on different antigens and antibodies were discovered along with their serological assays. In the 1980s, advances in the molecular biology techniques led to the development of hybridization assays and polymerase chain reaction (PCR) assays that permitted the detection of as little as 10 molecules of HBV-DNA per ml of serum. With the increasing awareness about the disease, more and more subjects are being detected who are clinically asymptomatic but positive for HBsAg. This entity of IDAHS is emerging, and it is important to look for the presence of any significant liver disease in them. Previously these subjects were called 'carriers'. This term may be misleading and of late the consensus is evolving to abandon the term 'carrier' and replace it by 'chronic HBV infection with or without liver disease'.[2]

The mere presence of HBsAg in the serum is not enough to make a diagnosis of hepatitis B and it needs to be combined with the clinical history and the other serological and/or hybridization assays. It is now possible to accurately diagnose the clinical disease, differentiate acute and chronic liver disease due to HBV, stage the chronic liver disease, to know replication status of the HBV, to assess the progression of the disease, and monitor the efficacy of antiviral drugs. Before we discuss the laboratory diagnoses, a brief background about the antigen and antibody systems of HBV is necessary.

ANTIGEN SYSTEMS

The HBV has four major components: its genomic DNA, the core capsid (HBcAg), a viral polymerase, and HBsAg (Table 1). There are mainly 3 different antigens in this hepatotropic DNA virus, namely HBsAg (hepatitis B surface antigen), HBcAg (hepatitis B core antigen), and HBeAg (hepatitis B e antigen).

Table 1. Components of the hepatitis B virus

HBV component	Function	Common name	Size
Membrane antigen	Coats viral core	HBsAg	20 nm lipoprotein particle composed of ca. 100 polypeptides of S, Pre-S2 + S, and Pre-S1 + Pre-S2 + S
HBcAg	Viral core capsid surrounds and bonds to viral DNA	HBcAg, capsid protein, core antigen	28 nm assembly of ca.100 core polypeptides 21 kD in size
DNA	Carries genetic information to make all HBV components	ds DNA, HBV-DNA	2100 kD, 3.2 kbp in size occurs as partially double stranded DNA
DNA polymerase	Enzyme synthesizes DNA on a single stranded template	DNA polymerase	70 kD

HBsAg

Although there are various subtypes of HBsAg, they are not important from diagnostic point of view. They are, however, important for two reasons, to study the epidemiology and mutant forms of HBV. The 'a' determinant is common to HBsAg, irrespective of its source.[3] There are four different subdeterminants; d, y, w, and r, making four major subtypes of HBsAg (adw, adr, ayw, ayr). The 'ayw' subtype is more common in the west and north of India and 'adr' in other parts of India.[4] At least 50% of the anti-HBs that develops after recovery from acute hepatitis B or immunization with hepatitis B vaccine are directed against the 'a' determinant, thus providing cross protection against other subtypes of HBV. Coexistence of HBsAg and anti-HBs has been reported in about 24% of HBsAg positive individuals. Antibodies are not able to neutralize the circulating virions as they are directed against one of the subtypic determinants.[5] Sequencing has shown that there are as many as 50 mutations in the 389 amino acids in the surface proteins. These mutations appear to serve as long as the intensity of the HBV persists. However, these subspecialities appear to have little or no immunological relevance to either convalescence or protection. However, a single amino acid mutation is reported[6] in the 'a' epitope of the S antigen at amino acid 145 in which glycine is replaced with arginine. This is induced by immune pressure exerted by vaccination used on a large scale and is also known as vaccine-escape mutant (VEM). This escapes detection by the routinely used HBsAg kits and can lead to HBV breakthrough infection. Several other studies demonstrated the occurrence of more diagnostic—escape mutants in different parts of the world leading to diagnostic and subtypic failures.[7,8] It is, therefore, important that detection of HBsAg assays should be adapted to the occurrence of local variant sequences.

HBcAg

Treatment of the virus particle with the detergents leads to the release of core particle which is known as HBcAg. While HBsAg circulates freely, HBcAg is not detectable in the serum.

HBeAg

The detection of this antigen is important as it reflects the replication of HBV, and in turn, a highly infectious state. If there is a mutation in the pre-C region at codon 28 or 29, the secretion of HBeAg is prevented. This is labeled as precore mutant infection, and is present in 15–20% of the total cases of HBV infection in India.[9]

Genome of HBV

Inside the core of the virion is present the viral genome consisting of HBV-DNA and DNA polymerase. HBV-DNA is partially double stranded, the genome being carried on the longer strand. The structure of the DNA (Fig. 1) may be analysed using the highly specific restriction endonucleases isolated from *E. coli* and *H. influenzae*. There are 4 major regions: P, S, C, and X. The S region comprising the pre-S region and the S gene, codes for the viral core proteins. The importance of the pre-S region is more for the HBV mutants and for the synthesis of new polypeptide vaccines. The pre-S regions have come under intensive study in the last about 10 years. There appears to be no prognostic significance of these antigens in the natural course of the disease. In general, presence of pre-S antigens correlates with detection of HBV-DNA and virus replication.[10] The pre-S1 antigen has been shown to be implicated in

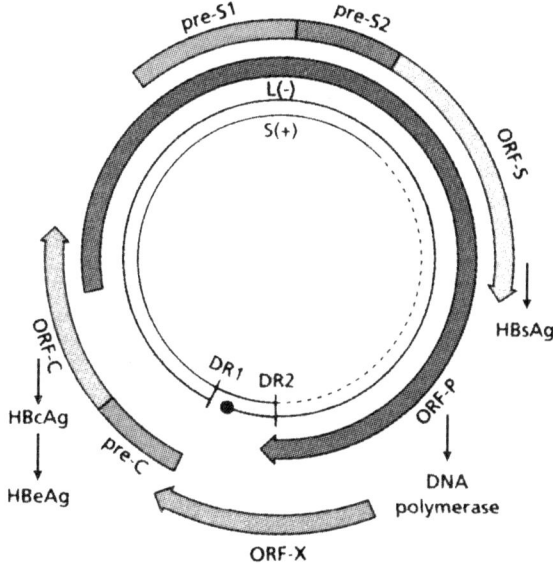

Fig. 1. Structure and organization of the genome of HBV

liver cell binding of HBV,[11] while the pre-S2 region has been implicated in assisting in an anti-HBs response to HBsAg vaccines containing only the S polypeptide.[12] The C-region codes for HBcAg and HBeAg. Region X codes for polypeptide of 154 amino acids, the HBx protein. Generally HBx protein is not detected in the serum of the patient because of its short half-life.[13] HBxAg appears to play a role in the regulation of HBV expression. Data suggest that it serves as a transcriptional transactivator, enhancing the transcription as well as the replication of HBV and other viruses. The data are emerging on the role of HBx protein in the hepatocarcinogenesis in India.[14] According to the homogeneity of the entire viral genome, HBV can be divided into seven genotypes, A-G.[15] In a recently published study, it was shown that genotype C is associated with more severe histological liver damage than genotype B.[16]

ANTIBODY SYSTEMS

Corresponding to each antigen, there is an antibody namely anti-HBs, anti-HBc, and anti-HBe.

Anti-HBs

It is generally found only after clearance of the HBsAg from the serum. Anti-HBs has been seen as conferring immunity against HBV. After vaccination, this is the usual antibody response. In patients who recover from acute hepatitis B, sero-conversion to anti-HBs occurs shortly after disappearance of HBsAg. There may be subjects who have an extended period between loss of antigenemia and appearance of anti-HBs, and this period is referred to as the 'core window',[17] a time when antibodies to HBcAg are the only serological indicators of HBV infection (Fig. 2). The anti-HBs antibody response after natural infection or after vaccination is protective against HBV infection.

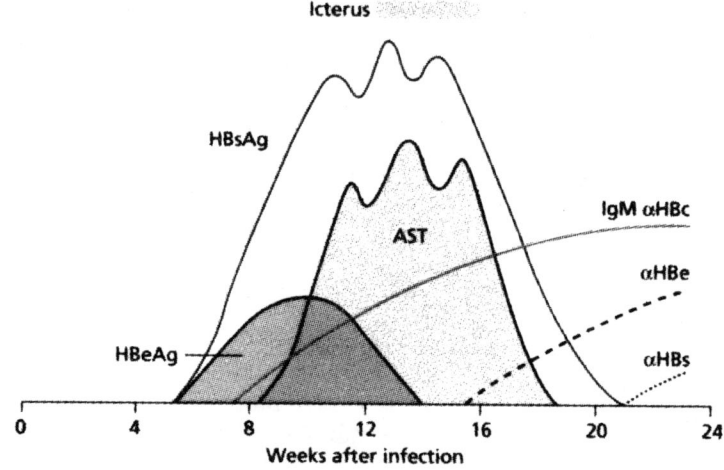

Fig. 2. Appearance of various antigens and antibodies after acute HBV infection.
ALT = alanine aminotransferase; PCR = polymerase chain reaction.

Anti-HBc

It develops within one month after the appearance of HBsAg, approximately 1–2 weeks before the liver enzymes start rising. In the acute phase, it is the IgM-anti-HBc, followed by IgG-anti-HBc which persists in the chronic state of the infection (Fig. 3).

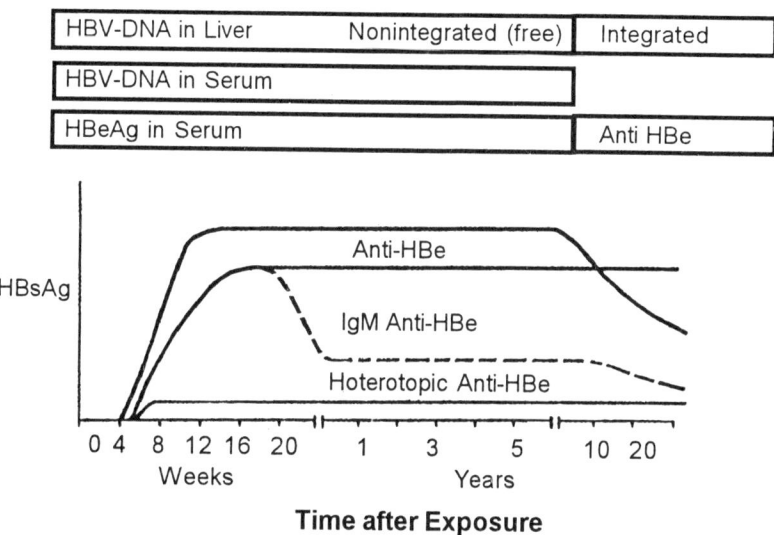

Fig. 3 Typical clinical and laboratory course of a patient with acute HBV infection that develops into chronic hepatitis B

Anti-HBe

As already stated, 'e' antigen denotes infectivity. The formation of anti-HBe usually denotes loss of infectivity and is considered to be the end-point of treatment of patients with chronic HBV infection on antiviral therapy.

METHODS TO DETECT HBV INFECTION

There are two types of tests to detect HBV infection, namely serological assays (to detect antigens and antibodies) and molecular assays (to detect the viral DNA). The technical details of the various tests is beyond the scope of this text and shall not be covered here.

Serological assays

By using the various serological methods, the different antigen and antibodies can be detected in the serum (Table 2). The sensitivity of the various modalities, however, is different (Table 3). The detection being highly dependent on the affinity or avidity of the antibody

Table 2. Sensitivity of serological assays

	Technique	Estimated sensitivity of detection (ng/ml)
First generation	* Immunodiffusion (ID)	5,000 – 10,000
	* Agar gel diffusion (AGD)	5,000 – 10,000
Second generation	* Counter immunoelectrophoresis (CIEP)	1,000 – 2,000
	* Complement fixation (CF)	200 – 400
	* Immune adherence hemagglutination assay (IAHA)	100 – 200
Third generation	* Passive hemagglutination assay (PHA)	5 – 20
	* Enzyme-linked immunosorbent assay (ELISA)	1.0 – 2.0
	* Radioimmunoassay (RIA)	0.5 – 1.0

Table 3. Hepatitis B serological assays

Name of the marker measured	Common name(s)	How measurement is made	Clinical utility
Hepatitis B surface antigen	HBsAg, Australia antigen	Sandwich RIA or EIA	Diagnose hepatitis B; assay HBsAg vaccines
Antibody to HBsAg	anti-HBs, anti-S, HBsAb	Sandwich RIA or EIA	Diagnose convalescence from disease; measure sero-conversion to vaccine
Antibody to core antigen (HBcAg)	anti-HBc, HBcAb	Competition of labelled anti-HBc and test serum for HBcAg	Identifies past hepatitis B disease and convalescence
IgM antibody to HBcAg	anti-HBc IgM, HBcAb-M	Human IgG capture assay Sandwich RIA	Measures current hepatitis B disease
Hepatitis B e antigen	HBeAg	using anti-HBe as the first and third layers	Indicates active disease and worse prognosis in chronic HBV infection
Antibody to HBeAg	anti-HBe, HBeAb	Neutralization followed by a sandwich assay	May be seen in active or past disease or optimistic prognosis in chronic HBV infection
Antibody to Pre-S2 antigen	anti-Pre-S2	Second antibody RIA	Unclear in disease and vaccine assays
Antibody to Pre-S1	anti-Pre-S1	Immunoblot or blocking EIA	Unclear in disease

being determined. The affinity constant is a measurement of the strength of binding of an antibody to a single distinct antigen, while avidity is defined as the net overall binding of a plurality of antibodies to complex antigen with more than one antibody binding domain. For the detection of these antigens and antibodies, the tests are now being carried out clinically, using more refined 3rd generation ELISA tests, for which the kits are commercially available.

HBsAg is the serologic hallmark of HBV infection. It can be detected by radioimmunoassay (RIA) or enzyme immunoassay (EIA). HBsAg appears in serum 1–10 weeks after an acute exposure to HBV and approximately 2–6 weeks before the onset of hepatitic symptoms or elevation of liver enzymes.[18] Initially, the HBsAg used to be detected by a method called agar gel diffusion (AGD) or counter immunoelectrophoresis (CIEP). These tests however, had low sensitivity and specificity. In 1972, a modified 'sandwich' radioimmunoassay (RIA) was developed.[19] Sandwich assays use anti-HBs that is bound to a solid phase to capture HBsAg from the specimen and a second labelled anti-HBs probe to identify the captured antigen. Sandwich assays have remained the method of choice for detecting HBsAg in the laboratory because of their long history of high sensitivity and specificity. In the last decade, enzyme sandwich immunoassays (EIAs) have largely replaced RIAs. Recent modified EIAs that use microspheres and computerized instrumentation produce very rapid and completely automated microparticle EIAs for HBsAg.[20, 21]

A negative test result for HBsAg with the current tests could be due to escape mutants,[22] – mutations in hepatitis B virus that produce changes in epitopes targeted by the detecting antibodies[23], and, mutations slowing the rate of virus replication thereby reducing the HBsAg to undetectable levels in the serum.[24] Due to the technical difficulties with RIA, EIA is most commonly used in clinical practice. It is based on a one step 'sandwich' principle. Antibody to HBsAg (anti-HBs) coupled to horseradish peroxidase (HRP) serves as the conjugate with tetramethyl benzidine (TMB) and peroxide as the substrate. Upon completion of the test, the development of color suggests the presence of HBsAg, and no or weak color development suggests the absence of HBsAg. Specifically, microelisa wells are coated with anti-HBs (murine monoclonal). Each microelisa well contains an HRP-labeled anti-HBs (ovine) conjugate sphere. The test sample or appropriate control containing HBsAg is inoculated in the microelisa wells. This test has the disadvantages of being expensive and more time consuming. The same test can be carried out using the 'card method' called "Hepacard", based on the same principle. The method uses monoclonal antibodies immobilized on a nitrocellulose strip in a thin line. The test sample is introduced to and from laterally through an absorbent pad where it mixes with the signal reagent. If the sample contains HBsAg, the colloidal gold antibody conjugate binds to the antigen, forming an antigen-antibody colloidal gold complex. The complex then migrates through the nitrocellulose strip by the capillary action. When the complex meets the line of immobilized antibody (test line), the complex is trapped, forming an antigen-antibody-colloidal gold complex. This forms a pink band indicating that the sample is positive for HBsAg. This gives the result within 20 minutes. False positive results can be obtained due to the presence of other antigen or elevated levels of rheumatoid factor. This occurs in less than 1% of the samples tested. A positive test by 'Hepacard' needs to be compared again with the usual kit or the well method. This is of significance for mass screening as it is a cheap method and results can be achieved faster. However, it shows overall agreement of 99% with RIA and EIA techniques.

Molecular methods

These are useful for detection of HBV-DNA and DNA polymerase. DNA in HBV was first detected in the infected serum by measuring the activity of the DNA polymerase enzyme present within the virion, but this method suffered from insensitivity, requiring a concentration of approximately 10^8 virions/ml to be detected. A number of tests have been developed to measure HBV-DNA in the serum of the infected individual. These tests differ in respect of their methodology, time to get results, their sensitivity and clinical utility (Table 4). Broadly, these tests can be divided into two groups.

Table 4. Different commercial assays for the measurement of serum HBV-DNA

Name	Company	Methodology	Lower limits of detection (genomes/ ml)	Time required in hours
Molecular hybridization assay	Abbott Laboratories	Liquid phase molecular hybridization with ^{125}I-labelled nucleic acid probe	40,000	24
Quantiplex HBV-DNA assay	Bayer Diagnostics Limited	Branched DNA signal amplification	700,000	24
Digene hybrid capture II hepatitis B DNA test	Digene Corporation	HBV-DNA: RNA hybridization	140,000 (standard assay) 5,000 (ultra-sensitive assay)	3.5 5.5
NAXCOR XLnt (cross-linking nucleotide) hepatitis B virus DNA quantitation assay	NAXCOR	Photoactive cross-linking hybridization	500,000	4
Amplicor HBV monitor test	Roche Diagnostics Limited	Competitive PCR assay	400 (standard assay) 200 (COBAS modification)	6

Molecular hybridization methods

It has become one of the principal diagnostic techniques for the detection of viral infection. In all the assays, the viral genome will be detected by hybridization in either solid or liquid medium.[25,26] Detection on solid supports can be performed using a filtration assay through a nylon membrane (referred to as spot or dot assays) or with the southern blot test. One of the most commonly used molecular hybridization methods is the branched DNA hybridization assay. The other methods are briefly described in Table 4.

Polymerase chain reaction (PCR)

PCR provides selective amplification of short DNA or RNA sequences. These sequences can be identified and cloned by conventional hybridization and recombinant DNA procedures. The technique has several advantages such as (a) only small quantities of material (serum / tissue) are required, as 1–5 gm of DNA or RNA is sufficient, (b) amplification is generally extremely efficient (10^6 to 10^9), (c) the procedure is quick, taking only 1-3 days, and (d) the amplified nucleic acid can readily be cloned and / or sequenced for fast and precise characterization. A PCR test involves a series (20–40) of amplification cycles (Fig. 4). Each cycle consists of 3 phases. The first is denaturation of the nucleic acid, the second is hybridization of short oligo nucleotides (20–30 bases; referred to as primers) to the target DNA, and the third is the extension of the primers using the Taq polymerase (a thermo-resistant DNA polymerase), which synthesizes complementary DNA molecules. It is a sensitive technique that can detect even minute quantities of DNA/RNA. While various in-house PCR assays

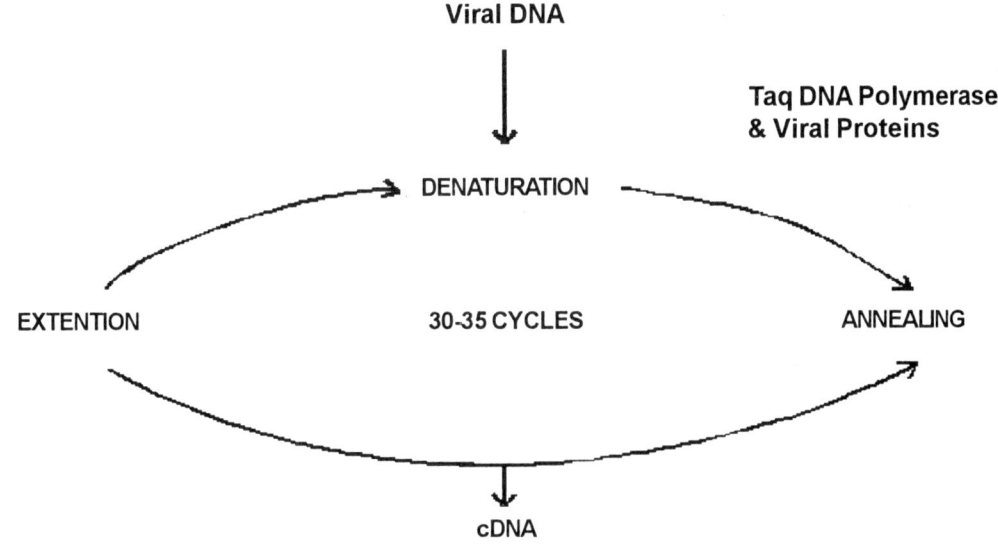

Fig. 4. Principle of polymerase chain reaction

have been utilized in research for a long time, the variation in detection standards and reproducibility of different laboratories render the test less than ideal for comparison purposes. This difficulty is involved with the availability of a commercial quantitative PCR assay, the amplicor HBV test. Refinement of this assay, the COBAS Amplicor HBV test, has recently become available. This is based on the principle of co-amplification of HBV target and an internal standard (IS) DNA which is added in a fixed known copy number to each specimen.[27] After amplification, the PCR ratio of the optical density of the HBV specific hybridization signal and of the IS- specific hybridization signal is calculated. The quantity of HBV-DNA in the specimen is obtained by reading this ratio against the calibration curve prepared from the standards. One major problem with these tests is the variability in the quantitative values assigned to the standard of the different assays. The values of HBV-DNA therefore measured in the different assays may vary by a factor of up to 120, making interpretation of the results from different clinical trials difficult. A new PCR assay has been developed recently,[28] the 'Light cycler' quantitative real time PCR assay. The authors evaluated a real-time PCR method performed in Light cycler TM analyser for quantitative HBV-DNA assay. HBV-DNA results with this method were compared with those obtained using a branched-chain DNA (b DNA) solution hybridization assay. The test was performed in 34 HBsAg positive, 93 anti-HBe positive and 66 asymptomatic subjects with chronic HBV infection. A linear standard curve was seen in the range from 10^3 to 10^8 copies/ ml. In the reproducibility analysis, intra-assay coefficient of variation (CVs) at the two known HBV-DNA concentrations were 4% and 2% and inter-assay CVs were 6% and 4%. The cut-off between chronic hepatitis patients and asymptomatic HBsAg positive subjects was found to be at a serum HBV-DNA concentration of 5×10^4 copies/ml. The authors concluded that the light-cycler quantitative real-time PCR is a practical, sensitive, reproducible, single tube assay with a wide range of detection. The assay is automatic except for DNA extraction and the running time is only 70 min. It is useful for identifying different states of HBV infection and for evaluating the efficacy of anti-viral therapy. HBV-DNA may be detectable by PCR and not by hybridization methods in patients after HBeAg sero-conversion, recovery from acute infection and 2–3 weeks before the appearance of HBsAg in acute HBV infection. The pathogenic significance of minute amounts of HBV-DNA that can be detected by PCR but not by hybridization assays is uncertain. Therefore, PCR assays for HBV-DNA should be reserved for research purposes and not for routine clinical practice.

One final assay which is not yet commercially available will be discussed. This is the semi-quantitative PCR assay of HBV supercoiled or covalently closed circular (ccc) DNA in the nuclei of infected hepatocytes. The technique described by Kock and his colleagues[29] utilizes an indigenous selection of primers. Primers that amplify across the non-interrupted part of HBV genome will detect both RC-DNA and ccc DNA. This technique has been further referred to measure the ccc DNA in the hepatocytes. Measurement of the ccc DNA of the hepatocyte may be the ultimate test for the efficacy of an antiviral treatment for chronic HBV infection in the future. With the fulcrum of internal standards (as in the Amplicor test mentioned above), the test can be made quantitative.[30]

In summary, the routine use of PCR for the detection of HBV-DNA is still limited to the following settings (Table 5): (a) detection of HBV replication in HBsAg positive, anti-HBe positive patients with active liver disease, despite a negative spot test for HBV-DNA; (b) approach to HBsAg negative liver disease; and (c) follow-up of HBV infection in liver transplantation programs. Other potential applications are follow up of antiviral treatment (using quantitative assays), detection of HBV-DNA in blood donors (pending automatization); analysis of the impact of the HBV-DNA variability; and investigation of nosocomial HBV transmission. Several studies have shown that PCR can be used for HBV-DNA detection in the serum, liver, and PBMCs.[31-33] The detection limit is 10-100 molecules / ml. It has been shown that about 50% of HBsAg positive and anti-HBc positive asymptomatic carriers who were HBV-DNA negative in a regular spot test had HBV-DNA identified by PCR. HBV-DNA has been shown to persist in the liver tissue despite clearence of serum HBsAg.[34] Detection of DNA in PBMCs after liver grafting indicates a 'window' during which the liver graft is not yet reinfected, although HBV-DNA is present in PBMCs. This is often followed by reinfection of the liver, probably from PBMCs.[35] Finally, although PCR is not necessary for routine diagnosis of HBV mother-to-child transmission, it can be used for a direct evaluation and to identify the HBV strains contaminating the newborns.[36]

Table 5. Main indications for HBV-DNA detection

Evaluation of HBV viremia:
Monitoring of therapy
Evaluation of infection
HBV-DNA detection by PCR: research protocols
Analysis of HBV genetic variability
HBsAg negative patients with chronic hepatitis "non-A–non-G"
Detection of HBV-DNA in biological fluids

DIAGNOSIS OF VARIOUS CLINICAL SITUATIONS

Acute hepatitis B

It is best diagnosed by the detection of IgM anti-HBc in the serum. Presence of HBsAg suggests the presence of HBV, but it should be confirmed with an IgM anti-HBc testing, as a chronic carrier may present for the first time with a superimposed bout of acute non-B hepatitis. Detection of IgM anti-HBc is especially important when serum is negative for HBsAg in acute hepatitis B infection. This can occur in two clinical situations (a) HBsAg has disappeared from the serum and anti-HBs has not yet appeared (window period)[37] and (b) in subfulminant and fulminant hepatic failure where because of strong immune response, the HBsAg is present in serum in low titers which evades detection by even the most sensitive techniques (Table 3).[38]

It has been shown that absence of HBsAg predicts a better survival.[39] The real diagnostic problem comes in differentiating acute hepatitis B from reactivation of chronic hepatitis B infection, especially in individuals who are not previously known to have chronic HBV infection. This may be detected by the titers of the antibody but may not always be possible. The typical course of acute hepatitis B infection is depicted in Fig. 2.

Incidentally detected asymptomatic HBsAg positive subject (IDAHS)

With the increasing awareness of hepatitis B, more and more HBsAg positive subjects are being picked up either in blood bank screening, routine health check up, health melas, etc. The rate of conversion from chronic hepatitis with active replication to clearence of infection (anti-HBc) has been estimated to be around 10% per year.[40] The rate of progression to cirrhosis is not linear, and the 1% per year risk of developing cirrhosis probably decreases over time. The annual risk of developing hepatocellular carcinoma is less than 1%.[41]

Chronic hepatitis B

It is known that an average of about 5–10% of HBV infected subjects fail to clear the virus from their body within 6 months period and develop chronic disease. The cornerstone of diagnosis is the presence of HBsAg. Total anti-HBc is present in almost every case of chronic HBV infection. IgM type is usually not seen in chronic infection, but interesting fact is that more sensitive tests can still detect it as a 7–8 S form of IgM anti-HBc whereas 19 S form predominates in acute infection. Titers of IgM anti-HBc are known to correlate with (a) liver enzymes and HBV-DNA in patients with chronic hepatitis, (b) monitoring response to interferon, and (c) risk of developing HCC, however this has not been confirmed by other studies. Anti-HBs is absent in 60–80% cases, however the remainder have detectable anti-HBs in the serum leading to co-existence of HBsAg and anti-HBs. This combination usually may not be of any clinical significance but sometimes represents disturbed immunologic response, immune complex formation, or an association with renal disease. These chronically infected individuals can be replicating (highly infectious) or non-replicating (low infectivity).

This can also be picked up by the specific tests (Table 6). It is said that once the virus stops replicating, the serum becomes much less infectious but simultaneously, the chances of the virus being integrated into the host genome are increased leading to the development of hepatocellular carcinoma. HBeAg tends to disappear in about 50% cases of chronic infection with subsequent appearance of anti-HBe. Lately, more and more reports are coming wherein HBV-DNA is present in the absence of HBeAg. This has been attributed to the infection by

Table 6. Features of replicative HBV

	Replicative virus	Non-replicative virus
HBV-DNA	+++	-ve
DNA polymerase	+++	-ve
HBeAg	+++	-ve
Anti-HBe	-ve	+++

precore mutants which are unable to synthesize precore/core protein from which HBeAg is derived. The usual course of chronic HBV infection is depicted in Fig. 3.

Efforts to classify the stage of chronic infection and the subsequent prognosis have become important with the availability of new therapeutic options. Presence or absence of symptoms fails to differentiate mild from progressive disease until patients are in advanced stage.[42] The accepted standard of current classification is the histological interpretation of a liver biopsy specimen. The information provided by this classification helps in monitoring of the patients on treatment.[43]

HBeAg negative chronic hepatitis B

It has been generally accepted that HBeAg-negative chronic hepatitis B (CHB) is not a separate disease and infection with precore mutants to begin with, but a late phase in the natural course of chronic HBV infection that develops after HBeAg loss and sero-conversion to anti-HBe.[44] Precore HBV mutants appear to exist from the early phase of HBeAg positivity being detectable in minute amounts together with the predominant wild type of HBV.[44,45] However, they are selected and predominate over the wild-type virus only during the seroconversion phase of HBeAg to anti-HBe.[46,47] About 25–30% of these HBeAg-negative cases develop reactivation or HBeAg negative CHB.[44,48]

Precore HBV mutants are associated with acute, fulminant, or chronic liver disease.[49,50] The diagnosis of the presence of precore HBV mutants in clinical practice can be made by fulfilling certain criteria (Table 7). The suggested cut-off level of HBV-DNA is 105 copies (cp)/ml.[51] In a recently reported study, a serum HBV-DNA level of 30,000 cp/ml estimated by a quantitative commercially available PCR assay, was shown to have a higher accuracy in the differentiation between cases of HBeAg negative CHB and asymptomatic carriers.[52] However, in clinical practice sequential ALT/AST estimation remain the basis for differentiation, considering the high cost of HBV-DNA determination. One practical problem is the fluctuating pattern in ALT/AST activity with long inactive periods in 45–65% of them.[53] Thus, even frequent ALT/AST determinations may miss flares of short duration. Semi-quantitative assessment of IgM class antibody to HBV core antigen has been suggested and is currently used in some countries as a supplementary marker for the diagnosis of HBeAg-negative CHB.[53,54] Documentation of HBcAg in the liver can also be used for the diagnosis.[44] How-

Table 7. Criteria for the diagnosis of HBeAg-negative chronic hepatitis B (e-CHB)

Positive serum HBsAg for at least 6 months,
Negative serum HBeAg (usually with positive anti-HBe) for at least 6 months or preferably 12 months,
Increased ALT (preferably ALT > 1.5 x upper limit normal on at least 2 monthly determinations) to establish hepatocellular damage,
Detectable HBV-DNA levels to establish active HBV replication,
Exclusion of other concomitant causes of liver disease such as superinfection with viruses (D or C), alcohol abuse, hepatotoxic drug use, or relatively rare liver diseases (autoimmune, metabolic, etc.).

ever, after the availability of molecular methods in the last 15–20 years for the detection of HBV-DNA, this method is not often required.

Reactivation of chronic HBV infection

This clinical situation is usually seen in patients with immunosuppressed status or in patients receiving chemotherapy or organ transplantation.[55] The clinical importance is to differentiate it from acute HBV infection, as the prognosis of both the conditions is entirely different. This may be difficult, in cases where the previous HBsAg status is not known. The markers of chronic infection such as IgG anti-HBc, anti-HBe, etc. shall be very useful in these cases. However, in a difficult case, a liver biopsy showing deposits of HBsAg in the hepatocytes confirms the diagnosis as presence of HBsAg is not expected in the liver tissue of patients with acute hepatitis B.

Follow-up of patients on antiviral therapy

It is generally agreed that the end-points of treatment for HBV are sero-conversion from HBeAg to anti-HBe along with the loss of HBV-DNA, improvement in the clinical condition, normalization of ALT, and improvement in liver histology by at least 3 points. However, it is known that even after sero-conversion, HBV-DNA may be detected in as high as 15–30% cases in the serum and more so, in the liver tissue. This is seen more so in Asian patients than in Caucasians.[56] It is, therefore, recommended that there may be a need to review the endpoint of treatment in Asian patients, as these patients who continue to harbor HBV-DNA detected by sensitive PCR assay, may go on to develop sequelae like cirrhosis and hepatocellular carcinoma.

The probability of a successful outcome to therapy is influenced by a number of variables, including duration of infection and gender differences, as well as levels of markers of viral replication and liver inflammation.[57] The two main characteristics of the HBV biology that affect the results of anti-viral therapy of chronic hepatitis B are the slow kinetics of viral clearance requiring long-term treatment to control or eradicate viral infection,[58,59] and the selection of HBV genome mutants that escape the pressure of anti-viral treatment.[60] It is, therefore, critical to monitor viral replication and study viral genome during the course of anti-viral therapy to tailor the anti-viral strategy to the virological situation of the patients.

Prior to antiviral therapy

Presence of HBeAg with raised ALT and an HAI of more than 3 on liver biopsy are sufficient criteria to start treatment. However, in a mutant infection (which may be seen in as high as 25% cases in India), HBV-DNA estimation is required to make a diagnosis of e Ag negative chronic hepatitis B (Table 8). Estimation of HBV-DNA may also have prognostic significance as patients with HBV-DNA <2.5 pg/ml are more likely to be benefited by anti-viral therapy. Most responders have HBV-DNA <10^9 genomes/ml, as defined by the Emokef standard (<10 pg/ml) and HBeAg less than 20,000 units/ml.[61] Testing for HBV-DNA and HBeAg during therapy permits an early differentiation between good and poor responses. Reports are now coming that monitoring with HBeAg (monthly assessment) is good enough to predict the response and routine HBV-DNA estimation may not be needed.[62,63]

Table 8. Rational approach to diagnosis of HBV infection

Indication	Serological tests	Molecular tests	Liver biopsy
Acute hepatitis B	HBsAg, anti-HBc IgM	Nil	Nil
Fulminant hepatitis B	-do-	Nil	Nil
Chronic hepatitis B	HBsAg, anti-HBc IgG, HBeAg, anti-HBe	HBV-DNA for 'e' –ve chronic hepatitis B	Rarely for demonstration of HBV particles
Hepatocellular carcinoma	HBsAg, anti-HBc	HBV-DNA in HBsAg –ve cases	Rarely for integration of HBsAg in host genome
Before anti-viral therapy	ALT, HBeAg	HBV-DNA for 'e' –ve cases	Only for immuno-compromised patients
Before blood donation	HBsAg	Nil	Nil
Pre-vaccination screening	HBsAg, anti-HBs (only when the prevalence is >20%)	Nil	Nil
Post-vaccination screening	Anti-HBs (only for immunocompromized patients)	Nil	Nil

Pre-vaccination screening

This is done by estimation of anti-HBs titers. Protective levels are usually taken as more than 10 mIU/ml. This is not only of significance in those who fail to seroconvert after full vaccination schedule, but also in those with vaccine escape mutants.

Isolated anti-HBc positivity

The isolated presence of anti-HBc in the absence of HBsAg has been reported in 0.4–1.7% of blood donors in low prevalence areas and in up to 22% of blood donors in endemic countries. This may also occur during the window period and years after recovery from chronic infection when HBsAg and/or anti-HBs are undetectable. The clinical significance of isolated anti-HBc is not clear, although HBV-DNA has been detected in 0–20% when detected by PCR assays. Transmission of HBV infection has been reported through blood and organ donation in donors with isolated anti-HBc positivity. About 50% of HIV positive individuals are also anti-HBc positive[64] and it is reassured that HIV positive donors are positive for anti-HBc before the onset of HIV infection. Despite the use of highly sensitive tests for HBsAg transfusion associated hepatitis B (TAH-B) remains a problem in some regions.[65,66] American blood banks implemented donor screening for anti-HBc and ALT in 1986. This has substantially reduced the incidence of TAH-B as studies have shown that cryptic HBV infections exist in subjects with isolated anti-HBc positivity.[67]

Cryptogenic chronic liver disease

In the majority of patients with chronic liver disease, the clinical data, pattern of abnormal liver profile, and serological markers along with histology will identify the etiology of liver disease. However, in 10–30% of cases, the cause remains obscure. These are labelled as idiopathic or cryptogenic. With the advent of PCR allowing detection of HBV-DNA and HCV-RNA in patients who lack antibodies, the problem of occult hepatitis infection is increasingly recognized. Data on this aspect have been highly variable depending on the region from which it is published and the prevalence of hepatitis B in that population.

Studies done from Europe have shown the occult HBV infection in 10–33% of cases.[68-70] This figure increases to 59% if the HBV is looked for in the liver biopsy specimen. Studies from Japan[71,72] and China,[73] which are hyperendemic zones for hepatitis B, have shown 70–90% of patients with 'idiopathic' liver disease to have HBV-DNA by PCR in their sera. Also, studies from various parts of the world in HBsAg-negative patients with hepatocellular carcinomas[74-76] suggest a significant contribution by occult hepatitis B infection.

From India, only 2 studies are available to address this issue. In one such study from Lucknow,[77] of the 35 patients initially labelled as cryptogenic, 57% tested positive for hepatitis B by PCR; in addition, one-third of patients thought to have alcohol related liver disease also were HBV-DNA positive. Liver tissues tested for HBV-DNA, in patients with negative serum HBV-

DNA, found an additional 4 cases to be positive. The authors concluded that hepatitis B was the most common cause associated with 'cryptogenic' liver disease in their patients. On the contrary Radhakrishnan et al,[78] showed a low rate of silent HBV infection among patients with chronic liver disease. Of the 62 HBsAg negative cases, 2 (3.2%) had detectable HBV-DNA. These two patients had evidence of past exposure to hepatitis B and were anti-HBc positive. Both had evidence of cirrhosis on histology. The difference in the two studies could be related to sample bias, different methodologies and definitions used for 'cryptogenic' liver disease, and small sample size especially in the second study.

There are several reasons postulated for HBV-DNA positivity in HBsAg negative sera. HBsAg could be present at a level too low for detection by conventional assays. Antigen could be hidden in the HBs antigen-antibody immune complexes. Deletion, mutation or rearrangement of HBV surface gene after viral integration could lead to HBsAg negativity. Hepatitis B variants with different antigenic and immunogenecity may exist. The only study available from India,[79] from Delhi, looking at DNA analysis in their cohort of HBV-DNA positive, HBsAg negative patients with chronic liver disease reported surface gene mutations previously described in vaccine escape mutants. We need more studies on cloning and sequencing of HBV-DNA from India to know the type of mutations our patients harbor.

What is not very clear as on today is the clinical relevance of patients with HBsAg negative chronic liver disease. In the light of available data, occult HBV infection should be looked for in the following situations: (a) in HBsAg-negative patients with continuing chronic hepatic inflammation when no other aetiologic factors have been identified, and not in those with normal liver function tests. This is more important in the transplantation context and in anti-HBc positive individuals, (b) before starting treatment for autoimmune hepatitis since positivity of autoimmune markers may be related to HBV infection, (c) co-infection by HCV and HBV may influence the course of HCV infection. HBV-DNA testing in an anti-HCV positive HBsAg-negative patient should, however, only be considered if liver inflammation is sustained despite repeated negative serum HCV-RNA tests and in absence of other pathogenic factors.[80-82] As virological techniques improve, we shall continue to redefine cryptogenic liver disease. We need to generate more data from our country on this issue before we can arrive at a consensus on how far to investigate these patients for the management of cryptogenic liver disease in India.

REFERENCES

1. Blumberg BS, Alter HJ, Visnuh S. A new antigen in leukemia sera. *JAMA* 1965;191:541-6.
2. Hepatitis B and C: Carrier to cancer—Asian perspectives. Consensus statements. *Indian J Gastroenterol* 1999; 18 (Suppl):S 16-20.
3. LeBouvier GL. The heterogeneity of Australia antigen. *J Infect Dis* 1971;123:671-5.
4. Chandra RK. Subtypes of hepatitis B antigen. *Indian J Pediatr* 1974;41:261-2.

5. Tabor E, Greety RJ, Smallwood LA, Basker LF. Co-incident hepatitis B surface antigen and antibodies of different subtypes in human serum. *J Immunol* 1977;118:369-70.
6. Carman WF, Zanetti AR, Karayiannis P, Waters J, Manzillo G, Tanzi E, Zuckerman AJ, et al. Vaccine induced escape mutant of hepatitis B virus. *Lancet* 1990;336:325-9.
7. Carman WF, Korula J, Wallace L, MacPhee R, Mimms L, Decker R. Fulminant reactivation of hepatitis B due to envelope protein mutant that escaped detection by monoclonal HBsAg ELISA. *Lancet* 1995;345:1406-7.
8. Wallace LA, Echevarria JE, Echevarria JM, Carman WF. Molecular characterization of envelope antigenic variants of hepatitis B virus from Spain. *J Infect Dis* 1994;170:1300-3.
9. Sarin SK. *Clinical spectrum of HBV in India.* In: Sarin SK, Singal AK. Eds. Hepatitis B in India: Problems and Prevention: CBS Publishers & Distributors, New Delhi, 1996;pp 51-63.
10. Thielmann L, Klinkert MQ, Gmelin K, Salfela J, Schaller H, Ptaff E. Detection of pre-S1 proteins in serum and liver of HBsAg positive patients: a new marker for hepatitis B. *Hepatology* 1986;6:186-90.
11. Neurath AR, Kent SB, Strick N, Pasher K. Identification and chemical synthesis of a host cell receptor binding site on hepatitis B virus. *Cell* 1986;46:429-36.
12. Milich DR, McNamara MK, Mchachlan A, Thornton GB, Chisari FV. Distinct H-2 linked regulation of T-cell response to the pre-S and S regions of the same hepatitis B surface antigen polypeptide allows circumvention of non-responsiveness to the S region. *Proc Natl Acad Sci USA* 1985;82:8168-72.
13. Schek N, Bartenschlager R, Kuhn C, Schaller H. Phosphorylation and rapid turnover of hepatitis B virus X protein expressed in Hep G2 cells from a recombinant vaccinia virus. *Oncogene* 1991;6:1735-44.
14. Katiyar S, Dash BC, Thakur V, Guptan RC, Sarin SK, Das BC. P53 tumor suppressor gene mutations in hepatocellular carcinoma patients in India. *Cancer* 2000;88:1565-73.
15. Stuyer L, De Gendt S, Van Geyt C, Zoulim F, Fried M, Schinazi RF, Rossau R, et al. A new genotype of hepatitis B virus: complete genome and phylogenetic relatedness. *J Gen Virol* 2000;81:67-74.
16. Chan HLY, Tsang SWC, Liew CT, Tse CH, Wong ML, Ching JYL, Leung NWL, et al. Viral genotype and hepatitis B virus DNA levels are corelated with histological liver damage in HBsAg-negative chronic hepatitis B virus infection. *Am J Gastroenterol* 2002;97:406-12.
17. Hoffnagle JH, Gerety RJ, Basher LF. Antibody to hepatitis B virus core in men. *Lancet* 1973;ii: 869-71.
18. Krugman S, Overy LR, Mushahwar IK, Ling CM, Frosner GG, Deinhardt F. Viral hepatitis type B. Studies on natural history and prevention re-examined. *N Engl J Med* 1979;300:101-6.
19. Overby LR, Miller JP, Smith ID, Decker RH, Ling CM, et al. Radioimmunoassay of hepatitis B virus associated (Australia) antigen employing ^{125}I antibody. *Vox Sang* 1973;24:102-13.
20. Decher RH. *New diagnostic technologies: automation of immunoassays for hepatitis markers and solution hybridization for HBV-DNA.* In: Hollinger FB, Lemon SM, Margolis HS. Eds. Viral hepatitis and Liver Disease. Williams and Wilkins, Baltimore, 1991:pp. 795-8.
21. Eble K, Clemans J, Krenc C, et al. Differential diagnosis of acute viral hepatitis using rapid, fully automated immunoassays. *J Med Virol* 1991;33:139-50.
22. Carman WF. *Vaccine associated mutants of hepatitis B virus.* In: Nishioka K, Suzuki H, Mishiora S, Oda T. Eds. Hepatitis and Liver Disease. Springer Verlag, Tokyo, 1994: pp 243-7.
23. Carman WF, Korula J, Wallace L, et al. Fulminant reactivation of hepatitis B due to envelope protein mutant that escaped detection by monoclonal HBsAg ELISA. *Lancet* 1995;345:1406-7.
24. Uchida T, Aye TT, Becker SO, Hirashima M, Shikata T, Komine F, Moriyama M, et al. Detection of

precore / core mutant hepatitis B genome in patients with acute or fulminant hepatitis without serological markers for recent HBV infection. *J Hepatol* 1993;18:369-72.

25. Brechot C. Hepatitis B virus (HBV) and hepatocellular carcinoma. HBV-DNA status and its implications. *J Hepatol* 1987;4:269-79.
26. Krogsgaard K, Wantzin P, Aldershvile J, Kryger P, Andersson P, Nielson JO, et al. Hepatitis B virus DNA in hepatitis B surface antigen positive blood donors: relation to the hepatitis B e system and outcome in recipients. *J Infect Dis* 1986;153:298-303.
27. Ranki M, Schatzl HM, Zachoval R, Uusi-Oulari M, Lehtovaara P. Quantification of hepatitis B virus DNA over a wide range from serum for studying viral replicative activity in response to treatment and in recurrent infection. *Hepatology* 1995;21:1492-9.
28. Jardi R, Rodriguez F, Buti M, Cortina M, Valdes A, Gelimany R, Esteban R, et al. Quantitative detection of hepatitis B virus DNA in serum by a new rapid real-time fluoroscence PCR assay. *J Viral Hepat* 2001;8:465-71.
29. Kock J, Theilmann L, Galli P, Schlicht HJ. Hepatitis B virus nucleic acids associated with human peripheral blood mononuclear cells do not originate from replicative virus. *Hepatology* 1996;23:405-13.
30. Dean J, Bomden DS, Angus P, Locarnini S. Development of quantitative PCR to detect hepatitis B virus cavalently closed circular DNA molecules in liver biopsy specimens. *Hepatology* 1998;28:481A (abstract).
31. Feray C, Zignego A, Samuel D, Bismuth A, Reynes M, Tiollais P, Bismuth H, et al. Persistent hepatitis B virus liver infection: the liver transplantation model. *Transplantation* 1990;49:1155-8.
32. Gerken G, Paterllini P, Manns M, Housset C, Terre S, Dienes HP, Hess G, et al. Assay of hepatitis B virus DNA by polymerase chain reaction and its relationship to pre-S and S encoded viral surface antigens. *Hepatology* 1991;13:158-66.
33. Keller GH, Huang DP, Shih JW, Manak MM. Detection of hepatitis B virus DNA in serum by polymerase chain reaction amplification and microtiter sandwich hybridization. *J Clin Microbiol* 1990;28:1411-6.
34. Marcellin P, Martinot-Peignoux M, Loriot MA, Giostra E, Boyer N, Thiers V, Benhamou JP, et al. Persistence of hepatitis B virus DNA demonstrated by polymerase chain reaction in serum and liver after loss of HBsAg induced by antiviral therapy. *Ann Intern Med* 1990;112:227-8.
35. Lanford RE, Michaeles MG, Chavez D, Brasky K, Fung J, Starzl TE, et al. Persistence of extrahepatic hepatitis B virus DNA in the absence of detectable hepatic replication in patients with baboon liver transplantation. *J Med Virol* 1995;46:207-12.
36. Liebermann HM, Labrecque DR, Kew MC, Hadziyannis SJ, Shafritz DA, et al. Detection of hepatitis B virus DNA directly in human serum by a simplified molecular hybridization test: comparison to HBeAg / anti-HBe status in HBsAg carriers. *Hepatology* 1983;3:285-91.
37. Perrillo RP, Chauk H, Overby LR, Deehar RH. Anti hepatitis B core immunoglobulin M in the serologic evaluation of hepatitis B virus infection and simultaneous infection with type B, delta agent, and non-A non-B viruses. *Gastroenterology* 1983;85:163-7.
38. Dudley FJ, Fox RA, Sherlock S. Cellular immunity and hepatitis associated Australia antigen liver disease. *Lancet* 1972;I:723-6.
39. Bernuau J, Goudeau A, Poynard T, Dubois F, Lesage G, Younnet B, Degott C, et al. Multivariate analysis of prognostic factors in fulminant hepatitis B. *Hepatology* 1986;6:648-51.
40. Wong JB, Koff RS, Tine F, Panker SG. Cost-effectiveness of interferon-alpha-2b treatment for hepatitis B e antigen-positive chronic hepatitis B. *Ann Intern Med* 1995;122:664-75.
41. McMahon BJ, Alberts SR, Wainwright RB, Bulkow L, Lanier AP, et al. Hepatitis B related sequelae.

Prospective study in 1400 hepatitis B surface antigen positive Alaska native carriers. *Arch Intern Med* 1990;150:1051-4.
42. Hoffnagle JH, Shafritz DA, Poffer H. Chronic type B hepatitis and the 'healthy' HBsAg carrier state. *Hepatology* 1987;7:758-63.
43. Malhotra V, Gondal R, Sakhuja P. *Role of liver biopsy in HBV infection.* In: Hepatitis B in India. Sarin SK, Singal AK. Eds. CBS Publishers & Distributors, New Delhi, 2003 (in press).
44. Hadziyannis SJ. Hepatitis B e antigen negative chronic hepatitis B. From clinical recognition to pathogenesis and treatment. *Vir Hep Rev* 1995;1:17- 36.
45. Chang MH, Hsu HY, Ni YH, Tsai KS, Lee PI, Chen PJ, Hsu YL, et al. Precore stop codon mutant in chronic hepatitis B virus infection in children: its relation to hepatitis B e sero-conversion and maternal hepatitis B surface antigen. *J Hepatol* 1998;28:915-22.
46. Okamoto H, Yotsumoto Y, Akahane T, Yamanaka T, Miyazaki Y, Sugai Y, Tsuda F, et al. Hepatitis B virus with precore defects prevail in persistently infected hosts along with sero-conversion to anti-HBe. *J Virol* 1990;64:1298-1303.
47. Hamasaki K, Nakata K, Nagayama Y, Ohtsuru A, Daikoku M, Taniguchi K, et al. Changes in the prevalence of HBeAg-negative mutant hepatitis B virus during the course of chronic hepatitis B. *Hepatology* 1994;20:8-14.
48. Hoofnagle JH, Shafritz DA, Popper H. Chronic type B hepatitis and the 'healthy' HBsAg carrier state. *Hepatology* 1987;7:758-63.
49. Carman WF, Jayna MR, Hadziyannis S, Mc Garvey M, Karayiannis P, Thomas HC. Mutation preventing formation of 'hepatitis B e antigen' in patients with chronic hepatitis B infection. *Lancet* 1989;ii: 588-90.
50. Omata M, Ehata T, Yahosuha O, Hosoda K, Ohto M. Mutations in the pre- core region of hepatitis B virus DNA in patients with fulminant and severe hepatitis. *N Engl J Med* 1991;324:1699-1704.
51. Lok AS, Heathcote J, Hoofnagle JH. Management of hepatitis B, summary recommendations. *Gastroenterology* 2001;120:1828-53.
52. Manesis E, Papatheodoridis GV, Sevastianos V, Cholagitas E, Papaionnou C, Hadziyannis SJ. Significance of HBV viremia levels estimated by a quantitative PCR assay in the evaluation of HBeAg negative chronic HBV infection. *J Hepatol* 2001;34(suppl 1):115 (abstract).
53. Hadziyannis S, Bramou A, Alexopoulo A, Makris A. *Immunopathogenesis and natural course of anti-HBe positive chronic hepatitis with replicating hepatitis B virus.* In: Hollinger FB, Lemon SM, Margolis HS, Eds. Viral Hepatitis and Liver Disease: Baltimore, Williams and Wilkins, 1991;pp. 673-6.
54. Hadziyannis SJ, Hadziyannis AS, Diurakin S, Alexopoulo A, Horsch A, Hess G. Clinical significance of quantitative anti-HBc IgM assay in acute and chronic HBV infection. *Hepatogastroenterology* 1993;40: 588-92.
55. Al-Taie OH, Mork H, Gassel AM, Wilhelm M, Weissbrich B, Scheurlan M, et al. Prevention of hepatitis B flare up during chemotherapy using lamivudine: case report and review of the literature. *Ann Hematol* 1999;78:247-9.
56. Yuen MF, Lai CL. Debates in hepatitis: how to assess HBV-DNA reductions in association with therapy. *Viral Hepat Rev* 1999;5:159-75.
57. Perrillo R. Interferon in the management of chronic hepatitis B. *Dig Dis Sci* 1993;38:577-93.
58. Nowak M, Bonhoeffer S, Hill A, Boehma R, Thomas H, Mc Dade H. Viral dynamics in hepatitis B virus infection. *Proc Natl Acad Sci USA* 1996;93:4398-4402.
59. Pichoud C, Barby F, Stuyer L, Petit MA, Trepo C, Zoulim F. Persistence of viral replication after anti-HBe sero-conversion during anti-viral therapy for chronic hepatitis B. *J Hepatol* 2000;32:307-16.
60. Allen MI, Deslauriers M, Andrews CW, Tipples GA, Walters KA, Tyrell DLJ, Brown N, et al.

Identification and characterization of mutations in hepatitis B virus resistant to lamivudine. *Hepatology* 1998;27: 1670-7.
61. Gerber MA, Thung SN. Biology of disease, molecular and cellular pathology of hepatitis B. *Lab Invert* 1985;52:572-90.
62. Perrillo R, Mimms L, Schechtman K, et al. Monitoring of antiviral therapy with quantitative estimation of HBeAg: a comparison with HBV-DNA testing. *Hepatology* 1993;18:1306-12.
63. Heijtink RA, Jansen HLA, Hop WCJ, Osterhaus ADME, Scalm SW. Interferon-alpha therapy in chronic hepatitis B: early monitoring of hepatitis B e antigen may help to decide whether to stop or to prolong therapy. *J Viral Hepat* 2000;7:382-6.
64. Dodd RY, Popovsky MA. Antibodies to hepatitis B core antigen and the infectivity of the blood supply. Scientific Section Coordinating Committee. *Transfusion* 1991;31:443-9.
65. Hoffnagle JH, Seeff LB, Bales ZB, Zimmerman HJ. Type B hepatitis after transfusion with blood containing antibody to hepatitis B core antigen. *N Engl J Med* 1978;298:1379-83.
66. Katchahi JN, Brouwar R, Siem TH. Anti-HBc and blood infectivity. *N Engl J Med* 1978;298:1421-2.
67. Parkinson AJ, McMahon BJ, Hall D, Ritter D, Fitzgerald MA, et al. Comparison of enzyme immunoassay with radioimmunoassay for the detection of antibody to hepatitis B core antigen as the only marker of HBV infection in a population with a high prevalence of hepatitis B. *J Med Virol* 1990;30: 253-7.
68. Brechot C, Degos F, Lugassy C, Thiers V, Zafrani S, Franco D, Bismuth H, et al. Hepatitis B virus DNA in patients with chronic liver disease and negative tests for hepatitis B surface antigen. *N Engl J Med* 1985;312: 270-6.
69. Cacciola I, Pollicino T, Squadiro G, Cerenzia G, Orlando ME, Raimondo G. Occult hepatitis B virus infection in patients with chronic hepatitis C liver disease. *N Engl J Med* 1999;341:22-6.
70. Berasain C, Betes M, Panizo A, Ruiz J, Herrero JI, Civeria MP, Preito J, et al. Pathological and virological findings in patients with persistent hypertransaminasemia of unknown etiology. *Gut* 2000;47:429-35.
71. Uchida T, Shimojima M, Gotoh K, Shikata T, Tanaka E, Kiyosawa K. "Silent" hepatitis B virus mutants are responsible for non-A, non-B, non-C, non-D, non-E hepatitis. *Microbiol Immunol* 1994;38: 241-5.
72. Fukuda R, Ishimura N, Kushiyama Y, Moriyama N, Ishihara S, Chowdhary A, Tokuda A, et al. Hepatitis B virus with X gene mutation is associated with the majority of serologically "silent" non-b, non-c chronic hepatitis. *Microbiol Immunol* 1996;40:481-8.
73. Zhang YY, Hansson BG, Kuo LS, Widell A, Nordenfelt E. Hepatitis B virus DNA in serum and liver is commonly found in Chinese patients with chronic liver disease despite the presence of antibodies to HBsAg. *Hepatology* 1993;17:538-44.
74. Yotsuyangi H, Shintani Y, Moriya K, Fujje H, Tsusumi T, Kato T, Nishiora K, et al. Virologic analysis of non-B, non-C hepatocellular carcinoma in Japan: frequent involvement of hepatitis B virus. *J Infect Dis* 2000;181:1920-8.
75. Sheu JC, Huang GT, Shih LN, Lee WC, Chou HC, Wang JT, Lee PH, et al. Hepatitis C and B viruses in hepatitis B surface antigen negative hepatocellular carcinoma. *Gastroenterology* 1992;103:1322-7.
76. Paterlini P, Driss F, Nalpas B, Pisi E, Franco D, Berthelot P, Brechot C, et al. Persistence of hepatitis B and hepatitis C viral genomes in primary liver cancers from HBsAg negative patients: a study of a low endemic area. *Hepatology* 1993;17:20-9.
77. Agarwal N, Naik S, Kini D, Somani SK, Singh H, Agarwal R, et al. Hepatitis B and hepatitis C infection contribute majority of cases of cryptogenic and alcoholic. *Indian J Gastroenterol* 2001;20(suppl 1):C5 (abstract).

78. Radhakrishnan S, Abraham P, Raghuraman S, Kabrawala M, Eapen CE, Sridharan G, et al. Infrequent occurrence of silent HBV infection among Indian patients with chronic liver disease. *Indian J Gastroenterol* 2001;20:87-9.
79. Guptan RC, Thakur V, Sarin SK, Banerjee K, Khandekar P. Frequency and clinical profile of precore and surface hepatitis B mutants in Asian-Indian patients with chronic liver disease. *Am J Gastroenterol* 1996;91:1312-7.
80. Brechot C, Thiers V, Kremsdorf D, Nalpes B, Pol S, Brechot PP. Persistent hepatitis B virus infection in subjects without hepatitis B surface antigen> clinically significant or purely "occult"? *Hepatology* 2001;34:194-203.
81. Mphahlele MJ, Moloto MJ. Detection of HBV-DNA from serologically negative or 'silent' HBV infections – viral or host factors? *S Afr Med J* 2002;92:613-5.
82. Torbenson M, Thomas DL. Occult hepatitis B. *Lancet Infect Dis* 2002;2:479-86.

19

Liver biopsy in chronic hepatitis B

Veena Malhotra, Puja Sakuja, Ranjana Gondal

Chronic hepatitis has been defined as continuing inflammation of the liver without improvement for at least 6 months based on a consensus conference of the International Association for the Study of the diver (IASL) and Fogarty foundation.[1] The main causes of chronic hepatitis are infection with hepatotropic viruses like HBV with or without HDV and HCV, autoimmune hepatitis, and hepatitis caused by drugs and toxic agents. Disorders like primary biliary cirrhosis, primary sclerosing chotangitis, metabolic liver disease, e.g., Wilson's and alpha-1-antitrypsin deficiency can show histological picture of chronic hepatitis.

Chronic hepatitis has been classified as chronic persistent hepatitis (CPH) and chronic active hepatitis (CAH).[2] CPH is considered to be a non-progressive disease. However, it is now understood that CPH and CAH are not distinct entities, but represent the continuing spectrum of the same disorder as CPH can occasionally progress to CAH. Several publications have now emphasized to abandon the widely used classification of chronic hepatitis into CPH and CAH.[3,4] Scheuer has commented that the separation of CPH and mild CAH are fundamentally not correct from the treatment as well as ethically point of view and it may deprive patient of effective treatment.[5]

Thus, the evolving consensus is that the final diagnosis of chronic hepatitis should have three primary components, i.e., etiology, grading, and staging. Grade expresses the degree of necroinflammation whereas stage quantitates the degree of fibrosis. The term CAH, CPH, and chronic lobular hepatitis (CLH) are now considered obsolete.[6]

ROLE OF LIVER BIOPSY IN CHRONIC HEPATITIS B

Following are the aims of liver biopsy in a patient of chronic hepatitis B.

(a) Confirming the diagnosis of chronic hepatitis;
(b) Comment on the etiology on chronic hepatitis based on histological, histochemical, and immunohistochemical studies and if required by performing *in situ* hybridization and PCR;

(c) Assessment of histological activity index (HAI);
(d) Staging of the disease depending on the fibrosis score, and comment on possible evolution of the disease;
(e) Comment on presence of iron overload;
(f) Comment on preneoplastic change or HCC;
(g) Presence of any concurrent disease like infection with other hepatotropic viruses, alcoholic liver disease, infection with HIV, etc.; and
(h) Evaluation of response to therapy by examining pre- and post-treatment biopsies.

Confirming the diagnosis of chronic hepatitis

Histological study of the liver biopsy in chronic hepatitis shows portal inflammation and periportal and lobular necroinflammatory changes. These may be accompanied by fibrosis. The degree of inflammation and lobular damage varies depending on the viral load and host factors. Portal and periportal changes dominate in chronic hepatitis in comparison to acute hepatitis where lobular changes predominate.

Portal changes

Portal area is infiltrated dominantly by lymphocytes. Few plasma cells, occasional neutrophils and PAS-positive-diastase-resistant macrophages can be present.

Periportal changes

Damage to the periportal hepatocytes accompanied by inflammation results in the destruction of the limiting plate. This is termed as piecemeal necrosis or interface hepatitis (Fig. 1, Colour plate 1). Piecemeal necrosis may not affect all the portal areas equally and only a single portal area or few portal areas may be involved. It can affect a small segment or entire perimeter of the portal area. Hepatocyte damage seen either by apoptosis or by cell lysis. Apoptosis results in formation of rounded eosinophilic bodies from the hepatocytes, which are extruded in the sinusoids (Fig. 2, Colour plate 1). These may occasionally contain degenerated nucleus or nuclear fragments. These can be phagocytosed by Kupffer cells or adjoining hepatocytes. Apoptosis may be mediated by Fas antigen. Expression of Fas antigen in the cytoplasm of liver cells has been shown in the area of piecemeal necrosis in chronic hepatitis C but it may have a role in other types of hepatitis as well.[7]

Lymphocytes have an important role in causing hepatocyte injury. Lymphocytes can be seen in close proximity to the hepatocytes. Lymphocytes present in the space of Disse may produce indentation in the cytoplasm of liver cell. This is termed as polesis. Lymphocytes may surround hepatocytes (peripolesis) or hepatocyte may encircle a lymphocyte or plasma cell (emperipolesis). There is loss of plasma membrane of hepatocyte facing the lymphocyte.

COLOUR PLATE 1

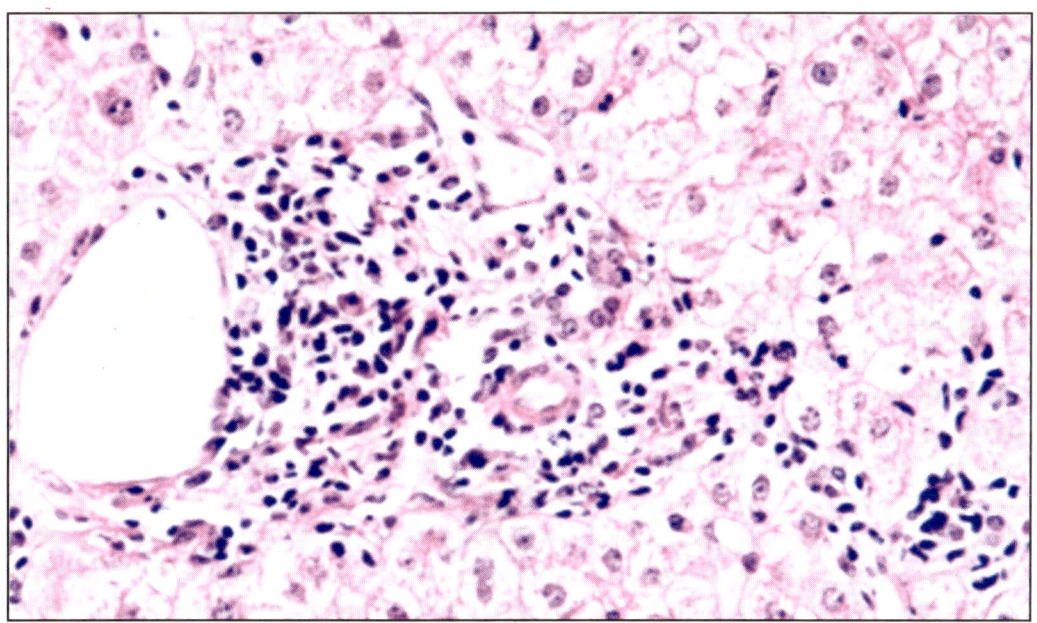

Fig. 1 Piece meal necrosis in chronic hepatitis B (hematoxylin & eosin × 160).

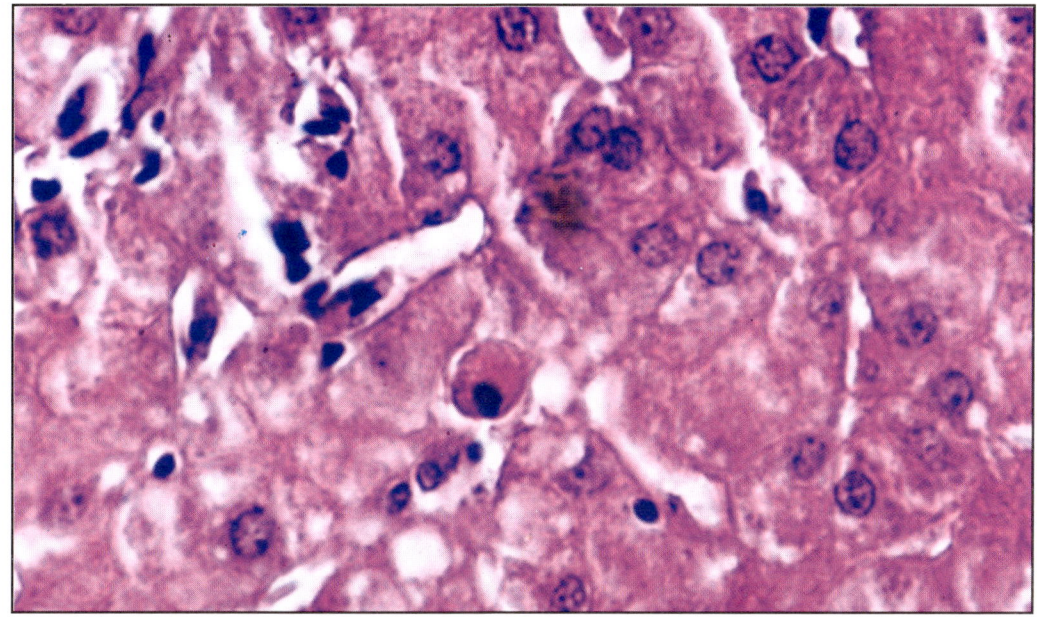

Fig. 2 Apoptotic body with nuclear fragment in chronic hepatitis B (hematoxylin & eosin × 400).

COLOUR PLATE 2

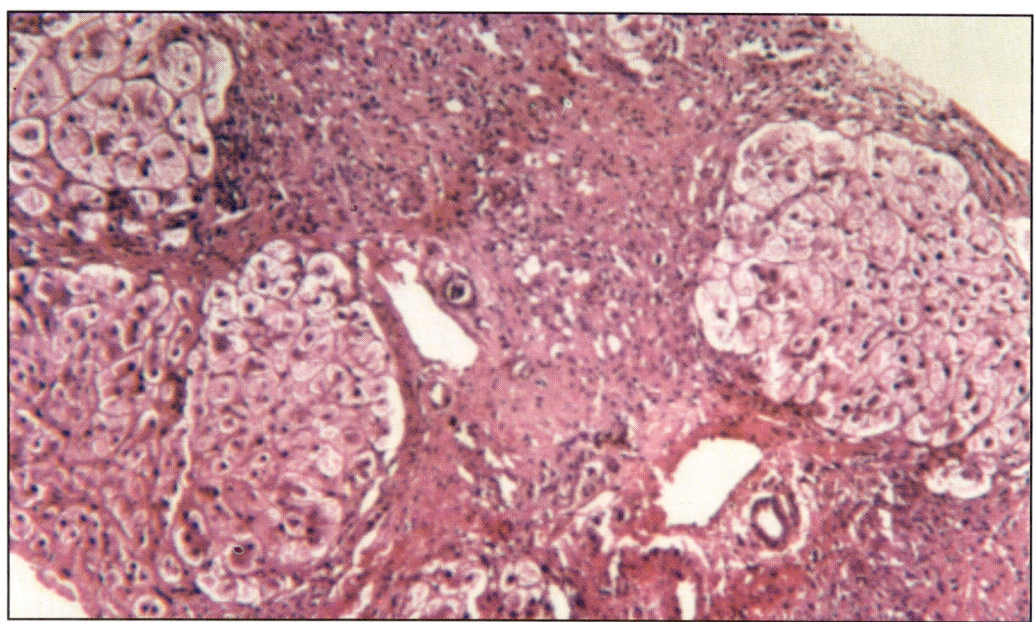

Fig. 3 Chronic hepatitis B with cirrhosis (hematoxylin & eosin × 63).

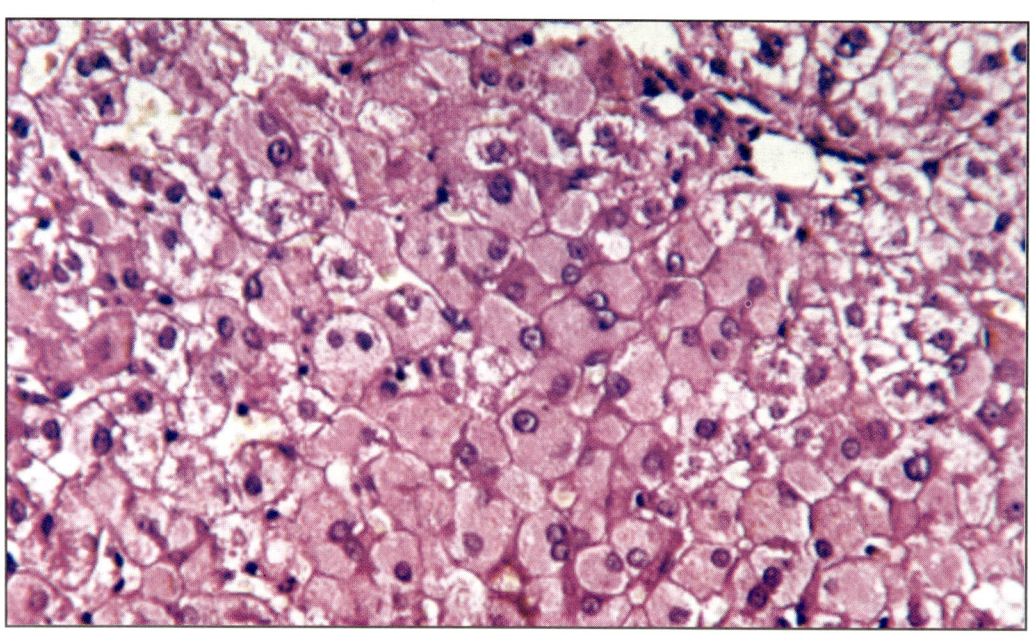

Fig. 4 Ground glass hepatocytes in chronic hepatitis B (hematoxylin & eosin × 160).

Hassan et al[8] observed that plasma cells in areas of interface hepatitis produce interleukin-1. Interleukin-1 along with other mediators may stimulate production of collagen in these areas.[8] Tumor necrosis factor-alpha is also activated in the liver in chronic hepatitis B and is thought to have an important role in the pathogenesis of liver damage and viral clearance.[9]

Lobular changes

Areas within the acinus may show isolated cell necrosis in the form of apoptosis, or focal necrosis represented by aggregates of lymphocytes, plasma cells, and Kupffer cells with loss of hepatocytes. Lymphocytes closely applied to hepatocytes as polesis, peripolesis and emperipolesis are commonly seen in the intraacinar area as well. Regeneration of hepatocytes may be present as binucleate and multinucleate cells. Proliferative activity of the hepatocytes can be assessed by immunohistochemical technique using antibody against proliferating nuclear antigen.[10] Ballooning degeneration, bridging necrosis, multiacinar necrosis are usually not seen but can be present during acute exacerbation. Cholestasis is not a feature of chronic hepatitis but may be seen occasionally when marked activity is present. Cholangiolar proliferation in portal area can also be seen in a few biopsies.

Fibrosis

Necroinflammatory changes in the periportal areas can be followed by fibrosis, which is initially laid down in the space of Disse. The fat storing 'Ito cell' plays a major role in laying down of extracellular matrix and subsequent fibrosis. Portal to portal fibrosis and portal - central fibrous bridges may form. Wide fibrous scars replace areas of multiacinar necrosis. Fibrous bands encircling groups of regenerating hepatocytes result in loss of architecture and subsequent cirrhosis (Fig. 3, Colour plate 2). Elastic fibers form a part of fibrous tissue and can be demonstrated by orcein stain. Positivity of orcein stain in areas of fibrosis in chronic hepatitis helps to differentiate from areas of collapse or bridging necrosis of acute hepatitis. Presence of bridging necrosis in acute hepatitis indicates likelihood of transition to chronicity.[10a]

Liver biopsy is not indicated in acute hepatitis B as diagnosis can be made by clinical, serological, and biochemical profile. However, in atypical cases, distinction has to be made from possible transition to chronicity and bile duct pathology. The histological features, which distinguish these conditions, are shown in Tables 1 and 2.

Confirming the etiology

Histological features distinctive of chronic hepatitis B

Liver biopsy can show certain features which are specific to hepatitis B (Table 3). Ground glass hepatocytes are seen in 50 to 80% of biopsies in chronic hepatitis B. Ground glass hepatocytes are randomly scattered and have pale granular cytoplasm (Fig. 4, Colour plate 2). The nucleus may be pushed to one side. These represent aggregates of excess hepatitis B surface antigen

Table 1. Histological features differentiating acute and chronic hepatitis

Histological features	Acute hepatitis	Chronic hepatitis
Zonal Involvement	Panlobular injury Dominant Zone III involvement	Periportal injury Dominant Zone I involvement
Piecemeal necrosis	Usually absent	Present
Fibrosis/Elastosis	Absent	Present
Ballooning degeneration	Usually present	Mild unless accompanied by acute exacerbation
Confluent necrosis		
Ground glass hepatocytes	Absent	Present
Plasma cells	Absent	Present

Table 2. Histological features differentiating acute cholestatic hepatitis and biliary pathology

Histological features	Acute cholestatic hepatitis	Biliary pathology
Hepatocellular damage	Present	Usually absent
Cholangitis	Usually absent	Usually present
Bile lakes	Absent	Usually present
Biliary piecemeal necrosis	Absent	Usually present
Rounded expansion of portal tract with oedematous fibrosis	Usually absent	Usually present
Copper in liver cells	Absent	Usually present

Table 3. Distinctive features of chronic hepatitis B*

- Ground glass hepatocytes
- Immunohistochemical staining for HBsAg and HBcAg
- Demonstration of HBV-DNA by *in situ* hybridization or PCR

*In addition to usual features of chronic hepatitis

admixed with smooth endoplasmic reticulum. Their presence indicates chronic infection, as they are not seen in acute hepatitis B. These cells can be recognized in routine haematoxylin eosin stained slides. However, they can be differentially stained by orcein stain or immunohistochemically by antibody against surface antigen.[11] Positivity with antibodies to surface antigen can be membranous or cytoplasmic. Membranous positivity is associated with presence of HBeAg expression and is indirect evidence of viral replication.[12] Cytoplasmic expression of HBsAg indicates excess surface antigen which cannot be secreted.[13] Immunohistochemically, core antigen can be demonstrated in the hepatocyte nuclei and its presence indicates active viral replication.[13] It is associated with the presence of HBeAg and HBV-DNA in the serum and failure of the host to eliminate cells with viral replication. Presence of core antigen in the cytoplasm indicates greater degree of viral replication. Sanded liver cell nuclei due to the presence of HBcAg can be delineated in the routine histological sections in HBV infection.[14] Presence of HBcAg in the hepatocytes on immunohistochemistry in HBeAg negative serum indicates infection with pre-core mutant.

In situ hybridization can also be used for demonstrating HBV and superinfection with HDV in hepatocytes.[15] Expression of pre-S1 and S2 peptides in hepatocytes in chronic hepatitis has been studied.[16] This expression is closely related to HBV replication. HBV genotypes A to D have been recognized, however, no correlation between HBV genotype and clinical and pathologic data has been observed.[17] Emperipolesis, characterized by the presence of lymphocytes in the cytoplasm of hepatocytes is frequently seen in chronic hepatitis due to HBV infection in comparison to other hepatotropic viral infections.[18]

Steatosis, portal lymphoid aggregates, or lymphoid follicles formation and bile duct injury are considered to be frequently associated with chronic hepatitis C.[19, 20] They are less commonly observed in chronic hepatitis B.[21] However, on evaluation of liver biopsies in our center we have not observed any significant difference in the incidence of these features in HBV and HCV infection (Table 4).[22] Peripolesis, emperipolesis were frequently associated with HBV infection and apoptosis with HCV infection in our patients.[22]

Histological picture of liver biopsy in patients infected with HBV mutants

Presence of HBV mutants, which can alter the course of natural infection, was first recognized

Table 4. Comparison of histological features in hepatitis B and C

Histological features	Hepatitis B (n = 30)	Hepatitis C (n = 30)	p value
Portal lymphoid aggregate/follicle (%)	36.6	33.3	NS
Bile duct damage (%)	26.6	30	NS
Steatosis (%)	66.6	70	NS
Apoptosis (%)	40	60	NS
Ground glass hepatocytes (%)	40	0	$p<0.001$
Peripolesis/emperipolesis (%)	10	0	NS
Histological Activity Index	8.6±3.5	7.4±3.3	NS
Cirrhosis (%)	30	33.3	NS

n number of cases, *NS* not significant
p value of <0.05 was taken as significant

by identification of HBeAg negative, HBA-DNA positive patients with active disease in liver biopsies. About one fourth of hepatitis B related chronic liver disease in India is caused by infection with HBV mutants.[23] The common mutants found in HBV-related chronic liver disease include HBsAg negative pre-core mutation (G1896→A), core mutation, and HBsAg mutation (G145→A). Infection with pre-core mutants was found to be associated with histologically more active disease than with wild type HBV at our center[23] and in other studies.[24] However, there are conflicting reports from Japan.[25] Fulminant hepatitis in association with pre-core mutants has been described in a number of reports.[26,27] However, it is observed that patients with fulminant hepatitis due to HBV do not share a specific mutation.[28] Fibrosing cholestatic hepatitis (FCH) has also been observed in biopsies of patients infected with pre-core variant and also with mutation in pre-S genome after transplant.[29,30] Histologically this is characterized by cytolytic hepatocellular necrosis, lobular collapse and prominent cytoplasmic expression of HBV antigens. This is probably due to the cytopathic effect of HBV rather than due to immune mediated injury. It is believed that pre-core mutants tend to respond poorly to interferon and if they do respond, they tend to relapse. Infection with surface mutants usually shows mild hepatitis, however, quiescent cirrhosis and higher incidence of HCC has been associated with this variant.[23]

Assessment of histological activity

The concept of scoring liver biopsies for histological activity was first proposed by Knodell et al.[31] This had wide acceptance and has been considered useful in giving a fairly accurate idea about the disease activity, in evaluation of response to treatment by examining pre- and post-treatment biopsies, and indicating a possible evolution of the disease process.

Knodell's scoring system is the most commonly used system (Table 5). This semiquantitative scoring system as described originally had four components, i.e., periportal necrosis, intralobular changes, portal inflammation, and fibrosis. This Knodell's scoring system has been subjected to criticism. The main drawback of this scoring system is that it includes fibrosis in activity score, which in fact represents the sequel of activity and not the activity as such.

Scheuer et al[32] proposed a simple grading system using portal and lobular necroinflammatory changes for grading the activity and fibrosis for staging the disease. Desmet et al[33] have suggested that only the first three components of Knodell's scoring system should be included for obtaining histological activity index whereas the fourth component, that is fibrosis, should be used for staging the disease. Ishak et al[34] responding to the criticism of their original Knodell scoring system have proposed a modified grading and staging system for chronic hepatitis. This complex system although permits detailed assessment, it generates fair degree of interobserver and intraobserver variability.

Ishak et al[34] have suggested that features like iron/copper overload, hepatocyte dysplasia although not included in the scoring should be commented on all biopsies separately. An

Table 5. HAI for numerical scoring of liver biopsy specimens (Knodell et al[30])

Periportal Bridging Necrosis	Score	Intralobular Degeneration and Focal Necrosis	Score	Portal Inflammation	Score	Fibrosis	Score
None	0	None	0	None	0	None	0
Mild piecemeal necrosis	1	Mild Acidophilic bodies Ballooning Degeneration and/or scattered foci of hepatocellular necrosis in <1/3 of lobules or nodules	1	Mild sprinkling of inflammatory cells in < 1/3 of portal tracts	1	Fibrous portal expansion	1
Moderate piecemeal necrosis involves < 50% of the circumference of most portal tracts	3	Moderate involvement of 1/3 - 2/3 of lobules or nodules	3	Moderate increased Inflammatory cells in 1/3-2/3 of the portal tracts	3	Bridging fibrosis (P-P or P-C linkage)	3
Marked piecemeal necrosis involves > 50% of circumference of most portal traits	4	Marked involvement of >2/3 of the lobules or nodules	4	Marked (dense packing of inflammatory cells in > 2/3 of portal tracts)	4	Cirrhosis	4
Moderate piecemeal necrosis plus bridging necrosis	5						
Marked piecemeal necrosis plus bridging necrosis	6						
Multilobular necrosis	10						

algorithmic approach based on piecemeal necrosis and lobular activity has also been proposed (Metavir scoring system).[35] This has advantage of simplicity and reproducibility (Table 6). This scoring system has been used dominantly for hepatitis C virus infection.

Table 6. Algorithm for the evaluation of histological activity

PMN	LN	A
PMN 0	LN 0	A 0
	LN 1	A 1
	LN 2	A 2
PMN 1	LN 0,1	A 1
	LN 2	A 2
PMN 2	LN 0,1	A 2
	LN 2	A 3
PMN 3	LN 0,1,2	A 3

Activity score
A = 0 No activity
A = 1 Mild activity
A = 2 Moderate activity
A = 3 Severe activity

Fibrosis scoring
F = 0 No fibrosis
F = 1 Portal fibrosis without septa
F = 3 Portal fibrosis with rare septa
F = 3 Numerous fibrous septae without cirrhosis
F = 4 Cirrhosis

PMN – Piecemeal necrosis, LN – Lobular necrosis

It is felt that while applying a scoring system, score for all the components, e.g. portal, periportal, lobular inflammation should be indicated separately, as the total score may not give exact picture of the pathological events. Presence of confluent necrosis has more serious implication for patient prognosis and evolution of the disease process than the portal inflammation.[36]

Staging of chronic hepatitis

The 'stage' of the disease refers to degree of fibrosis subsequent to necroinflammatory changes. Staging systems have been proposed by Scheuer et al[32] as well as in the modified histological HAI grading and staging system proposed by Ishak.[34] The Scheuer staging system uses the fibrosis score from 0 to 4, whereas the modified histological activity scoring and staging proposed by Ishak scores fibrosis from 0 to 6. Metavir scoring system scores fibrosis from F0 to F4.[35] Staging should be done in all the biopsies in chronic hepatitis B as it gives valuable information. It provides idea about disease progression.

Fibrosis progression index

Fibrosis progression index is estimated as ratio of fibrosis score in the biopsy and duration of the disease at the time of biopsy.[37] Thus it is useful in predicting the evolution of the disease and its likelihood of progression to cirrhosis.

Iron overload

Liver biopsies of patients with chronic hepatitis B must be stained for iron accumulation. Role of iron in modulating the course of viral hepatitis was first suggested by Blumberg et al fifteen years ago. Patients who had elevated serum ferritin had likelihood of developing disease, whereas those with lower values have often cleared the virus spontaneously. Since then, several workers have shown that increased grade of iron in the liver tissue correlates with severity of the disease and poor response to interferon therapy.[38] A study in chronic hepatitis B patients using desferrioxamine infusions has been reported to enhance the response to interferon-alpha treatment.[39] The mechanism by which iron renders liver cells more susceptible could be because of disease enhanced viral replication due to increased availability of iron or impaired immune response and oxidative stress produced by high iron concentration catalyzing toxic free radicals.[38] However, liver biopsies of chronic hepatitis B infection in our center, when stained for iron did not show significant iron overload.

Preneoplastic change and HCC

Preneoplastic change

While evaluating a liver biopsy from a patient of chronic hepatitis, the pathologist should provide information about the presence of any atypical changes in the hepatocytes such as small cell and large cell change earlier designated as small cell dysplasia and large cell dysplasia. In small cell change, there are clusters of hepatocytes which are considerably smaller than normal hepatocytes and appear as zone of nuclear crowding. There is no significant nuclear atypia. Large cell change, in comparison, consists of scattered foci within the cirrhotic liver of enlarged hepatocytes with large irregular nuclei and nucleoli but with a normal nuclear cytoplasmic ratio.[40] Anthony et al[41] have reported a high incidence (65.4%) of large cell dysplasia in the non-neoplastic but cirrhotic livers of HCC. The incidence was lower (19.3%) in cirrhotic livers with no HCC and even lower (6.9%) in non-cirrhotic livers with HCC.

The preneoplastic nature of these changes has been implicated but not proved. These changes may represent degenerative and regenerative process. However, when seen in clusters they are more compatible with preneoplastic change. Recently, an international working party[42] has recommended that the term dysplasia should be reserved for nodules that are thought to be preneoplastic in nature and the term small cell and large cell change should be used for cellular changes present in the liver, but not as nodular lesions.

Hepatocellular carcinoma

HBV infection is the most important etiological association for HCC in our country (Fig. 5).

In a study reported from our center, 85% of the patients with HCC had markers positive for HBV. Therefore, patients with chronic hepatitis B need constant monitoring for HCC. This is done by ultrasonography and serial estimation of alfa-fetoprotein levels. However, normal alfa-fetoprotein levels have been reported in as high as 38% patients of HCC.[43] If a space occupying lesion is detected on ultrasonography, it is subjected to fine needle aspiration biopsy. Fine needle biopsy is a simple procedure and gives definite result in 85 to 95 percent cases.[43, 44] The false negative rate is 5%. In rest of the patients an ultrasound guided trucut biopsy may be required.

There are several hypotheses regarding transformation of HBV associated chronic hepatitis to HCC[45]: (a) Integration of S- and X-genes of HBV into the host genome which may lead to insertional mutagenesis by turning on cellular growth genes, and (b) continuous cell death and regeneration due to persistent infection may trigger aberrant activation of cellular proto-oncogenes.

The persistent viral replication in the liver leads to progression of the disease to cirrhosis and subsequently may result in HCC. A very low incidence of p53 mutation found in these tumors at our center indicated that p53 gene mutation may not have a direct role to play in the development of HCC in India.[46]

Presence of concurrent disease

Liver biopsy is helpful in identifying presence of any concurrent disease in a patient with chronic hepatitis B infection. Presence of granulomas in a biopsy may indicate concurrent tuberculosis or any other granulomatous disease. Granulomatous hepatitis has been reported in a patient on interferon therapy.[47]

The commonest associated disease in patients of chronic hepatitis B is infection with HCV. Patients with dual infection tend to have severe disease although HBV replication as measured by HBV-DNA is suppressed.[48] Histologically, no specific features were associated with dual infection. In our center liver biopsies from patients with dual infection showed histological activity index comparable to that with isolated HBV infection. Thus, the severity of histologic lesion did not differ. Interpretation of biopsy in dual infection becomes difficult as on routine histological examination it is not possible to attribute the damage to any particular virus. Positive staining for HBcAg in this situation may indicate active contribution of HBV infection in the disease process.[36]

Infection with HBV and HDV is also associated with severe hepatitis.[49] Prominent microvesicular fatty change has been described in delta infection. Lymphoid follicles have been found in high proportion of HCV negative patients with HBcAg and HDAg in liver tissue. Immunostaining of liver biopsy with HDV antigen will indicate replication of HDV in HBV-HDV coinfection and thereby its role in progression of the liver disease.[49, 50] Association of alcoholism and

HBV infection has also been reviewed.[51] HIV infection can result in higher levels of HBV replication and greater risk of cirrhosis.[52]

Evaluation of response to therapy

The histological activity grading and staging of pre- and post-treatment liver biopsies is of great advantage in assessing the response to therapy. Number of studies have focussed on follow-up of patients treated with alpha-interferon. On applying Knodell's Scoring System, post-treatment biopsies in these patients have shown significant improvement in histological activity.[53, 54] However, there was no change in fibrosis as reported by Okuno et al.[53]

De Bisceglie[55] have reported clearance of HBeAg from the serum after interferon therapy followed by clearance of HBsAg and improvement in histology. However, HBV-DNA is detectable in the tissue by PCR indicating continuing low level replication of HBV. Patients on interferon therapy are considered responders if there is loss of HBeAg and HBV-DNA from the serum. Evaluation of pre- and post-treatment biopsies in responders have shown significant reduction in hepatic inflammatory activity as compared to non-responders and controls. Progression to cirrhosis was also not seen in patients on treatment with interferon as compared to controls.[54]

At our center, a controlled trial of alpha-interferon in chronic hepatitis B patients showed a significant improvement in the histological activity in responders in the post-treatment biopsies.[56] Lowering of fibrosis score was also observed in one out of 20 patients who responded to therapy, However, this can be due to sample variability.

In a meta-analysis of worldwide trials on alpha-interferon in chronic hepatitis B, Ruff et al[57] reported that patients with active disease and higher HAI scores in pre-treatment biopsies are likely to seroconvert. Similar observations have been made by other investigators also.[58] Non-cirrhotic patients on alpha-interferon therapy showed sero-conversion more frequently than the untreated controls, whereas cirrhotic patients did not show significantly higher sero-conversion as compared to controls. In a recent study, Hoofnagle et al[59] achieved complete response in 33 percent of patients with Child's A and B cirrhosis, but limited response in patients with Child's C cirrhosis.

Histological study of pre- and post-treatment biopsies in patients treated with nucleoside analogue, lamivudine, has also shown improvement in liver histology in more than two-thirds of post-treatment biopsies (Table 7).[60-67] A possible benefit in patients of active cirrhosis has also been reported.[61] Level of ALT prior to treatment has been considered to be an important determinant of response to therapy.[68] In a study on response to corticosteroid withdrawl therapy, decrease in periportal necroinflammatory activity and fibrosis was seen along with normalization of biochemical parameters and loss of HBeAg. However, long periods were needed for histological resolution of disease in a significant number of cases.[69]

Table 7. Pre- and post-therapy liver histology on lamivudine therapy

Author (year)	Histologic Improvement (%)
Lai et al[62] (1998)	56
Tassopoulas et al[63] (1999)	60
Dienstag et al[64] (1998)	52
Heathcore et al[65] (1998)	38
Lau et al[66] (2000)	81

Treatment induced mutation in the YMDD locus of the polymerase gene sequence has been associated with reduced susceptibility to therapy.[70] However, it has been observed that YMDD mutants replicate much less efficiently than wild type HBV. Thus, on continuing therapy, although these mutants continue to replicate at low levels, they induce little or no liver injury and patients maintain clinical control.[71] Significant histological and biochemical improvement has been observed in these patients compared to untreated controls.[72] In a study on pre-core mutants treated with lamivudine the histologic assessment revealed a >2 point reduction in Knodell score, both in patients with (55%, 6 of 11) and without (37%, 11 of 30) YMDD mutation.[63]

Liver biopsies from asymptomatic HBsAg positive patients with normal ALT have revealed varied histological picture. The biopsies can be normal or show mild disease in the form of chronic persistent hepatitis.[73, 74] However, some reports have indicated that CAH and cirrhosis may be present in a few cases.[75, 76] Koretz et al[73] have compiled liver histology data of asymptomatic HBsAg positive individuals from various countries including USA, Canada, Europe, Australia, and Taiwan. Normal nonspecific histology and CPH was reported in 232 out of 237 individuals. Only five of them showed CAH and cirrhosis. In view of these findings, the authors investigated the need for biopsy in such cases. In a study involving 88 asymptomatic HBsAg positive, anti-HBe positive patients with normal transaminases, progression to cirrhosis was not observed on follow-up for 130 months inspite of three patients showing CAH on initial biopsy.[76] However, in a study from Korea, liver biopsies from asymptomatic HBsAg positive subjects with normal liver function tests showed chronic liver disease in 46.4% cases.[77] This report is in conformity with our data on asymptomatic individuals with HBV infection which revealed significant liver disease (HAI>3) in 32.5% cases (Table 8).

Conflicting reports have appeared in the literature regarding relationship of ALT levels with liver histology. A linear relationship of liver enzymes with histology has been reported.[78] On the other hand, a large number of studies have indicated that normal ALT levels do not exclude presence of significant liver disease.[79, 80] A consensus conference on hepatitis B and C "Carrier to Cancer", provided valuable guidelines for the management of patients with asymptomatic hepatitis B infection.[81]

Table 8. Liver histology in Incidentally detected asymptomatic HBsAg positive subjects (IDAHS) with normal ALT

Serological profile	Liver histology	
	HAI<3	HAI>3
HBsAg+ (n=40)	27 (67.5%)	13 (32.5%)
HBsAg+, HBeAg+ (n=11)	6 (54.5%)	5 (45.5%)
HBsAg+, HBeAg- (n=29)	21 (72.7%)	8 (27.3%)

Limitations of liver biopsy

Liver biopsy represents a small piece of liver tissue and there can be limitations in interpretation. Even in a single biopsy, varied histological picture can be seen in different areas, e.g. extent of fibrosis may not be uniform throughout the biopsy. A fair amount of inter-observer variability is observed in assessing necrosis and inflammation in the biopsy. A number of histological grading and staging systems have been described but there is no universally accepted system. There is, however, agreement that the biopsies should be graded for activity and staged for fibrosis. Similar histological picture as seen in chronic hepatitis B can be seen not only in infection with other hepatotropic viruses, but also in autoimmune hepatitis and, injury by drugs and toxic agents. Even metabolic disorders and PBC may stimulate chronic hepatitis. Clinical, biochemical, serological picture as well specific histochemical techniques may be required for differentiation and accurate diagnosis.

REFERENCES

1. Leevy CM, Popper H, Sherlock S. Disease of the liver and biliary tract. Standardization of nomenclature, diagnostic criteria and diagnostic methodology, Washington. Fogarty International Centre Proceeding No. 22 DHEW. Publication (NIH), 1976.
2. DeGroote J, Desmet VJ, Gedigk P, Korb G, Popper H, Poulsen H, Scheuer PJ, et al. A classification of chronic hepatitis. *Lancet* 1968;ii:626-8.
3. Fattovich G, Brollo L, Alberti A, Giustina G, Pontisso P, Realdi G, Ruol G, et al. Chronic persistent hepatitis B can be progressive disease when associated with sustained virus replication. *J Hepatol* 1980;11:29-33.
4. Ludwig J. The nomenclature of chronic active hepatitis: an obituary. *Gastroenterology* 1993;105:274-8.
5. Scheuer P. Classification of chronic hepatitis a need for reassessment. *J Hepatol* 1991;13:372-4.
6. Desmet VJ, Gerber M, Hoofnagle JH, Manns M, Scheuer PJ, et al. Classification of chronic hepatitis, diagnosis, grading and staging. *Hepatology* 1994;19:1513-20.
7. Hiramatsu N, Hayashi N, Katayamo K, Mochizuki K, Kawanishi Y, Kasahara A, Fusamoto H, et al. Immunohistochemical detection of F as antigen in liver tissue of patients with chronic hepatitis C. *Hepatology* 1994;19:1354-9.
8. Hassan G, Moreno S, Massimi M, Di Biagio P, Stefanini S. Interleukin-1 producing plasma cells in close contact with hepatocytes in patients with chronic active hepatitis. *J Hepatol* 1997;27:6-17.

9. Marinos G, Naumov NV, Rossol S, Torre F, Wong PY, Gallati H, Portmann B, et al. Tumor necrosis factor in patients with chronic hepatitis B virus infection. *Gastroenterology* 1995;108:1453-63.
10. Nakamura T, Hayama M, Sakai T, Hotchi M, Tanaka E, et al. Proliferative activity of hepatocytes in chronic viral hepatitis as revealed by immunohistochemistry for proliferating cell nuclear antigen. *Hum Pathol* 1993;24:750-3.
10a. Tandon BN, Nayak NC, Tandon HD, Bijlani L, Joshi YK, Gandhi BM, Madanagopalan N, et al. Acute viral hepatitis with bridging necrosis. Collaborative study on chronic hepatitis. *Liver* 1983;3: 140-6.
11. Gerber MA, Thung SN. The diagnostic value of immunohistological demonstration of hepatitis viral antigens in the liver. *Hum Pathol* 1987;18:771-4.
12. Gudet F, Bianchi L. HBsAg: *A target antigen on the liver cell. In:* Popper H, Branch I, Reutten W, Eds. Membrane alterations as basis of liver injury. Lancaster MTP Press 1977; pp.171-8.
13. Bianchi L, Gudet F. *Chronic hepatitis, In:* MacSween RNM, Anthony PP, Scheuer PJ, Burt AD, Portman BC Eds. Pathology of Liver. 3rd ed Churchill Livingstone 1994; pp.349-95.
14. Bianchi I, Gudet F. Sanded nuclei in hepatitis B. *Lab Invest* 1976;35:1-5.
15. Nergo F, Pacchioni D, Mondardini A, Bussolati G, Bonino F, et al. In situ hybridization in viral hepatitis. *Liver* 1992;12(suppl):217-26.
16. Chu CM, Laiwd YF. Intrahepatic expression of pre-S1 and pre-S2 in chronic hepatitis B viral infection in relation to viral replication and delta virus superinfection. *Gut* 1992;33:1544-8.
17. Berasain C, Betés M, Panizo A, et al. Pathological and virological findings in patients with persistent hypertransaminasaemia of unknown aetiology. *Gut* 2000;47:429-35.
18. Scheuer PJ, Ashrafzadeh P, Sherlock S, Brown D, Dusheiko GM. *Chronic hepatitis. In:* Systemic Pathology, Ed. Symmers WSC. Liver biliary tract and endocrine pancreas Vol. ii. Ed DGD Wright 3rd ed. Churchill Livingstone UK 1994:156.
19. Scheuer PJ, Ashrafzaden P, Sherlock S, Brown D, Dusheiko GM, et al. The pathology of hepatitis C. *Hepatology* 1992;15:567-71.
20. Godman ZD, Ishak KG. Histopathology of hepatitis infection. *Semin Liver Dis* 1995;15:70-81.
21. Lefkowitch JH, Schiff ER, Davies GL. Pathological diagnosis of chronic hepatitis C, a multicentric comparative study with chronic hepatitis B. *Gastroenterology* 1993;104:595-603.
22. Malhotra V, Sakhuja P, Gondal R, Sarin SK, Siddhu M, Dutt N, et al. Histological comparison of chronic hepatitis B and C in an Indian population. *Tropical Gastroenterol* 2000;21:20-1.
23. Guptan RC, Thakur V, Sarin SK, Banerjee K, Khandekar P, et al. Frequency and clinical profile of pre-core and surface hepatitis B mutants in Asian Indian patients with chronic liver disease. *Am J Gastroenterol* 1996;91:1312-7.
24. Akasra US, Lok ASF. Naturally occurring hepatitis B virus core gene mutation. *Hepatology* 1995;22: 50-60.
25. Hamasaki K, Nakata K, Nagayama Y, Ohtsuru A, Daikoku M, Taniguchi K, Nagataki S, et al. Changes in the prevalence of HBeAg negative mutant hepatitis B virus during the course of chronic hepatitis. *Hepatology* 1994;20:8-14.
26. Kosaka Y, Takase K, Kojima M, Shimizu M, Inoue K, Yoshiba M, Tanaka S, et al. A hepatitis B virus mutant associated with an epidemic of fulminant hepatitis. *N Engl J Med* 1991;100:1087-94.
27. Karayiannis P, Alexopoulou A, Hadziyannis S, Thursz M, Watts R, Seito S, Thomas HC, et al. Fulminant hepatitis associated with hepatitis Be virus antigen negative infection: importance of host factors. *Hepatology* 1995;22:1628-34.
28. Sterneck M, Gunther S, Santantonio T, Fischer L, Broelsch CE, Greten H, Will H, et al. Hepatitis B virus genomes of patients with fulminant hepatitis do not share a specific mutation. *Hepatology* 1996;24: 300-6.

29. Booth JC, Goldin RD, Brown JL, Karayiannis P, Thomas HC. Fibrosing cholestatic hepatitis in a renal transplant recipient associated with the hepatitis B virus pre-core mutant. *J Hepatol* 1995;22: 500-3.
30. Trautwein C, Schrem H, Tillmann HL, Kubicka S, Walker D, Boker KH, Maschek, HJ, et al. Hepatitis B virus mutations in the pre-S genome before and after liver transplantation. *Hepatology* 1996;24:482-8.
31. Knodell RG, Ishak KG, Black WC, Chen TS, Craig R, Kaplowitz N, Kiernan TW, et al. Formulation and application of a numerical scoring system for histological activity in asymptomatic chronic active hepatitis. *Hepatology* 1981;1:431-5.
32. Lok AS, Lindsay L, Scheuer PJ, Thomas HC. Clinical and histological features of delta infection in chronic hepatitis B virus carrier. *J Clin Pathol* 1985;38:530-3.
33. Desmet VJ, Gerber M, Hoofnagle JH, Manns M, Scheuer PJ. Classification of chronic hepatitis, diagnosis, grading and staging. *Hepatology* 1994;19:1513-20.
34. Ishak K, Baptista A, Bianchi L, Callea F, De Geoote J, Gudat F, Denk H, et al. Histological grading and staging of chronic hepatitis. *J Hepatol.* 1995;22:696-9.
35. Metavir Cooperative group: Inter and intraobserver variation in assessment of liver biopsy of chronic hepatitis. *Hepatology* 1994;20:15-20.
36. Scheuer PJ, Dusheiko GM. *The histologist's role in diagnosis and management of chronic hepatitis. In:* Viral hepatitis. Zuckerman AJ, Thomas HC, Eds. Churchil Livingstone 1998; pp.617.
37. Poynard T, Bedossa P for Obsvirc, Metavir, Clinivar and Dosvirc groups. Natural history of liver fibrosis progression in patients with chronic hepatitis. *Lancet* 1997;349:825-32.
38. Bonkovosky HL, Banner BF, Rothman AL. Iron and chronic viral hepatitis. *Hepatology* 1997;25:759-68.
39. Bayraktar Y, Koseoglu T, Sommer C, Kayhan B, Temizer A, Uzunalimoglu B, DeMaria N, et al. The use of deferoxamine infusions to enhance the response rate to interferon-alpha treatment of chronic viral hepatitis B. *J Viral Hepat* 1996;3:129-35.
40. Crawford J. Pathologic assessment of liver cell dysplasia and benign liver tumors: differentiation from malignant tumors. *Sem Diagn Pathol* 1990;7:115-28.
41. Anthony PP, Vogel CL, Barker LF. Liver cell dysplasia: a premalignant condition. *J Clin Pathol* 1973;26: 217-23.
42. Ferrel LD, Crawford JM, Dhillon AP, Scheuer PJ, Nakanuma Y. Proposal for standardized criteria for diagnosis of benign, borderline and malignant hepatocellular lesions arising in chronic advanced liver disease. *Am J Surg Pathol* 1993;17:1113-23.
43. Sbolli G, Fornari F, Civardi G, Di Stasi M, Cavanna L, Buscarini E, Buscarini L, et al. Role of ultrasound guided fine needle aspiration biopsy in the diagnosis of hepatocellular carcinoma. *Gut* 1990;31:1303-5.
44. Bret PM, Labadie M, Bertagnolle M, Paliard P, Fond A, Valette PJ, et al. Hepatocellular carcinoma: diagnosis by percutaneous fine-needle biopsy. *Gastrointest Radiol* 1988;13:253-5.
45. Buendia MA, Paterlini P, Tiollais P. *Hepatocellular carcinoma: Molecular aspects. In:* Viral hepatitis. Zuckerman AJ. Thomas HC, Eds. Churchill Livingstone 1998, pp.192.
46. Katiyar S, Dash BC, Thakur V, Guptan RC, Sarin SK, Das BC. p53 tumor suppressor gene mutation in hepatocellular cacinoma patients in India. *Cancer* 2000;88:1565-73.
47. Propsi A, Propsi T, Dietze O, Katherin H, Judmeier G, Vogel W. Development of granulomatous hepatitis during treatment with interferon-alpha 2b. *Dig Dis Sci* 1995;40:2117-8.
48. Fong TL, Di Bisceglie AM, Waggoner JG, Banks SM, Hoofnagle JH. The significance of antibody to hepatitis C in patients with chronic hepatitis B. *Hepatology* 1991;14:64-7.
49. Colombari R, Dhillon AP, Piazzola E, Tomezzoli AA, Angelini GP, Capra F, Tomba A, et al. Chronic hepatitis in multiple virus infections: histopathological evaluation. *Histopathology* 1993; 22:319-25.

50. Smedile A, Farci P, Verme G, Caredda F, Cargnel A, Caporaso N, Dentico P, et al. Influence of delta infection on severity of hepatitis B. *Lancet* 1982;ii:945-7.
51. Lieber CS, Garro A, Leo MA, Mak KM, Worner T. Alcohol and cancer. *Hepatology* 1986;6: 1005-19.
52. Colin J-F, Cazals-Hatem D, Loriot MA, Mariot-Peignoux M, Pham BN, Auparein A. Influence of human immunodeficiency virus infection in chronic hepatitis B in homosexual men. *Hepatology* 1999;29:1306-10.
53. Okuno T, Shindo M, Arai K, Matsumoto M, Takeda M. Histological improvement of chronic hepatitis B, Non-A – Non-B with interferon treatment: application of a numerical scoring system for evaluating sequential morphological changes. *Gastroenterol Jpn* 1990;25:70-7.
54. Brook MG, Petrovic L, McDonald JA, Scheuer PJ, Thomas HC. Histological improvement after antiviral treatment for chronic hepatitis B virus infection. *J Hepatol* 1989;8:218-25.
55. Di Biscglie AM. Long-term outcome of interferon-alpha therapy for chronic hepatitis B. *J Hepatol* 1995;22(suppl):65-7.
56. Sarin SK, Guptan RC, Thakur V, Malhotra S, Malhotra V, Banerjee K, Khandekar P, et al. Etiology of low-dose alpha-interferon therapy in HBV-related chronic liver disease in Asian Indians: a randomized controlled trial. *J Hepatol* 1996:24:391-6.
57. Ruff JC. To treat or not to treat? The judicious use of interferon-alpha-2 for the treatment of chronic hepatitis B. *J Hepatol* 1993;17(suppl 3):542-6.
58. Nakano Y, Kiyosawa K, Sodeyama T, Tanaka E. Comparative study of clinical histological, immunological responses to interferon therapy in type non-A and non-B and type B hepatitis. *Am J Gasteroenterol* 1990:85:24-9.
59. Hoofnagle JH, Di Bisceglie AM, Waggoner JG, Park Y. Interferon-alpha for patients with clinically apparent cirrhosis due to chronic hepatitis B. *Gastroenterology* 1993;104:1116-21.
60. Pessoa MG, Wright TL. Update on clinical trials in the treatment of hepatitis B. *J Gasteroenterol Hepatol* 1999;14(suppl):S6-11.
61. Dusheiko G. Lamivudine therapy for hepatitis B infection. *Scand J Ghastroenterol* 1999;230(suppl): 76-81.
62. Lai CN, Chien RN, Leung NW, Chang TT, Guan R, Tai DI, Ng KY, et al. A one-year trial of lamivudine for chronic hepatitis B. Asia Hepatitis Lamivudine Study Group. *N Engl J Med* 1998; 339:61-8.
63. Tassopoulos NC, Volpes R, Pastore G, Heathcote J, Buti M, Goldin RD, Hawley S, et al. Efficacy of lamivudine in patients with hepatitis e antigen-negative/ hepatitis B virus DNA-positive (pre-core mutant) chronic hepatitis B. Lamivudine pre-core Mutant Study Group. *Hepatology* 1999;29:889-96.
64. Dienstag JL, Schiff ER, Wright TL, Perrillo RP, Hann HW, Goodman Z, Crowther, et al. Lamivudine as initial treatment for chronic hepatitis B in the United States. *N Engl J Med* 1999;341:1256-63.
65. Heathcote J, Schalm SW, Cianciara J. Lamivudine and Intron A combination treatment in patients with chronic hepatitis B infection. *J Hepatol* 1998;28:43 (abstract).
66. Lau DT, Khokhar MF, Doo E, Doo E, Ghany MG, Herion D, Park Y, Kleiner DE, et al. Long-term therapy of chronic hepatitis B with Lamivudine. *Hepatology* 2000;32:822-34.
67. Kweon YO, Goodman ZD, Dienstag JL, Schiff ER, Brown NA, Burkhardt E, Fried MW, et al. Decreasing fibrogenesis: an immmunohistochemical study of paired liver biopsies following lamivudine therapy for chronic hepatitis B. *J Hepatol* 2001;35:749-55.
68. Chien RN, Liaw YF, Atkins M. Pretherapy alanine transaminase level as a determinant for hepatitis B 'e' antigen sero-conversion during lamivudine therapy in patients with chronic hepatitis B. Asian Hepatitis Lamivudine Trial Group. *Hepatology* 1999;30:770-4.
69. Arase Y, Ikeda K, Murashima N, Chayama K, Tsubota A, Koida I, Suzuki Y, et al. Time course of

histological changes in patients with a sustained biochemical and virologic response to corticosteroid withdrawal therapy for chronic hepatitis B. *Am J Gastroenterol* 1999;94:3304-9.
70. Allen MI, Deslauriers M, Andrews CW, Tipples GA, Waltars KS, Tyrrell DL, Brown N, et al. Identification and characterization of mutations in hepatitis B virus resistant to lamivudine. *Hepatology* 1998;27:1670-7.
71. Schiff ER. Lamivudine for hepatitis B in clinical practice. *J Med Virol* 2000;61:386-91.
72. Atkins M, Hunt CM, Brown N. Clinical significance of YMDD mutant hepatitis B virus in a large cohort of lamivudine treated patients. *Hepatology* 1998;28:319.
73. Koretz RL, Lewin KJ, Rebhun DJ, Gitnick GL. Hepatitis B surface antigen carriers - to biopsy or not to biopsy. *Gastroenterology* 1978;75:860-3.
74. Vittal SB, Sourdourkas D, Shobassy D. Asymptomatic hepatic disease in blood donors with hepatitis B antigenemia. *Am J Clin Pathol* 1974;62:649-54.
75. Bolin TD, Davis AE, Liddelow AG. Liver disease and cell mediated immunity in hepatitis associated antigen (HBsAg) carriers. *Gut* 1973;14:365-8.
76. De Franchis R, Meucci G, Vecchi M, Tatarella M, Colombo M, Del Ninno E, Rumi MG, et al. The natural history of asymptomatic hepatitis B surface antigen carriers. *Ann Int Med* 1993;118:191-4.
77. Chon CY, Han KH, Lee KS, Moon YM, Kang JK, Park IS, Park C, et al. Peritoneoscopic liver biopsy findings in asymptomatic chronic HBsAg carriers with normal liver function tests and no hepatomegaly. *Yonsei Med J* 1996;37:295-301.
78. Russell RJ, Goldberg DM, Allan JG, Macsween RN, Wallace J, et al. A study of hepatic disease in Australia antigen and antibody positive blood donors. *Am J Dig Dis* 1974;19:113-21.
79. Reincki V, Dybkjaer E, Poulsen H, Banke O, Lylloff K, Nordenfelt E. A study of Australia antigen positive blood donors and their recipients with special reference to liver histology. *N Engl J Med* 1972;286: 867-70.
80. Villeneuve JP, Richer G, Cote J, Guevin R, Marleau D, Jolly JF, Viallet A. Chronic carriers of hepatitis B antigen (HBsAg): histological, biochemical, and immunological findings in 31 voluntary blood donors. *Am J Dig Dis* 1976;21:18-25.
81. Proceedings of the Single Theme Consensus Conference on Hepatitis B and C: carrier to cancer, Asian Perspectives. *Indian J Gastroenterol* 1999;18(suppl):S15-17.

Fig. 1. Piece meal necrosis in chronic hepatitis B (hematoxylin & eosin × 160).
Fig. 2. Apoptotic body with nuclear fragment in chronic hepatitis B (hematoxylin & eosin × 400).
Fig. 3. Chronic hepatitis B with cirrhosis (hematoxylin & eosin × 63).
Fig. 4. Ground glass hepatocytes in chronic hepatitis B (hematoxylin & eosin × 160).

Section III
Hepatocellular carcinoma and hepatitis B virus infection

20

Pathogenesis of hepatocellular carcinoma in hepatitis B virus infection

Bhudev C Das

Hepatocellular carcinoma (HCC) is one of the major causes of death in sub-Saharan Africa, Southern China and South-East Asian region. This cancer ranks eighth in the world's top ten cancers.[1] In India, hepatocellular carcinoma is one of the major cancers in both sexes along with cervical carcinoma in women. Epidemiological studies have identified several undisputable risk factors such as hepatitis B virus (HBV) and/or hepatitis C virus (HCV) infection, intake of alcoholic beverages, exposure to dietary aflatoxins and genetic alterations. The relative contribution of each of these factors is not very clear because of differential distribution of these factors in various geographic regions of the world. The two major causative agents that have been strongly implicated in the development of liver cancer in humans are HBV infection and aflatoxin B_1 exposure.[2,3]

Recently, several studies have also identified specific genetic alterations that often occur in HCC. The most prominent of them is the p53 tumor suppressor gene which is found to be frequently mutated in majority of HCC. Mutation of the p53 gene is also the most commonly detected genetic change found in most of the cancers affecting human beings.

In 1991 two groups[4,5] first described a mutational "hot spot" at codon 249 of the p53 gene ($ACG^{Arg} \rightarrow AGT^{Ser}$) in hepatocellular carcinoma. Interestingly, mutant p53 with codon 249 substitution (arginine to serine) is shown to enhance mitotic activity suggesting that such mutation may directly promote carcinogenesis. Soon it was also demonstrated that this specific codon 249 mutation could be induced by a liver specific carcinogen, aflatoxin B_1.[6] More than 50% of HCC patients living in high aflatoxin areas show this specific p53 mutation 'hot spot' but this mutation is very rare from low aflatoxin areas.[7] Interestingly in India, where aflatoxin exposure is high, a low frequency of p53 mutation in HCC patients has been reported.[8]

HEPATITIS B VIRUS (HBV) AND HCC

Hepatitis B virus (HBV) is considered to be the major causative agent of blood borne hepatitis in humans. There are about 350 million cases of chronic HBV infection all over the world. These individuals may either be healthy and asymptomatic or suffer from chronic hepatitis which often leads to serious sequlae such as cirrhosis and HCC. In spite of the successful vaccination programs, at least one million subjects succumb to HBV-related disease and HCC every year.

HBV is the prototype of hepatotropic (hepadna) DNA viruses whose genome is composed of a double stranded DNA genome with a complete coding (minus) strand paired with an incomplete non-coding (plus) strand and is maintained on an open circular conformation. The HBV genome is the smallest (3.2kb) among mammalian viruses with four overlapping open reading frames (ORFs) which encode a number of structural and non-structural proteins (Fig. 1). They are: the surface (S), the core (C), the polymerase (P), and the X-protein (HBX) which code for the surface protein (HBsAg), core protein (HBcAg/HBeAg), DNA polymerase/ reverse transcriptase and transactivation protein, HBX respectively.

Although, it is not clearly understood how HBV enters the hepatocyte following the infection and gets integrated with the host cell genome, interaction between cell membrane and viral envelope is thought to play a major role during integration. Once the virus enters the cell, incomplete viral genome is repaired to form a closed covalently circular (ccc) DNA which exists as a mini chromosome in the nucleus and acts as template for transcription of the pregenomic RNA, the precursor of replication and synthesis of viral proteins. The mRNAs thus synthesized encode the envelope and HBX transactivator proteins. HBV–induced HCC has been ascribed to the transcriptional deregulation of cellular growth control genes by the viral transactivating protein, the hepatitis B virus X-protein or HBX.

The role of HBX protein

HBX a protein of about 17kD, is derived from mRNA transcript of about 0.8 kb arising from X promoter. Generally, HBX protein is not detected in patient's sera because of its short half-life.[9, 10] Observation of anti-HBX antibodies in circulation is generally considered to

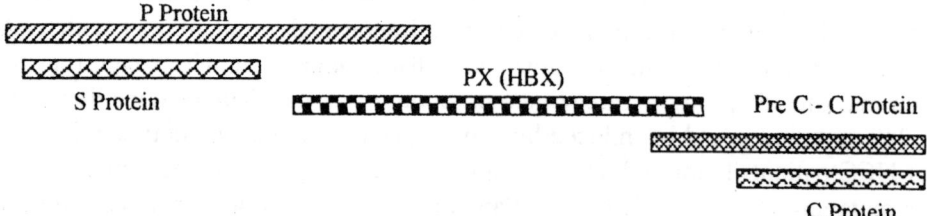

Fig. 1. Overlapping ORF (protein) of HBV

be indicator of HBX expression.[11] HBX protein has been implicated in virus replication and pathogenicity. It has been suggested that HBX gene products derived from integrated viral DNA may promote hepatocarcinogenesis.

HBX is a multifunctional protein which seems to use several major signalling pathways for gene expression. It can also interact directly with transcription factors.[12] By activating the binding of inducible transcription factor AP-1 (activator protein–1) and NFkB, HBX can stimulate RAS-GTP complex and activates the ras-raf mitogen activated protein (MAP) kinase signal transduction pathways.[13,14] Most importantly, HBX can complex with p53 protein and inhibits sequence specific DNA binding and p53–mediated transcriptional transactivation activities.[15,16] Similar to p53 binding and its inactivation demonstrated for the products of other DNA tumor viruses,[17] HBX protein can also bind with p53 to inactivate it. It is suggested that HBX-mediated p53 inactivation may be important in those HCC lacking mutation of the p53 gene leading to interference with DNA repair and apoptosis.

Although, infection of HBV is essential for the development of HCC, it does not directly involve in regulating the expression of cellular oncogenes or tumor suppressor genes[18] which have been often linked to development of this disease. Several lines of evidence suggest that one of the viral genes, the HBX protein plays a pivotal role in cellular transformation and uncontrolled cell growth.[19] It is considered to be an oncogenic protein encoded by HBV. It can transactivate cellular genes and can cause neoplastic transformation of rodent cells *in vitro*.[20] It is also shown that transgenic mice carrying human HBX gene can develop liver cancer.[21] Furthermore, HBX can induce cell proliferation in quiescent fibroblasts and deregulate cell cycle check points.[22]

Functional domains of HBX protein

The X gene is located downstream to enhancer I (Enh I) overlapped by P and the N-terminal of pre-C at the C-terminal and also by several cis-elements plus enhancer II (Enh II) and promoters (Fig. 2). X-gene is transcribed independently of other viral transcripts. Enh I and X-promoter are considered as the transcriptional regulatory unit of X-gene.[23] Enhancer I

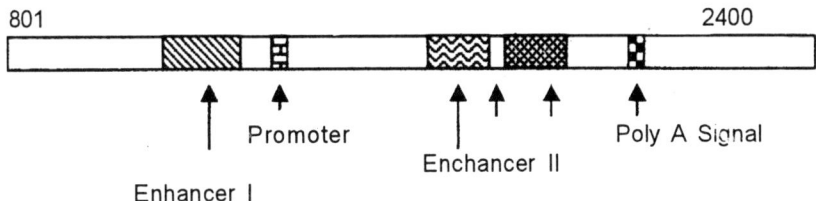

Fig. 2. DNA cis-element of HBV

consists of multiple cis elements of liver-specific or non-specific transcriptional regulators (Fig. 3).[24-27] The X-gene is transcribed independently of other transcripts and this can be detected in liver tissues of humans. The X ORF is nearer to enhancer I which along with X-promoter is the transcriptional regulator of X-gene. The HBV Enh 1 core is highly conserved and includes a PMA or TPA responsive elements like sequence, C-stretch and NF-1 binding sites (Fig. 3), Enh 1 harbours many cis-elements for liver-specific transactivator such as HNF1, HNF3, RXR. The wide variety of cis-elements have been documented to be responsive to HBX designated as XRE which include binding sites for transcription factors such as AP2, APL, NFkB, SRE, C/EBP, Ets, ATF1, and CREB. The transactivating factors were demonstrated in transient expression system as well as in stable HBX expressing cell lines or in transgenic cells.[28]

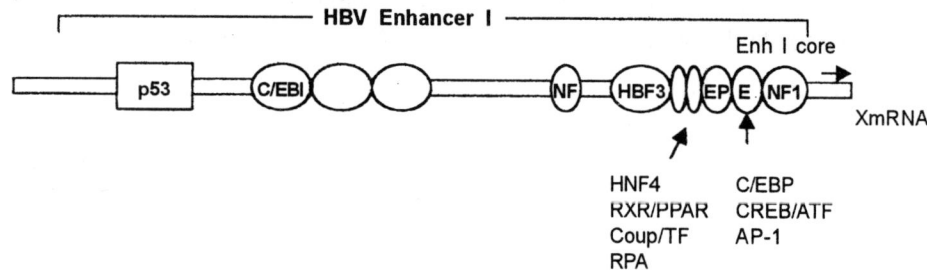

Fig. 3. HBV Enhancer I

The interaction of X-protein and p53 is highly conserved. The direct interaction between p53 and HBX has been reported by several authors. P53 binds in the c-terminal region of HBX but it is mapped within the transactivation domain. The interaction between p53 and HBX may interfere with their functions such as binding of p53 to Enh 1 and DNA repair of p53 (Fig. 3). HBX also plays a role in DNA repair processes in a p53 independent manner.

Recently, attempts are being made to study the actual impact and mechanism of HBX during malignant transformation of hepatocytes. Also, specific domains responsible for growth arrested apoptosis have been mapped to HBX (Fig. 4). Sirma et al[29] compared the effects of HBX and its naturally occurring mutants on cell growth and viability and showed that HBX inhibits clonal outgrowth and induces apoptosis. But, mutations in the HBX abolish both HBX-induced growth arrest and apoptosis. This seems to render hepatocytes susceptible to uncontrolled growth leading to HCCs.

To establish that HBX plays a major role in the events that lead to tumorigenic transformation, a transgenic mouse model has been developed for hepatocellular carcinoma There are conflicting results regarding the development of liver-specific tumours in HBX-transgenic mice. This could be because of promoter strength and duration of HBX expression, etc. Recently, Jameel and his group (Annual report ICGEB, 1998)[30] have developed interesting

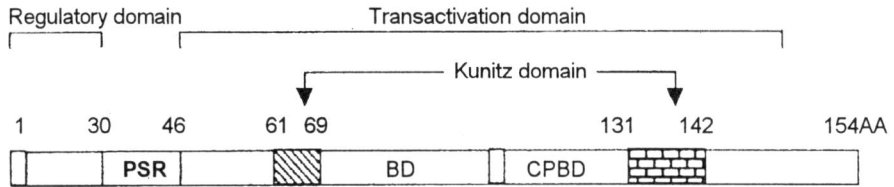

BD=basic domain, PSR = protein-serine rich region, CPBD=cellular protein-binding domain

Fig. 4. Functional domain of HBV protein

transgenic mouse model of human HCC using a novel construct called X15-myc. This construct expresses a truncated X-protein (amino acid 58 to 154) which encompasses a minimal transactivation domain of HBX (Fig. 4) along with a full length c-myc protein. C-myc is often known to selectively amplify in HBV-induced HCC. This construct when microinjected to transgenic mice has been found to develop large tumours over a period of 10 to 12 months. The expression of both HBX and c-myc has been confirmed in these tumors.

p53 mutation and HCC

Mutations or deletions of the p53 tumor suppressor gene located on the short arm of chromosome 17 is critical for the induction of apoptosis. It is, therefore, not surprising that p53 mutation is most common in HCC. It has been also shown that HCC cells with mutant p53 can induce apoptosis following restoration of wild type p53 gene into it.

In contrast to wide spectrum of p53 mutations identified in a variety of human cancers, more than 50% of liver cancers show a specific G to T transversion at codon 249 of the p53 gene. Epidemiologic studies have indicated that exposure to aflatoxin B_1 causes the p53 mutations. Specific G to T transversions at codon 249 have been shown to be most common in HCC patients from Central China, Africa, Mexico, and Mozambique where aflatoxin contamination of food is high but less or rare in Hongkong, Singapore, Japan, Europe, and USA (Table 1). It has also been shown in an *in vitro* study that aflatoxin B_1 can induce this specific 249 codon mutation. In contrast, an ingenious experiment[31] has been carried out using tree shrews which show 92% and 93% homologies with human wild type p53 DNA and amino acid sequence respectively. This animal model was used for the development of HCC after either HBV infection or HBV infection plus aflotoxin B_1 (AFB-1) treatment. Five HCCs which developed following either HBV infection or HBV and AFB-1 treatment, showed no change in p53 gene except one which showed point mutation at codon 275. But tree shrews exposed to AFB1 and/or HBV showed no codon 249 mutation or significant level of other mutations in the p53 gene.

Recently, p53 mutation pattern in hepatocellular carcinoma in workers exposed to vinyl

Table 1. Mutations reported in 'Hot Spot' codon 249 from different regions of the world

Aflatoxin exposure	Status of mutation	Place
High exposure	High / exon 7/249	China, Africa, Mexico
Low exposure	Low / other exons but not exon 7	Beijing
Low/no exposure	Low / other exons 4, 5, 8	USA, Europe, Hong Kong, Singapore
Low/no exposure	Low / other exons plus exon 7 codon 249	Germany and Japan
High exposure	Low / exon 7 codon 249	India

chloride in Germany was analysed. P53 mutations were found in 11 of 18 HCCs examined but the mutations were at CpG sites comprising several codons (codons 175, 245, 248, 273, and 282) exons codon 249.[32] Occurrence of different frequency of p53 mutations from different geographic regions may be attributed to various factors such as ethnic variations in susceptibility to aflatoxin B_1 polymorphisms and variations in carcinogen detoxifying enzymes, glutathione S-transferase epoxide hydrolase including cytochrome P450.[33-38] But in these places more than 78% tumors were also positive for HBV-DNA. It indicates that inactivation of p53 may occur by mechanisms other than point mutations, i.e. by hepatitis B virus X-protein-mediated inactivation. However, p53 mutations are equally prevalent in X-negative and X-positive HCC.

Observation of differential distribution of p53 mutations in HCC from different geographic regions indicate that p53 mutations cannot be considered as a sole factor for development of HCC (Table 2). p53 mutation as such may not be directly associated with the development of HCC, and HBV along with p53 should interact in the carcinogenic process in the liver. Recent demonstration that wild type p53 can inhibit transcription from the HBV core promoter indicates that wild type p53 can protect against the carcinogenic process in liver.[39] Studies have also indicated that progressive risk of HCC may be due to accumulation of multistage genetic mutations in target cells and several new loci have been implicated in hepatocarcinogenesis.[40,41] It is suggested that persistent HBV infection is essential for inducing these genetic mutations or alterations through immune-mediated injury of the hepatocytes. Active immuni-

Table 2. Mutations of the p53 gene as revealed by PCR-SSCP and sequencing in HCCs in India

No.	Exon	Codon	Nucleotide change	Amino acid change	Type
9	7	249	AGG → AGT	Arg → Ser	Transversion
15	7	249	AGG → AGT	Arg → Ser	Transversion
16	7	249	CCC → TCC	Pro → Ser	Transition

zation or treatment of chronic hepatitis B by interferon or other antiviral agents can control HBV but whether they can control HCC is not known. Therefore, there is a need for a multidisciplinary approach to unravel the role of important viral and host genes during development of hepatocellular carcinoma. This will help in developing new approaches to diagnosis and treatment of HCC.

CONCLUSIONS

Although the infection of hepatitis B virus (HBV), exposure to dietary aflatoxin B_1 or high consumption of alcohol, all important risk factors, are known to contribute in the development of hepatocellular carcinoma, none of them can cause cancer directly. These factors must bring about changes in the genes responsible for growth and differentiation. One of the growth regulating genes which have strongly been implicated in almost all human cancers and specifically in liver cancer is the p53 gene which either by mutation or by binding to the hepatitis B virus X-protein or by yet unknown mechanisms, seems to be important in multistep hepatocarcinogenesis. The variable incidence of p53 mutations from different geographic regions reflect a different genetic background in the etiology of HCC. High prevalence of HBV irrespective of exposure to dietary carcinogens such as aflatoxin or alcohol indicates an important role of viral and host cell genes in hepatocarcinogenesis. Possibly the HBV X-protein and HCV core protein interact with variety of cellular proteins such as NFkB, AP-1 and p53 leading to alterations in signal transduction and transcriptional activity. These events facilitate malignant progression by promoting hepatocyte survival, escape immune surveillance and acquisition of genetic alteration. Regions like India where in spite of high aflatoxin exposure, the p53 hot-spot mutation is much lower, the reason could be ethnic variation either in susceptibility to aflatoxin B_1 or variation in metabolic/dextoxifying enzymes such as P-450, HST m-1 and epoxide hydrolase. Understanding functional interactions between viral genes and host cell genes would throw light in developing approaches for early diagnosis and better management of patients with HCC.

REFERENCES

1. Parkin DM, Bray F, Firlay J, Pisani P. Estimating world cancer burden: globoscan 2000. *Int J Cancer* 2000;94:153-6.
2. IARC. IARC monographs on the evaluation of carcinogenic risk to humans. Some naturally occurring substances: food items and constituents, heterocyclic aromatic amines and mycotoxins. Lyon, France: *IARC*, 1993;56:245-345.
3. IARC. IARC monographs on the evaluation of carcinogenic risk to humans. Hepatitis viruses. Lyon, France: *IARC*, 1994;59.
4. Bressac B, Kew M, Wands J, Ozturk M. Selective G to T mutations of p53 gene in hepatocellular carcinoma from southern Africa. *Nature* 1991;350:429-31.
5. Hsu IC, Metcalf RA, Sun T, Welsh JA, Wang NJ, Harris CC. Mutational hot-spot in the p53 gene in human hepatocellular carcinoma. *Nature* 1991;350:427-8.

6. Aguilar F, Hussain PP, Cerutti P. Aflatoxin B1 induces the transversion of G-T in codon 249 of the p53 tumor suppressor gene in human hepatocytes. *Proc Natl Acad Sci USA* 1993;90:8586-90.
7. Ozturk M. *Chromosomal aberrations and tumor suppressor genes in primary liver cancer. In:* Brechot C, Ed. Primary liver cancer etiological and progression factors: CRC Press, USA 1994;pp.269-81.
8. Katiyar S, Das BC, Thakur V, Guptan RC, Sarin SK, Das BC. p53 tumor suppressor gene mutations inhepatocellular carcinoma patients in India. *Cancer* 2000;88:1565-73.
9. Henkler F, Koshy R. Multiple functions of the hepatitis E virus X-protein. *Viral Hepatitis Rev* 1996;2:143-59.
10. Schek N, Bartenschlager R, Kuhn C, Schaller H. Phosphorylation and rapid turnover of hepatitis B virus X-protein expressed in Hep G2 cells from a recombinant vaccinia virus. *Oncogene* 1991;6:1735-44.
11. Pfaff E, Salfeld J, Gemelin K, Schallewr H, Theilmann C. Synthesis of the X-protein of hepatitis E virus in vitro and detection of anti-X antibodies in human sera. *Virology* 1987;158:456-60.
12. Maguire HF, Hoeffler JP, Siddiqui A. HEV X-protein alters the DNA binding specificity of CREP and A TF-2 by protein interactions. *Science* 1991;252:842-4.
13. Eenn J, Schneider RJ. Hepatitis E virus HEx protein activates Ras-GTP complex formation and establishes a Ras, Raf, MAP kinase signaling cascade. *Proc Natl Acad Sci USA* 1994;91:10350-3.
14. Natoli G, Avantaggiata ML, Chirillo P, Puri PL, Lanni A, Ealsano C, Lavrero M, Ras-and Rat Dependent activation of c-jun transcriptional activity by hepatitis E virus trans activator pX oncogene. *EMEOJ* 1994;9:2837-43.
15. Wang XW, Forrester K, Yeh H, Feitelson MA, Gu JR, Harris CC. Hepatitis E virus X-protein inhibits p53 sequence specific DNA binding transcriptional activity and association with transcription factor ERCC3. *Proc Natl Acad Sci USA* 1994;91:2230-4.
16. Ueda H, Ullrich SJ, Gangemi JD, Kappel CA, Ngo L, Feitelson MA, Jay G. Functional inactivation but not structural mutation of p53 causes liver cancer. *Nat Genet* 1995;9:41-7.
17. Neil JC, Cameron ER, Baxter EW. p53 and tumor viruses catched the guardian off-guard. *Trends Microbiol* 1997;5:115-20.
18. Ganem D, Varmus HE. The molecular biology of the hepatitis B viruses. *Annu Rev Biochem* 1987;56:651-93.
19. Yen TS. Hepadnaviral X Protein: Review of Recent Progress. *J Biomed Sci* 1996;3:20-30.
20. Kim CM, Koike K, Saito I, Miyamura T, Jay G. HBx gene of hepatitis B virus induces liver cancer in transgenic mice. *Nature* 1991;351:317-20.
21. Shirakata Y, Kawada M, Fujiki Y, Sano H, Oda M, Yaginuma K, Kobayashi M, et al. The X gene of hepatitis B virus induced growth stimulation and tumorigenic transformation of mouse NIH3T3 cells. *Jpn J Cancer Res* 1989;80:617-21.
22. Benn J, Schneider RJ. Hepatitis B virus HBx protein deregulates cell cycle checkpoint controls. *Proc Natl Acad Sci USA* 1995;92:11215-9.
23. Guo WT, Bell KD. Ou JH. Characterization of the hepatitis B virus Enh I enhancer and X promoter complex. *J Virol* 1991;65:6686-92.
24. Faktor O, Budlovsky S, Ben-Levy R, Shaul Y. A single element within the hepatitis B virus enhancer binds multiple proteins and responds to multiple stimuli. *J Virol* 1990;64:1861-3.
25. Dikstein R, Faktor O, Ben-Levy R, Shaul Y. Functional organization of the hepatitis B virus enhancer. *Mol Cell Biol* 1990;10:3682-9.
26. Huan B, Siddiqui A. Retinoid X receptor RXR alpha binds to and trans activates the hepatitis B virus enhancer. *Proc Natl Acad Sci USA* 1992;89:9059-63.
27. Garcia AD, Ostapchuk P, Hearing P. Functional interaction of nuclear factors EF-C, HNF-4 and RXR alpha with hepatitis B virus enhancer I. *J Virol* 1993;67:3940-50.

28. Murakami S. Hepatitis B virus X-protein structure, function and biology. *Intervirology* 1999;42: 61-99.
29. Sirma H, Giannini C, Poussin K, Paterlini K, Paterlini P, Kremsdorf D, Brechot C. Hepatitis B virus X mutants, present in hepatocellular carcinoma tissue aclorograte both the antiprolifeative and transactivation effects of HBX. *Oncogene* 1999;26:4848-59.
30. Annual Report International Centre for Genetic Engineering and Biotechnology, New Delhi, 1998.
31. Park US, Su JJ, Ban KC, Qin L, Lee EH, Lee YI. Mutations in the p53 tumor suppressor gene in tree spread hepatocellular carcinoma associated with hepatitis B virus infection and intake of aflatoxin B_1. *Gene* 2000;251:73-80.
32. Weihrauch M, Lehnert G, Kocherling F, Wittekind C, Tannapfel A. p53 mutation pattern in hepatocellular carcinoma in workers exposed to vinyl chloride. *Cancer* 2000;88:1030-6.
33. Scorsone KA, Zhou YZ, Butel JS, Slagle BL. p53 mutations cluster at codon 249 in hepatitis B virus positive hepatocellular carcinomas from China. *Cancer Res* 1992;52:1635-8.
34. Ozturk M, Bressac B, Puisieux A, Kew M, Volkmann M, Bozcall S, Mura JS, et al. p53 mutation in hepatocellular carcinoma after aflatoxin exposure. *Lancet* 1991;338:1356-9.
35. Slagle BL. p53 mutation and hepatitis B virus: co-factors in hepatocellular carcinoma. *Hepatology* 1995;21:597-9.
36. Liu YH, Taylor J, Linko P, Lucier GW, Thomson CL. Glutathione S-transferase mu in human lymphocyte and liver, role in modulating formation of carcinogen derived DNA adducts. *Carcinogenesis* 1991;12:2269-75.
37. McGlynn KA, Rosvold EA, Lustbader ED, Hu Y, Clapper ML, Zhou T, Wild CP, et al. Susceptibility to hepatocellular carcinoma is associated with genetic variation in the enzymatic dextoxification of aflatoxin B_1. *Proc Natl Acad Sci USA* 1995;92:2384-7.
38. Hall AJ, Wild CP. *The toxicology of aflatoxins: human health: veterinary and agricultural significance*. In: Eaton DL, Groopman JD, Eds. Academic Press, New York, 1994;pp. 233-58.
39. Uchida T, Takahashi K, Tatsuno K, Dhingra U, Eliason JF. Inhibition of hepatitis B virus core promoter by p53: Implications for carcinogenesis in hepatocytes. *Int J Cancer* 1996;17:892-7.
40. Chen PJ, Chen DS. Hepatitis B virus infection and hepatocellular carcinoma: molecular genetics and clinical perspectives. *Sem Liver Dis* 1999;19:253-62.
41. Satoh S, Varmaoka Y. Multi step carcinogenesis of HCC. *Nippon Rensho* 2001;59(suppl):40-4.

21

Epidemiology of hepatitis B associated hepatocellular carcinoma in India

K M Mohandas

Hepatocellular carcinoma (HCC) is the fourth most common cause of death from cancer worldwide.[1,2] It is estimated that by the year 2000, there will be 4,30,000 deaths per year from liver cancer all over the world.[2] Approximately 77% of all deaths due to liver cancer occur in developing countries and China alone contributes to 44% of these deaths.[2] In sub-Saharan Africa, HCC is the leading cause of cancer deaths in men.[2] The prognosis in symptomatic HCC is dismal. The five year survival after the onset of symptoms of HCC in developing countries is 0.8% in men and 4.4% in women.

DESCRIPTIVE EPIDEMIOLOGY

The estimate of prevalence of HCC in India is available from autopsy studies in teaching hospitals. The incidence at autopsy varied from 0.2% to 1.6% which was markedly lower than the rates in east asia.[3,4] Corroborating the autopsy data was the population-based incidence data that was available in early 1970s.[4] The age-adjusted incidence of HCC is low in all Indian cancer registries compared to the incidence in China, Japan, and other South East Asian countries (Table 1).[1,4-9] The incidence rates are a little higher than in western countries like USA, UK, and Australia. The mean age adjusted incidence of HCC in 6 Indian populations is 2.77 for males and 1.28 for females.[4] We have projected that there will be 13,039 patients with HCC in India in 2001. This would constitute 1.8% of all new incident cancer cases in India in 2001.[6]

Age and sex distribution

As reported worldwide, the incidence of HCC in India increases after the fifth decade and peaks in the sixth decade (Tables 2 and 3).[1,4] Referral bias and skewed age distribution of Indian population creates a false impression that HCC in India occurs a decade earlier.[4] Very rarely a variant called the fibrolamellar HCC may occur in infants and children in India.[11] The

Table 1. Number of incident cases of HCC recorded in 8 population-based registries[1,5]

Place	Population (all ages)		Total cases		Years
	Male	Female	Male	Female	
Actual population incidence					
Mumbai	5350952	4354682	506	226	88-92
Delhi	4225192	3489858	110	66	88-89
Bangalore	2103290	1897352	185	80	88-92
Chennai	1965810	1836022	161	32	88-92
Trivandrum	523853	541543	23	9	91-92
Barshi	226969	215541	15	6	88-92
Bhopal	509795	453067	13	5	88-89
Karunagapally	191149	193954	9	6	91-92
All 8 registries	15,097,010	12,982,019	251	112	1-year (average)
India	53,00,00000	49,00,00000	8812	4227	2001 (estimated)

Table 2. Incidence of HCC in different age groups and age standardized male population

Place of Registries	Age groups specific rates*					ASR* (0-74)	CIR
	30-34	40-44	50-54	60-64	70-74		
Japan, Osaka	1.4	12.1	71.6	288.3	286.3	46.7	5.97
Hong Kong	10.0	36.6	88.7	146.9	197.3	36.2	4.27
Singapore: Chinese	2.7	10.8	31.8	115.7	167.0	22.1	2.78
Singapore: Malay	4.8	13.4	12.5	42.4	62.4	11.6	1.31
Singapore: Indian	–	3.0	4.6	21.5	86.3	6.3	0.97
India, Madras	0.3	1.7	8.0	10.5	9.3	2.5	0.29
India, Bombay	0.4	1.6	6.1	15.9	34.9	3.9	0.51
UK, Scotland	0.4	1.2	3.2	13.4	28.8	3.1	0.38
UK, England & Wales	0.3	0.7	2.5	8.6	16.0	2.0	0.25
US, (SEER): Black	0.9	5.6	13.6	33.0	45.6	6.5	0.81
US, (SEER): White	0.2	1.5	4.0	11.3	21.3	3.0	0.35

* Per 100,000 population. ASR, age standardized rates. CIR, cumulative incidence rates
Note: The cumulative risk is the probability that an individual will develop the disease in question during a certain age period (e.g. 0–74), in the absence of any competing cause of death. If the cumulative risk is less than 10%, which is the case for most cancers, it can be approximated very well by the cumulative rate (CIR). The cumulative rate is like the standardized rate a weighted sum of age specific incidence rate. The cumulative rate as an approximation to cumulative risk has a greater intuitive appeal, and is more directly interpretable as a measurement of lifetime risk, ignoring mortality from other diseases.[1]

sex distribution of HCC reveals preponderance of men over women as seen worldwide.[1,4] However, the male–female ratio in population-based data is about 3:1 to 2:1 as compared to 10:1 to 5:1 in hospital data.[1,4] This is most probably due to gender bias in seeking medical treatment among Indians.

Table 3. Age standardized incidence* of HCC in immigrants from south and north India[3, 4]**

Place	Men	Women
South Indians		
Chennai	2.5	0.5
Singapore	6.3	2.8
North Indians		
Delhi	2.2	1.1
British Indians	6.2	2.4

* Per 100,000 population **Age standardized to world population

Time trends

The incidence of HCC has been declining gradually in most parts of the world.[1-2, 4] The incidence of HBV associated HCC is declining fast with introduction of safe blood transfusions and the use of HBV vaccination.[12-13] Time-trends over the past three decades in the population-based registry of Mumbai reveal a gradual increase in the incidence of HCC in both males and females.[4] While some of this increase may be due to better registration and improved diagnosis, there appears to be a genuine increase in the incidence of HCC due to unknown reasons.

Immigrant studies

Studies on Indian immigrants from several developed countries provide very reliable and yet contradictory data. Bias is possible as some Indians might return to their native places in India after being diagnosed to have a terminal illness. Paradoxically, the incidence of HCC is much higher in immigrant Indians when compared to the rates in most parts of India.[1, 8-10] However, these rates are lower than in the Singapore Chinese.[1] The mortality rates from HCC are significantly higher in Indian immigrants compared to the native British population in UK.[9] Interestingly the HCC mortality ratio in Whites who were born or had lived in India during the Raj was higher than that in the native white population.[10] These observations provide a strong circumstantial evidence that the environment in India does favour the development of HCC.

Role of chronic viral hepatitis

Globally about 57% of all liver cancer deaths can be attributed to hepatitis B alone.[2] However, there are no large case-control studies on HCC from India. Prevalence of HBV surface antigen (HBsAg) in Indian HCC patients has varied from 36% to 74% with an average of 47%.[4, 14-17] It is estimated that nearly 42.5 million Indians are HBsAg positive.[18] We have estimated that in the year 2001 there will be 4935 patients with HCC associated with hepatitis

B.[6] The estimated relative risk of developing HCC in HBsAg positive Indians would be 17.9.[6] Few studies from India have shown serological evidence of combined hepatitis B and C infection in patients with chronic liver disease and HCC.[4] A north Indian study reported HCV seropositivity in 15.1% of patients with HCC, half of who also had evidence of hepatitis B infection. There is no prospective data from India to support cost-effectiveness of HBV vaccination to prevent HCC in India. In theory, universal HBV vaccination program is unlikely to be cost effective due to the lower incidence of HCC and the large population of subjects with chronic HBV infection who would not benefit from vaccination. Longitudinal studies must be undertaken before we can recommend either primary prevention by vaccination or secondary prevention by ultrasound screening as done in most developed countries.

Role of aflatoxin

Aflatoxins are metabolites of the fungi *Aspergillus flavus* and *Aspergillus parasiticus* that contaminate foodstuffs like maize, parboiled rice, coconut, and groundnuts. Environmental exposure to aflatoxin is strongly associated with the development of HCC.[19-20] Few studies have shown independent hepatic carcinogenesis by aflatoxins. However, most studies reveal a marked amplification of the hepatic carcinogenesis of HBV infection.[19-24] Aflatoxins act as co-carcinogen with HBV.[19] The role of reducing aflatoxin exposure to prevent the development of HCC in subjects with chronic HBV infection. Acute hepatitis following poisoning by aflatoxins has been reported from India.[23] There is little epidemiological data on the exposure of HCC patients to aflatoxins in India.

MOLECULAR EPIDEMIOLOGY OF HBV ASSOCIATED HCC

There are no studies on Indian sub-types of HBV associated with HCC. Mutations of p53 tumor suppressor gene are reported in over 50% hepatoma cells in endemic regions of the word.[21,22] Specific p53 mutations are considered to be a marker of exposure to aflatoxin. In a study from New Delhi, only a very small percentage of Indian hepatoma cells had mutations in the p53 genes.[26] HBx gene of the HBV is known to transactivate a variety of cellular genes associated with cell proliferation. Unpublished results reveal a high frequency of full-length HBx transcripts in patents with chronic viral hepatitis. In the tumor tissues of HCC patients, truncated HBx transcripts along with full length HBx transcripts have been observed (personal communication, Dr. Chiplunkar SV, Cancer Research Institute, Mumbai).

CONCLUSIONS

Incidence data from eight population based registries reveal that HCC is not a common cancer in India. From preventive viewpoint we have estimated that half to three fourth of all HCC in India are associated with HBV. Theoretically, most of the HCC in India is amenable to primary prevention by immunization, safe blood transfusion practices and life style changes.[27-29] However, there is a large burden of subjects with chronic HBV infection who will remain at risk for several decades to come. Indian clinicians should consider screening of all patients who have chronic HBV infection with at least once a year ultrasound examination. This would help to diagnose small HCC when simple techniques such as percutaneous ethanol injection can be used.[30] More epidemiological studies are needed to assess true risk of HCC in chronic liver disease of viral etiology and unravel the role of aflatoxin in the development of HCC in India.

REFERENCES

1. Parkin DM, Whelan SL, Ferlay J, Raymond L, Young J. *Cancer Incidence in Five Continents*, Vol. VII. Lyon: International Agency for Research on Cancer, 1997.
2. Pisani P, Parkin DM, Ferlay J. Estimates of the worldwide mortality from eighteen major cancers in 1985. Implications for prevention and projections of future burden. *Int J Cancer* 1993;55:891-3.
3. Okuda K, Beasley RP. *Epidemiology. In:* Okuda K, Mackay I, Eds. Hepatocellular carcinoma: UICC Technical Report Series, Vol. 74, 1982; pp. 9-30.
4. Dhir V, Mohandas KM. Epidemiology of digestive cancer in India-III. Liver. *Indian J Gastroenterol* 1998;17:100-3.
5. Annual report 1987. *National Cancer Registry Program.* Indian Council of Medical Research, New Delhi. 1990.
6. Mohandas KM, Jagannath P. Epidemiology of digestive cancer in India-VI, Projected burden in the new millennium and the need for primary prevention. *Indian J Gastroenterol* 2000;19:74-8.
7. Parkin DM, Muir CS, Whelan SL, Gao YT, Ferlay J, Powell J. *Cancer Incidence in Five Continents*, Vol. VI. Lyon: International Agency for Research on Cancer, 1992.
8. Grulich AE, Mcredie M, Coates M. Cancer incidence in Asian migrants to New south Wales Australia. *Br J Cancer* 1995;71:400-8.
9. Winter H, Cheng KK, Cummins C, Maric R, Silcocks P, Varghese C. Cancer incidence in the south Asian population of England (1990-92). *Br J Cancer* 1999;79:645-54.
10. Swerdlow AJ, Marmot MG, Grulich AE, Head J. Cancer mortality in Indian and British ethnic immigrants from the Indian subcontinent to England and Wales. *Br J Cancer* 1995;72:1312-9.
11. Borges A, Santhi Swaroop V, Desai PB. Fibrolamellar carcinoma. *Am J Gastroenterol* 1991:86:789-90.
12. Chang MH, Chen CJ, Lai MS, Hsu HM, Wu TC, Kong MS, et al. Universal hepatitis B vaccination in Taiwan and the incidence of hepatocellular carcinoma in children. *N Engl J Med* 1997;336:1855-9.
13. Tanaka K, Hirohata T, Koga S, Sugimachi K, Kanematsu T, Ohryoji F, Nawata H, et al. Hepatitis C and hepatitis B in etiology of hepatocellular carcinoma in the Japanese population. *Cancer Res* 1991; 51:2842-7.
14. Dhir V, Swaroop VS, Mohandas KM, Dinshaw KA, Desai DC, Nagral A, Sharma V, et al. Combination chemotherapy and radiation for palliation of hepatocellular carcinoma. *Am J Clin Oncol* 1992;15: 304-7.
15. Durga R, Muralikrishna P, Ali N. Viral markers in hepatocellular carcinoma. *Indian J Gastroenterol* 1994;13:A89.
16. Kumar A, Sreenivas DV, Nagarjuna YR. Hepatocellular carcinoma: The Indian scenario. *Indian J Gastroenterol* 1995;14:A100.
17. Ramatilakhan B, Dinkaran N, Balasubramaniam V, Madangopalan N, Jayanthi V. Pattern of primary liver cancer in Madras. *Indian J Gastroenterol* 1995;14:A95.
18. Thyagarajan SP, Jayaram S, Mohanavalli B. *Prevalence of HBV in the general population of India. In:* Sarin

SK, Singal AK, Eds. Hepatitis B in India: Problems and Prevention. CBS Publishers & Distributors, New Delhi. 1996; pp. 5-16.
19. Ross RK, Yuan JM, Yu MC, Wogan GN, Qian GS, Tu JT, Groopman JD, et al. Urinary aflatoxin biomarkers and the risk of hepatocellular carcinoma. *Lancet* 1992;339:943-6.
20. Qian GS, Ross RK, Yu MC, Yuan JM, Gao YT, Henderson BE, Wogan GN, et al. A follow-up study of urinary markers of aflatoxin exposure and liver cancer risk in Shangai, Peoples Republic of China. *Cancer Epidmiol Biomarkers Prev* 1994;1:3-10.
21. Hsia CC, Kleiner DE Jr., Axiotis CA, Di Bisceglie A, Nomura AM, Stemmerman GN, Tabor E. Mutations of p53 gene in hepatocellular carcinoma: roles of hepatitis B virus and aflatoxin contamination in the diet. *J Natl Cancer Inst* 1992;84:1638-41.
22. Lunn RM, Zhang YJ, Wang LY, Chen CJ, Lee PH, Lee CS, Tsai WY, Santella RM. p53 mutations, chronic hepatitis B virus infection and aflatoxin exposure in hepatocellular carcinoma in Taiwan. *Cancer Res* 1997;57:3471-7.
23. Henry SH, Bosch FX, Bowers JC. Alfatoxin, hepatitis and worldwide liver cancer risks. *Adv Exp Med Biol* 2002;504:229-33.
24. Smela ME, Currier SS, Baitex EA, Essigmann JM. The chemistry and biology of alfatoxin B(1): from mutational spectrometry to carcinogenesis. *Carcinogenesis* 2001;22:535-45.
25. Krishnamachari KAVR, Bhat RV, Nagarajan V, Tilak TBG. Hepatitis due to aflatoxicosis. *Lancet* 1975;11061-3.
26. Katiyar S, Dash BC, Thakur V, Guptan RC, Sarin SK, Das BC. p53 tumor suppressor gene mutations in hepatocellular carcinoma patients in India. *Cancer* 2000;88:1565-73.
27. Zoli M, Magalotti D, Bianchi G, Gueli C, Marchesini G, Pisi E. Efficacy of surveillance program for early detection of hepatocellular carcinoma. *Cancer* 1996;78:977-85.
28. Collier J, Sherman M. Screening for hepatocellular carcinoma. *Hepatology* 1998;27:273-8.
29. Sarin SK, Thakur V, Guptan RC, Saigal S, Malhotra V, Thyagarajan SP, Das BC. Profile of hepatocellular carcinoma in India: an insight into the possible etiologic associations. *J Gastroenterol Hepatol* 2001; 16:666-73.
30. Tang ZY. Hepatocellular carcinoma-cause, treatment and metastasis. *World J Gastroenterol* 2001; 7:445-54.

Screening for hepatocellular carcinoma in patients with chronic hepatitis B virus infection

Ashok K Jain

Hepatocellular carcinoma (HCC) is one of the commonest cancer world wide, accounting for an estimated one million deaths annually.[1] Hepatitis B virus (HBV) infection appears to be one of the important causes, particularly in Asia and Africa, where HBsAg positivity among HCC patients is 85–95%, compared to 10–25% HBsAg positivity among the HCC patients in United States and Western Europe. In a study from Taiwan, 100-fold higher risk of developing HCC was noted in HBsAg positive subjects than in HBsAg negative individuals.[2] Moreover, a significant reduction in the incidence of childhood HCCs along with decrease in the prevalence of chronic HBV infection have been noted in Taiwanese children following universal hepatitis B vaccination in the newborn.[3]

PATHOGENESIS OF HCC

The mechanism by which HBV infection causes HCC is not clear. However, various mechanisms have been postulated.

Cirrhosis related

Chronic liver injury usually results in inflammatory changes, regeneration and fibrosis. In some cases, large regenerative nodules (>1 cm) can develop areas of atypia and progress to low grade dysplastic nodules, and subsequently high grade dysplastic nodules (synonym - adenomatous hyperplasia), finally well differentiated HCC. This may be a pathway in development of HCC. Genesis of dysplastic nodules is debatable. These may be overgrown cirrhotic nodules than adjacent ones or may represent clonal expansion of transformed hepatocytes, which have risen outside cirrhotic nodule. Nearly half of HCCs in children do not have accompanying cirrhosis, even with the background of HBV infection.[1] This suggests that HBV by itself has hepatocarcinogenic properties.

HBV related

Hepatitis B virus DNA (HBV-DNA) can be integrated within the genome of the host hepatocyte. The integration site of the circular HBV genome is variable. The integrated HBV-DNA is damaged and may contain deletions, rearrangement, duplication, or inversion of normal DNA sequence. However, in clinical studies, the risk of development of HCC is minimal with non-replicating virus.[9,10] Activation of growth factors and oncogenes – integration of HBV-DNA adjacent to genes related to IGF-II, cyclin-A, TGF-α and oncogene (c-myc) leads to rearrangement, activation and expression of the growth factors and oncogenes. HBV X-protein may function as a transcriptional transactivator, thereby activating other growth related genes.

NEED FOR HCC SCREENING

Symptomatic HCCs, when present clinically, are usually at an advanced stage of the disease. These are not amenable to surgical resection or non-surgical tumor ablative therapy. Diagnosis at a pre-symptomatic stage, when the tumor is small and readily treatable can improve the survival significantly. A study conducted in Japan substantiated this contention. The median survival time from diagnosis of 229 symptomatic HCCs was only 1.6 months, in contrast to 25.6 months in stage I HCC, who underwent surgical resection.[4] During recent years still better survival (100% at 5 years,[5] and 83% disease free survival at 4 years)[6] have been observed in stage 1 ($T_1N_0M_0$) HCCs.

Availability of a curative therapy with high possibility of return to work in early HCC argues in favor of routine screening of all subjects at high-risk of developing HCC. However, to undertake mass screening, other prerequisites have to be fulfilled like the availability of non-invasive highly accurate diagnostic methods, reasonable cost of detection of an early cancer, and easy identification of subjects at high-risk. These issues have been discussed below and these conditions by and large have been satisfied, justifying the need for screening in subjects at high-risk of developing HCC.

Identification of high-risk infected subjects

First requirement for evolving a proper screening strategy is recognition of subjects who are at high-risk of developing HCC. Chronic HBV infection is one of the known high-risk factors for development of HCC. Other factors include HCV infection (HCC risk is higher than HBV infection), ethanol ingestion, α_1-antitrypsin deficiency, hemochromatosis, etc. Risk being higher among HBV plus HCV dual infections and HCV infection plus ethanol ingestion, and lower with cryptogenic cirrhosis.

There are two subsets of presentation of chronic HBV infection with varied risk of HCC development and ultimate outcome. Chronic HBV infection with normal transaminases, normal or near normal liver histology and non-replicating virus, the risk of developing HCC is minimal and the prognosis is excellent. On a mean follow-up of 130 months in such cases, histologic progression of the disease was noted only in 2%.[7] Another study reports a five year survival of 97% in such cases.[8] Occasional development of HCC on screening of subjects with chronic HBV infection with minimal histologic change, has also been attributed to sampling error of initial liver biopsies, missing chronic active hepatitis, and picking tissue from areas of chronic persistent hepatitis or minimal change.[9,10] The second group of patients present with chronic HBV infection with evidence of liver disease in the form of raised transaminases, histologic evidence of liver injury (HAI >3), and evidence of HBV replication. Risk of HCC is 300-fold high in these subjects compared to those without chronic HBV infection.[2] In contrast, overall risk of HCC with HBV infection in high endemicity areas has been 100–200 folds.[3,11] Regular screening for detection of small HCC and early effective therapy are likely to give most cost-effective benefit in this group of subjects.

Genotype B of HBV has been noted more frequently in young Taiwanese with HCC, whereas genotype C is more common in elderly (> 50 years) subjects with HCC. However, due to considerable overlap, it lacks clinical utility in recognizing subjects at high-risk.[12]

Screening modalities

Modalities presently available for screening include serum alfa-fetoprotein and ultrasonography as these are inexpensive, informative, non-invasive, and easily available. Other techniques are employed if results of the above tests are suspicious or inconclusive.

Alfa-fetoprotein (AFP)

It has often been argued that the sensitivity of AFP is higher in HBsAg negative HCCs than in HBsAg positive cases. However, this contention could not be substantiated and in a recently conducted study on 1069 subjects with chronic HBV infection the sensitivity of AFP (>20ng/ml) was 64% and specificity 91% in detection of HCC on regular screening.[13] This is comparable to reported AFP sensitivity of 30–79% and specificity of 76–91% in detection of HCC on screening of high-risk cases of chronic hepatitis and cirrhosis.[14,15] Using higher cut-off value (>50ng/ml) the specificity has been improved to 85%, however, the sensitivity reduced to only 30%.[16] As the aim for cancer screening is not to miss out any case, the cut-off level of 15 to 20ng/ml appears appropriate. Very few studies on screening of HCC are available from India. In one such study, 50% AFP positivity using counter immuno-electrophoresis has been reported.[17,18] There were no false positive results as the test system used gives positive result usually when the AFP titer is >200 ng/ml.

AFP is not very specific for HCC, titers can also rise and give false positive result in acute or chronic hepatitis, during sero-conversion, pregnancy and in the presence of hepatoblastoma, tumors of endodermal origin and undifferentiated teratocarcinomas, or embryonal cell carcinomas of ovary and testis. Some of the benign events like exacerbation of hepatitis and HBeAg sero-conversion are common in HBV infected patients and levels are mostly <100ng/ml. Since the rise is usually transient, follow-up estimations might be useful. Moreover, follow-up studies may also be of value for subjects with high-risk for HCC development or suspected HCC, with low or normal AFP values on initial testing. Progressive increase in AFP titers was noted in 46% of those cases where initial level was low.[19] Frequent transient rise in AFP were also found to be associated with HCC.[20] However, in subjects with borderline elevations, more specific alternative modalities could be used to establish the diagnosis.

Lower level of AFP (111 ng/ml) with significantly better survival (22 months) have been noted in subclinical HCC detected on screening than in symptomatic HCC (mean AFP level 824 ng/ml; survival 5 months).[21] Still, no linear correlation exists between the serum levels of AFP and survival time after diagnosis, tumor size, metastasis, and the extent of liver disease.[22] AFP positivity in resectable and unresectable tumor has been comparable. In a study from Europe,[10] AFP positivity (>20 ng/ml) in tumors of >5 cm size was 60%, which was comparable to 66% overall positivity. Even with very small tumors of less than 2 cm size, the AFP levels of >20 ng/ml was noted in 68%, whereas, larger tumors (>2 cm) had 87% positivity.[23] Thus, the difference in positivity with the size of the tumor, if any, was only marginal.

Other tumor markers

Apart from AFP, there are other substances produced by HCC in sufficient amount and are present in the serum. These have been used to facilitate the detection of HCC. However, these tumor markers have not been used for HCC screening because of the limited availability, high cost and low sensitivity. These tumor markers are:

Fucosylated AFP : Small well differentiated HCC produce AFP which is glycosylated with fucose. These fucosylated variants have propensity to bind with lectins. This lectin binding pattern of AFP improves the sensitivity of detection of HCC. The specificity of detection can be improved by monoclonal AFP assays or evaluating for AFP having abnormal gel motility pattern. However, none of these tests have been developed to the level of clinical application.

Des-gamma-carboxyprothrombin (DCP) : It is also known as prothrombin produced by vitamin K absence or antagonism II (PIVKAII) and is raised in 58–91% subjects with HCC, having 84% specificity. It is an easy and a rapid test but much more expensive than AFP. The sensitivity and specificity for DCP is reported to be low as compared to AFP. In high-risk black African population, DCP may be of particular use in low incidence population where the sensitivity of AFP is only 50–70%.[24]

α-L-fucosidase : It has 75% sensitivity and 75–90% specificity in detection of HCC. Although it is easy, rapid, and inexpensive test, it has lower diagnostic yield than AFP, particularly in high-risk black African population.[24]

γ Glutamyl transferase isoenzymes : Three tumor associated isoenzymes of γ glutamyl transferase have been noted in HCC patients. These have 60% sensitivity and 96% specificity. Isoenzyme I' is present in 60%, I" in 27% and II' in 30%.[24] The test is relatively simple and quick, but is expensive.

Tumor markers like CA-125, tissue polypeptide antigen, and tumor associated isoenzyme of 5-nucleotide phosphodiesterase have high sensitivity and poor specificity. Ferriitin, CEA, CA19-9, and calcitonin have poor sensitivity as well as poor specificity. Variant akaline phosphatase has high specificity but poor sensitivity. Abnormal vitamin B_{12} binding protein and neurotensin almost confirm the diagnosis of fibrolamellar HCC but have low sensitivity.

Ultrasonography

Limitations in sensitivity and specificity of AFP have led to the use of ultrasonography (US) which is as reproducible, widely available, and is relatively inexpensive. Among subjects with chronic HBV infection, it has been found to have a sensitivity of 71% to 79% and specificity of over 90% in the detection of HCC.[13,14,25] US has a better accuracy than AFP in detecting smaller HCCs (<3 cm); 61% of tumors identified were less than 3 cm and in 60% of such cases AFP levels were normal.[10] Findings of a hepatic mass on US suggestive of HCC include a peripheral halo around the mass, hypoechoic character of the mass (occasionally hyper-echoic), and a mosaic pattern. Color doppler US may assist in both the diagnosis and the patency of the vessels in anticipation of potential resection. However, US many a times fails to discriminate between small-well differentiated HCC, regenerating nodule, nodular hyperplasia, and hemangioma for which other imaging modalities may be more useful (Table 1).

Advanced screening modalities which can give more precise diagnosis of HCC have recently been reviewed by Kudo.[26] These can also reveal extent of the lesions, vascular involvement, grade of differentiation (without histology), post-treatment follow-up and can also discriminate small HCC from nodular hyperplasia and dysplastic nodules. On US angiography, HCC shows peripheral arterial supply with homogeneous or mosaic hypervascular pattern. On the other hand, adenomatous hyperplasia or dysplastic nodule shows central hypervascular supply with centrifugal filling to the periphery in the arterial phase and a uniform or lobulated dense stain in the parenchymal phase. CT angiography and CT aorto-portography also provide useful information in this context. These modalities are not readily available and are expensive and hence occasionally used for HCC screening. One or more of these techniques can be used to establish the diagnosis when results of AFP and US studies are equivocal.

Combination of tomography and angiographic techniques

These have greatly improved the yield of imaging. Usefulness of these procedures is listed in Table 2.

Table 1. Usefulness of regular imaging modalities in HCC screening

Imaging modalities	Focal nodular hyperplasia	Adenoma	Hemangioma	HCC
US	Non-specific (nodular, well marginated, variable echogenicity, central scar)	Non-specific (well demarcated, smooth lesion with variable echogenicity)	Demarcated, hyperechoic and homogenous	Initially hypoechoic, later hyperechoic with hypoechoic rim
Color Doppler	Arterial signals within the tumor	Venous signals within the tumor	–	–
CT	Hypo- or iso-attenuated short-lived arterial enhancement	Peripheral arterial enhancement, precontrast hypo/hyperdense areas	Early peripheral/progressive centripetal enhancement, delayed venous phase	Hypoattenuated, arterial phase prominence
MRI (Unenhanced)	Iso/hypointense in T_1, Slight hyperintense in T_2	Hyperintense on T_1 & T_2 (hemorrhages)	Low signal on T_1, characteristic high signal on T_2	High intensity on T_1, low intensity on T_2
Angiography	Hypervascular/dense blush ventral vascular supply (spoke wheel)	Hypervascular, peripheral vascular supply	Venous lakes, delayed venous phase arterial supply	Hypervascularity with puddling of contrast, peripheral

Table 2. Usefulness of advanced imaging modalities in HCC screening

Imaging techniques	Intranodular arterial and portal blood flow	Tumour	Malignancy grading	Remarks
US Angiography	Highly sensitive	Accurate	Possible	Invasive and angiographic technique using CO_2 bubbles. Early HCC in dysplastic nodule appear as vascular spot with hypovascular back ground (nodule in nodule)
CT Arteriography (CTA)	Highly sensitive	Accurate	Possible	Invasive angiographic technique.
CT Arterial portography	Highly sensitive	Accurate	Possible	Invasive angiographic technique.
Colour Doppler US	Low sensitivity	Good	–	Non-invasive and easy to perform useful in D/D of early HCC and benign nodule
Power Doppler US	Highly sensitive	Accurate	–	Non-invasive, D/D dysplastic (constant wave from) and HCC nodules (pulsatile wave form)
Enhanced Doppler US	Highly sensitive	Accurate	–	Non-invasive (using IV contrast)
US-tissue harmonic imaging	–	Good	–	Better spatial resolution and contrast resolution useful in detection of cyst, and HCC in obese patients.
US perfusion Imaging:				
a. Contrast enhanced second harmonic Imaging	–	Accurate	Possible	Using micro-bubbles HCC confirmation and staging, and post-treatment follow-up possible.
b. Flash echo Imaging	–	Accurate	Possible	May be used for therapeutic procedures if viable cancer cells are accurately imaged.
Three dimensional US	Highly sensitive	Accurate	–	Can demonstrate continuity of intranodular vessels.

Helical dynamic CT

Triphasic helical dynamic CT provides all the information obtained by angiography. It helps to detect the lesion, establish the diagnosis, stage tumor and evaluate therapeutic response.[26] In a recent study on pre-transplant cases, where HCC was not suspected, helical CT could detect small HCC in 59% on prospective evaluation and 68% on retrospective evaluation. Prevalence of HCC was highest (27%) in HBV infected cases. AFP estimation in this study was of no value in detection of small HCC, as AFP positivity was comparable in cases, where explanted liver revealed HCC or was free from HCC.[27]

Lipiodol CT

It is a very sensitive method (only next to US angiography and CTA) for detecting small hypervascular HCC. The limitation of this technique is that it requires a week and lipiodol does not accumulate in early well differentiated HCC. Lipiodol CT, is positive in only 78% cases with early well differentiated HCC as compared to 95% positivity of CTA. Even angiography (conventional or DSA) in such cases has much lower yield (62–65%).[26]

SPIO-MRI

Super paramagnetic iron oxide (SPIO) is taken up by Kupffer cells reducing signal intensity on MRI. Hence, overt HCC (where Kupffer cells are deficient) show high signal intensity whereas early well differentiated HCC and dysplastic nodules (having abundance of Kupffer cells) become unclear on SPIO-MRI. It can ascertain histologic grade of HCC.[26]

Nuclear medicine imaging

A late phase seen in hepatobiliary imaging suggests early well differentiated HCC and focal nodular hyperplasia. Colloid imaging can also be useful for the diagnosis of dysplastic and well differentiated HCC. Asialoglycoprotein receptor imaging can demonstrate functional hepatocytes, and therefore, can differentiate between dysplastic nodule (hot accumulation) and overt HCC (cold defect).[26]

Choice of Modalities

Ultrasound is a preferred technique, as it is widely available, inexpensive, and has better yield (i.e., sensitivity and specificity) than AFP. Whether US should be used alone or combined with AFP estimation is often debated. Available results of screening studies indicate that AFP improved the detection yield of US by 15 to 29%.[10,23,25] Moreover, AFP is also a noninvasive test, commercially available at cost comparable to US. Hence both these techniques should be used in combination for periodic screening of HCC. Following plan of screening appears appropriate for chronic HBV patients (Fig. 1).

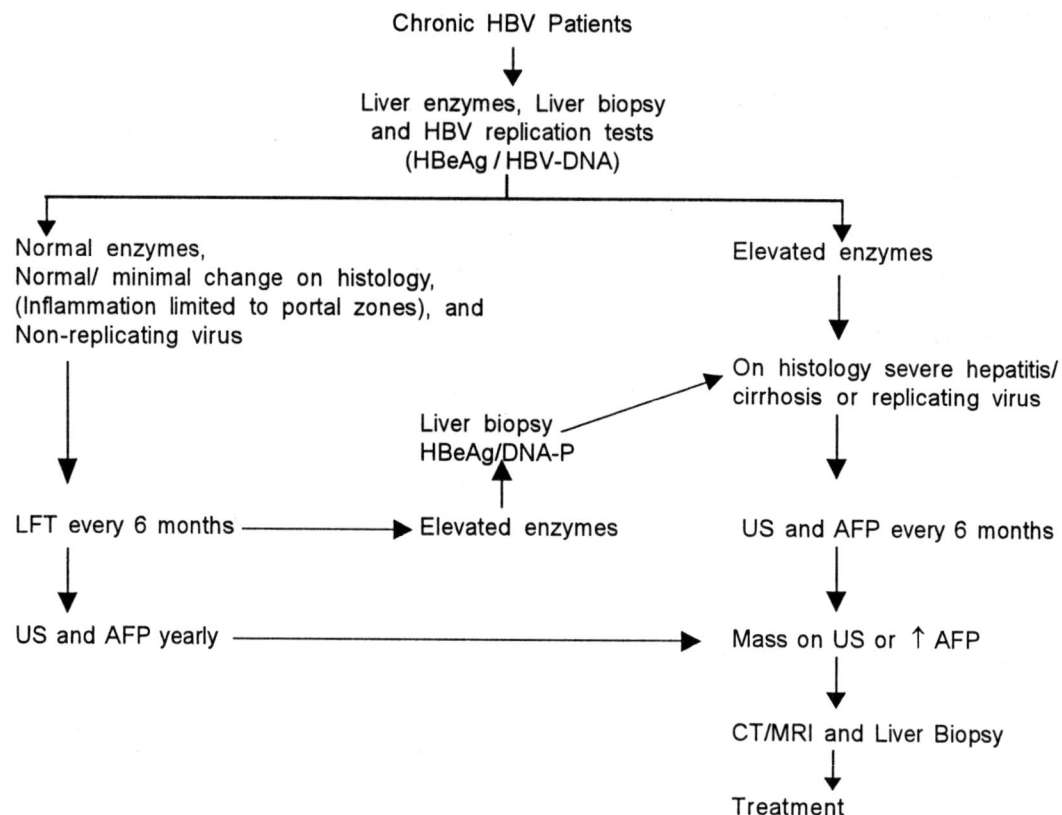

Fig. 1. Algorithm for HCC screening of patients with chronic HBV infection

Screening Interval

Median doubling time for HCC is 3 to 4 months (varies widely),[28] and HCC of 3 to 4 cm size are usually amenable to effective therapy. Hence, six monthly screening schedule appears appropriate for subjects with chronic HBV infection at high-risk of developing HCC.[13, 16, 25, 29-31] Screening approach can be tailored according to the severity of hepatic injury. In some studies, an aggressive screening approach of US and AFP estimation every 3 months has been performed in HBV infected individuals with histology showing severe chronic active hepatitis or cirrhosis as the incidence of HCC in these subjects has been reported to be as high as 25%. However, HCC detection rates and their resectability was comparable to every 6 months screening.[13, 16, 25, 30, 31] Estimation of AFP every three months and US every six months has recently been advocated for subjects with cirrhosis due to HBV.[32] However, such a strategy appears to increase the cost of extra visit and without any additional benefit in the detection of HCC. Hence, US examination and AFP estimation every six month is considered most appropriate.[16, 29] For HBV infections at lower or modest risk, yearly screening[24, 29] with

US and AFP[10] has been advocated. Although, the risk of HCC development in such cases is negligible (0.4%) and 5 year survival is 97%.[8] In a recent consensus statement from New Delhi, regular six-monthly screening has been proposed for males with age over 50 years and yearly screening for those under 50 years of age.[29] These approaches are based on higher incidence (M:F:2:1) in males[16,19] and elderly age group.[31,33] Although HCC detected on screening had only marginally higher mean age (57–63 years) than those who were free from cancer (54–59 years),[19,27] but only few with HCC were under 50 years,[19] hence preceding screening strategy according to age may be appropriate and more cost effective.

Cost-effectiveness of screening

Treatability

Screening program in high-risk subjects with chronic liver disease has resulted in detecting tumors at the rate of 2.5–5.8% per annum.[16,20,25,33] About two-third of these tumors are detected early when these are small and potentially treatable using either surgical resection or non-surgical ablative therapies.[10,16,25] Among non-resectable tumors, many a times (upto two-third instances) these are due to advanced liver disease rather than large size of the tumor or distant metastases.[10] In such cases, alternatives like liver transplantation are still available.

Survival

Subclinical HCC detected on screening had a median survival of 22 to 47 months, this was significantly better than 5 to 8 months survival noted in symptomatic HCC detected on clinical presentation.[21,34] Even small tumors detected on clinical presentation had lower mean survival (18 months) than those detected on screening (47 months).[34,35] This substantiates that screening significantly improves the survival. However, in terms of life expectancy the benefits have been marginal in a study even when the incidence of HCC was high (6% per annum).[30] Overall, average life prolongation was <3 months, but in a subset of patients with well compensated disease (80% predicted survival rate at 5 years), the increase in life expectancy was 3–9 months. This group of patients with chronic liver disease is the ideal one for screening for HCC.[30]

Cost involved

Since most of the screening studies are available from the West and the Far East, the cost calculations have been made in terms of US$. The cost to identify a case has been $1,167 and for diagnosis of treatable case $1,667.[21] Each life year gained costs between $26,000 and $55,000.[30] The cost of AFP estimation and US examination accounted in these studies is $26 and $.58 respectively. This cost in our set up is about seven times in Indian Rupees. Using this multiplication factor, the cost of detecting a treatable case works out to be about Rs. 12,000 and the cost of a life year gained between Rs. 2,00,000 to 4,00,000. At present, screening strategies for HCC fulfils 9 out of the 10 criteria for cost effective screening program put forth by the World Health Organization.[21, 36]

REFERENCES

1. Di Bisceglie AD. *Malignant neoplasms of the liver. In*: Schiff ER, Sorrel MF, Mackfrey WE. Eds. Schiff's Diseases of the liver Philladelphia: Lippincott-Raven Publishers. 1999; pp. 1281-1304.
2. Beasley RP. Hepatitis B Virus. The major etiology of hepatocellular carcinoma. *Cancer* 1988;61: 1942-56.
3. Change MH, Chen CJ, Las Ms, Hsu HM, Wu TC, Kong MS, Liang DC, et al. Universal hepatitis B vaccination in Taiwan and the incidence of hepatocellular carcinoma in children. Taiwan Childhood Hepatoma Study Group, *N Engl J Med* 1997;336:1855-9.
4. Okuda K, Ohtuski T, Obata H, Tomimatsu M, Okazanki N, Husegawa H, Nakajima Y, et al. Natural history of hepatocellular carcinoma and prognosis in relation to treatment. *Cancer* 1985;56: 1918-28.
5. Zhous XD, Tang ZY, Yu YQ, Ma Sc, Yang BH, Lu JZ, Lin XY, et al. Solitary minute hepatocellular carcinoma: a study of 15 patients. *Cancer* 1991;67;2855-8.
6. Mazzaferro V, Regalia E, Doci R, Andreda S. Liver transplantation for the treatment of small hepatocellular carcinoma in cirrhotic patients. *N Engl J Med* 1996;334:693-9.
7. de Franchis R, Meucci G, Vecchi M, Tatarella M, Colombo M, Ninno ED, Rumi MG, et al. The natural history of asymptomatic hepatitis B surface antigen carriers. *Ann Intern Med* 1993;118:191-4.
8. Weissberg JI, Andres LL, Smith CI, Weick S, Nichols JE, Garcia G, Robinson WS, et al. Survival in chronic hepatitis B: an analysis of 379 patients. *Ann Intern Med* 1984;10:613-6.
9. Takanos, Yokosuka O, Imazeki F, Tagawa M, Omata M. Incidence of hepatocellular carcinoma in hepatitis B and C: a prospective study of 251 patients. *Hepatology* 1995;21:650-5.
10. Curley SA, Izzo F, Gallipoli A, Bellis M, Cremona F, Parisi V. Identification and screening of 416 patients with chronic hepatitis at high-risk to develop hepatocellular cancer. *Ann Surg* 1995;222: 380-3.
10a. Yang HI, Lu SN, Liaw YF, You SL, Sun CA, Wang LY, Hsiao CK, et al. Hepatitis B e antigen and the risk of hepato cellular carcinoma. *N Engl J Med* 2002;347:168-74.
10b. Okoshi S, Igarashi M, Suda T, Iwamatsu H, Watanabe K, Ishihara K, Ogata N, et al. Remote development of hepato cellular carcinoma in patients with liver cirrhosis type b serologically cured for HBs antigenemic with long-standing normalization of ALT values. *Dig Dis Sci* 2002;47:2002-6.
11. Beasley RP, Hwang LY, Lin CC, Chien CS. Hepatocellular carcinoma and hepatitis B virus: a prospective study of 22,707 men in Taiwan. *Lancet* 1981;2:1129-33.
12. Kao JH, Chen PJ, Lai MY, Chen DS. Hepatitis B genotypes correlates with clinical outcomes in patients with chronic hepatitis B. *Gastroenterology* 2000;118:554-9.
13. Sherman M, Peltekian KM, Lee C. Screening for hepatocellular carcinoma in chronic carriers of hepatitis B virus: Incidence and prevalence of hepatocellular carcinoma in North American Urban Population. *Hepatology* 1995;22:432-8.
14. Whang-Peng J, Chao Y. Clinical Trials of HCC in Taiwan. *Hepatogastroenterology* 1998;45:1937-43.
15. Reddy KR. Screening and work-up of hepatocellular carcinoma (symposium-hepatocellular carcinoma). *Program and abstracts of the American College of Gastroenterology* 64th Annual Scientific Meeting, 1999;16-20.
16. Cottone M, Turi M, Caltagirone M, Parisi P, Orlando A, Firentino G, Virdone R, et al. Screening for hepatocellular carcinoma in patients with Child's A cirrhosis: an 8 years prospective study by ultrasound and alpha-fetoprotein. *J Hepatol* 1994;21:1029-34.

17. Panchanadam M, Madangopalan N, Thyagrajan SP, Hill PG, Arumugam S. Corelated clinical, histopathological, HBV and AFP studies of primary carcinoma liver. *Ann Acad Med Singapore* 1980;9: 210-4.
18. Hill PG, Johnson S, Madanagopalan N. Serum alfa-fetoprotein and hepatitis B-antigen in subjects with hepatoma in South India. *Ind J Med Res* 1977;65:482-7.
19. Zoli M, Magalotti D, Bianchi G, Gueli C, Marchesini G, Pisi E, et al. Efficacy of a surveillance program for early detection of hepatocellular carcinomas. *Cancer* 1996;78:977-85.
20. Oka H, Tamori A, Kuroki T, Kobayashi K, Yamamoto S. Prospective study of alfa-fetoprotein in cirrhotic patients monitored for development of hepatocellular carcinoma. *Hepatology* 1994;19:61-6.
21. Yuen MF, Cheng CC, Lauder IJ, Lam SK, Ooi CGC, Lai CL. Early detection of hepatocellular carcinoma increases the chances of treatment. Hong Kong experience. *Hepatology* 2000;31:330-5.
22. Thung SN, Gerber MA, Sarna E, Popper H. Distribution of five antigens in hepatocellular carcinoma. *Lab Invest* 1979;41:101-8.
23. Oka H, Kurioka V, Kim K, Kanno T, Kuroki T, Mizoguchi Y, Kobayashi K. Prospective study of early detection of hepatocellular carcinoma in patients with cirrhosis. *Hepatology* 1990;12:680-7.
24. Kew MC. *Hepatic tumors and cysts. In:* Feldman M, Sleisenger MH, Scharschmidt. Eds. Sleisenger and Fordtran's Gastrointestinal and Liver disease. Philadelphia: WB Saunders 1998; pp.1364-87.
25. Pateron D, Granne N, Trinchet JC, Aurousseau MH, Mal F, Meicler C, Coderc E, et al. Prospective study of screening of hepatocellular carcinoma in caucasian patients with cirrhosis. *J Hepatol* 1994;20: 65-71.
26. Kudo M. Imaging diagnosis of hepatocellular carcinoma and premalignant/borderline lesions. *Sem Liver Dis* 1999;19:297-309.
27. Peterson MS, Baron RL, Marsh JW, Oliver JH, Confer SR, Hunt LE. Pre-transplantion surveillance for possible hepatocellular carcinoma in patients with cirrhosis. Epidemiology and CT based tumor detection rate in 430 cases with surgical pathologic correlation. *Radiology* 2000;217:743-9.
28. Sheu JC, Sung JL, Chen DS, Yang PM, Lai MY, Lee CS, Hsu HC, et al. Growth rate of asymptomatic hepatocellular carcinoma and its clinical implications. *Gastroenterology* 1985;89:259-66.
29. Indian association for study of the Liver. Changing terminology of hepatitis B and C carrier: Consensus statement. *Indian J Gastroenterol* 1999;18(suppl 1):S15-20.
30. Sarasin FP, Giostra E, Hadengue A. Cost effectiveness of screening for detection of small HCC in Western patients with child–pugh class A cirrhosis. *Am J Med* 1996;101:422-34.
31. Benvegn L, Fattovich G, Noventa F, Chemello L, Cecchetto A, Alberti A. Concurrent hepatitis B and C virus infection and risk of hepatocellular carcinoma in cirrhosis. A prospective study. *Cancer* 1994;74: 2442-8.
32. Zitternman RK. Caring for the patients with hepatocellular carcinoma. 64th Annual Scientific Meeting American College of Gastroenterology, (October 16-20, 1999). Conference Summary Index *Medscape Gastroenterology* (*http:ll gastroenterology.medscape.com*) November 3, 1999.
33. Ikeda K, Saitoh S, Koida I, Arase Y, Tsubota A, Chayama K, Kumada H, et al. A multivariate analysis of risk factors for hepatocellular carcinogenesis: a prospective observations of 795 patients with viral and alcoholic cirrhosis. *Hepatology* 1993;18:47-53.
34. Wong LL, Limm WM, Severino R, Wong LM. Improved survival with screening for hepatocellular carcinoma. *Liver Transplantation* 2000;6:320-5.
35. Chen TH, Chen CJ, Yen MF, Lu SN, Sun CA, Huang GT, Yang PM, et al. Ultrasound screening and risk factors for death from hepatocellular carcinoma in a high-risk group in Taiwan. *Int J Cancer* 2002;98:257-61.
36. Okano H, Shiraki K, Inoue H, Ino T, Xamanaka T, Deguch M, Sugimoto K. Comparison of screening methods for hepatocellular carcinoma in patients with cirrhosis. *Anticancer Res* 2001;21: 2979-82.

23

Prevention of hepatocellular carcinoma in reference to hepatitis B virus

Maniyalath Narendranathan

Hepatocellular carcinoma (HCC) is the fourth most common cancer in the world[1] and causes 3,00,000 to one million deaths per year worldwide. Infection with hepatitis B virus (HBV) accounts for 80% of cases of HCC seen in the world. The other major etiological factors are hepatitis C virus (HCV) and exposure to the mycotoxin – aflatoxin-B_1. The incidence of HCC in individuals with chronic hepatitis B is as high as 0.46% per year.[2,3]

The different levels of prevention,[4] as applied to HCC in hepatitis B virus infection, are given in Table 1. Primary prevention refers to manuvers which prevent the disease from occurring by removing the risk factors. Secondary prevention is the detection of early disease when it is still asymptomatic so that early detection and treatment will prevent the disease from progressing. Tertiary prevention refers to those clinical activities that prevent further deterioration or reduce complications after the manifestations of the disease.

PREVENTION OF HEPATITIS B INFECTION

Chronic viral hepatitis is a major risk factor for the development of HCC. Therefore, prevention of viral hepatitis would have a significant impact on diminishing the incidence of HCC. Currently available medical treatment modalities cannot cure chronic HBV infection completely and thus eliminate the source of new infections. Therefore, immunizing susceptible persons with hepatitis B vaccine is the best available option to prevent new infections. It is currently recommended to vaccinate all the infants with the HBV vaccine at birth, 1 month, and at 6 months of age. As the chances of developing chronic liver disease are maximum when the infection is acquired early in life, prevention of vertical transmission is the most important step in the prevention of HCC (Table 1).

Prevention of perinatal hepatitis B virus infection

The recommendations[5] of the Centre for Disease Control published in MMWR (1998) are given in the footnote.*

A nationwide hepatitis B vaccination program was implemented in Taiwan in July 1984. To assess the effect of the program on the development of hepatocellular carcinoma, the incidence of HCC in children in Taiwan from 1981 to 1994 was studied.[6] Data were collected on liver cancer in children from Taiwan's National Cancer Registry. The average annual incidence of hepatocellular carcinoma in children 6 to 14 years of age declined from 0.70 per 1,00,000 children between 1981 and 1986 to 0.57 between 1986 and 1990, and to 0.36 between 1990 and 1994 ($p<0.01$). The corresponding rates of mortality from hepatocellular carcinoma also decreased. The incidence of hepatocellular carcinoma in children 6 to 9 years of age declined from 0.52 for those born between 1974 and 1984 to 0.13 for those born between 1984 and 1986 ($p<0.001$). This study concluded that after the institution of program of universal hepatitis B vaccination in Taiwan, the incidence of hepatocellular carcinoma in children has declined. This study also suggests that given the resources and necessary funds, the elimination of the vertical transmission of HBV and HCC is possible.

---

1. *All pregnant women should be routinely tested for HBsAg during an early prenatal visit in each pregnancy along with the other routine prenatal laboratory tests. HBsAg testing should be repeated late in the pregnancy for women who are HBsAg negative but who are at high risk of HBV infection (e.g. a injecting drug users, those with intercurrent sexually transmitted diseases) or who have had clinically apparent hepatitis. Tests for other HBV markers are not necessary for the purpose of maternal screening. However, HBsAg-positive women identified during screening may have HBV-related liver disease and should be evaluated.
2. Infants born to mothers who are HBsAg positive should receive the appropriate doses of hepatitis B vaccine and 0.5 ml of hepatitis B immunoglobulin (HBIg) within 12 hours of birth. Both should be administered by intramuscular injection. Hepatitis B vaccine should be administered concurrently with HBIg but at a different site. Subsequent doses of the vaccine should be administered according to the recommended schedule.
3. Women admitted for delivery who have not had prenatal HBsAg testing should have blood drawn for testing. While test results are pending, the infant should receive hepatitis B vaccine within 12 hours of birth, in a dose appropriate for infants born to HBsAg-positive mothers.
   - If the mother is later found to be HBsAg positive, her infant should receive the additional protection of HBIg as soon as possible and within 7 days of birth, although the efficacy of HBIg administered after 48 hours of birth is not known. If HBIg has not been administered, it is important that the infant receives the second dose of hepatitis B vaccine at 1 month and not later than 2 months of age because of the high risk of infection. The last dose should be administered at the age of 6 months.
   - If the mother is found to be HBsAg negative, her infant should continue to receive hepatitis B vaccine as part of routine vaccinations and, in the dose appropriate for infants born to HBsAg-negative mothers.

Table 1. Levels of prevention of hepatocellular carcinoma in hepatitis B infection

Primary prevention
    Immunization of all newborns and at risk individuals
    Screening of all pregnant women and active-cum-passive immunization of newborns of HBsAg positive mothers
    General precautions against hepatitis B
Prevention of HCC in chronic HBV infection
    Treatment of Infection
        Treatment when indicated–Interferon, Lamivudine (?)
        Herbal remedies (?) *Phyllanthus amarus*, Japanese herbal preparations
    Prevention of aflatoxin-induced hepatic damage
        Improving food storage and distribution
        Oltipraz
    Chemoprevention
        Sulindac
        Cox-2 inhibitors
        Polyprenoic acid
Secondary prevention
    Screening and early detection
    Aggressive management of lesions, if indicated
Prevention of second primary

General measures for preventing transmission of hepatitis B

Immunization of high-risk groups, education of the public, safe sex, use of disposable needles and syringes, and general blood and body fluid precautions are necessary to prevent the spread of the disease.

PREVENTION OF HCC IN CHRONIC HBV INFECTION

Once chronic liver disease has set in, the best method to prevent complications like cirrhosis and HCC is to give specific treatment for the disease. Interferon and lamivudine are the two approved drugs for the treatment of chronic HBV infection.

Interferon therapy

Interferon therapy for patients with HBV-related cirrhosis has been shown to decrease the incidence of HCC significantly, especially in patients with a high level of serum HBV-DNA.[7] Three hundred and thirteen consecutive patients with cirrhosis were analyzed by Ikeda et al. Ninety-four patients underwent long-term intermittent administration of interferon for 6 months or more, and the remaining 219 patients received no interferon or any other antiviral drug. Cumulative occurrence rates of HCC in the group treated with interferon and the untreated group were 4.5% and 13.3%, respectively, at the end of 3 years; 7% and 19.6%, respectively at the end of 5 years; and 17% and 30.8%, respectively, at the end of 10 years.[7] The study shows that interferon therapy reduces the occurrence of HCC in patients with chronic HBV infection.[7a]

Lamivudine

The role of lamivudine in preventing HCC has not been well established. This is an area which warrants further trials. The therapeutic goals in chronic hepatitis B are to prevent or decrease cirrhosis and hepatocellular carcinoma in patients with early cirrhosis and to stabilize patients with end-stage chronic liver disease. Lamivudine is an oral nucleoside analogue that suppresses HBV replication and, hence, may achieve both these treatment objectives.[8-9a] There is some concern that by exerting a selection pressure on the virus to integrate into the host genome, lamivudine may actually foster the development of hepatocellular carcinoma. Viral integration has been implicated in the oncogene production and carcinogenesis. Studies in woodchucks seem to refute this concern when woodchucks were initiated on lamivudine very early in life. Treatment of established infection in adults may however behave differently.[9]

Herbal remedies

The antiviral activity of many herbal remedies is well established. But their role in prevention of HCC has not been documented in humans. *Phyllanthus amarus*[10] and a Japanese herbal preparation[11] are some of the preparations which may be useful in the prevention of HCC in chronic HBV infection.

Prevention of aflatoxin-induced hepatic injury

There is evidence from both epidemiological studies and animal models that the HBV and aflatoxin can act synergistically to increase the risk of HCC. One possible mechanism is that chronic liver injury alters the expression of specific carcinogen metabolising enzymes thus modulating the binding of aflatoxin to DNA in the hepatocytes. The high levels of aflatoxin exposure, which occur in many areas of the world where chronic HBV infection is endemic, indicate that measures to reduce aflatoxin exposure would contribute in reducing the incidence of HCC.[12] A community-based intervention to improve post-harvest processing and storage of the groundnut crop, a major source of aflatoxins, is one of the methods that has been tried. An alternative measure is to modulate the metabolism of aflatoxins once ingested using chemopreventive agents, e.g. oltipraz.[13]

Chemoprevention

Another option available for prevention of HCC in patients with chronic HBV infection is chemoprevention. The drugs available are discussed below.

Cyclooxygenase-2 (COX-2) inhibitors

Increased expression of COX-2 in the hepatocellular carcinoma (HCC) cells has been demonstrated. Furthermore, COX-2 expression was upregulated in both small-sized and well-differentiated HCC, indicating that this enzyme may play a role in the early stages of hepatocarcinogenesis. Whether a chemopreventive strategy using selective COX-2 inhibitors will be applicable for hepatocarcinogenesis remains unknown, but recent findings suggest that precisely targeting COX-2 with specific inhibitors may represent a viable therapeutic option for HCC in the future.[14]

Sulindac and exisulind

Antiproliferative effect of both sulindac and exisulind on hepatocellular carcinoma cell lines have been described.[15] The growth inhibition and cytotoxicity of sulindac in human hepatocellular carcinoma cell lines were investigated by studying cell growth, cell cycle distribution, and induction of apoptosis. In the presence of sulindac, there was a marked time- and dose-dependent decrease in cell proliferation and viability. The findings of this study suggest that sulindac exhibits a growth-inhibitory effect on human hepatocellular carcinoma cell lines. Therefore, these drugs might serve as an effective tool for the prevention of hepatocellular carcinoma.

Indomethacin

A study from Turkey[16] showed that indomethacin given in a dose of 75 mg per day was significantly more effective than placebo in eliminating HBeAg and sero-conversion to anti-HBe. The authors conclude that prostaglandin pathway may be involved in the pathogenesis of immune response against hepatitis B and that may be the reason for the effect of indomethacin seen in their patients. Based on this they suggest that indomethacin may be a potentially useful drug for the chemoprevention of HCC. This data needs to be confirmed further.

Polyprenoic acid

Oral polyprenoic acid, an acyclic retinoid, has been shown to prevent second primary hepatomas after surgical resection of the original tumor or after percutaneous injection of ethanol.[17]

SCREENING AND EARLY DETECTION

Screening is the one-time application of a test that allows the detection of a disease at a stage when intervention may significantly improve the natural course and outcome. In contrast, surveillance is the repeated application of such tests over time. The objective of both is to reduce the disease-specific mortality.[18] This review will deal only with screening in HBV infections.

Target population to be screened

The target population for screening includes all the subjects with chronic hepatitis B infection. This includes both the asymptomatic (those diagnosed as HBsAg positive in other screening programs) and symptomatic subjects with chronic HBV infection. Twenty to 56% of patients presenting with HCC have previously undiagnosed chronic liver disease and it is certain that these persons will not be included in a surveillance program.[19]

Screening interval

Reported surveillance intervals vary from 3 to 12 months. A 6-month surveillance interval may be a rational choice, based on data from China. Sheu et al studied the tumor doubling time in asymptomatic HCC's less than 5 cm.[20] They found a median tumor doubling time of 117 days. Alfa-fetoprotein (AFP) levels corresponded with tumor doubling time in 17 of 31 tumors studied. The most rapidly dividing tumor took 5 months to increase in size from 1 to 3 cm. Therefore, 6-month surveillance interval appears to be justifiable.

Screening tests

The most commonly used screening tests are serum alfa-fetoprotein (AFP) and ultrasonography (US). In evaluating these tests, it is important to note that the performance characteristics of a test that is used for diagnosis may differ when used for screening/surveillance and when used in different populations with varying prevalence. So the data relating to AFP and US should be interpreted cautiously.

Alfa-fetoprotein

The sensitivity of AFP in detecting HCC varies widely in both the HBV-positive and HBV-negative populations. The specificity was 50% in HBV-positive patients compared to a specificity of 78% in HBV-negative patients.[21] In high-risk populations, AFP has a sensitivity of 39 to 64%, a specificity of 76 to 91% and a positive predictive value of 9 to 32%.[22,23] Patients with other malignancies like germ cell carcinoma, pancreatic, and gastric cancer may also have elevated levels. Titers also rise with flares of acute hepatitis.[24] In one study, the cause of elevated AFP was found to be exacerbation of underlying liver disease rather than HCC in about 41% of cases. Only 14% of those with high AFP had HCC.[25] In individuals with viral hepatitis who do not have HCC, AFP levels may be transiently, persistently, or intermittently elevated. Increases are most likely caused by viral hepatitis when they parallel elevations in transaminases, and may be due to active hepatitis or HBeAg sero-conversion. There is no consensus on the issue of the level of AFP at which one should start investigations to rule out HCC. There is a trade-off between sensitivity and specificity as the levels are increased. When the level is raised from 20 to 100 ng/l the sensitivity falls from 39 to 13% while the specificity increases.[26]

Other tumor markers

Other tumor markers used for detection/screening for HCC are fucosylated alfa-fetoprotein (FAP), desgamma carboxy prothrombin (PIVKA II), alpha-l-fucosidase (ALF), and isoenzyme of gamma-glutaryl transferase (iso-γ-GT).[27] FAP is useful in differential diagnosis of HCC when AFP concentration is less than 500ng/l. The estimation of FAP involves a complex procedure and is not useful as a screening test. Iso-γ-GT has been thoroughly studied in Japanese and in black populations. The sensitivity is 60% and specificity is 96%, however, its estimation is very expensive. The levels of PIVKA II are raised in majority of the HCC. The specificity is 70–90% and sensitivity varies from 58 to 91%. The measurement is easy but expensive. ALF was reported to have a sensitivity of 75% and specificity of 90% but later studies did not confirm this. The algorithm for screening and follow-up of cases with high AFP are given in Fig. 1.

Ultrasound scan (US)

The poor performance of AFP has led to the introduction of US as an additional screening

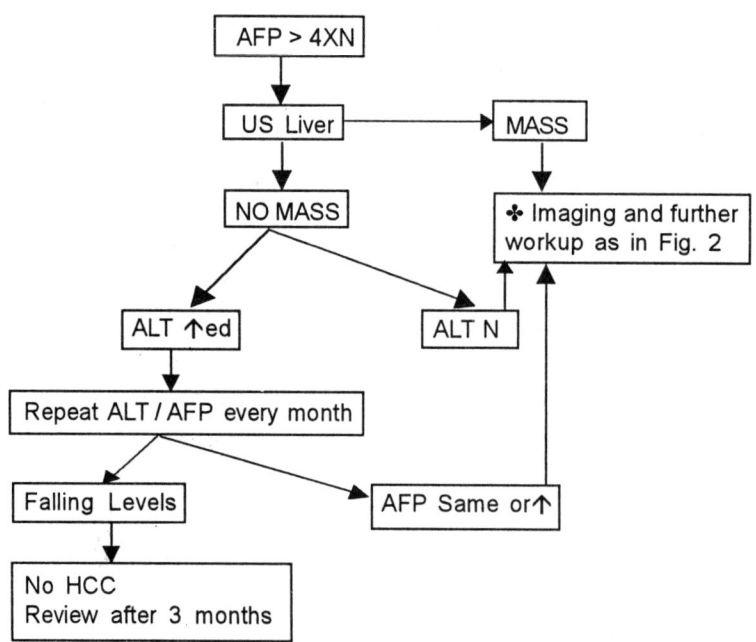

Fig. 1. Algorithm for work-up of cases with raised AFP after screening

tool. The sensitivity of US varies from 71% in HBsAg positive subjects without cirrhosis to 78% in patients with cirrhosis. The specificity is 93%.[23,28] The algorithm for screening and follow-up are given in Fig. 2.

Dealing with abnormal screening results

Suspected lesions on screening are confirmed by a variety of tests. These include computerized tomography (CT), spiral CT, magnetic resonance imaging (MRI), lipiodol-CT, hepatic angiography, and CT during arterial portography (CTAP). For lesions greater than 3 cm, the overall sensitivity and specificity of contrast-enhanced CT are 68% and 81%, respectively.[29] Smaller tumors are better detected by MRI, with 81% sensitivity for tumors less than 2 cm.[30] Spiral CT scanning is even more sensitive, with 87% of tumors less than 1 cm being detected compared with 64% by MRI.[31] Sensitivity can be improved still further by using techniques such as lipiodol-CT scanning. Sensitivities of 93% to 97% have been reported,[32,33] although it falls to 86% for tumors less than 1 cm. All of these radiological techniques are also subject to false-positive rates.

Liver imaging techniques basically play four roles in the management of HCC.[34] These are: (a) confirmation or differentiation of HCC from other tumors, (b) evaluation of the grade of malignancy or borderline (hyperplastic) lesions, (c) staging of HCC, and (d) evaluation of the therapeutic response and detection of recurrence of HCC. These techniques have contributed considerably in the differentiation of overt (advanced) hepatocellular carcinoma from benign or premalignant/borderline lesions. Recently, noninvasive ultrasonographic vascular imaging techniques have been developed, such as color Doppler, power Doppler, and enhanced Doppler imaging. In particular, gray-scale contrast second harmonic imaging may prove useful in the management of HCC and will replace some of the roles of magnetic resonance

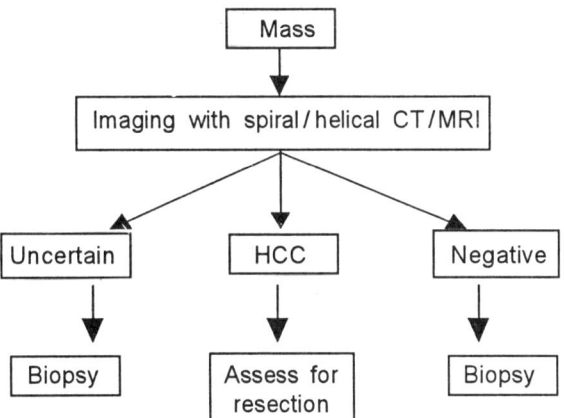

Fig. 2. Work-up of cases with mass lesion on ultrasound

imaging (MRI) and CT in the near future. Ultrasonographic visualization of the vascularity of viable cancer cells is essential for the US-guided interventional therapy of HCC.

Tissue diagnosis

The use of biopsy to confirm HCC is controversial. It is difficult to differentiate large cirrhotic nodules from well differentiated HCC. Low grade dysplastic nodules also pose problems in the differential diagnosis.[35] Liver biopsy does carry a small risk of tumor spread along the needle track.[36] Fine-needle aspirates provide cells without some of the architectural abnormalities that are important in making a diagnosis. Therefore, fine-needle aspiration is not recommended for distinguishing cirrhotic nodules from small neoplastic lesions that are likely to have subtle abnormalities.

Does screening improve survival?

This issue was addressed in one study[37] where cases of HCC were retrospectively reviewed from 1993 to 1998 for demographic data, risk factors, symptoms, stage, treatment, and survival. Patients were divided into 3 groups according to presentation: symptomatic (S), asymptomatic (A), and asymptomatic but screened for disease (A/Sc). Kaplan-Meier analysis was performed on overall survival by group. Ninety-one patients were referred for HCC. There were 56 patients in group S, 19 patients in group A, and 16 patients in group A/Sc. Patients in group A/Sc survived significantly longer than those in group S ($p = .009$), with the former group being 1,399 days compared with 234 days for group S. Median survival for group A was 545 days and it did not differ significantly from the other groups. Patients who were asymptomatic and screened for HCC had an increased survival compared with those patients who presented with symptoms. The authors conclude that this study may justify the use of a formal screening program for HCC in Hawaii.

Can the results be explained by "lead time" or "length-time" bias?

The issue of *"lead time bias"* needs attention. It is likely that the tumors detected by screening are identified before they present clinically and if left without intervention they would have manifested after a variable period of time and the survival is overestimated because the lesions identified by screening are detected very early.[38] Another possibility is that rapidly growing tumors have a lesser chance of being detected in surveillance programs and that tumors with lesser malignant potential are preferentially detected in a screening program. This is called *"length time bias"*. The possibility that lead-time and length-time bias operate in studies of screening in hepatocellular carcinoma cannot be completely excluded.

Cost-effectiveness of screening

The cost of finding HCC while screening HCV- or HBV-infected patients has been determined to be approximately $ 25,000–$ 72,000/tumor detected. When assessed by quality life year gained, screening those with Child-Pugh Class A cirrhosis is associated with a cost of $ 25,000–$ 55,000/life year gained. In comparison, screening at risk populations for colon cancer has a cost of approximately $ 25,000/life year gained.[39, 40]

In another study, the cost-effectiveness ratios of systematic surveillance range between $ 48,000 and $ 2,84,000 for each additional life-year gained. However, for a minority of patients with a predicted cirrhosis-related survival rate above 80% at 5 years (the "ideal" candidates) screening may increase mean life expectancy by 3 to 9 months depending on age, cancer incidence (1.5% to 6% per year), and survival rate after surgery (40% to 60% at 3 years). In this clinical setting, the cost-effectiveness ratios range between $ 26,000 and $ 55,000 for each additional life-year gained.[41] These studies have to be interpreted taking into account the regional problems and views. In a country like India, this may be too much of a burden to be taken up by the government or followed as a policy.

A US survey of practicing clinicians regarding their screening practices for patients with end-stage liver disease showed that only 36% screened non-transplantation candidates for HCC while 80% screened their liver transplantation candidates. Is this level of surveillance sufficient for the pre-transplant patient? While it is critical to know if a patient being considered for transplantation has HCC, the improved ability to provide adequate therapeutic options to those with small HCC lesions suggests that screening should be offered to all 'at-risk' patients.

Management of HCC detected at screening

For malignant liver neoplasms in the absence of extrahepatic disease, resection with negative pathological margins is the mainstay of treatment.[42] Major typical or atypical anatomical resections can now be carried out with low morbidity and minimal mortality. Extended resections (up to 75%) can be safely performed in patients if the liver function is not compromised by underlying liver disease (e.g., cirrhosis, steatosis), hypotension, infection, or ischemic injury. Many other treatment options are available for patients with hepatocellular carcinoma ranging from percutaneous alcohol injection in small tumors to arterial embolization or chemoembolization in advanced hepatocellular carcinoma. The role of transplantation is controversial. A three-year disease-free survival of 83% was seen after transplantation for uninodular and binodular tumors of less than 3 cm. The overall five-year survival for patients with small tumors (0 to 5 cm) was 75% vs. 36% for patients with tumors greater than 5 cm. Today, resection remains the mainstay of treatment for most patients with HCC arising in a non-cirrhotic liver or Child-Pugh A class of patients with cirrhosis.

PREVENTION OF SECOND PRIMARY

Knowledge of the risk factors for post-operative recurrence provides a basis for logical approaches to prevention of second primary tumors occurring after surgery or percutaneous ethanol injection. Minimal surgical manipulation of tumors to prevent tumor cell dissemination, avoidance of perioperative blood transfusion, and suppression of chronic hepatitis activity in the liver remnant are strategies that may be useful in preventing recurrence. The efficacy of postoperative adjuvant regional chemotherapy deserves further evaluation. New concepts on the influence of tumor biologic factors such as angiogenic activity on recurrence of HCC suggest a potential role of novel approaches such as antiangiogenesis for adjuvant therapy in the future. Currently, the most realistic approach in prolonging survival after resection of HCC is early detection and aggressive management of recurrence.[43-45] Chemoprevention (e.g. oral polyprenoic acid) appears to be promising, but further trials are needed before it can be put to routine clinical practice.

REFERENCES

1. Parkin DM, Muir CS, Whelan SL, Eds. *Cancer incidence in five continents:* Vol. VI. New York, NY: Oxford University Press, 1992.
2. Villeneuve JP, Desrochers M, Infante-Rivard C, Willems B, Raymond G, Bourcier M, Cote J, et al. A long-term follow-up study of asymptomatic hepatitis B surface antigen-positive carriers in Montreal. *Gastroenterology* 1994;108:1000-5.
3. McMahon BJ, Alberts SR, Wainwright RB, Bulkow L, Lanier AP. Hepatitis B-related sequelae. Prospective study of 1400 hepatitis B surface antigen-positive Alaska native carriers. *Arch Intern Med* 1990;150:1051-4.
4. Fletcher R, Fletcher SW, Wagner EH, Eds. *In: Clinical Epidemiology* – the essentials. Williams and Wilkins, Baltimore. 1988; pp.158.
5. Recommendations of the Immunization Practices Advisory Committee (ACIP) Hepatitis B Virus: A Comprehensive Strategy for Eliminating Transmission in the United States Through Universal Childhood Vaccination: *MMWR* 1991;40:1-19.
6. Chang MH, Chen CJ, Lai MS, et al. Universal Hepatitis B Vaccination in Taiwan and the Incidence of Hepatocellular Carcinoma in Children *N Engl J Med* 1997;336:1855-9.
7. Ikeda K, Saitoh S, Suzuki Y, Kobayashi M, Tsubota A, Fukuda M, Koida I, et al. Interferon decreases hepatocellular carcinogenesis in patients with cirrhosis caused by the hepatitis B virus: a pilot study. *Cancer* 1998;1:827-35.
7a. Ikeda K. Prevention of hepatocellular carcinogenesis by interferon. *Nippon Rinsho* 2001;59:755-63.
8. Lai CL, Yuen MF. Profound suppression of hepatitis B virus replication with lamivudine *J Med Virol* 2000;61:367-73.
9. Peek SF, et al. "3í Thiacytidine (3TC) delays development of hepatocellular carcinoma (HCC) in woodchucks with experimentally induced chronic woodchuck hepatitis virus (WHV) infection: preliminary results of a lifetime study," *Hepatology* 1997;26(S):368A.
9a. Franco J, Saeian K. Role of antiviral therapy in prevention of hepatocellular carcinoma. *J Vasc Interv Radiol* 2002;13(suppl):S191-6.
10. Blumberg BS, Millman I, Venkateswaran PS, Thyagarajan SP. Hepatitis B virus and hepatocellular carcinoma—treatment of HBV carriers with Phyllanthus amarus. *Cancer Detect Prev* 1989;14:195-201.
11. Shimizu I. Sho-saiko-to: Japanese herbal medicine for protection against hepatic fibrosis and carcinoma. *J Gastroenterol Hepatol* 2000;15(suppl):D84-90.
12. Sylla A, Diallo MS, Castegnaro J, Wild CP. Interactions between hepatitis B virus infection and

exposure to aflatoxins in the development of hepatocellular carcinoma: a molecular epidemiological approach. *Mutat Res* 1999;428:187-96.
13. Wild CP, Hall AJ. Primary prevention of hepatocellular carcinoma in developing countries. *Mutat Res* 2000;462:381-93.
14. Shotaro Sakisaka, Hironori Koga. Hepatocarcinogenesis: Is there Chemopreventive Potential for a COX-2 Inhibitor? *Medscape Gastroenterology* 2000.
15. Rahman MA, Dhar DK, Masunaga R, Yamanoi A, Kohno H, Nagasue N. Sulindac and exisulind exhibit a significant antiproliferative effect and induce apoptosis in human hepatocellular carcinoma cell lines. *Cancer Res* 2000;60:2085-9.
16. Kapicioglu S, Sari M, Kaynar K, Baki A, Ozoran Y. Effect of indomethacin on hepatitis B virus replication in chronic healthy carriers. *Scand J Gastroenterol* 2000;35:957-9.
17. Hepatoma Prevention Study Group, Japan. Prevention of second primary tumors by an acyclic retinoid, polyprenoic acid in patients with hepatocellular carcinoma. *N Engl J Med* 1996;334:1561-7.
18. Collier J, Sherman M. Screening for Hepatocellular Carcinoma. *Hepatology* 1998;27:273-8.
19. Zaman SN, Johnson PJ, Williams R. Silent cirrhosis in patients with hepatocellular carcinoma. Implications for screening in high-incidence and low-incidence areas. *Cancer* 1990;65:1607-10.
20. Sheu JC, Sung JL, Chen DS, Yang PM, Lau MY, Lee CS, Hsu HC, et al. Growth rates of asymptomatic hepatocellular carcinoma and its clinical implications. *Gastroenterology* 1985;89:259-66.
21. Lee HS, Chung YH, Kim CY. Specificities of serum alfa-fetoprotein in HBsAg+ and HBsAg– patients in the diagnosis of hepatocellular carcinoma. *Hepatology* 1991;14:68-72.
22. Oka H, Tamori A, Kuroki T, Kobayashi K, Yamamoto S. Prospective study of alfa-fetoprotein in cirrhotic patients monitored for development of hepatocellular carcinoma. *Hepatology* 1994;19:61-6.
23. Sherman M, Peltekian KM, Lee C. Screening for hepatocellular carcinoma in chronic carriers of hepatitis B virus: incidence and prevalence of hepatocellular carcinoma in a North American urban population. *Hepatology* 1995;22:432-8.
24. Bisceglie AM, Hoofnagle JH. Elevations of serum alfa-fetoprotein levels in patients with chronic hepatitis B. *Cancer* 1989;64:2117-20.
25. Lok ASF, Lai CL. Alfa-fetoprotein monitoring in Chinese patients with chronic hepatitis B virus infection: role in the early detection of hepatocellular carcinoma. *Hepatology* 1989;9:110-5.
26. Sherman M, Pateron D, Ganne N, Trinchet JC, Aurousseau MH, Mal F, Meicler C, et al. Prospective study of screening for hepatocellular carcinoma in Caucasian patients with cirrhosis. *J Hepatol* 1994; 20:65-71.
27. Michael CK. *Hepatic tumors and cysts*. In: Feldman M, Sleisenger MH, Scharschmidt BF, Klein S, Eds. WB Saunders Company, London. 1998;pp.1364-87.
28. Pateron D, Ganne N, Trinchet JC, Aurousseau MH, Mal F, Meicler C, Coderc E, et al. Prospective study of screening for hepatocellular carcinoma in Caucasian patients with cirrhosis. *J Hepatol* 1994;20: 65-71.
29. Miller WJ, Baron RL, Dodd GD, Federle MP. Malignancies in patients with cirrhosis: CT sensitivity and specificity in 200 consecutive transplant patients. *Radiology* 1994;193:645-50.
30. Hirai K, Aoki Y, Majima Y, Abe H, Nakashima O, Kojiro M, Tanikawa K. Magnetic resonance imaging of small hepatocellular carcinoma. *Am J Gastroenterol* 1991;86:205-9.
31. Murakami T, Kim T, Oi H, Nakamura H, Igarashi H, Matsushita M, Okamura J, et al. Detectability of hypervascular hepatocellular carcinoma by arterial phase imaging of MRI and spiral CT. *Acta Radiol* 1995;36:372-6.
32. Ngan H. Lipiodal computerized tomography: how sensitive and specific is the technique in the diagnosis of hepatocellular carcinoma? *Br J Radiol* 1990;63:771-5.
33. Takayasu K, Moriyama N, Muramatsu Y, Makuuchi M, Hasegawa H, Okazaki N, Hirohashi S. The

diagnosis of small hepatocellular carcinomas: efficacy of various imaging procedures in 100 patients. *AJR* 1990;155:49-54.
34. Kudo M. Imaging Diagnosis of Hepatocellular Carcinoma and Premalignant/Borderline Lesions. *Sem Liv Dis* 1999;19:297-309.
35. International working party. Terminology of nodular hepatocellular lesions. *Hepatology* 1995;22: 983-93.
36. John TG, Garden OJ. Needle track seeding of primary and secondary liver carcinoma after percutaneous liver biopsy. *Surgery* 1993;6:199-203.
37. Wong LL, Limm WM, Severino R, Wong LM. Improved survival with screening for hepatocellular carcinoma. *Liver Transpl* 2000;6:320-5.
38. *Early diagnosis. In:* Clinical Epidemiology – A basic science for clinical Medicine. Sackett. DL, Haynes RB, Guyatt GH, Tugwell P, Eds. Little Brown and Company. London 1991;pp.153-70.
39. Mima S, Sekiya C, Kanagawa H, et al. Mass screening for hepatocellular carcinoma: experience in Hokkaido, Japan. *J Gastroenterol Hepatol* 1994;9:361-5.
40. Kang JY, Lee TP, Lun KC. Analysis of cost-effectiveness of different strategies for hepatocellular carcinoma screening in hepatitis B virus carriers. *J Gastroenterol Hepatol* 1992;7:463-8.
41. Sarasin FP, Giostra E, Hadengue A. Cost-Effectiveness of screening for detection of small hepatocellular carcinoma in western patients with Child-Pugh class A cirrhosis: *Am J Med* 1996:101: 422-34.
42. Jean-Nicolas Vauthey, Hepatobiliary Cancer. Cancer Control: *JMCC* 1998:5:32-3.
43. Tung-Ping Poon R, Fan ST, Wong J. Risk factors, prevention and management of postoperative recurrence after resection of hepatocellular carcinoma. *Ann Surg* 2000;232:10-24.
44. Tang ZY. Hepatocellular carcinoma-cause, treatment and metastasis. *World J Gastroenterol* 2001;7: 537-41.
45. Dominguez-Malagon H, Gayatar Graham S. Hepatocellular carcinoma: an update. *Ultrasound Pathol* 2001;35:497-516.

24

Surgical resection in hepatitis B virus related hepatocellular carcinoma

Adarsh Chaudhary, Rajesh Bhojwani

With the advances in technology for pre-operative evaluation and "improvement in technical skills", the short-term outcome of surgery for hepatocellular cancer (HCC) has significantly improved. The biological behaviour of the tumor and its associated etiology are the major factors which affect the long-term results. Development of HCC is generally more frequent in patients with hepatitis C virus (HCV) infection than in those with hepatitis B virus (HBV) infection. Although there are several studies which have addressed the prognosis after resection of HCC, there are only a few which have evaluated it specifically in patients with HCC associated with hepatitis B virus infection.

SURGICAL TREATMENT OF HCC

Surgical treatment of HCC is either resection of the tumor or liver transplantation.

Resection of HCC

Most of the studies pertaining to results of resection of HCC are from Europe where alcoholic cirrhosis is very common or from Japan where hepatitis C has been the leading cause of HCC. Very few studies have analyzed the various issues of surgery specifically in relation to HBV-related HCC. Hepatitis B surface antigen positivity is closely related to the mode of growth of HCC and therefore has implications on the treatment of these tumors.[1]

The oncogenic mechanism of HBV is thought to be based on the genetic damage associated with chronic inflammation and with the integration of HBV-DNA into the host genome.[2,3] When severity of the liver disease is estimated, most of the patients with HBV infection show Child's A grading whereas patients with HCV show Child's B or C grading. Moreover, 50% of HCC associated with HBV sprout at the moderate stage of chronic hepatitis as compared to HCV positive cases, in which 70% have liver cirrhosis. This is because HBV-DNA gets integrated into cancer cells, which induces carcinogenesis even in early stages of the disease.[4]

Hepatic resections for HCC in a cirrhotic liver usually entails a segmental resection of the tumor bearing area with a reasonable tumor free margin. Major hepatic resections are indicated only in patients with good liver functions (Child's grade A). Bleeding during surgery is the major risk in patients with cirrhotic livers not only because of deficiency of coagulation factors and deranged platelet functions but also because of the coexisting portal hypertension. Moreover, the hard fibrotic liver prevents retraction of vessels during the phase of parenchymatous transection. Strategies to decrease bleeding during surgery include inflow occlusion, selective clamping and hepatic vascular exclusion. The duration of the 'safe limit' of inflow occlusion in cirrhotic livers is still undetermined. Hannoun et al[5] reported the use of hypothermic perfusion of the remnant liver using University of Wisconsin solution cooled to 4 degrees Celsius. Hepatic vascular exclusion has conventionally been avoided in patients with cirrhosis because of the fear of increased chances of post-operative liver failure and other complications. Emond et al[6] compared surgical outcome in 12 patients with abnormal liver function who had hepatic vascular exclusion during hepatic resection with 48 patients with normal liver parenchyma and showed no significant difference in the outcome in these two groups. A useful adjunct to surgery for HCC is the use of laparoscopy. Lo et al reported their experience with laparoscopy performed before laparotomy to assess the nature of the lesion, presence of extra hepatic disease and the adequacy of the liver remnant.[7] This simple investigation prevented unnecessary laparotomy in 63% patients with unresectable disease and allowed the non-operative treatment of the tumor to be initiated earlier. Subsegmentectomy for small peripheral tumors has also been performed laparoscopically with the aid of laparoscopic ultrasound.[8] The procedure is still in evolution and needs considerable skill and experience in both hepatic and minimally invasive surgery.

Complications of resection

The operative mortality depends on the extent of resection and the presence of associated cirrhosis. The mortality in cirrhotics ranges from 7–25% and in non-cirrhotics from 3–7.3%.[9-11] However, some series have reported no post-operative deaths.[12,13] Intra-operative deaths usually are caused by uncontrollable bleeding from hepatic veins or injury to the IVC. Post-operative deaths usually result from hepatic failure, haemorrhage, sepsis, or ascites. The morbidity ranges from 17–50% and hepatic failure is the most common post-operative complication.

Hepatic failure : The risk correlates with pre-operative liver function, extent of parenchymal resection and to peri-operative haemorrhage. Liver failure as a cause of death is usually precipitated or compounded by the addition of a complication of liver resection, such as sepsis, bile fistula, renal dysfunction, gastrointestinal bleeding, ascites, or portal thrombosis. Hepatic insufficiency as the cause of death in patients with impaired liver function has been reported in 1.4–2.9% of patients.[14-16] However, Makkuchi et al[17] reported zero mortality in their series of 277 patients out of which 185 patients had HCC with cirrhosis. They attributed their success to careful selection of patients and the extent of resection based on the status of serum bilirubin, ascites and Indocyanine green retention at 15 minutes. The importance of pre-operative intra-venous nutritional support, portal venous embolisation when indicated, intra-operative use of hydrocortisone and fresh frozen plasma (FFP) and minimising intra-operative loss of blood has also been stressed.

Post-operative hemorrhage : It has been reported to be in the range of 1.7–20.9%.[18, 19] In patients with cirrhosis, various factors contributing to it include liver dysfunction, thrombocytopenia, coagulopathy, and portal hypertension. Post-operative variceal bleeding may be induced by acute portal hypertension after major liver resection and Pacquet et al[10] recommended prophylactic sclerotherapy to prevent this complication.

Post-operative ascites : The incidence ranges from 36–50% and causes wound dehiscence, fluid leakage and secondary sepsis leading to multiple organ failure.

Infective complications : These constitute significantly to the morbidity. Multiple immunologic defects in cirrhotic patients, cavity remaining after resection and the presence of an ischaemic margin of liver tissue at the resection line are presumed to be the contributing factors.

Bile leakage : The incidence of bile leakage ranges from 3.1%–10.8%.[15, 19] No difference has been reported in the occurrence between the cirrhotic and non-cirrhotic patients. Operative technique and appropriate drainage are considered important in avoiding this complication.

Liver transplantation for HCC

Initially OLT (orthotopic liver transplantation) was considered as a treatment option only for unresectable malignancy or in presence of multiple tumor nodules. Expectedly it showed poor results both due to the high mortality associated with the procedure and also due to the high rate of recurrence of tumors. Now it has been shown that if the extrahepatic disease can be excluded, the results of OLT are significantly better in patients with small HCC (< 3 cm) and those with only one or two tumors. The survival at 3 years in these patients with OLT has been reported to be around 83%, while surgical resection had a survival of 18% in the same subgroup.[20] The OLT appears to be the most radical therapy since it removes both the tumor and the underlying cirrhosis. The OLT reduces the risk of hepatic recurrence at the same time as avoiding the complications such as hepatocellular failure and portal hypertension.

It was believed that the prognosis following transplantation for HCC in patients with chronic hepatitis B was poor. Recurrence of hepatitis B was the cause of death in many of these patients before they developed recurrence of HCC. However, in recent years, this attitude has changed as recurrence of HBV has been low (<15%) with the administration of hepatitis B immunoglobulin with or without lamivudine. The OLT has been established as a treatment option in patients with cirrhosis and HCC < 5 cm. Some centres also advocate transplantation as the treatment of choice for small HCC complicating cirrhosis, even for patients with Child's C cirrhosis because of the poor survival results obtained with surgical resection.[21-23] However, for tumors >5 cm, the outcome is poor and OLT is generally considered unjustified.[24-26]

LONG-TERM RESULTS AND PROGNOSIS

Poon et al[27] recently published their study on long-term prognosis in HCC specifically related to HBV. One hundred forty-six patients with HBV-related cirrhosis who had undergone resection of HCC over a 10-year period were prospectively evaluated for long-term results. These patients were compared with 155 non-cirrhotic patients with HBV-related HCC resected in the same period. The overall survival results of cirrhotic patients after resection of HCC were comparable to those of non-cirrhotic patients (5-year survival 44.3% vs. 45.6%) but the cirrhotic patients had smaller tumors. When stratified according to tumor size, the survival results were similar in patients with tumors of <5 cm irrespective of presence or absence of cirrhosis, but in patients with HCC of >5 cm size, the results were worse in those having cirrhosis compared to noncirrhotic patients. The authors feel that with the current shortage of organ donors, surgical resection should be the first line of treatment for patients with tumors < 5 cm and compensated cirrhosis. The high recurrence rate after resection is one of the main factors in the poor outcome for patients with HCC. Apart from the inherent invasiveness of the tumor, factors for tumor recurrence include vascular invasion, positive resection margins, tumor free interval, tumor size and degree of differentiation.

The significance of resection margin for HCC remains controversial. It is generally accepted that a 1 cm margin from the palpable edge of the tumor may be sufficient. Intra-hepatic recurrence cannot be prevented by increasing this margin. A review from Hong Kong[28] revealed that the inability to obtain a resection margin of 1 cm should not be regarded as a contraindication to resection of HCC. In patients with limited hepatic reserve, preservation of hepatic parenchyma should take priority over a wide resection margin. Jeng at al[29] showed that the biological behaviour of the mutant p53 gene is strongly related to invasiveness of the HCC and may also influence the post-operative course. These authors also suggested that the immunopositivity of the mutant p53 gene has a predictive value in the prognosis of patients with resected HCC. In another study, intra-hepatic recurrence in HCC due to hepatitis B and C were found to be higher than in non-B and non-C related HCC.[30] Fibrosis staging, pathological grade of the tumor, and serum AFP levels were found to be significantly linked to the intra-hepatic recurrence in univariate analysis and fibrosis staging was the strongest in the multivariate analysis for HCC related to hepatitis C. In contrast, fibrosis staging did not affect the recurrence of HBV-related and non-B non-C-related HCC.

REFERENCES

1. Shijo H, Okazaki M, Koganemaru F, Higashi M, Sakaguchi S, Okumara M. Influence of hepatitis B virus infection and age on mode of growth of heptocellular carcinoma. *Cancer* 1991;67:2626-32.
2. Okuda K. Hepatocellular carcinoma: recent progress. *Hepatology* 1992;15:948-63.
3. Shafritz DA, Shoval D, Sherman HI, Kew MC. Integration of hepatitis B virus DNA into the genome of liver cells in chronic liver disease and hepatocellular carcinoma. Studies in percutaneous liver biopsies and post mortem tissue specimens. *N Engl J Med* 1981;305:1067-73.
4. Shiratori Y, Shina S, Imamura M, Kato N, Kanai F, Okudaira T, Teratani T. Characteristic difference of HCC between hepatitis B and C viral infection in Japan. *Hepatology* 1995;22:1027-33.
5. Hannoun L, Delriviere L, Gibbs P, Borie D, Vaillant JC, Delva E. Major extended hepatic resections in diseased livers using hypothermic protection: Preliminary results from the first 12 patients treated with this new technique. *J Am Coll Surg* 1996;183:597-605.
6. Emond J, Wachs ME, Renz JF, Kelley S, Harrio H, Roberts JP, Ascher NL, et al. Total vascular exclusion for major hepatectomy in patients with abnormal liver parenchyma. *Arch Surg* 1995;130:824-31.
7. Lo CM, Lai EC, Liu CL, Fans S, Wong J, et al. Laparoscopy and laparoscopic ultrasonography avoid exploratory laparotomy in patients with hepatocellular carcinoma. *Ann Surg* 1998;227:527-32.
8. Ken CG, Chen HY, Juan CC, Chang WS, Trai CY, Lo HW, Yau MT. Laparoscopic subsegmentectomy for hepatocellular carcinoma with cirrhosis. *Hepatogastroenterology* 2000;47:1260-3.
9. Bismuth H, Houssin D, Ornowski J, Meriggi F. Liver resections in cirrhotic patients: a western experience. *World J Surg* 1986;10:311-5.
10. Pacquet KJ, Koussouris P, Mercado MA. Limited hepatic resection for selected cirrhotic patients with hepatocellular or cholangiocellular carcinoma: a prospective study. *Br J Surg* 1991;78:459-62.
11. Gozzeti G, Maziotti A, Cavallari A, Bellucci R, Bolondi L, Grigioni W, Bragaglia R, et al. Clinical experience with hepatic resections for HCC in patients with cirrhosis. *Surg Gynecol Obstet* 1988;166:503-10.
12. Ringe B, Pichlamyr R, Witterand L, Rusch G. Surgical treatment of HCC: experience with liver resection and liver transplantation in 198 patients. *World J Surg* 1991;15:270-4.
13. Franco D, Smadja C, Kahwaji F, Grange D, Kemeney F, Traynor O. Segmentectomies in the management of liver tumors. *Arch Surg* 1988;123:519-22.
14. Takenaka K, Shimada M, Higashi H, Adachi E, Nishizaki T, Yanaga K, Matsemata T, et al. Liver resection for hepatocellular carcinoma in the elderly. *Arch Surg* 1994;129:846-50.
15. Wu CC, Ho WL, Lin MC, Yeh DC, Wu HS, Hwang CJ, Liu TJ, et al. Hepatic resection for bilobar multicentric hepatocellular carcinoma. Is it justified? *Surgery* 1998:123:270-7.
16. Iwatsuki S, Starzl TE. Personal experience with 41 hepatic resections. *Ann Surg* 1988;208:421-34.
17. Yutaka Midorikawa, Makkuchi M. A comparative study of post-operative complications after hepatectomy in patients with and without chronic liver disease. *Surgery* 1999;126:484-91.
18. Farid H, O'Conell T. Hepatic resections, changing mortality and morbidity. *Am Surg* 1994;60:748-52.
19. Thompson HH, Tompkins RK, Longmire WP. Major hepatic resection: a 25 year experience. *Ann Surgery* 1983;197:375-88.
20. Bismuth H, Chiche L, Adam R, Castaing D, Diamond T, Dennison A. Liver resection vs. transplantation for hepatocellular carcinoma in cirrhotic patients. *Ann Surg* 1993;218:145-51.
21. Mazzaferro V, Regalia E, Doci R, Andreola S, Pulvirenti A, Bozzetti F, Montalto F, et al. Liver transplantation for treatment of small HCC in patients with cirrhosis. *N Engl J Med* 1996;334:693-9.
22. Michel J, Suc B, Montpeyroux F, Hachemanne S, Blane P, Domergue J, Mouiel J, et al. Liver resection

or transplantation for hepatocellular carcinoma? Retrospective analysis of 215 patients with cirrhosis. *J Hepatol* 1997;26:1274-80.
23. Balsells J, Charco R, Lazaro JL, Murio E, Vargas V, Allende E, Margarit C, et al. Resection of hepatocellular carcinoma in patients with cirrhosis. *Br J Surg* 1996;83;758-61.
24. Figueras J, Jaurrieta E, Valls C, Benasco C, Rafecas A, Xior X, Fabregat J, et al. Survival after liver transplantation in cirrhotic patients with and without hepatocellular carcinoma: a comparative study. *Hepatology* 1997;25:1485-9.
25. Mor E, Kaspa RT, Sheiner P, Schwartz M. Treatment of hepatocellular carcinoma associated with cirrhosis in the era of liver transplantation. *Ann Intern Med* 1998;129:643-53.
26. Klintmann GB. Liver transplantation for HCC. A registry report of the impact of tumor characteristics on outcome. *Ann Surg* 1998;228;479-90.
27. Poon RT, Fan ST, Lo CM, Liu CL, Ng IO, Wong J. Long-term treatment after resection of Hepatocellular carcinoma associated with hepatitis B-related cirrhosis. *J Clin Oncology* 2000;18:1094-1101.
28. Poon RTP, Fan ST, Wong J. Risk factors, prevention, and management of post-operative recurrence after resection of hepatocellular carcinoma. *Ann Surg* 2000;222;10-24.
29. Jeng KS, Sheen JS, Chen BF, Wu JY. Is the p53 gene mutation of prognostic value in HCC after resection. *Arch Surg* 2000;135:1329-33.
30. Koike Y, Shiratori Y, Sato S, Obi S, Teratani T, Imamura M, Hamamura K, et al. Risk factors for recurring hepatocellular carcinoma differ according to infected hepatitis virus–an analysis of 236 consecutive patients with a single lesion. *Hepatology* 2000;32:1216-23.

25

Newer non-surgical modalities for the treatment of hepatocellular carcinoma

Ching L Lai, Man F Yuen

Hepatocellular carcinoma (HCC) remains one of the world's major health problems. The annual incidence of HCC is estimated to be 530,000 cases globally.[1] Chronic viral hepatitis infection is the main aetiological cause, contributing to 82% of cases who develop HCC. Hepatitis B virus (HBV) and hepatitis C virus (HCV) infections cause 3,16,000 and 1,18,000 cases per annum respectively.

HCC is notorious for its poor prognosis. There are four factors which may account for this:[2]

(a) Patients present late because they usually experience no symptoms until the tumor grows to more than 8 cm in diameter,
(b) Approximately 85% of patients with HCC have co-existing liver cirrhosis. This would affect the outcome of both surgery and chemotherapy,
(c) HCC is multifocal. This may be present at the initial presentation or may develop as early 're-occurrence' (i.e. occurrence of new tumors at new foci) after resection, and
(d) HCC is prone to early haematolocial spread, portal vein infiltration, and/or thrombosis.

To improve upon the prognosis of this dermal problem, the lesions need to be picked up early enough, when they are still small and amenable to treatment (Fig. 1).

While surgical resection remains the treatment of choice, the operability of patients with subclinical HCC diagnosed by screening remains less than 30%.[3] The recurrence rate is also high after surgery. Intraarterial injection of 1850 MBq of ^{131}I–lipiodol through selective cannulation of hepatic artery after resection can prolong disease-free interval and survival.[4] Intrahepatic recurrence after surgery can also improve survival.[5]

Liver transplantation can also be contemplated provided the tumor is less than 5 cm in diameter, the portal vein is not infiltrated, and there are less than 3 tumor nodules

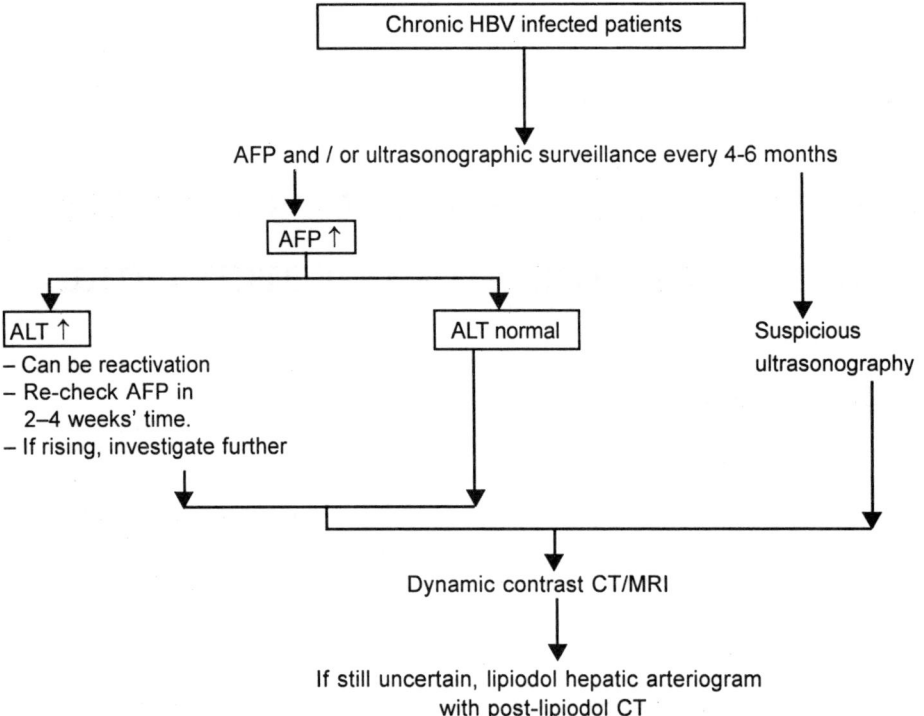

Fig. 1. Algorithmic approach for the early detection of hepatocellular carcinoma

(Fig. 2). However, transplantation as a treatment for hepatocellular carcinoma is limited by the availability of donor organs and the cost of the procedure. There is also the problem of recurrence of hepatitis B and C in the transplanted liver, though the risk for the former is now lessened with the availability of nucleoside analogue therapy, e.g. lamivudine.

Because of the scarcity of randomized controlled trials and conflicting results from different trials, the benefit of medical treatment for HCC is still controversial. Moreover, it is difficult to perform meta-analyses because of the heterogeneity of patient population.[6] Medical treatment can be divided into systemic and local/regional therapy. Systemic therapy comprises the use of doxorubicin, alpha-interferon (IFN-α), combination therapy, and tamoxifen. Doxorubicin is the only agent for the treatment of HCC approved by the Food and Drug Administration. There are only two controlled trials till date to assess the use of doxorubicin for the treatment of HCC.[7,8] Only 3.3% patients showed more than a 50% tumor regression. More importantly, 25% had fatal neutropenia and cardiotoxicity. Cardiotoxicity can occur even if the dose of doxorubicin does not exceed the recognized cardiotoxic dose of 500 mg/m^2.

Apart from the antiviral and immunomodulatory effects of IFN-α, its anti-proliferative effect on HCC was assessed in two controlled trials.[8,9] In dosages of 50×10^6 U/m^2 three times a

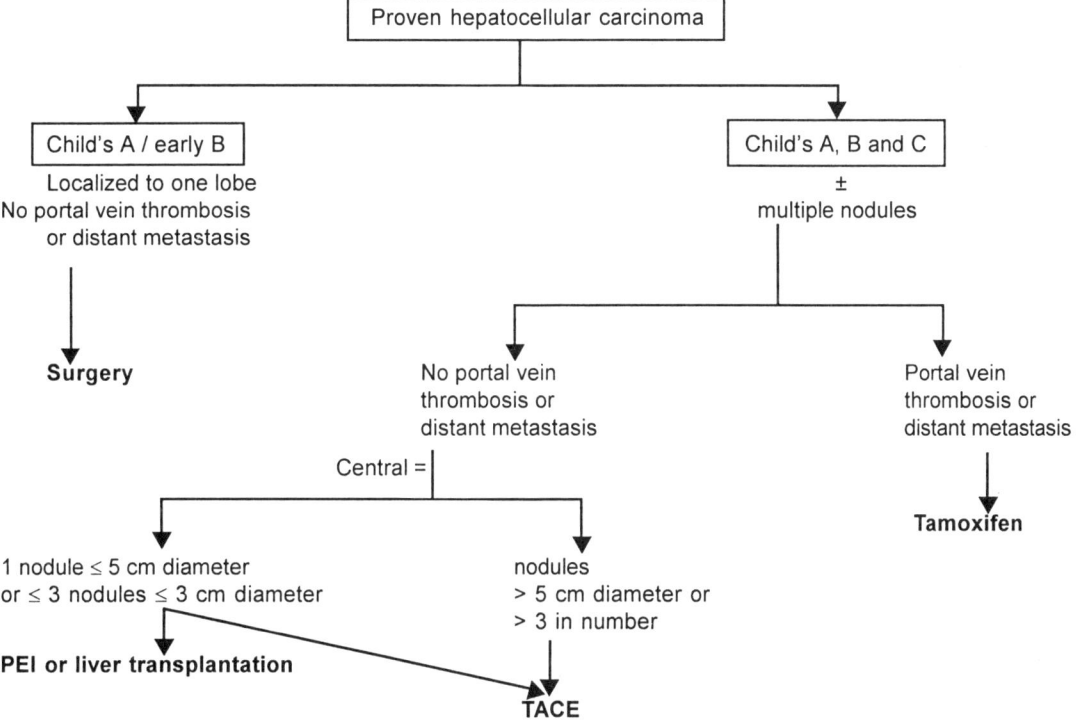

Fig. 2. Algorithm for the management of hepatocellular carcinoma

week, IFN-α can prolong the median survival of patients with HCC from 7.5 to 14.5 weeks ($P=0.0471$). In addition, 31.4% of patients had more than 50% tumor regression. As expected, the side effects were quite severe with such a high dose. However, they were tolerable by the majority of patients after the reduction of the dose. One major drawback is the prohibitively expensive cost for the treatment (approximately US$ 2000/week).

Various combination therapies are currently being assessed. One of these trials, combining cisplastin (20 mg/m^2), low-dose IFN-α (5 MU/m^2), doxorubicin (adriamycin) (40 mg/m^2), and 5-fluorouracil (400 mg/m^2) given for 4 days every 3 weeks to a maximum of 6 cycles showed that none had a complete response and only 26% had partial response.[10] The overall median survival was 8.9 months.

The efficacy of tamoxifen in the treatment of HCC was evaluated in four randomized controlled trials.[11-14] The significance for survival benefit is borderline and controversial. A randomized controlled trial involving 496 patients has shown that tamoxifen does not prolong survival of patients with HCC.[14] Whether a subgroup of patients in whom the HCC expresses estrogen receptors may respond to this hormonal therapy is worthy of investigation.

For the local/regional therapy, alcohol injection,[15] cryotherapy,[16] and transcatheter arterial chemoembolization (TACE) with lipiodol[17-19] have been assessed in multiple trials. Alcohol injection given for 6–14 sessions performed once or twice weekly (a mean total of 36 ml alcohol given in one series) is an effective curative treatment for tumors less than 5 cm in diameter.[15] It is associated with minimal side effects. Cryotherapy also is only useful for tumors of less than 5 cm in diameter. In one centre in China, its use in 80 patients is associated with a 5-year survival of 55.4%.[16]

Lipiodol (iodized oil) allows the chemotherapeutic agent to remain selectively in tumors for a comparatively longer period of time since it is removed in the normal liver tissue by lymphocytes and Kupffer cells, and tumor cells contain neither of these. The chemotherapeutic agent being used differs in different centres. Cisplatin is the commonly used agent. The dosage used varies from 10 mg[17] to 70 mg.[18] The interval between each session of TACE is usually 8 weeks. The number of courses given varies in different centres from a maximum of four[18] to unlimited number of courses depending on the patient's response to the treatment.[17] In a randomized trial of 96 patients (50 with TACE given for a maximal of four courses and 46 with conservative treatment), TACE reduced tumor growth but did not improve survival.[17] It caused liver failure (defined as the presence of encephalopathy, ascites, or an increase in serum bilirubin concentration of 15 μmol/l) after 47 courses of treatment in 30 patients. There was one death due to liver failure. The authors concluded that TACE may be beneficial in a select group of patients only.

A similar but uncontrolled study including 132 patients was conducted in Hong Kong.[17] One hundred and four patients received TACE; 28 patients had transarterial chemotherapy without gel foam embolization. There was no limit to the number of courses. It was found that transarterial chemotherapy decreased the tumor size in 72% of patients having tumors less than 9 cm in diameter, irrespective of whether embolization was given or not. For tumors more than 9 cm in diameter, the response rate to transarterial chemotherapy without gelfoam embolization was 0%, whereas adding gel embolization to chemotherapy increased the response rate to 41%. The appearance of new daughter nodules occurred in 30% of patients, but the nodules were equally responsive to TACE. The side effects were usually tolerable; these included vomiting (62%), pain (55%), fever (53%), bleeding peptic ulcer (1.5%), liver abscess (1.5%), liver failure (1.5%), and septicemia (<1%). The relatively low rate of liver failure in this series is in contrast to the series from Groupe d'Etude.[18] This may be related to the more careful selection of patients in the series of Ngan et al[17] where all patients with a bilirubin above twice the upper limit of normal were excluded.

A recent uncontrolled study using intra-arterial ^{90}(yttrium) microspheres showed that 26.7% patients had 50% reduction in tumor volume after the first session of treatment.[20] In addition, there was an 89% response in terms of the reduction of alpha-fetoprotein levels. The median survival of the studied population ($n=71$) was 9.4 months. There was no bone marrow toxicity nor any clinical evidence of radiation hepatitis or of pneumonitis.

The authors of this chapter are currently conducting a dose-defining trial of transcatheter arterial interferon-embolization (TAIE) in their own centre.[21] To date, 15 patients (12 males and 3 females) have been recruited. They were randomized to receive IFN-α mixed with lipiodol given intraarterially in the dosages of 10×10^6, 30×10^6, or 50×10^6 units at interval of 8 weeks intervals. Six patients had more than 50% tumor regression and four others had no change in tumor size. The main side-effect was fever lasting for 1–25 days. The only other possible IFN-related side-effect was the development of hypothyroidism in one patient.

Overall, the 3- and 5-year actuarial survival rates of HCC for different modalities of treatment from one centre are as follows: surgical resection – 60% and 40%; liver transplantation –72% and 68%; percutaneous ethanol injection – 55% and 35%; and TACE – 30% and 20% respectively.[22] In evaluating these survival rates, one must bear in mind that patients given TACE are inoperable patients with the largest number of tumours and/or poorest liver reserve.

Treatment for HCC at present is still far from satisfactory because of the low resection rate, the high recurrence/new occurrence rate and the high prevalence of background cirrhosis. Randomized controlled trials are relatively rare and urgently needed to assess the efficacy of various medical treatments.[23, 24]

REFERENCES

1. World Health Organisation. Geneva: World Health Organisation, 1996.
2. Yuen MF, Lai CL. Hepatocellular carcinoma: Screening and non-screening treatment. *Ann Coll Surg* 1999;4:107-11.
3. Yuen MF, Cheng CC, Lauder IJ, Lam SK, Ooi CGC, Lai CL. Early detection of hepatocellular carcinoma increases the chance of treatment: Hong Kong experience. *Hepatology* 2000;31:330-5.
4. Lau WY, Leung TWT, Ho SKW, Chan M, Machin D, Lau J, Chan ATC, et al. Adjuvant intra-arterial iodine-131-labelled lipiodol for respectable hepatocellular carcinoma: a prospective randomized trial. *Lancet* 1999;353:797-801.
5. Poon RT, Fan ST, Lo CM, Liu CL, Wong J. Intrahepatic recurrence after curative resection of hepatocellular carcinoma: Long-term results of treatment and prognostic factors. *Ann Surg* 1999;229:216-22.
6. Mathurin P, Rixe O, Carbonell N, Bernard B, Cluzel P, Bellin MF, Khayat D, et al. Review article: overview of medical treatments in unresectable hepatocellular carcinoma – an impossible meta-analysis? *Aliment Pharmacol Ther* 1998;12:111-26.
7. Lai CL, Wu PC, Chan GCB, Lok AS, Lin AJ. Doxorubicin versus no antitumour therapy in inoperable hepatocellular carcinoma: a prospective randomized trial. *Cancer* 1988;62:479-88.
8. Lai CL, Wu PC, Lok ASF, Lin HJ, Ngan H, Lau JY, Chung HT, et al. Recombinant a_2 interferon is superior to doxorubicin for inoperable hepatocellular carcinoma: a propective randomized trial. *Br J Cancer* 1989;60:928-33.
9. Lai CL, Lau JYN, Wu PC, Ngan H, Chung HT, Michell SJ, Corbett TJ, et al. Recombinant interferon-alpha in inoperable hepatocellular carcinoma: a randomized controlled trial. *Hepatology* 1993;17: 389-94.
10. Leung TW, Patt YZ, Lau WY, Ho SK, Yu SC, Chan AT, Mok TS, et al. Complete pathological

remission is possible with systemic combination chemotherapy for inoperable hepatocellular carcinoma. *Clin Cancer Res* 1999;5:1676-81.
11. Castells A, Bruix J, Bru C, Ayuso C, Roca M, Boix L, Vihana R, et al. Treatment of hepatocellular carcinoma with tamoxifen: a double-blind placebo-controlled trial in 120 patients. *Gastroenterology* 1995;109:917-22.
12. Elba S, Glannuzi V, Misciagna G, Manghisi OG. Randomized controlled trial of tamoxifen versus placebo in inoperable hepatocellular carcinoma. *Ital J Gastroenterol* 1994;26:66-8.
13. Marinez Cerezo FJ, Tomas A, Donoso L, Enriquez J, Guarner C, Balanzo J, Marinez Nogveras A, et al. Controlled trial of tamoxifen in patients with advanced hepatocellular carcinoma. *J Hepatol* 1994;20: 702-6.
14. CLIP Group (Cancer of the Liver Italian Program). Tamoxifen in treatment of hepatocellular carcinoma: a randomized controlled trial. *Lancet* 1998;352:17-20.
15. Lencioni R, Paolicchi A, Bartolozzi C. Percutaneous alcohol administration for hepatocarcinoma: Long-term results. *Radiol Med Torino* 1997;94:8-13.
16. Zhou XD, Tang ZY. Cryotherapy for primary liver cancer. *Semin Surg Oncol* 1998;14:171-4.
17. Ngan H, Lai CL, Fan ST, Lai EC, Yuen WK, Tso WK. Transcatheter arterial chemoembolization in inoperable hepatocellular carcinoma: four-year follow-up. *J Vasc Intern Radiol* 1996;7:419-25.
18. Groupe d'Etude et de traitement du carcinome hepatocellulaire. A comparison of lipiodol chemoembolization and conservative treatment for unresectable hepatocellular carcinoma. *N Engl J Med* 1995;332:1256-61.
19. Harris M, Gibbs P, Cebon J, Jones R, Sewell R, Schelkmann T, Angus P. Hepatocellular carcinoma and chemoembolization. *Intern Med J* 2001;31:517-22.
20. Lau WY, Ho S, Leung TW, Chan M, Ho R, Johnson PJ, Li AK, et al. Selective internal radiation therapy for nonresectable hepatocellular carcinoma with intraarterial infusion of ^{90}yttrium microspheres. *Int J Radiat Oncol Biol Phys* 1998;40:583-92.
21. Yuen MF, Ooi C, Wong WM, Chan OO, Wong BCY, Lai CL. A pilot study of transcatheter arterial interferon-embolization for hepatocellular carcinoma. *Gastroenterology* 2000;118:A915 (abstract).
22. Colella G, Bottelli R, Carlis L De, Sansalone CV, Rondinara GF, Alberti A, Belli LS, et al. Hepatocellular carcinoma: comparison between liver transplantation, resective surgery, ethanol injection, and chemoembolization. *Transpl Int* 1998;11(suppl 1):S193-6.
23. Wong ET, Chew YP, Lee LA, Lee CG. Therapeuticd strategies for hepatitis B virus – associated hepatocellular carcinoma. *Curr Drug Targets* 2002;3:369-78.
24. Rabe C, Pilz T, Allegaier HP, Halm U, Strasser C, Wettstein M. Sauerbruch T, et al. Clinical outcome of a cohort of 63 patients with hepatocellular carcinoma treated with octeotide. *Z Gastroenterol* 2002; 40:395-400.

26

Liver transplantation in the developing world

Magaral R Rajasekar, Arvinder S Soin, Anupam Sibal, Durairajan Vijayarajkumari

Liver transplantation is now the established mode of treatment for end-stage-liver disease. While it is performed routinely in the developed nations, it is still in its infancy in the developing world. Orthotopic liver transplantation (OLT) was first performed successfully in 1963. With the advent of cyclosporin, the eighties saw a rapid growth in this field. Now, with the availability of better immunosuppressive agents such as Tacrolimus, improvement in the surgical technique, and post operative critical care, the 1-and 5-year survival rates after liver transplantation are 85% and 80% respectively.

Liver transplantation is usually done for either irreversible acute or chronic liver failure, or metabolic diseases that predispose to liver malignancy or result in life-threatening extrahepatic end-organ damage. The commonest form of chronic liver disease accounting for 50–80% of all liver transplants in children is biliary atresia. On the other hand, chronic liver disease due to viral hepatitis B or C and alcoholic liver disease are the commonest indications for liver transplantation among adults.

THE NEED IN INDIA

Approximately 2–3 per million pediatric and over 6 per million adult population liver transplants are done annually in the West. At that rate, around 2000 children and 8000 adults would need liver transplant in India annually. This estimate is likely to be representative since the incidence of biliary atresia (1/12,000 to 1/18,000), viral hepatitis and metabolic diseases is similar all over the world. Even if 10–15% of the patients can actually afford this procedure, at least 200–300 children and twice that number of adults could be saved each year by liver transplantation. This necessitates the establishment of at least 8–10 liver transplant centres across the country.

Do we need our own program?

A developing country like India needs to develop its own program for two reasons. First, our patients even if accepted onto a foreign transplant program will always be the last to be considered as there is always a shortage of suitable organs. Second, the exhorbitant cost of Rs. 60–80 lakhs for a liver transplant in a western center cannot be afforded by the majority. Add to this the cost of living abroad for several months, and that too, away from family support which is very vital. In India, a liver transplant can be performed at the cost of Rs. 10 lakhs. Although, this is beyond the reach of the majority of Indians, it might well be the only hope for some patients. The sceptics might argue that a poor country like India should concentrate only on basic health care issues rather than transplantation. However, we should be looking at the positive aspects of this, which are as follows:

(a) enormous saving of foreign exchange that some recipients would otherwise spend on treatment abroad,
(b) concomitant with the development of a liver program in an institution, the level of facilities and expertise in allied specialities (critical care, radiology, histology, viral diagnosis, blood bank, etc.) increase appreciably. This shall help in elevating the level of health care in these hospitals to an international standard, and
(c) this could bring back the smile to a family with a member who faces certain death from liver failure.

Prerequisites for setting up a program in India

Development of a successful liver transplant program requires adequate infrastructure, trained staff, and availability of cadaver donors. Infrastructural requirements include a dedicated ICU, a blood bank with state-of-the-art facilities, and comprehensive round the clock laboratory support. Laboratory facilities should include transplant immunology, pathology with availability of rapid paraffin and immunohistochemistry techniques, microbiology with provision for diagnosis of fungal and viral infections, and a full biochemistry support including drug level monitoring. In addition, advanced theatre facilities with laminar flow operating rooms is mandatory. This also requires equipment such as microscope, argon beam coagulator, monitors for invasive monitoring, and measurement of cardiac indices, cell saver, rapid fluid infuser, veno-venous bypass pump, blood gas, electrolyte, and coagulation analyzers.

In order to manage all the aspects of patient care, it is recommended to develop a multi-disciplinary team comprising trained transplant surgeon, anesthetist, intensivist, radiologist, gastroenterologist, pathologist, nurses, psychologist, transplant co-ordinator, nutritionist and social worker. Certified training of at least the key members like the surgeons and anaesthetists is strongly recommended.

Lack of pediatric donors has been the bottleneck in most pediatric liver transplant programs.

However, with increasing experience and technical refinement in the use of segmental liver grafts, many surgical options are now available for pediatric liver transplantation. In the case of cadaveric donors, the use of reduced whole grafts, and split liver transplantation has eased the situation somewhat. In addition, use of partial livers from living donors now has an established place in pediatric liver transplantation and living donor right lobe transplants is now done routinely in nearly 10 centers around the globe including the one in New Delhi. Globally more than 350 adult to adult living donor right lobe liver transplants are done each year.[1,2] The prerequisites for living related liver transplantation are listed in Table 1.

Table 1. Prerequisites for living related liver transplantation

Two fully qualified transplant surgeons with expertise in microsurgery
Two fully equipped operating theatres
Two sets of trained theatre staff
Two teams of anaesthetists
Two sets of major liver surgery instruments
Operating microscope
Intraoperative Doppler facility and a trained radiologist
3-D CT spiral or MR volumetry, and
All other requirements as for liver transplants in general.

Are we ready in India?

There are now at least a few centres in India where all the above infrastructure requirements are met to international standards. However, not many trained surgeons with expertise in OLT are available in India. Only 10–15 cadaver organ donors materialize annually in India. The Human Organ Transplant Act passed in 1994, legalizes declaration of brain death and subsequent donation of organs from such donors on the basis of consent obtained from the next of kin. Brain death can be declared based on international criteria by a panel of doctors approved by the government. Further organ retrieval, preservation, and transplantation can be performed only by the surgeons at centers approved by medical board appointed by the Union Health ministry. Cadaver organ donation requires enormous amount of public awareness and education. The cadaver organ donation rates are presently very low in India and this is not likely to improve significantly in the near future. As efforts in promoting organ donation will take another decade to bear fruit, a parallel living donor transplant program is mandatory for all the aspiring centers in the country. However, the demand on technical expertise and infrastructure is several fold greater with a pediatric and adult living donor program. In depth assessment of strengths and weakness of the center will be called for. Though donor hepatectomy is safe in trained hands, serious donor related morbidity and even mortality is a distinct possibility, if suitable expertise is not available in live donor hepatectomy.

Selection of recipients

Selection of patients for transplantation requires consideration of not only medical criteria (see above), but also the socioeconomic and educational background of the family. This is of paramount importance because in addition to the initial expenditure, this also involves a lifelong commitment on the part of the patient and the family to spend around Rs.10,000 per month on immunosuppression, and long-term medication. Moreover, if a graft is lost due to poor patient compliance, it is a colossal waste of efforts of the treating team, of the donor resources, and the expenses incurred on the procedure. The indications for liver transplantation have increased exponentially. These are as follows:

Pediatric: Extra-hepatic biliary atresia, biliary hypoplasia, hepatoblastoma, metabolic disorders such as alpha-1 antitrypsin deficiency, Wilson's disease, etc.

Adult: Alcoholic liver disease, primary biliary cirrhosis, sclerosing cholangitis, primary liver tumor with cirrhosis (selected cases)

Common to pediatric and adult patients: Hepatitis B and C associated end stage liver disease, cryptogenic cirrhosis, fulminant liver failure

The liver transplantation cannot be performed in certain situations such as patients with concomitant HIV infection, disseminated primary HCC or liver secondaries, thrombosis of portal and mesenteric veins, multi-centric HCC and/or HCC >5 cm, severe pulmonary hypertension, and severe hypoxia (hepatopulmonary syndrome).

Selection and timing

The timing of OLT is dictated by the natural history of the underlying disease, evidence of decompensation of hepatic function, and quality of life. All the patients suffering from chronic liver disease who develop refractory ascites, one or more episodes of spontaneous bacterial peritonitis, variceal bleeding, vitamin K resistant prolongation of prothrombin time, hypoalbuminemia less than 2.5 gm/l, refractory itching, severe cholestasis, recurrent cholangitis, respiratory compromise due to cirrhosis and portal hypertension, and growth failure in case of children, should be referred expeditiously for transplant evaluation and counseling. Delay in referral adversely affects immediate and long-term outcome after OLT.

Optimal timing of liver transplantation is important to ensure the best chances for survival. All children with chronic liver disease who have growth retardation and/or an expected survival less than one year should be considered for transplantation. Such a prognosis may be indicated by the presence of refractory ascites, spontaneous bacterial peritonitis, gastrointestinal bleeding not controlled by conservative measures, prothrombin ratio (INR) >1.4, indirect bilirubin >6 mg/dl, hypoxia, and encephalopathy. All children with advanced liver disease should be referred to the transplant center to ensure timely assessment and pre-transplant management.

In the case of acute liver failure, urgent liver transplantation should be considered in the presence of poor prognostic indicators. The poor prognostic indicators are age under 10 years, non A-E hepatitis, rising prothrombin time (> 30 seconds), rising bilirubin (> 10mg/dl), worsening encephalopathy, a shrinking liver, worsening renal function, and hypoglycemia despite infusion of IV dextrose.[3,4]

All patients with fulminant hepatic failure should be managed in specialized liver units in close consultation with the transplant team, since a proportion of them will need life-saving emergency liver transplantation. Indications for liver transplantation in fulminant hepatic failure are more complex. In general, worsening coagulopathy (prothrombin time), increasing glucose requirements to maintain euglycemia, falling liver enzymes with shrinking liver, acidosis, onset of renal insufficiency, and worsening encephalopathy are some of the parameters which indicate urgent liver transplantation. Since cadaver organ availability is unpredictable, living partial liver donation from one of the family members is usually required. Results following liver transplantation for fulminant hepatic failure are generally poor (65%), as compared with liver transplantation in stable patients with chronic liver disease (85%). Children grafted for fulminant hepatitis have a worse prognosis, with survival rates of about 60 per cent.

Pre-transplant assessment/counselling

This involves assessment of the following parameters.

(a) Liver disease
    Liver function tests
    Doppler ultrasonography
    Esophago-gastro-duodenoscopy
    Liver biopsy (selected cases)
    Infection/cancer markers
(b) Nutritional status
(c) Cardiac and respiratory function
(d) Surgical and anesthetic risks
(e) Social, psychological and economic issues
(f) Patient and family counselling.

The transplant

The type of OLT, i.e. cadaveric or live related (LROLT) depends on patient preference, policy of the transplant program, local legislation, and urgency for transplant. The recipient receives either a whole liver of appropriate size or a reduced size graft. The advantages of LROLT are many. It almost guarantees an organ for each child with a suitable parent donor. The donor will not have undergone trauma or shock, and the implanted liver shows better function. We can choose the date of the operation, so that the patient receives it in a good condition. Knowing the operation dates removes the uncertainty of the conventional transplant and allows the family to plan. The risk, however, with strict donor selection is small. There is always the risk that the newly donated liver, or even the recipient may be lost. There may be more emotion attached to complications of LROLT. The blood group must be the same or compatible to that of the patient own group.

The development of orthotopic auxiliary liver transplantation is of particular relevance to patients with acute liver failure or inherited metabolic disorders. In this technique, the left lateral segments of the patient's liver are replaced with the same segments from a donor liver. Although there are some surgical complications, this method has the advantage that the native liver is retained and can function in the event of graft failure.

The operation usually lasts for 4–8 hours. The blood loss during the operation is on an average 4 liters. The complexity of the operation is increased with previous abdominal surgery, portal vein thrombosis, recurrent spontaneous bacterial peritonitis, and severe portal hypertension. The patient is usually ventilated post-operatively for 24–48 hours. The patient is weaned from the ventilator in 72 hours and allowed to take oral feeds, if everything goes on smoothly. The average hospital stay is 2–3 weeks. Initial immunosuppression is with cyclosporin, steroids and azathioprine, however, cyclosporin is required for life-long.

Post-transplant-care

Post-operatively the patient is returned to the intensive care unit (ICU), intubated and ventilated with central venous access. An arterial line is placed for monitoring blood pressure and blood gas analysis. Meticulous hygiene is essential in the management of catheters and intravenous lines. If the new graft is functioning well, the early post-operative recovery is fast, however, early impaired graft function may rapidly result in a hemodynamically unstable patient with severe metabolic disturbances and multi-organ failure.

Good early graft function can be predicted by hemodynamic stability of the patient, early bile production, progressive improvement in base excess, arterial pH, falling serum lactate, and INR with a normal blood glucose. Serum aspartate transaminase (AST) levels on day one should be less than 1000 IU/L, with a reduction of the AST levels by 50% daily until normal values are reached.

The blood pressure should be well maintained and inotropes may be required in some patients with significant vasodilatation. Subcutaneous heparin (50 IU/kg bid) and venesection to maintain a hemoglobin of 10–12 g/dl and hematocrit below 35% may reduce the risk of hepatic artery thrombosis. Doppler ultrasound examination of the hepatic vasculature is carried out on the first post-operative day and daily until liver function is satisfactory. A chest X-ray is performed on return to ICU and on subsequent days if the ICU stay is prolonged to exclude fluid overload, pleural effusion, atelectasis, or pulmonary infiltrates.

Nutritional support has a significant effect on morbidity and mortality. It is usual to provide a high protein (3 g/kg) and high carbohydrate intake using glucose polymers. The fat content of the feed should be balanced to provide 50 per cent medium chain triglyceride and 50 per cent long-chain triglyceride to reduce steatorrhoea and to prevent essential fatty acid deficiency. It is essential to make sure before the transplantation that the routine immunizations are complete in children. If necessary, advance immunization dates for MMR and vaccinate against varicella for a child of > 2 years.

Outcome after liver transplant and result

Early complications following OLT include primary non-function, vascular thrombosis, sepsis, biliary leak/obstruction, and acute rejection. Late complications include biliary stricture, chronic rejection, infections, and occasionally malignancy. Recurrence of primary disease may be a problem in patients with hepatic tumors and hepatitis C infection. Hepatitis B recurrence is rare after transplantation for fulminant liver failure. In those with positive hepatitis B status and chronic liver disease, recurrence can be reduced from 70% to 10–15% with the peri- and post-operative use of combination of hepatitis B immunoglobulin and lamivudine.

Liver transplantation remains a high risk procedure with a mortality of 10–20% with high perioperative morbidity. The survival rates have been reported to be about 85% at one year with a five year survival rate of about 80%.

SPECIAL ISSUES RELATED TO LIVER TRANSPLANT

Metabolic disorders in children

Inherited metabolic disorders

This group of disorders includes those diseases in which (a) there is a specific hepatic enzyme deficiency that leads to acute or chronic liver failure and the potential development of hepatic cancer (antitrypsin deficiency, tyrosinemia type I, or glycogen storage disease type IV), (b) the precise metabolic defect is unknown but the main clinical features are hepatic (Wilson's disease, Byler's disease, neonatal hemochromatosis), and (c) the hepatic enzyme deficiency leads to acquired liver disease (factor VIII and IX deficiency and subsequent chronic viral hepatitis).

Inherited metabolic disorders leading to extrahepatic disease

These inherited diseases include Crigler-Najjar type I, primary oxalosis, familial hypercholesterolaemia, the urea cycle defects and propionic acidaemia. Successful management of this condition requires liver transplantation before the development of renal failure. If renal failure is advanced, a combined liver and kidney transplant is mandatory. As the metabolic defect is associated with a relative deficiency of low density lipoprotein receptors on the hepatocytes, liver transplantation successfully corrects the abnormal cholesterol metabolism. It is for this reason that auxiliary heterotopic liver transplantation, in which the segmental liver graft is placed close to the native liver, has been considered.

More recently, technical advances have encouraged the development of orthotopic auxiliary liver transplantation in which the left lateral segments of the patient's liver are replaced with the same segments from a donor liver. Recent reports of successful auxiliary liver transplantation for Criglar-Najjar type I disease are encouraging despite the development of both acute and chronic rejection in the auxiliary liver. Although, this form of transplantation would seem most appropriate for those disorders in which the liver is normal (Criglar-Najjar type I, urea cycle defects, familial hypercholesterolemia), it may not be appropriate treatment for all metabolic disorders.

Likewise, it is not yet clear whether adequate liver tissue would be available from segmental auxiliary transplant to correct the enzyme defects in urea cycle or replace the abnormal low density lipoprotein receptors in familial hypercholesterolaemia.

Correction of the metabolic defect

In alpha-1 antitrypsin deficiency, Byler's disease, Wilson's disease, and neonatal hemochromatosis, there is both phenotypic and functional cure. In tyrosinaemia type I, liver transplantation corrects the hepatic enzyme deficiency and cures the liver failure, although the kidney continues to produce toxic metabolites. In Criglar-Najjar type I, and the urea cycle defects, the metabolic defect is completely corrected. In primary oxalosis, although the metabolic defect is corrected, the perioperative course is determined by the extent of preoperative oxalate deposition and renal function particularly after a combined liver/kidney transplant.

Orthotopic liver transplantation (OLT) is a therapeutic option that should be considered at an early stage in any child with a life-threatening liver disease. The majority of recipients can expect to enjoy a good quality of life with normal growth and development. Liver transplantation should be performed before growth is retarded by liver disease. The results are better, however, in children transplanted after 1 year of age or when weighing more than 10 kg. The procedure is best done electively rather as an emergency. The aim of liver transplantation in this clinical situation is to cure the inherited metabolic defect both phenotypically and functionally. It is indicated in children with inborn errors of metabolism due to a primary hepatic enzyme deficiency that leads to either liver disease and/or hepatic cancer, or severe extrahepatic disease when complete resolution of the disease may be anticipated after transplantation.

Cure of these metabolic diseases may require liver transplantation alone, or in combination with kidney, heart, or bone marrow transplantation. The current indications for transplantation when the liver is structurally normal but the patient is at risk from irreparable damage to vital tissues (for example, the brain, heart, or kidneys), caused by a hepatic based defect in metabolism, has been the subject of recent reviews. In two rapidly developing fields close liaison between hepatologists and specialists in metabolic disorders is mandatory. OLT has not been effective in erythropoietic protoporphyria and Niemann-Pick disease type II.

Liver transplant for hepatitis B induced cirrhosis

Before the advent of hepatitis B immunoglobulin (HBIg) and lamivudine, hepatitis B infection used to be an absolute contraindication for liver transplant. With the availability of HBIg and lamivudine, even patients with HBV-DNA positive status can be taken up for a liver transplant.[5-10] If time permits, pre-transplant treatment with lamivudine is recommended to achieve HBV-DNA to negative status.[5] During transplant, 10,000 mIU/ml of HBIg is given during the anhepatic phase followed by a similar dosing daily for 1 week, then weekly for one month, and subsequently every month. The further dosing is based on monitoring the anti-HBs levels, which is maintained at 500 mIU/ml. Usually lamivudine therapy is combined with the HBIg therapy.[6,7] The cost implications for an Indian patient is to the tune of Rs. 2.5 million for the first year alone. There are several cost saving modifications of this regimen, but the HBV recurrence rates are higher with such regimens. Patients with fulminant hepatitis have very low recurrence rates and can be treated with lower dose HBIg therapy in the post-transplant period. Any sudden deterioration in hepatic reserve should arouse the suspicion of either flare up of hepatitis or a new co-infection.

Liver transplant for HCC

Active surveillance for HCC is indicated for all patients listed for liver transplantation, especially for those with hepatitis-induced cirrhosis.[11] Our approach is to do alfa-fetoprotein (AFP) estimation every 3 months and ultrasound examination every 6 months. CT scan and T2 weighted imaging with MRI can help to differentiate a regenerating nodule from HCC.[8] Fine needle aspiration cytology (FNAC) of lesions is considered only when the diagnosis is likely to influence the decision to transplant especially if the lesion in the liver is not accompanied by a significant elevation of serum AFP. Occasionally a biopsy may be preferable to FNAC to differentiate between HCC and cholangiocarcinoma or a metastatic deposit. Research tools such as Aldolase mRNA expression in liver tissue may indicate early onset HCC.[12]

Presence of incidental small HCC (<2 cm) in the diseased liver has no impact on post-transplant survival. Patients with HCC which are unifocal measuring 2–5 cm, with no extra-hepatic spread or portal vein invasion are now being transplanted with pre-transplant adjuvant chemotherapy. The 1, 3, and 5 years survival are 77%, 68% and 68% respectively. Liver transplantation for multicenteric HCC or tumors >5 cm with adjuvant chemotherapy are proving to be promising with reasonable survival figures of 51%, 25% and 25% at 1, 3, and 5 years respectively.[13-15] Stage 4a tumors are also being treated with chemoembolization followed by transplantation in a few centers with appreciable results.[16] Stage 4b HCC remains an absolute contraindication for OLT.

Quality of life after liver transplantation

The change in the quality of life of a patient after a transplant is truly amazing. Most people resume their normal activities including work within three months of the transplant. Apart from the fact that they need lifelong immunosuppressive medication (as is the case with any organ transplant) to prevent rejection of their new liver, they can expect a life which is normal in all respects including longevity, reproductive function, and physical activity.

At present, what has been documented is that patients with growth failure secondary to liver disease will resume their growth. There appears to be an improvement in the general condition and health. A small study indicates that some children show delayed development for upto one year after the transplant. Overall, it appears that liver transplantation in children improves the quality of life, however, this needs to be studied in greater detail.

Is liver transplantation affordable?

Liver transplantation entails not only the initial expenditure of the procedure, but also the lifelong commitment of a recurring expenditure of around Rs. 10,000 per month on immunosuppression. This factor must always be considered when the suitability of a potential transplant candidate is determined. Although, it is not feasible to extend this treatment to all the patients due to economic reasons, there are an appreciable number of patients who could benefit from it. As the procedure becomes established, it is likely that a number of patients from lower socioeconomic background will also be transplanted as charities and funds are set up to support such people.

LIVER TRANSPLANT CENTERS IN ASIA

Seol in South Korea, Kyoto and Tokyo in Japan, Taiwan, and Hong Kong have large live donor liver transplant programs, while Singapore, Bangkok, and Saudi Arabia have largely cadaver liver transplant programs. The cost of liver transplantation in any of the above programs would be more than Rs. 6 million. For the live donor programs it will be mandatory to take a suitable relative to donate. The cadaver transplant centers do not guarantee any time frame for cadaver organ availability due to low donation rates and large waiting list of local population in need of such a service.

CURRENT STATUS IN INDIA AND FUTURE OUTLOOK

Several centers have attempted liver transplantation in India with little success until

November 1998, when the first Indian aged 45 years received a successful cadaver graft at Indraprastha Apollo Hospital, New Delhi. Within a week of this procedure the first child aged 18 months suffering from biliary atresia underwent a successful living donor liver transplant from his father at the same hospital. Both these recipients are live and well 24 months after the transplant. Apollo Hospital has carried out over 15 liver transplants, eight cadaver and seven live related transplants since then. Among these 8 patients are alive and well after their transplant. Among the living related group, three were pediatric recipients and two were adult right lobe recipients. The two adult live donor right lobe recipient are live and well 1 year and 6 months respectively after transplant. Three among the eight survivors experienced rejection which was treated successfully. The failures are attributed mainly to the marginal grafts, advanced disease state and sepsis, and occasionally to GI hemorrhage and portal vein thrombosis.

The centers apart from Apollo Hospital, New Delhi, which have reported successful liver transplants include: Apollo Hospital, Chennai (1 cadaveric OLT-current status not known), St. Johns Hospital, Bangalore (one survivor out of two pediatric LROLT), Jaslok Hospital, Mumbai (1-Paediatric OLT), and CMC Hospital, Vellore (1 out of two alive after cadaveric OLT). The other hospitals which have attempted liver transplants in India include AIIMS, New Delhi; SGPGI, Lucknow; SRMC Hospital, Chennai; and Sir Gangaram Hospital, Delhi.

Major thrust to liver transplantation will occur only if both the patient and physician confidence in the procedure increases which is a catch-22 situation for most start-up programs. Another major bottleneck seems to be non-availability of cadaver organs of good quality (exemplified by the fact that only one of the five cadaver organs transplanted at our center had pristine histology). In spite of the waiting list for liver transplant, we at Indraprastha Apollo Hospital are helpless due to organ shortage. In order to overcome this stalemate, we are promoting live donor liver transplantation for adult recipients. Eight other centers in the world carrying out this procedure have published very encouraging results. We see this as the future of liver transplantation in India for the next decade.

REFERENCES

1. Marcos A. Right lobe living donor liver transplantation: a review. *Liver Transpl* 2000;6:3-20.
2. Marcos A, Fisher RA, Ham JM, Shiffman ML, Sanyal AJ, Luketic VA, Sterling RK, et al. Right lobe living donor liver transplantation. *Transplantation* 1999;68:798-803.
3. Panwels A, Mostefa-Kara N, Florent C, Lang VG. Emergency liver transplantation for acute liver failure: evaluation of London and Clichy criteria. *J Hepatol* 1993;17:124-7.
4. Schafer D, Shaw B. Fulminant hepatic failure and orthotopic liver transplantation. *Semin Liver Dis* 1989;9:189-94.
5. Dodson SF, Bonham CA, Geller DA, Cacciarelli TV, Rakela J, Fung JJ. Prevention of de novo hepatitis B infection in recipients of hepatic allografts from anti-HBc positive donors. *Transplantation* 199;68:1058-61.
6. Bzowej NH, Wright TL. Viral hepatitis and liver transplantation. *J Gastroenterol Hepatol* 1999;14(suppl):S53-60.

7. Markowitz JS, Martin P, Conrad AJ, Markmann JF, Seu P, Yersiz H, Goss JA, et al. Prophylaxis against hepatitis B recurrence following liver transplantation using combination lamivudine and hepatitis B immune globulin. *Hepatology* 1998;28:585-9.
8. Caholin C, Olausson M, Friman S. Orthotopic liver transplantation in patients with hepatitis B-related liver disease. *Transplant Proc* 2001;33:2465-6.
9. Chu CJ, Fontana RJ, Moore C, Armstrong DR, Punch JD, Su GL, Lok AS, et al. Outcome of liver transplantation for hepatitis B: report of a single center's experience. *Liver Transpl* 2001;7:724-31.
10. Teo EK, Han SH. Terrault N, Luketic V, Keeffe EB, Lok AS. Liver transplantation in patients with hepatitis B virus infection: outcome in Asian versus white patients. *Hepatology* 2001;34:126-32.
11. Gambarin-Gelwan M, Wolf DC, Shapiro R, Schwartz ME, Min AD, et al. Sensitivity of commonly available tests in detecting hepatocellular carcinoma in cirrhotic patients undergoing liver transplantation. *Am J Gastroenterol* 2000;95:1535-8.
12. Castaldo G, Calcagno G, Sibillo R, Cuomo R, Nardone G, Castellano L, Del Vecchio Blanco C, et al. Quantitative analysis of Aldolase mRNA in liver discriminates between HCC and cirrhosis. *Clin Chem* 2000;46:901-6.
13. Bismuth H, Majno PE, Adam R. Liver transplantation for hepatocellular carcinoma. *Semin Liver Dis* 1999;19:311-22.
14. Yokoyama I, Todo S, Iwatsuki S, Starzl TE. Liver transplantation in treatment of primary liver cancer. *Hepatogastroenterology* 1990;37:188-93.
15. Stone MJ, Klintmalm GB, Polter D, Husberg BS, Mennel RG, Ramsay MA, Flemens ER, et al. Neoadjuvant chemotherapy and liver transplantation for HCC: A pilot study in 20 patients. *Gastroenterology* 1993;104:196-202.
16. Harnois DM, Steers J, Andrews JC, Rubin JC, Pitot HC, Burgart L, Weisner RH, et al. Preoperative hepatic artery chemoembolization followed by orthotopic liver transplantation for hepatocellular carcinoma. *Liver Transpl Surg* 1999;5:192-9.

Section IV
Prevention of hepatitis B virus infection in India

27

Universal guidelines for health care workers in prevention of hepatitis B

Archana Thakur

Health care personnel are frequently exposed to the infectious agents in the course of their duties through occupational exposure to blood and blood contaminated objects.[1] Hepatitis B, C, and HIV pose a great threat and are of special concern. However, the infectivity of HBV is 100 times more than that of HIV.[2]

Health care workers (HCW) have a prevalence rate of HBV infection that is three- to five-fold higher than that of the general population. In the USA, 4% of the HCW are chronically infected with HBV as compared to 0.3 % of the general population.[3] The risk of transmission of HBV, HCV, and HIV[4] is shown in Table 1.

Table 1. Risk of transmission of blood-borne viruses to health care workers

Human immunodeficiency virus (HIV)	
Percutaneous exposure	0.4%
Mucocutaneous exposure	0.05%
Hepatitis B virus (HBV)	
Percutaneous exposure	9–30%
Hepatitis C virus (HCV)	
Percutaneous exposure	3–10%

HBV INFECTION IN HCW

The risk of acquiring HBV infection in HCW depends on the following factors.[3-7]

(a) Degree of exposure to blood, body fluids, or sharps.[3]
(b) The presence and titre of virus in blood and various body fluids. Risk of transmission is 30% after needle stick exposure from HBeAg positive source and < 6% from HBeAg negative source.[5]

(c) Duration of employment[6] in an occupational category with frequent blood / needle exposure (two-fold higher prevalence in physicians, surgeons, laboratory technicians, blood bank workers, anaesthetists, etc. than in other HCW).
(d) Underlying prevalence of HBV infection in patient population. Acute and chronic infection in many admitted patients is unrecognized.[7]
(e) Risk of infection in HCW is more in urban hospitals compared with rural hospitals and in tertiary care hospitals compared with primary care hospital as patients coming to these hospitals are at a higher risk for hepatitis B (e.g. drug users).[7]

Routes of transmission

Possible pathogen transmission pathway in health care setting is from patient to the HCW, from patient to patient, or from HCW to patient. Transmission from patient to HCW is through direct contact of pierced skin or mucocutaneous membrane of HCW with blood, blood products, excretions, secretions, and tissues of infected patients.[2] Transmission by saliva occurs only after bite and not by oral inoculation.

HBV is stable on environmental surfaces and retains its infectivity in dried blood for at least one week. Therefore, another route of transmission is indirect person to person through contamination of environmental surfaces.[8] This is an important route of transmission in hemodialysis centers. The various procedures and the risk they carry of transmission of blood-borne agents[4] are given in Table 2.

GUIDELINES FOR PREVENTION OF INFECTION

These guidelines[9-14] describe precautions which health care personnel should take to avoid bringing their skin and mucous membranes in direct contact with blood, blood products, excretions, secretions, and tissues of patients potentially infected with infectious diseases.

Universal precautions

Precautions are the most effective and efficient method of preventing hepatitis B and other infections and are based on the assumption that all blood and body fluids are potentially infectious regardless of whether they are from any patient or HCW. The principles of universal precautions are the use of protective barriers, prevention of accidents, and proper use of disinfection and sterilization techniques.

Use of protective barriers

Appropriate barriers should be worn where exposure to blood and other potentially infectious fluid is anticipated. The type of protection selected depends on the type of exposure[4] as shown in Table 3.

Table 2. Procedures carrying potential risk of HBV, HIV, and other blood-borne agents

Procedure	Person at risk	Mode of infection
Collection of blood sample	Patient	• Contaminated needle • Contaminated hands or gloves of HCW
	Health care worker	• Skin puncture by needle or broken specimen container • Contamination of hands by blood
Transfer of specimens (within laboratory)	Laboratory personnel	• Contaminated exterior of specimen container
	Transport worker	• Broken container
HIV serology and virology	Laboratory personnel	• Skin puncture or contamination of skin or mucous membrane • Spill or splash of specimen • Broken specimen container • Perforated gloves
Cleaning and maintenance	Laboratory personnel Support staff	• Skin puncture or skin contamination • Splash or spills • Contaminated work surfaces
Waste disposal	Laboratory personnel Support staff Transport worker Public	• Contact with contaminated waste • Puncture wounds
Shipment of specimens (to other centers)	Transport worker Postal worker Public	• Broken or leaking specimen containers and packages

Table 3. Selection of protective barriers

Type of exposure	Protective barriers	Examples
Low risk Contact skin, no visible blood	• Gloves helpful but not essential	Injections, minor wound dressing
Medium risk Probable contact with blood, splashing unlikely	• Gloves • Gowns and apron may be necessary	Vaginal examination, insertion or removal of I/V cannulae, handling of laboratory specimens, large open wounds dressing, venipuncture, spills of blood, etc.
High-risk Probable contact with blood, splashing, uncontrolled bleeding	• Gloves • Waterproof gown or apron • Eyewear • Mask	Major surgical procedures particularly in orthopedic and oral surgery; vaginal delivery

(a) Use of double gloves is not recommended because this practice is no more protective than use of one glove. It may rather lead to more accidents due to clumsiness.
(b) Latex or vinyl gloves should be used for direct contact with blood or infective body fluids. Heavy duty rubber till elbows should be used by cleaners.
(c) Plastic aprons or waterproof gowns to be worn underneath sterile gown where splash of blood is expected during surgery/procedures.
(d) Proper use of eyewears as ordinary spectacles may not provide adequate protection in some situations.
(e) Any reusable protective barrier contaminated with blood or body fluids should be cleaned by washing thoroughly after use and sterilized as indicated.

Prevention of accidents through safe handling and disposal of sharps

The greatest risk of transmission of blood-borne pathogens in health care setting is by percutaneous exposure through needles and other sharps.[15] They commonly occur when needles are recapped, cleaned, disposed off, or inappropriately discarded. The following precautions should be followed to avoid needle stick injuries.

Rational injection practice Reducing unnecessary injections and limiting blood transfusions is essential for decreasing infections through blood-borne route. Injections should be used when absolutely indicated. Injectable antibiotics should be avoided if an equally effective preparation is available for oral administration or if one injection can be given instead of multiple doses.[16] Adequate number of disposable syringes and needles must be arranged. Boiling and autoclaving of reusable syringes and needles must be avoided.

Instructions[17] for handling syringes and needles Following are the do's and dont's for handling syringes and needles.

Do's	*Don'ts*
Pass syringes and needles in a tray preferably cut it with needle cutters	Never pass syringes and needles directly to the next person
Put needles and syringes in 1% hypochlorite solution if needle cutter is not available	Do not bend or break used needles with hands
Remove cap of needle near the site of use	Never test the fineness of the needle tip before use with bare or gloved hand
Pick-up open needle from tray/drum with forceps	Never pick-up open needle by hand
Destroy syringes by burning their tips if cutters are not available	Never dispose it off by breaking it with hammer/stone.

Recapping needles Recapping of needles is discouraged. Recapping a needle with two hands increases the likelihood of sustaining a sharp injury. If recapping is unavoidable, following steps may be undertaken: (a) place the needle cap on a hard flat surface, (b) with one hand hold the syringe and use needle to scoop up the cap, and (c) when the cap covers the tip of the needle, use the other hand to place cap firmly on the needle hub.

Good practices for safe handling and disposal of sharps can be achieved by the following steps:

(a) Always dispose of your own sharps.
(b) Never pass used sharps directly from one person to another.
(c) During exposure-prone procedure, the risk of injury should be minimized by ensuring that the operator has the best possible visibility, e.g. by positioning the patient, adjusting good light source, and controlling bleeding.
(d) Protect fingers from injury by using forceps instead of fingers for guiding suturing.
(e) Never recap, bend or break disposable needles.
(f) Directly after use place needles, syringes and sharps in a puncture resistant container and disinfect before disposal.
(g) Locate sharps disposal containers close to the point of use, e.g., in patient's room, on the medicine trolley, and in treatment room, etc.
(h) Never place used sharps in other waste containers.
(i) Keep all sharps and sharp disposal containers out of the reach of children.
(j) Sharps containers are often overfilled with sharps sticking out from the top which increases the risk of accidents. So replace the sharps container when it is three-quarters full.
(k) Wear heavy duty gloves and take care when transporting sharps containers.

Proper use of disinfection and sterilization techniques

Hepatitis B and other blood-borne infections can be transmitted via needles, syringes, and other equipments contaminated with body fluids. These items should be cleaned and sterilized or disinfected before use. The method depends on the procedures for which they are used and associated level of risk of transmission (Table 4).

Table 4. Selecting the methods of decontamination

Level	Items	Decontamination method
High-risk	Instruments which penetrate the skin and the body	Sterilization Single use of a disposable item
Moderate risk	Instruments which come in contact with mucous membrane or non-intact skin	Sterilization Boiling Chemical disinfection
Low-risk	Equipments which come in contact with intact skin	Thorough washing

Sterilization : This can be achieved by the following two methods.

(a) All forms of sterilization destroy HIV, HBV and HCV. Steam under pressure (autoclave) is the most effective method. If sterilization by autoclaving is not possible then disinfection by boiling for 20 minutes is acceptable,[18] and

(b) Dry heat sterilization should be used for thermostable material which cannot be sterilized by steam such as oils, powders and glassware.

Disinfection : Two methods[18, 19] are used commonly. (a) Boiling of equipments which have already been cleaned for 20 minutes and (b) chemical disinfection for heat sensitive equipments. Most disinfectants are effective against limited range of microorganisms. There are certain rules which should be followed up while using disinfectants:[17] (a) Follow the manufacturer's instructions; (b) check the expiry date of the solution; (c) ensure that the optimum dilution is used; (d) chemical disinfectants are unstable and chemical breakdown can occur so it should be changed at prescribed intervals; (e) do not refill disinfectant containers without sterilizing the containers between each use, topping up is not allowed; (f) always wash and clean articles before disinfection, these should be dismantled and fully immersed in the disinfectant; (g) care must be taken to rinse off the disinfected items with sterile water as the residual disinfectant left may be corrosive and irritant; and (h) open containers of disinfectant should not be tolerated as there is a serious risk of contamination with multiple antibiotic resistant bacteria such as *Pseudomonas* and spores.

The disinfectants used commonly in health care facilities include the following.[17]

(a) 1% Bleach or sodium hypochlorite (distributed throughout the hospital in plastic recyclable bottles for disinfection of materials contaminated with blood and body fluids).
(b) Bleaching powder (for toilets, bathrooms, etc.).
(c) Methylated spirit –70% (for disinfecting surfaces on which bleach cannot be used, e.g. smooth metal surfaces, table tops, etc.).
(d) Alcoholic handwash (70% methyl alcohol to which 1% glycerin is added, available in all clinical settings).
(e) Glutaraldehyde 2% (disinfection of surfaces and instruments that are destroyed by bleach).
(f) Detergent with enzyme (for cleaning endoscopes, theatre instruments and obstetric instruments before disinfection).
(g) Savlon 1% (for cheatle forceps – solution to be changed daily).

HIGH-RISK PROCEDURES

Certain activities/techniques/procedures can be said to be of high-risk.

Surgical procedures

All surgical procedures are invasive involving a break in the continuity of the skin and/or mucus membrane. There is a lot of handling of tissues, organs, and body fluids during these procedures.[20-23] Microorganisms get directly inoculated into the body if there is a lapse in aseptic precautions. Therefore, it is absolutely essential that all the instruments, equipments, and material used during surgery are sterile.

During surgery, different surfaces (table tops, floors, walls, lights, etc.), materials (sponges, swabs), linen (mask, gown, caps) equipments, gloves, etc. get contaminated with blood and body fluids. They must be disinfected before disposal or sterilization. Spill on the floor or any surface of an infected or potentially infected material should be covered with an absorbent material. A disinfectant fluid (0.5% sodium hypochlorite) should be poured around contaminated area and then over the absorbent material and left for more than 10 minutes before removal.[18] The surface then should be wiped with soap and water.

Dressing of wounds

Wounds can be surgical, accidental, due to purulent infection, or due to underlying disease like fistula and piles. They require dressing for proper healing and prevention of super infections. The dressing should be done in two separate areas, one should be for clean wound or clean contaminated wounds and other for contaminated and dirty wounds. Only sterile instruments and material (cotton, gauze, etc.) should be used for dressing. After dressing, all materials and instruments should be taken as contaminated with blood. Therefore, it should be disinfected before disposal and reusable instruments should be sterilized.

Endoscopic procedures

Most of the body cavities like rectum, intestine, oral cavity, lungs, vagina, etc. are colonized with commensals or pathogens. Instruments used for endoscopic examination (such as endoscopes, bronchoscopes, urethroscopes, cystoscopes, pharyngoscopes, laparoscopes, arthroscopes, etc.) get contaminated with blood or mucous membranes if they are not sterilized properly. Several infectious organisms can crossinfect the other patients or HCWs. Commonly transmitted infections through these equipments are HIV, HBV, HCV, HAV, HEV, *M. tuberculosis*, *E. coli*, *Salmonella*, *Staph. aureus*, *Pseudomonas*, *H. pylori*, fungi like *Candida* and *Trichosporon*, and parasites like *Amoeba*, *Giardia*,[20] etc. These equipments are best decontaminated with 2% glutraldehyde for 30 minutes followed by 3–4 times rinsing with sterile water.

Laboratory investigations

The clinical specimens are collected for different laboratory tests. Most of these specimens are highly infective and on occasions can cause life-threatening diseases like hepatitis and AIDS. Hence, great care must be taken in collection, transportation, processing, discarding, and disposal of these specimens. Following are the guidelines for collecting blood samples.

(a) Use gloves and take special care if there are cuts or scratches on the hands,
(b) take care to avoid contamination of hands and surrounding area with the blood,
(c) use disposable syringes and needles,
(d) use 70% ethanol or isopropyl alcohol swabs or sponges for cleaning the site of needle puncture,
(e) tourniquet must be removed before the needle is withdrawn,
(f) place dry cotton swab and flex the elbow to keep this in place till bleeding stops,
(g) place used needles and syringes in a puncture-resistant container containing disinfectant, and
(h) do not recap used needles.

Other specimens can be tissue, pus, body fluid (CSF, pleural and pericardial fluids, bronchial washings), urine, sputum, and swabs from mucous membrane and skin. All clinical specimens should be treated as potentially infectious and be transferred to the laboratory in spill-proof screw-capped bottles. Blood suspected to be from patients of hepatitis or AIDS should be transported in leak-proof polythene bags. Following are the standard biosafety regulations for handling and processing these specimens:

(a) Wear gloves when handling infectious material,
(b) discard gloves whenever they are thought to have become contaminated or perforated—wash hands and put on new gloves,
(c) do not touch eyes, nose or other exposed membrane with gloved hands,
(d) do not leave workplace or walk around the laboratory while wearing gloves,
(e) wear a laboratory gown or uniform when in the laboratory, remove this protective clothing before leaving the laboratory,
(f) when work with material that is potentially infected with HIV is in progress close the laboratory door and restrict access to the lab, the door should have "Bio-hazard, No admittance" sign.
(g) any blood or blood contaminated specimen can be positive for HIV or hepatitis virus investigation. Therefore it must not spill on the table tops and floor, etc. In case of such spilling the surface must be disinfected, and
(h) under no circumstances mouth pipetting should be permitted for carrying out any test.

These basic practices and procedures are designed to keep laboratory accidents to a minimum by: (a) prevention of puncture wounds, cuts and abrasions and protection of existing wounds, skin lesions, conjunctiva and mucosal surfaces, (b) application of simple protective devices designed to prevent contamination of the person and his clothing, (c) control of surface contamination by containment and disinfection procedures, and (d) safe disposal of contaminated waste.

REFERENCES

1. Shanks NJ, Al-Kalai D. Occupational risk of needlestick injuries among health care personnel in Saudi Arabia. *J Hosp Infect* 1995;29:221-6.
2. Culver J. Preventing transmission of blood-borne pathogens: a compelling argument for effective device-selection strategies. *Am J Infect Control* 1997;25:430-3.
3. Sharpio CN. Occupational risk of infection with Hepatitis B and Hepatitis C virus. *Surg Clin N Am* 1995;75:6:1047-53.
4. World Health Organization. *Guidelines for preventing HIV HBV and other infections in health care settings.* 1996: New Delhi, India.
5. Grady GF, Lee VA, Prince AM, Gitrick GL, Fawaz KA, Vyas GN, Levitt MD, et al. Hepatitis B immune globulin for accidental exposures among medical personnel: Final report of a multicenter controlled trial. *J Infect Dis* 1978;138:625-38.
6. Hadler SC, Margolis HS. *Hepatitis B immunization: vaccine types, efficacy, and indications for immunization.* In: Remington JS, Swartz MN. Eds. Current Topics in Infectious Diseases. Boston, Blackwell Scientific Publications, 1992; p. 282.
7. Harris JR, Finger RF, Kobayahsi JM, Hadler SC, Murphy BL, Berkelman RL, Bussell KE. The low-risk of hepatitis B in rural hospitals: Results of a seroepidemiologic survey. *JAMA* 1984; 252:3270-2.
8. Bond WW, Favero MS, Petersen NJ, Gravelle CR, Ebert JW, Maynard JE. Survival of hepatitis B virus after drying and storage for one week. *Lancet* 1981;1:550-1.
9. CDC. Recommendations for prevention of HIV transmission in health-care settings. *MMWR* 1987;36:(suppl 2S)S1-18.
10. CDC. Update: Universal precautions for prevention of transmission of human immunodeficiency virus, hepatitis B virus, and other blood-borne pathogens in health-care settings. *MMWR* 1988; 377:82-8.
11. CDC. *Hepatitis Surveillance Report* No. 48. Atlanta: U.S. Department of Health and Human Services, Public Health Service, 1982;2-3.
12. CDC. *CDC Guideline for Infection Control in Hospital Personnel,* Atlanta, Georgia; Public Health Service, 1983. 24 pages (GPO #6ARO31488305).
13. CDC. Guidelines for prevention of transmission of human immunodeficiency virus and hepatitis B virus to health-care and public-safety workers. *MMWR* 1989;38:(suppl):1-37.
14. Aarnio P, Laine T. Glove perforation rate in vascular surgery—a comparison between single and double gloving, *Vasa* 2001;30:122-4.
15. Nelsing C, Neilsen TC, Dronnum Hansen H, Neilsen JB. Incidence and risk factors of occupational blood exposure: a nationwide survey among Danish doctors. *Eur J Epidemiol* 1997;13:1-8.
16. O'Neill TM, Abbot AV, Radecki SE. Risks of needle-sticks and occupational exposures among residents and medical students. *Arch Intern Med* 1992;152:1451-6.
17. *Manual for Control of Hospital Associated Infections – Standard Operative procedures.* National AIDS Control Organization, Ministry of Health & Family Welfare Government of India.
18. Bond WW. *Sterilization, disinfection and antisepsis in the hospital.* In: Balows A, Hausler WJ, Eds. Manual of Clinical Microbiology. American Society of Microbiology, Washington DC, 1991. Fifth edition. pp.183-200.
19. Payan C, Co Hin J, Lemarie C, Ramaont C. Inactivation of hepatitis B virus in plasma bym hospital in-use chemical disinfectants assessed by a modified HepG2 cell culture. *J Hosp Infect* 2001;36:212-3.
20. Wenzal RW. *Epidemiology of hospital acquired infection.* In: Balows A, Hausler WJ, Eds. Manual of Clinical Microbiology. American Society of Microbiology, Washington DC, 1991. Fifth edition. pp. 147-51.

21. Gerberding JL, Little C, Tarkington T, Brown A. Schecter WP. Risk of exposure of surgical personnel to patients' blood during surgery at San Francisco General Hospital. *N Engl J Med* 1990;522:1788-93.
22. Johanet H, Antona B, Bouvet E. Risks of accidental exposure to blood in the operating room. Results of a multicenter prospective study. *Ann Chir* 1995;49:403-10.
23. CDC. *Guidelines for the prevention and control of nosocomial infections: guideline for hand washing and hospital environmental control.* Atlanta, Georgia: Public Health Services, 1985; 20 pages. (GPO# 544-436/24441).

28

Disposal of waste in hospitals with special reference to hepatitis patients

Anandita Mandal

Biomedical waste is defined as any solid, fluid or liquid waste including its container or any intermediate product, which is generated during the diagnosis, treatment or immunization of human beings or animals, in research pertaining thereto, or in the production or testing of biological and the animal waste from slaughter houses or any other similar establishments.[1]

SOURCE OF HEALTH CARE WASTE

It is ironical that hospitals which provide treatment to the ailing, can also create health hazards. Indiscriminate disposal of waste may be a major source of hospital-associated infections and spread of pollution and infections in the community at large. The quantum of average hospital waste at a glance has been highlighted (Table 1) in *Vatavaran Report* in Feb 1996.[2] About 85% of the waste is non-hazardous, around 10% is infectious, and around 5% is non-infectious but still hazardous. Waste is generated by all hospitals, nursing homes or clinics, and associated supportive services, viz. blood banks, central sterilised supply department (CSSD), laundry, laboratories, mortuary, etc. The quantum of waste varies from country to country and types of hospital services rendered. On an average, 1–5 kg per patient per day waste is generated. The basic approach to waste management is to reduce the quantity of waste at source as much as possible. Use of large number of disposables has added to the bulk of wastes to the modern day practice. Every hospital must develop suitable, practicable and specific guidelines for effective waste management.

RISK OF HOSPITAL WASTE

Health care workers

Three main categories of people are liable to be exposed to health hazards associated with medical waste. Patients on dialysis, with immunosuppression or with bleeding/clotting disorders are at special risk. Personnel handling blood soaked objects contaminated with body

Table 1. Average hospital waste at a glance

Biomedical waste		Recycleable waste		Biodegradable waste	
Items	%	Items	%	Items	%
O.T.	1.7	Card board boxes Thermocol		Left over food	
IV sets, uro bags, catheters	2.1	Paper boxes, loose toilet papers Medicine wrappers			
Blood vials	2.8	Medicine bottles Milk sachets		Horticulture waste	20
Sputum, blood clotted	4.7	Plastic bags Coffee cups Pepsi/coke glasses			
Syringes	6.6	Potato chips/wafers	32.8	Flowers wrappers	
Gloves	6.8	Pan masala sachets			
Glucose bottles	9.8	Razors Cigarette boxes and X-rays			
Cotton swabs, plaster, bandages	12.7	Mineral water plastic bottles Rags			
Total	47.2				52.8

Source: Hospital waste. A dangerous infusion by Dr. Iqbal Malik and Rajinder Singh, Ajay Kumar, Meenu Ratanai, Alka Tomar, Vijay Bhan, Dr. Jagjit Kaur, A Vatavarn report, February, 1996.

fluids are directly exposed to infections. Table 2 shows risk of transmission of blood-borne viruses to the health care workers.[3] Personnel working in a laboratory, laundry, incinerator or engaged in garbage disposal are equally at danger. Patients / personnel involved in home-care, e.g. dialysis are also at risk. All categories of hospital staff should be made aware of the

Table 2. Risk of transmission of blood-borne viruses to health care workers

Human immunodeficiency virus (HIV)	
Percutaneous exposure	0.05–0.4%
Mucocutaneous exposure	0.006–0.05%
Hepatitis B virus (HBV)	
Percutaneous exposure	9–30%
Hepatitis C virus (HCV)	
Percutaneous exposure	3–10%

potential risks of mishandling waste by regular training. Health care waste may be classified into 10 categories (Table 3)[4] and these are to be handled differently.

Table 3. Categories of biomedical waste

Category No.	Waste Category	Treatment and disposal
1	**Human anatomical waste** Human tissues, organs, body parts	Incineration[#] / deep burial[*]
2	**Animal waste** Animal tissues, organs, body parts carcasses, bleeding parts, fluid, blood and experimental animals used in research waste generated by veterinary hospitals colleges, discharge from hospitals, animal houses	Incineration[#] / deep burial[*]
3	**Microbiology and biotechnology waste** Wastes from laboratory cultures, stocks specimens of microorganisms live or attenuated vaccines, human and animal cell culture used in research and infectious agents from research and industrial laboratories, wastes from production of biologicals, toxins, dishes and devices used for transfer of cultures	Local autoclaving/ or microwaving incineration[#]
4	**Waste sharps** Needles, syringes, scalpels, blades, glass, etc. that may cause puncture and cuts; this includes both used and unused sharps	Disinfection/chemical treatment[**]/ autoclaving/ micro-waving and mutilation/shredding[##]
5	**Discarded medicines and cytotoxic drugs** Wastes comprising of outdated, contaminated medicines	Incineration[#] /destruction medicines and drugs disposal in secured landfills
6	**Soiled waste** Items contaminated with blood, and body fluids including cotton, dressings, soiled plaster casts, line, beddings, other material contaminated with blood	Incineration[#], autoclaving/ microwaving

Contd.

Contd.

Category No.	Waste Category	Treatment and disposal
7	**Solid waste** Wastes generated from disposable items other than the waste sharps such as tubing catheters, intravenous sets, etc.	Disinfection by chemical treatment** autoclaving/ microwaving and mutilation shredding##
8	**Liquid waste** Waste generated from laboratory and washing, cleaning, housekeeping and disinfecting activities	Disinfection by chemical treatment** and discharge into drains
9	**Incineration ash** Ash from incineration of any bio-medical waste	Disposal in municipal landfill
10	**Chemical waste** Chemicals used in production of biologicals, chemicals used in disinfection, as insecticides, etc.	Chemical treatment** and discharge into drains liquids and secured landfill for solids

\# There will be no chemical pretreatment before incineration. Chlorinated plastics shall not be incinerated.
\## Multilation/shredding must be such so as to prevent unauthorized reuse.
* Deep burial shall be an option available only in towns with population less than five lakhs and in rural areas.
** Chemicals treatment using at least 1% sodium hypochlorite solution or any other equivalent chemical reagent. It must be ensured that chemical treatment ensures disinfection.

Patients

A large number of patients are housed under one roof, some are already infected with virulent and resistant microbes. The patients are subjected to various diagnostic (invasive/ noninvasive) and therapeutic interventions. So there is every chance of cross-contamination from patient to personnel and vice versa. Through contaminated equipments, body fluids (blood, urine, salvia aspirates, etc.), many patients/ blood donors are chronically infected by HBV, HCV or AIDS. Screening of donor blood for HCV was not mandatory before 1990. HCV circulates in blood at a concentration of 10^2–10^7 particles/ml and prevalence around the world ranges from 0.4–2%, sero-prevalence in India being around 1.85%. HBV is the most widely prevalent blood-borne agent for acute and chronic hepatitis and is also associated with cirrhosis and HCC. All pathological and infectious waste must be segregated. Syringes, needles, IV transfusions, urobags, ascitic taps, dialysis items are potentially contaminated. All sharps should be packed in puncture-proof plastic or cardboard containers before further handling. High-risk infectious waste may initially be autoclaved, preferable at source to reduce risk. All syringes or needles are destroyed after use after disinfection in 1% sodium hypochlorite and collected separately. The color coding of bags for different categories of waste is very important. Table 4 shows the types of containers and bags to be used for segregation at

Table 4. Color coding and type or container for disposal of biomedical wastes

Color Coding	Type of container	Waste Category	Treatment options
Yellow	Plastic bag	1, 3, 6	Incineration/deep burial
Red	Disinfected container Plastic bag	3, 6, 7	Autoclaving/microwaving/ chemical treatment
Blue/White translucent	Plastic bag/puncture proof container	4, 7	Autoclaving/microwaving/ chemical treatment and destruction/shredding
Black	Plastic	5, 9, 10 10 (solid)	Disposal in secured landfill

Color coding of waste categories with multiple treatment options shall be selected depending on treatment option chosen.
Waste collection bags for waste types needing incineration shall not be made of chlorinated plastics.
Categories 8 and 10 (liquid) do not require containers/bags.
Category 3 if disinfected locally need not be put in containers/bags.

source. These bags/containers are for single use, moisture proof, labeled with appropriate biohazard symbol (Fig. 1). All plastic/ metal bins are lined with bags. Random audit of collected waste is done to check if segregation is proper or not. All containers are sealed before transport to the treatment site.

HANDLING OF WASTE

All waste is transported in trolleys and or handcarts, which should be cleaned regularly with detergents and should not be used for any others purpose. There are 5 broad medical waste treatment categories such as (a) mechanical, (b) thermal, (c) chemical, (d) irradiation, and (e) biological.

BIOHAZARD SYMBOL   CYTOTOXIC HAZARD SYMBOL

BIOHAZARD   CYTOTOXIC
HANDLE WITH CARE

Fig. 1. Label for biomedical waste containers/bags

Mechanical

The mechanical process includes compaction and shredding to reduce volume but is not considered an acceptable system unless coupled with prior decontamination. General waste like food remnants, paper, glass, plastic needs no special measures and can be dealt with as municipal waste (burning and dumping), but it has disadvantages of smoke and bad odor.

Thermal

The thermal treatment process includes mainly (a) incinerators, (b) autoclaves, (c) hydroclaving, and (d) microclaving.

Incineration

Incineration burns down waste into inert ash.[5] A standard incinerator must have 3 "Ts, temperature, time and turbulence." It must have a secondary gas phase combustion chamber and minimum stack height shall be 30 meters. Waste impurities, lack of O_2, low temperature in combustion chamber may cause formation of toxic fumes and gases. Chlorinated plastics (PVC) liberate dioxins and furans. Unburnt particulate matter can cause respiratory distress. Incinerators with combustion efficiency (CE) of 99.9% and temperature of $1050 \pm 50°C$ in the secondary combustion chamber with minimum of 3% O_2 in the stack gas should be installed at appropriate location to avoid nuisance to patient, staff and neighbourhood. Proper personal safety equipments (mask, boot, gloves) must be provided to persons handling incinerators.

Autoclaving

Autoclaving is a better way of treatment of infectious waste (except human body parts). Tuttnauer medical waste steam sterilizers have no toxic emissions, no toxic liquid discharge and treats over 97% of regulated medical waste. Since there is no reduction in volume, shredders are installed simultaneously. Shredded material can be disposed off safely.

Hydroclaving

The newer technologies include hydroclaving, microwaving and high temperature pyrolysis by plasma torch. Hydroclaves have also been found to be very useful for sharp, PVC, pathological waste. Waste can be disposed off by using microwaving technology. It applies steam (which is stored in a double wall/jacket) as an indirect heat source, allowing total dehydration of the waste at 130°C and 36 psi. Also the waste is internally agitated and fragmented to attain a high sterilization level of all components. In this technique, no pretreatment of waste is required. The volume of the waste is reduced upto 85% and the weight is reduced upto 60%. It is considered to be an environment responsible technology as no dioxins/furans are emitted. Waste can be disposed off by using microwaving technology.

Microwaving

This involves using a part of electromagnetic radiation spectrum between the frequency of 300 and 300,000 MHz. There is total destruction of all microbial activities due to thermal effects of radiation. The process involves pre-shredding the waste, injecting it with steam and heating for 25 minutes at 95°C in series of microwave units. Microwave heating occurs inside the waste material. The biological indicator employed is *Bacillus subtilis* spore strips (1×10^4 spores per ml). The technology is complex, requires automation, and skilled persons. It is not recommended for cytotoxic, hazardous, and radioactive wastes.

Plasma technology is based on high temperature (2000–3000°C or more) pyrolysis process using plasma torch. The plasma-fired chambers operate in an oxygen deficient mode and the off gases need to be combusted separately. Plasma is a sort of a meta-gas at a very high temperature. The advantage is transformation of all hydrocarbonated process into combustible gas without solid residues. The ashes from inorganic material are melted and vitrified into a glass like substance. There is substantial reduction in the volume of the non-hazardous residue. There is no release of harmful gas as in incinerator and does not require any segregation. It is an environment friendly technology.

The main problem in wards, OTs, diagnostic laboratories are contaminated sharps and items soiled with blood/blood products and soiled lines. All these items are to be kept soaked in disinfectant (sodium hydrochlorite) for 30 minutes. Syringes/needles are to be destroyed with the help of destroyers. All materials to be packed in puncture proof or leak-proof bags and sent for final disposal. Waste disposal protocols of general ward/ICU is same as for any other ward and must be done once in 24 hours. Efficient management of the solid waste in heath care set up needs selection of a proper technology, monitoring of segregation, monitoring of the treatment site, and final disposal of treated waste. For liquid waste, efficient treatment plants are to be installed in sewer lines.

REFERENCES

1. *Parivesh*, Newsletter, Central Pollution Control Board, ISSN: 0971-6025, 1998, Vol. V(iv).
2. Hospital Waste Management, An integrated approach by Sulabh International, Institute of Health and Hygiene, 1998; p. 9.
3. NACO Manual for control of hospital associated infections; standard operative procedures, Govt. of India, 1999.
4. Hospital Waste management (National guidelines, draft) prepared by GOI/WHO project Ind. EHH 001, 1998.
5. First workshop on Hospital Waste Management Source book, Ministry of Health and Family Welfare, Govt. of India and Maulana Azad Medical College, Govt. of NCT of Delhi.

29

Prevention of hepatitis B in the endoscopy units

Vineet Ahuja, Rakesh K Tandon

Flexible endoscopes have been used for a wide range of therapeutic and diagnostic procedures for more than three decades. Earlier, the usual procedure of reprocessing of the instruments consisted only of minimal flushing of the channels and wiping of the exterior surface, sometimes, with water only. However, progress has been made over the decades and now it is customary to state that endoscopes undergo high level disinfection. In practical terms, standard cleaning and disinfection processes do not decontaminate the endoscopes of all the bacterial spores. Endoscopes subjected to full decontamination regimes, which then have their channels filled with culture media and stored in sterile bags, may still grow bacteria after several days, if there are any irregularities at junctions such as cracking or splitting of the surface of internal channels. At present, the main aim of disinfection of endoscopes is to (a) prevent transmission of the pathogen from one patient to another and (b) prevent transmission of hospital environmental contaminants from the endoscope or accessories to the patients.[1]

Low infective dose has been reported for many human pathogenic viruses but in spite of that the viral infections can spread easily and relatively little is known about interrupting the spread of viral disease with biocides. Biocides used against viruses are variously termed as disinfectants, germicides, and virucides. The importance of biocidal inactivation of viruses was reemphasized only after the advent of human immunodeficiency virus and the recognition of the spread of viruses through blood, blood products, and tissues. Relatively few systematic studies have been performed on the potency of disinfectants against viruses.

The virucidal property of a disinfecting agent often depends upon (a) nature of the virus, e.g. morphology, size, etc. (b) parameters inherent to the disinfectant, and (c) the manner in which a viral particle is exposed to the disinfectant, e.g. presence or absence of the organic matter. The factors influencing the interaction between the disinfectant and the virus have been listed in Table 1.

Table 1. Factors that influence disinfectant–virus interaction

Disinfectant factors
    Chemical composition
    Concentration
    Mode of action
    Time
    Temperature
    pH
    Organic matter or other interfering substances
    Methods of exposing virus to disinfectant
Virus factors
    Concentration of virions in reaction mixture
    Degree of aggregation
    Enveloped or non-enveloped
    Lipid affinity
    pH stability
    Size
Sensitivity of detection methods determines reliability of results

DISINFECTION PRACTICES IN INDIA

A survey conducted in 1990 obtained responses from 32 of 60 endoscopy centers. Mechanical cleaning of the endoscope with some sort of detergent followed by a 10 minute exposure to 2% glutaraldehyde was considered adequate. Using these criteria, 12 (37.5%) centers performed adequate disinfection at the beginning of the endoscopy session but only 4 (12.5%) centers did so in between cases. The remaining 20 centers (62.5%) either did not use any disinfection procedure or used inadequate disinfection practices. Four centers claimed to have followed up their patients for 2 weeks to 6 months during a follow up period of 1–3 months, but none noticed any case of endoscopically acquired symptomatic hepatitis B virus (HBV) infection.[2] A questionnaire sent to 435 endoscopy centers in India revealed that only 2 (1.5%) centers reported occurrence of infections following upper gastrointestinal endoscopic examinations. Only 8 (18%) of the 44 centers performing endoscopic retrograde cholangiopancreatography (ERCP) reported infections, primarily cholangitis in patients with obstructive jaundice.[3]

Problems with HBV

Hepatitis B virus cannot be grown in tissue culture. Hence strategies to verify disinfection have been derived retrospectively by (i) studies involving human volunteers, (ii) instances where blood products treated chemically or with heat resulted in infection of recipients, and (iii) experimental evidence to determine HBV inactivation by inoculation of chimpanzees with the treated material. Moreover, detection of HBsAg on environmental surfaces does not indicate the simultaneous presence of viable HBV. However, it does serve as an indicator of contamination with potentially infective material.

Magnitude of HBV transmission by endoscopes

Hepatitis B infected patients present clinical manifestations of variable severity. They require a variety of diagnostic and therapeutic procedures. Medical personnel handling these patients are, therefore, exposed to the risk of acquiring hepatitis B infection from these patients. Also, subsequent patients examined with the same instrument, e.g., gastrointestinal (GI) endoscopes, may get cross-infected if the instruments are not properly sterilized or disinfected. The risk of transmission of HBV is, however, more through needle pricks or cuts than through endoscopic procedures. Whereas clinical infection follows in at least 1 in 20 exposed to hepatitis B positive blood by needle stick injury,[4,5] only a single case of HBV transmission by endoscope has been reported worldwide.[6] A number of clinical studies have evaluated the possible risk of HBV infection due to endoscopic procedures, but the risk of transmission was found to be negligible.[7,8]

A possible reason of the low rate of hepatitis B transmission may be the high susceptibility of this lipid containing virus to disinfectants (Fig. 1). Pooled human plasma with 10^8 hepatitis B

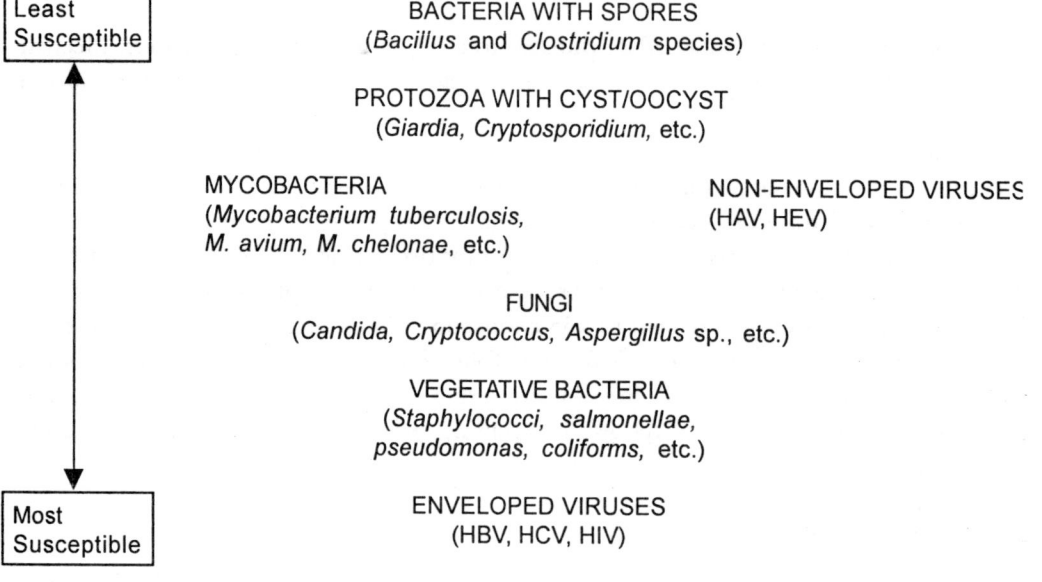

Fig. 1. Comparative susceptibility of microorganisms to biocides
(HAV – Hepatitis A virus, HBV – Hepatitis B virus, HCV – Hepatitis C virus, HEV – Hepatitis E virus, HIV – Human immunodeficiency virus)

virus infectious doses/ml failed to infect chimpanzees after exposure to 1% and 0.1% aqueous glutaraldehyde at 24°C for 5 minutes.[9] In similar studies, 80% ethyl alcohol at 11°C for two minutes inactivated HBV.[10] Nonetheless, viral particles can remain protected from chemical inactivation in coagulums of blood or body secretions underlining the need for scrupulous mechanical cleansing before disinfection. Hansen et al, while evaluating endoscopes used on AIDS patients, found that scrupulous mechanical cleansing alone removed the HIV.[11]

Interaction of glutaraldehyde with HBV

Glutaraldehyde is widely used for high level disinfection Thraenhart et al developed a system called morphological alteration and disintegration test (MADT) to measure the virucidal activity of disinfectants against the HBV.[12,13] The hypothesis of this test was that the physical destruction of intact HBV particles correlated with the loss of infectivity as evaluated in chimpanzees. It was observed that the morphology of Dane particles was severely altered by succinaldehyde. Disintegration of the outer membrane and asymmetric enlargement of the space between the outer membrane and the HBV core resulted in loss of characteristic substructure. It has been shown that 2% alkaline glutaraldehyde alters the HBV surface (HBsAg) and core (HBcAg) antigens.[14] Although the exact physical and chemical mechanism of action of glutaraldehyde has not been explained, it has been suggested that glutarldehyde probably reacts chemically with HBsAg and HBcAg sites containing lysine residues. Howard et al[15] showed that aldehyde based disinfectant reduced the activity of HBV-DNA polymerase and possibly denatured HBcAg. It was suggested that chemical antigens of markers (DNA polymerase, HBsAg) may precede gross morphological changes. In 1993, Prince et al[16] demonstrated that HBV in dry human plasma is also inactivated by any of the three proprietary germicide products used primarily for routine housekeeping purposes. Hepatitis B nucleic acid has been detected by polymerase chain reaction in improperly cleaned endoscopes, but the significance of this is unclear.[17] The possible sites of action of glutaraldehyde on HBV are shown in Table 2.

Table 2. Viral target sites in HBV for glutaraldehyde

Alteration of the viral envelope
Interaction with viral proteins
Alteration of viral markers
    HBsAg and HBcAg
    HBV-DNA
Structural alterations
Σ amino acid of lysine residues

Disinfection of endoscopes

There is no way to identify with certainty all the patients who are immunocompromised or who are a potential source of hepatitis B and other infections. This is especially true in emergency situations, like gastrointestinal bleeding or acute cholangitis when there is no time to do the relevant tests. It is, therefore, advisable to adhere to the use of the universal precautions and to ensure that every patient is examined with an endoscope which has been properly cleaned and disinfected. Ideally there is no need for HBV screening before endoscopic procedures, however, in a survey conducted in Asia Pacific region it was observed that 47.2% of the centres are carrying out such a screening.[18]

The endoscopes should ideally be sterilized, as they come in close contact with the mucosa and with the patient's blood all the time. This is more so when there is breach of the mucosa during procedures like biopsies, polypectomy, and papillotomy. It is, however, not possible to sterilize gastrointestinal endoscopes because of the following reasons and hence high level disinfection is being recommended for them.

(a) Flexible fiberoptic endoscopes (FFEs) are delicate instruments and will be destroyed by steam autoclaving or may be severely damaged by repeated or prolonged immersion in liquid chemical disinfectants.

(b) Most FFEs are also damaged to some extent by repeated ethylene gas cycles and this method of sterilization has the added disadvantage of removing the instruments from service for hours or even days because of the necessary process and aeration time.

(c) Another important reason why the FFEs cannot be properly cleaned and disinfected is that they have many crevices, channels, and valves all of which tend to harbour proteinacious material, a potential source of bacterial growth.

Many of the accessories used during the endoscopy, e.g. biopsy forceps, cannulae, and other endoscopic accessories can, however, tolerate sterilization procedure and should therefore be regularly sterilized before use.

A definite protocol of cleaning and disinfection must be followed strictly prior to each endoscopy. Following are the major steps of the process of reprocessing.

(a) *Mechanical cleaning of endoscope* This is the most important step and all efforts should be made to clean the outside and inside of the endoscope immediately after the procedure. Initial cleaning should be with water and then a mild detergent may be used but the final cleaning of the internal channels as well as outside must be with clean water. For cleaning the channels, the cleaning brush provided by the manufacturers should be passed at least three times both through the endoscope as well as its umbilical cord.

(b) *Disinfection* The present recommendations are to immerse the endoscope completely in 2% glutaraldehyde for a period of 10 minutes. It must be ensured that the disinfectant goes through the channels also. Such an exposure to the disinfectant is believed to be sufficient for preparing it for use in any patient about to undergo endoscopy irrespective of his/her immune status. Prolonged periods of disinfection can be done now by an automatic disinfecting machine. The advantages of these are: (a) Certain standard of disinfection is assured and (b) the vapours of the disinfectants remain within the closed system of the machine. The initial manual cleaning of the surface and channels of the FFE must however, be done scrupulously before placing the endoscope in the automatic disinfector.

(c) *Rinsing of endoscope* After disinfection has been done, it should be ensured that all the disinfectant is removed by repeated rinsing with quality drinking water. Even small amounts of disinfectant left in the endoscopic channels may injure the mucosa.

(d) *Drying* The outside as well as the inside (channels) of the endoscope should be dried by wiping and flushing air. In the final stage of drying, the endoscope should be connected to the light source and fitted with valves and distal hoods. The air/water channel is dried by simultaneously occluding the water bottle connector of the endoscope and depressing the air/water valve. Finally, the instruments should be connected to the suction machine and dried completely by depressing the suction valve several times. The endoscope is now ready for use or storage.

(e) *Storage* The endoscope should be hung on special racks in such a way that their channels dry up completely. They should not be stored coiled up in their original boxes.

Endoscopic accessories

All accessories which come in contact with blood, have been classified as "critical" items and hence should be used either as single use disposable or reused after sterilization. An accessory which has been used must not be used again except after thorough cleaning followed by reliable sterilization. Such a practice as washing biopsy forceps with water after use, then wiping it off with alcohol and immediately using it for the next patient must be strictly prohibited. As reprocessing can be cumbersome, the trend has been to market accessories as single use disposables. The single use accessories suffer from the disadvantage of cumulative cost and cumulative medical waste. The advantage offered is assured sterility. The ideal solution would be to establish a program which can provide reprocessed single-use devices as equally safe and effective as reusable devices after processing.

The divergent views of the various infection control committees, the complex issues, and scanty data to arbitrate among polarizing views reinforces our opinion that it is impossible for individual hospitals to assess in isolation if reuse of accessories is safe, equally efficient, and cost effective. This issue was also discussed by a working party on endoscope disinfection and their report[19] favored formation of a central body with adequate resources and expertise to make a decision on reuse applicable as minimum standard. This decision should be based on a full and accurate cost analysis and stringent quality assurance studies.

It was tentatively recommended that considering all the view points, accessories like injection sclerotherapy needles, cytology brush, stents, and biliary balloon dilators should not be reused and others may be reused if the following guidelines were followed.

(a) Strict adherence to cleaning and sterilization standards,
(b) Continuous quality control, and
(c) Patients informed and consent taken for reuse.

As recommendations were 'minimal requirements', they need to be followed up in India also.

Protection of endoscopy personnel

All endoscopy personnel should be immunized against hepatitis B. All those who assist in the endoscopy procedure must wear gloves, gowns or aprons, and masks. Protective eye wears and X-ray resistant shields should be available for use during special procedures. To avoid needle stick injury, all sharp equipment should be disposed off in special containers immediately after use without being recapped.

Staff training and supervision

The disinfection of endoscopes and other safety measures can only be done properly by trained and motivated personnel. Therefore, regular training of the endoscopy staff is very essential. A constant supervision check should be done to ensure that the protocols of disinfection are strictly followed. Cultures should be obtained periodically from the surface of endoscopes as well as from the channels. Finally, an audit of the number of infections occurring after endoscopy must be done on a regular basis.

RECOMMENDATIONS

Recommendations for reprocessing of endoscopes are revised at regular intervals. The latest of these recommendations came from a working party formed during the Asia Pacific Congress held at Hong Kong in March 2000.[19] The salient features of the recommendations as applicable to Asia Pacific region are as follows.

1. Manual cleaning of endoscopes is the most vital step in the chain of disinfection and needs to be reiterated repeatedly. There is universal agreement by all the societies that emphasis should be given on cleaning and disinfection rather than increasing the immersion time. Despite this knowledge, the focus has been on increasing the immersion time. We have no replacement to manual cleaning and a 'good clean is half the work done'.
2. Cleaning and disinfection should be carried out before the start of the session, in between the cases, and at the end of the day's session. Often, disinfection at the start of the session is neglected, even though it is most important as bacterial proliferation in residual dampness is at its peak after overnight storage.
3. Two or more scopes should be alternated for consecutive cases. This reduces the time pressure for proper disinfection.

4. Sterile water which is bacteriologically safe (passed through a 0.2 μm filter) should be used for ERCP procedures. Hospital tap water, if used, should be examined for contamination on a regular basis.
5. Water bottles should be autoclaved and only sterile water should be used in them.
6. Glutaraldehyde (2%) is the most widely used disinfectant. It is an effective agent but there is a need to follow the guidelines for safety of glutaraldehyde handlers which include: (i) wearing long nitrile gloves which should be changed regularly as they absorb glutaraldehyde, (ii) using disposable waterproof aprons, and (iii) monitoring of glutaraldehyde concentration by test strips, so that it does not fall below 1–1.5%.
7. While defining minimal standards which can be applied all over the world, especially in developing countries, we recommend a minimum of 10 minutes soak time in 2% glutaraldehyde at 25°C. Based on national and legislative concerns, the maximum time of immersion can vary from region to region. The immersion time while using duodenoscopes should be 20 minutes. There is no necessity to change the immersion time after performing endoscopy on HIV patients, immunodeficient patients, or open cases of pulmonary tuberculosis.
8. Automated disinfectors have gained acceptability and where the endoscopy load is high, these disinfectors would be the preferred choice. There is a need to exercise caution while using them. These are: (i) endoscopes still need to be manually cleaned before being subjected to mechanical disinfection and (ii) wherever automated disinfectors are used, there is a heavy responsibility on the unit to monitor its efficacy and performance.
9. Drying of the channels by forced air drying or by instilling alcohol is a must at the end of the day's session.

REFERENCES

1. Tandon RK, Ahuja V. Non United States guidelines for endoscope reprocessing. *Gastrointest Endosc Clin N Am* 2000;2:295-314.
2. Arora A, Seth S, Tandon RK. Gastrointestinal endoscope disinfection practices in India: Results of a survey. *Indian J Gastroenterol* 1992;11:62-4.
3. Tandon RK. Endoscope disinfection: Practices and recommendations. *J Gastroenterol Hepatol* 1991;6:37-9.
4. Hoofnagle JH, Seeff LB, Bales ZB, Wright EC, Zimmerman HJ. Type B hepatitis after needle stick exposure. Prevention with hepatitis B immune globulin. Final report of the Veterans Administration Cooperative study. *Ann Intern Med* 1979;91:813-8.
5. Grady GF, Lee VA. Prevention of hepatitis from accidental exposure among medical workers. *N Engl J Med* 1975;293:1067-70.
6. Birnie GG, Quigley EM, Clements GB, Follet EA. Watkinson G. Endoscopic transmission of hepatitis B virus. *Gut* 1983;24:171-4.
7. Villa E, Pasquinelli C, Rigo G, Ferrari A, Perini M, Ferrati I, Gandolfo M, et al. Gastrointestinal endoscopy and HBV infection: no evidence for a causal relationship: A prospective controlled study. *Gastrointest Endosc* 1984;30:15-7.
8. Ayoola EA. The risk of type B hepatitis infection in flexible endoscopy. *Gastrointest Endosc* 1981;2:60-2.

9. Bond WW, Favero MS, Petersen NJ, Ebert JW. Inactivation of hepatitis B virus by intermediate to high level disinfectants chemicals. *J Clin Microbiol* 1983;18:535-8.
10. Kobayashi H, Tsuzuki M. The effect of disinfectants and heat on hepatitis B virus. *J Hosp Infect* 1984;5(suppl A):93-4.
11. Hansen PJV, Gor D, Clarke JR, Chadwick MV, Nicholson G, Shah N, Gazzard B, et al. Contamination of endoscopes used in AIDS patients. *Lancet* 1989;2:86-8.
12. Thraenhart O, Kuwert EK, Dermietzel R, Scheiermann N, Wendt F. Influence of different disinfection conditions on the structure of hepatitis B virus (dane particle) as evaluation in the morphological alteration and disintegration test (MADT). *Zentralbl Bakteriol* 1978;242:299-314.
13. Thraenhart O, Kuwert EK, Scheiermann N, Dermietzel R, Paar D, Maruhn D, Alberti A, et al. Comparison of the morphological alteration and disintegration test (MADT) and the chimpanzee infectivity test for determination of hepatitis B virucidal activity of chemical disinfectants. *Zentralbl Bakteriol* 1982;176:472-84.
14. Adler-Storthz K, Sehulster LM, Dreesman GR, Hollinger FB, Melnick JL. Effect of alkaline glutaraldehyde on hepatitis B virus antigens. *Euro J Clin Microbiol* 1983;2:316-20.
15. Howard CR, Dixon JL, Young P, van Eerd P, Schellekens H. Chemical inactivation of hepatitis B virus: the effect of disinfectants on virus associated DNA polymerase activity, morphology and infectivity. *J Virol Methods* 1983;7:135-48.
16. Prince DL, Prince HN, Thraenhart O, Muchmore E, Border E, Pugh J. Methodological approaches to disinfection of human hepatitis virus. *J Clin Microbiol* 1993;31:3296-304.
17. Deva AK, Vickery K, Zou J, West RH, Selby W, Benn RAV, Harris JP, et al. Detection of persistent vegetative bacteria and amplified viral nucleic acid from in house testing of gastrointestinal endoscopes. *J Hosp Infect* 1998;39:149-57.
18. Ahuja V, Tandon RK. A survey of the GI endoscope disinfection and accessory reprocessing practices in the Asia pacific region. *J Gastroenterol Hepatol* 2000;15(suppl):G78-81.
19. Tandon RK. Aim of the working party and summary of recommendations. *J Gastroenterol Hepatol* 2000;15(suppl):G69-72.

Prevention of hepatitis B in the nephrology units

Sanjay K Agarwal

For a nephrologist, hepatitis B virus (HBV) infection has been a major cause of concern in the past. Despite advances in the prevention and treatment, it has still remained an important infection to be controlled in the nephrology units. The association between HBV and renal diseases can be two fold: (a) HBV directly producing glomerular disease, and, (b) HBV infection occurring in patients with end-stage renal disease (ESRD) on renal replacement therapy (RRT), i.e., hemodialysis (HD), chronic ambulatory peritoneal dialysis (CAPD), and renal transplantation (RT).

In patients with chronic renal failure being treated with RRT, HBV infection is an important cause of mortality and morbidity. The high incidence and mortality due to HBV related liver disease in these patients is due to high-risk of HBV infection in the hemodialysis patients. In these patients, number of blood transfusions and the duration of chronic hemodialysis are correlated with the prevalence of infection.[1] HBV infection in RT patients is primarily continuation of infection from the dialysis period to the RT period. The infection can also be acquired through the organs being transplanted. However, as all the donors are now being screened for HBV infection, transplanted organs as a source of HBV infection is currently unlikely. In the last three decades, HBV infection has been extensively studied during RRT. Course of HBV infection in these patients is altered due to characteristic immunological dysfunction that develops in renal failure interfering with the patient's ability to eliminate the virus. Even with the active HBV disease, elevated serum alanine aminotransferases (ALT) levels are seen in only 10 to 44% of patients on maintenance hemodialysis (MHD) and 7 to 24% of transplant recipients. Thus, transaminases are not the reliable markers to assess the disease activity in these patients.[2] About 90% of patients with normal renal function eliminate the virus with only little and reversible hepatic damage. In patients with chronic renal failure, immune defect results in a varying spectrum of clinical disease ranging from complete immune unresponsiveness towards the virus with an asymptomatic HBsAg positive state to chronic active hepatitis (CAH). The acute course of the infection is often anicteric and peak transaminase concentration is significantly less than in patients with normal renal function. Upto 60% of patients on regular dialysis with HBV infection develop chronic hepatitis with persistence of HBsAg and infectivity. While patients with chronic hepatitis B and normal renal function eliminate the HBsAg at the rate of 1–2% annually, in patients on dialysis, elimination of the virus beyond ten months is rare. Asymptomatic subjects with chronic HBV infection probably have more favourable prognosis. However, they remain a potential reservoir for transmission of infection to other dialysis patients and staff.

MAGNITUDE OF PROBLEM

Hemodialysis patients and staff are at a high-risk of acquiring hepatitis B infection. In 1978, 28.8% of these patients had been positive in France. With prophylactic measures, the incidence has come down and in 1990, 6.1% of dialysis patients in the European Dialysis and Transplantation Association (EDTA) registry were positive for HBsAg. However, even today, in Eastern Europe, Central America and Asia, prevalence of HBV infection in patients with chronic renal failure ranges between 20–30% in certain centres. The prevalence of HBV in the MHD and in RT patients in India is reported to range between 3.4% to 42%,[3-12] much higher than that in the general population (Table 1).[13] As CAPD in India is still in infancy, there is no data on the prevalence of HBV in our country in patients on CAPD.

Studies of higher prevalence of HBV infection in the staff of the dialysis units have been available in India from Vellore, Delhi, Mumbai, and Chennai confirming that hepatitis is one of the important occupational hazards in the nephrology units.[4, 6, 14] In a study reported from

Table 1. Prevalence of HBV in hemodialysis (HD) and renal transplant (RT) patients in India

Author	Year	HD patients (%)	HD staff (%)	RT patients (%)
Gunasekran et al[4]	1979	25	28.5	NA
Acharya et al[5]	1983	3.4	10.5	NA
Thomas et al[3]	1987	40	23	NA
Thomas et al[9]	1991	45.5	NA	83.3
Sharma et al[10]	1991	9	NA	NA
Vijay Kumar et al[11]	1993	NA	NA	12.8
Bhaskaran et al[7]	1994	7.7	NA	NA
Roy et al[12]	1994	NA	NA	35.2
Jyothi et al[8]	1999	4.5	NA	NA
Agarwal et al[UP]	2001	4.2	0	15

NA–not available, UP–unpublished

K.E.M. Hospital, Mumbai, wherein 76 staff members of hemodialysis unit were tested longitudinally during their stay in the unit. It was noted that 6.5% had developed HBsAg positive hepatitis. Amongst them, the staff nurses had the highest incidence of HBsAg positive hepatitis (23%), followed by dialysis technicians (13%). During the same period, amongst 471 hemodialysis patients, 62 (13.1%) developed HBsAg positive hepatitis. Looking at the severity of hepatitis, it was noted that morbidity due to hepatitis B was much greater among the staff as compared to the patients. Undoubtedly, the staff needs protection as much as the dialysis patients do.

TRANSMISSION

There are three modes of transmission of HBV infection in the dialysis unit.

Percutaneous needle-stick

Risk of HBV infection following a percutaneous needle-stick exposure to such contaminated blood is 45 to 125 times greater than that of HIV infection (45% vs. 0.3%).[15] This is because the HBV circulates at higher biological concentration with more than 100 million viral particles per ml of blood as compared to HIV which has viral load of 10–1000 infectious particles per ml of blood.

Transmission through blood and blood products

Transmission through blood and blood products is a major source of HBV transmission. However, ever since the HBsAg testing in the blood has been made mandatory, role of this mode of transmission has become negligible. This is still possible in special situations such as acquiring infection in the window period, infection with HBV mutants, and low level viremia that escapes detection.

Nosocomial transmission through environment

Hepatitis B subjects amongst hospital personnel and patients are a major source of infection. Moreover, equipment in the hospitals as well as the environmental surfaces become contaminated with HBV when they come in contact with infected patients. Hence, hepatitis B is a significant occupational hazard amongst the hospital personnel. The risk of transmission of HBV infection through blood from one patient to another is mostly because of inadequate precautions taken by the dialysis staff. Transmission via the dialysis membrane and through dialysis machine is rare. In patients on peritoneal dialysis, the rate of sero-conversion is much low (0.01/patient year) in comparison to patients on hemodialysis (0.19/patient year),[16] suggesting the role of hemodialysis centre in the transmission of hepatitis B. One multivariate analysis report revealed an association of positivity of the HBV with the duration of renal replacement therapy, number of previous blood transfusions, and past history of hemodialysis treatment.[17]

PREVENTION OF HEPATITIS B

Prevention of HBV infection in the nephrology units is primarily concentrated on prevention in the hemodialysis unit. In nephrology ward and in peritoneal dialysis setting, general guidelines for prevention are sufficient. In hemodialysis unit, two issues involved are:

(a) Prevention of HBV infection from patient to patient, and (b) prevention of HBV infection from health care worker (HCW) to the patients.

Prevention of hepatitis B in patients from other patients

It is of utmost importance to prevent transmission of infectious blood from one patient to another. The use of separate rooms and separate dialysis machines is recommended for the patients with evidence of HBV replication as suggested by HBeAg positivity and definitely for patients in whom HBV-DNA is detected by PCR. Most important measure for prevention of transmission is to follow "universal precautions". In a recent study, 59 patients on MHD who were potentially exposed to a strongly positive HBV patient did not develop infection on follow-up for 9 months despite the fact that 29 of them were fully unprotected as detected by the absence of anti-HBs.[18] It is recommended that universal precautions (UP) need to be stressed again and again. In a survey conducted at the AIIMS, it was shown that 100% of nurses know about UP but only 70% follow them in their day to day practice. More importantly, nearly half of them comment that hospital and the department in which they are working have not done much to make them aware of UP. About two-thirds of these nurses agree that hospital does not provide adequate facilities to follow-up. Almost all wish that hospital should do "more" regarding this aspect of health care.[19] Apart from the use of universal precautions, the prevalence of hepatitis B has been reduced significantly in these patients by the effective use of hepatitis B vaccine.[20]

The blood transfusion as a source for HBV transmission can be decreased by the regular use of erythropoietin, which decreases the need for blood transfusion. However, the therapy with erythropoietin is costly, and many patients cannot afford this especially in a developing country like India. In this scenario, we must follow "voluntary blood donation" program and regular screening of all the blood units for HBsAg.

Universal precautions in a dialysis unit

Aseptic precautions while inserting intravascular catheter and construction of AV fistulae
    Skin cleaned with antiseptic containing soap solution,
    skin painted with 10% povidon Iodine for 10 minutes, and
    ensure sterility of intravascular items.

Ensuring proper handling and disposal of sharps
    Re-usable sharps to be treated with gluteraldehyde and washed with saline/distilled water before use,

all sharps before discarding to be put in puncture proof containers with 3% sodium hypochlorite solution,

no recapping of needles should be done,

additional precautions, when caring for known HBsAg positive patients,

use of gloves, high efficiency masks, proper eye protection, boots, impervious gowns, and closed wound drainage,

HBsAg positive cases should be taken as a last case in the theatre with use of disposable anesthetic circulatory or use appropriate method of decontamination (use of 2% gluteraldehyde for 60 min.),

disinfecting theatre floor and walls with 5% sodium hypochlorite, and

air-conditioning ducts to be fumigated with 5% formaldehyde with the use of aerosol spray.

Other guidelines specific for hemodialysis units

No eating, drinking and smoking in dialysis unit,

linen should be changed for every patient,

cleaning of machine surface and disinfection of machine with proper disinfectant must be done after every dialysis,

medication during dialysis should be given in the drip chamber directly,

pippetting of blood should be done with rubber treat,

HBsAg negative patients and staff should be adequately vaccinated,

infected patients should be dialysed in a separate room, and

in infected patients, dialyser should not be re-used.

Prevention of hepatitis B from health care workers to patients

Current data suggests that the risk for transmission of HBV from health care worker (HCW) to patient is small. However, a precise assessment is not clearly documented. It is shown that infected HCW, who adheres to the use of universal precautions[21, 22] and who does not perform 'invasive procedure' poses no risk for transmission of HBV to the patient. But, if HCW performs "invasive procedure", it poses a small risk for HBV transmission. From nephrology point of view, all the cannulations, both temporary and permanent vascular access, renal biopsy, and peritoneal dialysis will be included in the list of "invasive procedures". The risk of transmission increases if the HCW is HBeAg positive also.[15] The risk of transmission further increases, if the "invasive procedure" is an exposure prone procedure" [EPP]. These are the procedures which involve digital palpation of a needle tip in a body cavity or simultaneous presence of HCW's finger and needle or other sharp instrument or object in a poorly visualised anatomical site in the body. In nephrology practice, EPP is not generally performed. Following are the recommendations for HCW working in nephrology units.

(a) strict adherence to the use of universal precautions,

(b) infected HCW should not perform invasive procedures,
(c) who perform EPP should know their HBsAg and HBeAg status, and
(d) HBeAg positive HCW should not perform EPP.

REFERENCES

1. Szmuness W, Prince AM, Grady GF, Mann MK, Levine RW, Friedman EA. Hepatitis B infection: a point prevalence study in 15 US hemodialysis centers. *JAMA* 1974;227:901-6.
2. Guh JY, Lai YH, Yang CY, Chen SC, Chuang WL, Hsu TC, Chen HC, et al. Impact of decreased serum transaminase levels on the evaluation of viral hepatitis B in hemodialysis patients. *Nephron* 1995;69: 459-65.
3. Thomas P, Kirubakaran MG, Jacob CM, Srinivasa NS, Hariharan S, John TJ, Shastry JS. Hepatitis B infection in a dialysis unit in South India. *J Assoc Phys Ind* 1987;35:284-5.
4. Gunasekaran, Kirubakaran MG, Johny KV, Shastry JCM, John TJ. Hepatitis B virus infection in a renal unit in India. *Ind J Med Res* 1979;70:1-4
5. Acharya VN, Chawla KP, Ravichandran R, Rao RS. Study of Australia antigen (HBsAg) and hepatitis in patients and staff of dialysis unit in Bombay. *Proceedings of 13th Annual Indian Society of Nephrology Conference held at Cuttack* 1983.
6. Malhotra KK, Prabhakar S, Sharma RK, Dash SC. Hepatitis B in a hemodialysis unit in New Delhi. *J Assoc Phys Ind* 1985;33:216-7.
7. Bhaskaran S, Mani MK, Prakash KC. A study of hepatitis B surface antigen positive patients on hemodialysis and following transplantation. *J Assoc Phys Ind* 1994;42:363-5.
8. Jyothi R, Padma G, Georgi A, Soundararajan P, Panicker. Hepatitis B and C in ESRD on RRT. *Proceedings of 1st National Conference on hepatitis & Renal Medicine* held at New Delhi, 1999.
9. Thomas PP, Samuel BU, Jacob CK, John TJ, Shastry JCM. Low prevalence of hepatitis D (Delta) virus infection in a nephrology unit in south India. *Trans R Soc Trop Med Hyg* 1991;85:652-3.
10. Sharma RK, Elhence R, Kher V, Naik SR, Bhandari M. Liver disease in renal transplant recipients. *Ind J Nephrol* 1991;4:136.
11. Vijaykumar R, Ismail TSMS, Rajendan S, Jayakumar M, Shivakumar S, Muthusethupathy MA. Hepatitis in renal transplant recipients. *Ind J Nephrol* 1993;3:84.
12. Roy DM, Thomas PP, Dakshinamurthy KV, Jacob CK, Shastry JCM. Long-term survival in living related donor renal allograft recipients with hepatitis B infection. *Transplantation* 1994;58:118-9.
13. Thyagarajan SP, Jayaram S, Mohanvalli B. *Prevalence of hepatitis B in the general population of India.* In: Sarin SK, Singal AK, Eds. Hepatitis B in India: Problems and Prevention. CBS Publishers & Distributors, New Delhi 1996; pp.5-16.
14. Thyagarajan SP, Subramanian S, Sundervelu T, Shivkumar S, Prasad PR, Thiruvengadam KP. HBsAg carrier amongst hospital personnel – A serostudy of Govt. general hospital, *Madras Journal of API* 1981; 29:941.
15. Alter H, Seeff L, Kaplan PM, McAuliffe VJ, Wright EC, Gerin JL, Purcell RH, et al. Type B hepatitis. The infectivity of blood positive for e antigen and DNA polymerase after accidental exposure. *N Eng J Med* 1976;295:909-13.
16. Cendoroglo Neto M, Draibe SA, Silva AE, Ferraz ML, Granato C, Pereira CA, Sesso RD, et al. Incidence of and risk factors for hepatitis B virus and hepatitis C virus infection among hemodialysis and CAPD patients: evidence for environment transmission. *Nephrol Dial Transplant* 1995;10:240-6.
17. Cendorglo Neto M, Mangano SI, Canziani ME, Silva AE, Ciranza LF, Sesso RD, Azzen H, et al.

Environmental transmission of hepatitis B and hepatitis viruses within the hemodialysis unit. *Artif Organ* 1995;19:251-5.
18. Kores AC, Van Bommel EF, Kluytoman JA, Weiner W. Hepatitis B and hemodialysis the impact of universal precaution in preventing the transmission of blood borne viruses. *Infect Control Hosp Epidemiol* 1998;19:508-10.
19. Agarwal SK, Mohan MP, Varghese M. Assessment of awareness regarding universal precautions among the nursing staff of AIIMS in 1997. A hospital based study. *J Assoc Phys Ind* 1998;46:1061.
20. Ly D, Yee HF Jr. Brezma M, Martin P, Gitnick G, Saab S. Hepatitis B surface antigenemia in chronic hemodialysis patients: effect of hepatitis B immunization. *Am J Gastroenterol* 2002;97:138-41.
21. CDC Update. Universal precautions for prevention of transmission of HIV, hepatitis B virus and other blood-borne pathogens in healthcare setting. *MMWR* 1988;37:377-82,387-8.
22. Zuckerman M. Surveillance and control of blood-borne virus infections in hemodialysis units. *J Hosp Infect* 2002;50:1-5.

Routine screening for hepatitis B virus before surgery or intervention

Chittoor M Habibullah, Mohammed A Habeeb, Mohammed M Hussain, Mohammed N Khaja, Viral Patrawala, Sharad Shah

Hepatitis B virus (HBV) infection has emerged as a major public health problem in our country. The prevalence of HBsAg is about 4–5%. In this background the necessity of formulating the comprehensive hospital policy for managing HBV infection is being felt. Routine screening before surgery or intervention for HBV is necessary now. The debate on which tests should be performed before surgery to identify HBV is going on. The following article provides information about the above question after analysing various publications and authors' interaction with various specialists and superspecialists involved in surgery.

HEPATITIS B

The discovery of HBV in 1967[1] heralded a new era in identification and management of transfusion associated hepatitis. Within 33 years of the discovery, significant advances have been made in the understanding of the pathobiology of HBV infection. However, hepatitis B virus infection still remains an important cause of morbidity and mortality worldwide. The prevalence of this infection is highest in areas of Sub-saharan Africa and South east Asia. The average HBsAg prevalence in our country is about 4–5%, placing India in the intermediate zone for hepatitis B endemicity.[2] Out of 400 million subjects with chronic HBV infection worldwide, roughly 35–40 million are in India.[3] Thus hepatitis B remains a significant public health problem in India. One recent study has shown hepatitis B prevalence rate of more than 20% among primitive tribes of Andaman and Nicobar islands.[4]

This recent finding raises the issue of the need for detailed epidemiological studies about prevalence of hepatitis B infection in our country. The hepatitis B virus infection is responsible for chronic hepatitis, cirrhosis of the liver and hepatocellular carcinoma (HCC). The term hepatitis B "carrier" has been replaced by a term "chronic hepatitis B virus infected" person, at the Single theme conference on "Carrier to Cancer" – New Delhi 1998. Of all the subjects with chronic HBV infection, about 40–70% have active viral replication and this group is at the highest risk of developing progressive liver disease.[5] Hepatitis B e antigen (HBeAg) positivity, which denotes viral replication and high infectivity, has been reported in 7.8 to 47% of HBsAg positive subjects in different regions of India with wide variations in social, economic and health factors.[6] Around 5–10% of adult patients exposed to HBV fail to clear the virus and develop chronic infection. In about one-third of these patients, chronic hepatitis and cirrhosis may develop after 5–30 yrs.[7,8] In patients with HBV-related cirrhosis, there is an increased risk of developing HCC, the risk is higher in men than in women.[8] As high as 80% of the cases of cirrhosis of the liver are due to chronic HBV infection.[9] More than 60% of patients with HCC seen at Madras were positive for markers of HBV infection.[6] Around 57% of patients with HCC seen at Osmania General Hospital (OGH) over a four-year period between 1989–1992 were positive for HBV.[10]

It is clear from the above statistics (which represent only tip of the iceberg), that the HBV infection and its sequelae are of great medical significance in our country. In this context, screening for HBV infection before any surgery or intervention is not only necessary but should also be made mandatory.

Transmission of hepatitis B and its significance

There are several modes of transmission for HBV infection. Of these, perinatal transmission appears to be the most important. This includes both vertical transmission from infected mother to the newborn and horizontal transmission after birth up to 6 months of age from mother or other close contacts. Another important mode of transmission is through transfusion of infected blood and blood products. In addition to blood and blood products, HBV has been detected in a wide variety of human secretions like semen, saliva, nasopharyngeal secretions, menstrual fluid, bile, pancreatic juice, pleural fluid, ascitic fluid, cerebrospinal fluid, urine, tears, etc. However, the relative contribution of these secretions in the epidemiology of HBV infection is not known. Other important modes include: sexual transmission (both homosexual and heterosexual), tattooing, needle stick exposure, etc. We have chosen to discuss transmission modes because any patient who will be evaluated for surgery might have been exposed to any or all of above transmission modes during his/her life time.

We also should keep in mind the fact that the practice of using disposable syringes was introduced in our country only about 10 years ago. Earlier, syringes and needles were reused after sterilizing them by boiling in water. We should be aware that this might have been one of the possible ways of HBV transmission earlier. Keeping above points in view, any patient being prepared for surgery or intervention should be evaluated for the presence of HBV infection.

SCREENING FOR LIVER DISEASE BEFORE SURGERY

All patients undergoing surgery should undergo a careful history and physical examination to exclude findings or risk factors for liver disease. This should include history of prior blood transfusions, tattoos, illicit drug use, sexual promiscuity, a family history of jaundice or liver disease, a history of jaundice or fever following anesthesia, alcohol use, and a complete review of current medications. Findings on physical examination suggestive of liver disease (such as fatigue, pruritus, increased abdominal girth, jaundice, palmar erythema, spider telangiectasias, splenomegaly, gynaecomasia, and testicular atrophy) should be evaluated.[11] HBV infection and its sequelae can adversely affect the outcome of surgery/intervention due to its insidious nature. There are certain advantages (Table 1) of screening for HBV before surgery. Hence, patients undergoing evaluation for surgery should be checked for presence of HBsAg.

Table 1. Advantages of routine screening for HBV before surgery

For patients
Unmasking of chronic liver disease
Evaluation for possible treatment
For doctors
Medico-legal aspects
Prevention of spread amongst HCW
For general population
Taking care of family contacts

Screening for HBV-current status

Currently HBV infection is detected by third generation ELISA test for the presence of HBsAg. This test is extremely reliable provided it is done with a good quality kit. The test detects hepatitis B virus except surface mutants (hepatitis B virus deficient in secretion of surface antigen), the significance of which will be discussed later.

Screening before surgery / intervention and testing

When we discuss about screening for HBV before surgery, we should keep two important factors in mind. These are: (a) type of surgery involved and (b) patient health and life-style profile. As discussed earlier, patients who had any of the risk factors for HBV transmission should be tested for HBsAg using third generation ELISA kits. In addition to HBsAg, other tests are suggested under two circumstances: (a) for major surgery or surgery involving large volume infusion of blood or blood products and (b) for surgeries involving high quantity blood transfusion as these expose the patient to the risk of acquiring transfusion association hepatitis (TAH). Recent study has shown that the incidence of HBV seems to be about 4 per 1000 units transfused. The higher the quantity of blood transfused, the higher is the risk of contracting TAH. HBsAg negativity does not mean absence of HBV infection. Three recent studies have shown high frequency of HBV-DNA positivity (5, 10, 25%) in HBsAg negative blood units.[12-14]

The knowledge about the patient's HBV status is also important for the protection of the surgeon, as the risk of HBV infection is highest due to needle-stick injuries during surgical procedures. The risk of infection of the surgeon following a hollow needle-stick injury is about 30% for HBV, 10% for HCV, and 0.3% for HIV.[15] This knowledge helps the surgeons to take extra caution during the surgical procedures.

Patients being evaluated for surgeries of solid malignancies should also be comprehensively tested for HBV infection. These patients may subsequently undergo radiation therapy or chemotherapy. These therapies are known to bring down immune response making the patient more susceptible for HBV infection. The patients who need emergency surgeries (trauma patients and cases requiring immediate surgical care, e.g. appendicitis) should also be tested for HBsAg so that postoperative care can be taken keeping in mind their HBsAg status.

Complete screening for HBV

The prevalence of HBV in the dialysis population in India is reported to range between 3.4% to 42%, much higher than that in general population and upto 60% of dialysis patients with HBV infection develop chronic hepatitis with persistence of HBsAg.[16] The sero-conversion rate after vaccination is as low as 50–60% in these patients. The reasons for this are still not very clear. However, uremia is reported to be one major contributory factory.[17] Hence, these patients should be tested for IgM anti-HBc, HBeAg, and anti-HBe in addition to HBsAg (Fig. 1). This is essential in view of immunocompromised condition of these patients. These patients have multiple exposures to needle-stick injuries. These patients are usually tested for HBsAg as soon as CRF is diagnosed and are given hepatitis B vaccine if negative for HBsAg. However, a significant percentage of them become positive for HBsAg during dialysis. These patients require a complete work-up of their HBV replication status and should be treated before transplant surgery. This is extremely important in view of immune suppressant therapy needed after the transplantation. Patients waiting to undergo bone marrow transplant (BMT) should also be evaluated for all HBV replication markers. If replication is identified, they should be treated aggressively before the transplant. Patients undergoing elective cardiac procedures involving high volume blood transfusion should also be evaluated for HBV replication status, as these patients already have a risk of contracting TAH.[12-14]

Patients undergoing procedures associated with large amount of blood loss should also be evaluated for HBV replication status as this can aggravate ischemic hepatic injury. Patients

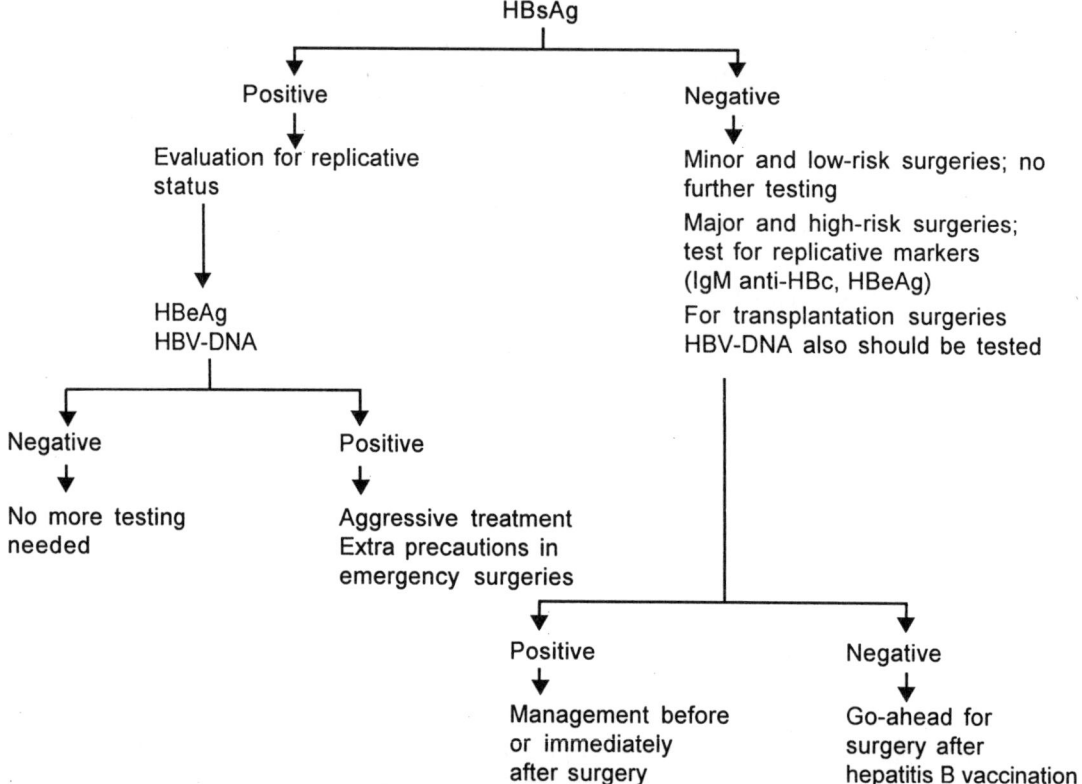

Fig. 1. Suggested algorithm for routine HBV screening before surgery

with liver disease who require surgeries are at a greater risk for surgical and anesthesia related complications than those with a healthy liver.[17,18] The magnitude of the risk depends on the type of liver disease and its severity, the surgical procedure, and the type of anesthesia. As a general rule, most inhalation anesthetics are associated with reduction in portal blood flow and cardiac output.[19] Hence, the presence of HBV in the liver and its sequelae on liver histology and physiology can further aggravate the surgical and aneasthesia-related complications. In view of this, testing for HBV infection is mandatory to adjust the settings and selection of anesthesia.

Special population of patients such as patients with a history of intravenous drug abuse should also be tested for presence of other HBV replicative markers apart from HBsAg to ensure that the patient is not at a high-risk during surgery. Patients with a history of blood transfusion such as hemophiliacs and thalassiemics should also be tested in the above manner. Patients with a history of diabetes should also be tested for other HBV replicative markers as diabetes is known to lower body's immune response and make the patient susceptible to infections during and after surgery.

Significance of HBV mutants

Existence of HBV mutant forms, in variable frequency, has been recognised well in the different populations around the world. Now, it is well known that HBV mutants could alter the course of a natural HBV infection in an unfavourable way such as development of severe hepatitis, immune escape phenomenon, vaccine failure, and a higher potential for causing HCC.[20]

During the past decade, two clinically important variants of HBV have been characterized, the pre-core mutant (PM) and the surface mutant (SM) forms. In the former, a mutation in codon 28 of the open reading frame generates a stop codon and prevents the synthesis of HBeAg but not HBcAg and HBV-DNA (HBsAg positive, HBeAg negative, anti-HBe positive and HBV-DNA positive). Nearly 12 subtypes of pre-core mutants have been described; the 1898, 1896 and 1856 are common in the Indian continent.[21] These cannot be detected by routine HBsAg ELISA test. Use of anti-HBc, anti-HBs and anti-HBe could help in determining the presence of surface mutants.[21] These tests are only essential for patients evaluated for surgery needing high volume blood transfusion to avoid further complications. However, there are certain disadvantages of such screening practices, e.g., cost of screening and possibility of discrimination, although problem is not as alarming as for HIV patients.

Cost of screening

Every patient before surgery is assessed by a number of tests including tests for liver functions. In addition to these, if the patient is tested for HBsAg (in case of low-risk surgeries) the cost involved is miniscule, Rs. 150–250 depending on various factors. Complete panels of HBV tests are required in special group of patients as mentioned above. These patients are naturally at high-risk and testing them for presence of HBV by IgM anti-HBc, HBeAg, anti-HBe is safer as it clearly indicates the presence/absence of HBV and their immune status. These reports will be useful in managing the patient during and after surgery.

The cost involved in the treatment of HBV infection (acute as well as chronic) is very high. Not only we should take cost into consideration, we also should calculate the time lost, and other valuable resources including human resources used in managing these infections. All the above steps are to ensure that the patient does not harbour HBV prior to surgery. In an ideal condition where universal vaccination against HBV is available, all the above steps are not necessary except in patients with CRF and patients waiting for BMT. However, in our country we are struggling to get HBV vaccine included in the list of vaccines given to children. We have a long way to go in managing to vaccinate against HBV all high-risk subjects. Till that state is reached, the above steps to identify HBV infected patients before surgery should be made mandatory after consultations and discussions with other specialists.

HBV infection and management

If the patient being evaluated for elective surgery is found to be having replicating HBV (HBeAg positive, HBV-DNA positive with elevated ALT levels > 1.5 times the upper limit of normal), he should be considered for antiviral therapy. The dosage for Interferon is 5 mIU daily for at least 4 months. If the ALT levels are more than 5 times elevated, the patient should be treated with lamivudine. The duration of both the therapies should be determined depending on the patient's condition and also the discretion of the treating physician. If the surgery is an emergency one, the therapy should be initiated once the surgery is over and the patient is in a condition to tolerate the treatment. In any condition the patient should be made to understand the implications of replicating HBV and its possible impact on his health.

HBV, SURGERY, AND HEALTH CARE WORKERS

HBV infection from the patient to the HCW is also an important issue. Although, most of the HCW are vaccinated, there still remains a risk for acquiring HBV infection. However, as a prophylactic measure, vaccination status of all health care workers should be known as this shall take care of laxities that lead to increased risk of transmitting virus from patients to the HCW.[22] The data about transmission of HBV infection from patient to the HCW is not available in our country. Occupational safety and health administration (OSHA) has recommended that all high-risk employees should be offered immunization. However, in 1994 about 400 HBV infections were estimated to occur in health care workers in USA. More than 250 health care workers still die each year from acute and chronic HBV infection.[23] These figures speak for themselves about the risk faced by the HCWs from HBV. Hence, extra precautions are necessary when surgery on an HBV infected patient is to be undertaken. This should include change of gloves every 30 minutes as perforated gloves seem to be the highest risk factor for infection during the surgical procedures.[24]

REFERENCES

1. Blumberg BS, Gerstley BJS, Hungerford DA London WT, Sutnick AI. A serum antigen, Australia antigen in down's syndrome, lukemia and hepatitis. *Ann Intern Med* 1967;66:924-31.
2. Suzuki H, Woodfield G. *Viral Hepatitis in Asia: Summary of a Planery Session. In:* Nishioka K, Suzuki H, Mishiro S, Oda T, Eds. Viral hepatitis and liver disease: Springer Verlag, Tokyo, 1994;pp. 385-402.
3. Agarwal R, Naik SR. Prevention of hepatitis B infection: the appropriate strategy for India. *Natl Med J India* 1994;7:216-20.
4. Ganapati M. Research finds high hepatitis brake in Indian Island tribes. *Br Med J* 2000;321:440.
5. Wong DK, Cheung AM, O'Rourke K, Naylor CD, Detsky AS, Heathcote J. Effect of alpha-Interferon in patients with hepatitis B e antigen positive, chronic hepatitis B, a meta-analysis. *Ann Intern Med* 1993;119:312-23.
6. Tandon BN, Acharya SK, Tandon A. Epidemiology of hepatitis B infection in India. *Gut* 1996;38 (suppl 2):S56-9.
7. Benhamou JP. Chairman's introduction: Viral hepatitis; Management; Standards for the future, Proceedings of a symposium in Cannes, France on 22, 23 May 1992, *Gut* 1993;(suppl):4-8.

8. Liaw YF, Tal DI, Chu CM, Chen TJ. The development of cirrhosis in patients with chronic type B hepatitis: a prospective study. *Hepatology* 1988;8:493-8.
9. Nayak NC, Dhar A, Sachdeva R. Association of HCC and cirrhosis with hepatitis B virus surface and core antigens in the liver. *Int J Cancer* 1977;20:643-54.
10. Data on file. HCC and viral etiology: OGH experience.1989-1992.
11. Friedman LS. Assessing surgical risk in patients with liver disease. *Harvard Medical School Update* 2000;1:1-12
12. Banerjee K, Sharma G, Upadhyaya S, Anand BS, Raju GS, Khandekar PS. Detection of hepatitis B virus in blood samples negative for surface antigen by DNA probe hybridization assay. *J Biosol* 1989;14:279-87.
13. Nandi J, Banerjee K. Detection of hepatitis B virus DNA in donor blood by the polymerase chain reaction. *Natl Med J India* 1992;5:5-7.
14. Nagaraju K, Misra S, Saraswat S, Choudhary N, Masih B, Ramesh V, Naik S. High prevalence of HBV infectivity in blood donors detected by the dot blot hybridization assay. *Vox Sang* 1994; 67:183-6.
15. Guidelines for prevention of surgical site infection (SSI)–prepared by CDC's Hospital Infection Control Practice Advisory Committee–*Infection in the OR: Best practices for the next millennium*–October 11, 1999 – San Francisco, CA.
16. Sharma RK, Sural S. Hepatitis B and C in dialysis: presentation at symposium on hepatitis and renal medicine held at AIIMS, New Delhi on 13th February 1999.
17. Friedman LS, Maddrey WC. Surgery in the patient with liver disease. *Med Clin N Am* 1987;71:453-76.
18. Friedman LS. The risk of surgery in patients with liver disease. *Hepatology* 1999;29:16-7.
19. Klemperer JD, Ko W, Krieger KH, Connolly M, Rosengart TK, Attorki NK, Lang S, et al. Cardiac operations in patients with cirrhosis. *Ann Thorac Surg* 1998;65:85-7.
20. Guptan RC, Thakur V, Sarin SK. *Hepatitis B Virus Mutants: Indian experience. In:* Sarin SK, Hess G. Eds. Transfusion Associated Hepatitis: CBS Publishers & Distributors, New Delhi 1998; pp. 39-48.
21. Sarin SK. Hepatitis B Mutants: Prevalence, Significance and Therapy *Hepatitis World* 1998;3.
22. Mishra A, Sarin SK. Transmission of hepatitis B from health care workers to patients. *J Assoc Phys India* 1997;45:392-5.
23. Statement on the Surgeon and Hepatitis by American College of Surgeons. *Bull Am Coll Surgeons* 1999;84:21-4.
24. Kralj N, Beie M, Hoffmann F. Health care workers and Gloves study. *Gesundheitswesen* 1999;61: 398-403.

32

HBsAg positive health care worker: the rational policy?

Subhash R Naik

Hepatitis B virus (HBV) is among the major pathogens that are transmitted through contact with infected blood and blood products.[1,2] The infectivity of HBV is several times higher than that of the dreaded human immunodeficiency virus (HIV).[3] HBV infection is generally diagnosed by demonstrating the presence of hepatitis B surface antigen (HBsAg) in the serum of the infected individual. This article deals with the issue of significance of infection of health care workers (HCW) with HBsAg.

HBV INFECTION IN HEALTH CARE WORKERS: SIGNIFICANCE

It has long been known that the HCW are at a higher risk of acquiring hepatitis B than general population, mainly because of occupational blood exposure.[4,5] Indeed, HCW have a higher proportion of HBV infected persons.[6,7] Observations of higher prevalence of HBV infection among HCW have led health authorities of many countries to consider measures to protect HCW. These measures include passive immunoprophylaxis,[8] vaccination against HBV,[9] and the well publicized universal precautions[10] against the spread of infection in hospitals. Protection against HBV is particularly justified because of the high rate of chronicity of infection and the well-known sequelae of chronic hepatitis, cirrhosis and the hepatocellular carcinoma. In spite of all this knowledge, what seemed to escape widespread attention of the medical profession and the health authorities for a long time is that the HCWs can transmit infection to patients, a situation that should ordinarily be much less ethically acceptable than that of patients transmitting infections to the HCW.

Exposure-prone invasive procedures (EPIP)

Although the reports of HCW infecting patients with HBV have appeared in medical literature regularly for the last quarter century,[11-14] the impetus to energetically document such cases was provided by the 1987 report[15] from the Centers for Disease Control (CDC), USA. This report sought to prevent HCW infected with HIV from performing exposure-prone invasive procedures. This report was followed by recommendations[16] that were later extended by CDC to cover HCW with HBV infection.[17] This report defined the EPIP and detailed precautions, notification procedures and recommendations for testing of HIV and HBV infections (Table 1).

Table 1. Recommendations for US health care workers for preventing transmission of hepatitis B to patients during exposure-prone invasive procedures*

1. Universal precautions
   Hand washing
   Protective barriers
   Care in the use and disposal of needles and other sharp instruments
   HCW with exudative lesions or weeping dermatitis to refrain from direct patient care or handle patient-care equipment or devices to be used during EPIP
   Comply with guidelines for disinfection and sterilization of reusable devices used in EPIP
2. Infected HCW may carry out invasive procedures classified as non-EPIP provided they comply with universal precautions and guidelines for disinfection/sterilization
3. EPIP must be identified by medical, surgical and dental organizations and institutions where EPIP are performed
4. HCW must know the results of their previous hepatitis B vaccination and their current HBsAg/HBeAg status
5. HBeAg positive HCW must not perform EPIP unless his case is examined by expert review panel and the conditions of permissible procedures are defined. Such conditions may include notifying prospective patients of HCW's positivity status
6. Mandatory testing of HCW for hepatitis B markers is not recommended on cost-efficacy analysis.# Compliance of HCW should be increased through education, training and appropriate confidentiality safeguards

* Adapted from recommendations of the Center for Disease Control, USA[17]
\# Recent Canadian regulations recommend mandatory testing of all HCW and prevention of HBeAg positive from performing EPIP[24]

Exposure-prone invasive procedure (EPIP) has been defined as those procedures which involve digital palpation of a needle tip in a body cavity or simultaneous presence of the HCW's fingers and a needle in a poorly visualized or highly confined anatomic site. Further, EPIP were characterized as procedures that present a recognized risk of percutaneous injury to the HCW, and, if such an injury occurs, the HCW's blood is likely to contact the patient's body cavity, subcutaneous tissues and/or mucus membranes. Since there could be several other factors influencing a reasonable categorization of EPIP, such as the surgeon's technique and skill, the equipment, and the surgical appliances and material available, it was considered inappropriate to devise a standard list of EPIPs. Eventually, it was therefore decided[18] to consider an EPIP on a case-to-case basis to be decided by local hospital authorities taking into consideration various factors. These recommendations eventually were supported by legislations and are in vogue now in the USA.[18]

Determinants of HBV infectivity of HCW

As mentioned earlier, several reports in the 70's and 80's have described that HCW positive for HBV can infect their patients.[11-14] The earliest evidence to demonstrate the potential of HCW to infect their patients with HBV came from the USA leading to CDC recommendations.[15-17] As the need for clear regulatory measures to prevent the spread of infection from HCW to the patients was felt, it became necessary to characterize the criteria for infectivity. Early recommendations were based on hepatitis B e antigen (HBeAg) positivity.[17] More recently, in an important systematic investigation[19] conducted by the Incident Investigation Teams and others in the United Kingdom between 1984 and early 1993, the authors tracked down the source of infection of ten clusters of patients. They showed that the patients were infected from the gynecologists, cardiovascular surgeons, general surgeons, colorectal surgeons and neuroanesthetists. Besides establishing that the HCW in those specialities are most prone to transmit the HBV infection to their patients, the report also showed that all these infecting HCW were HBeAg negative.

The concept that HBeAg was the sole determinant of infectivity was challenged by Caspari and Gerlich[20] who suggested that it was more useful to do a quantitative estimation of HBV-DNA. They suggested that if $>10^6$ copies of HBV-DNA are present, these HCW should not perform EPIP. It is expected that in near future these recommendations will be assessed more critically and simpler techniques to assess the infectivity of the HCW will be developed.

Regulatory efforts to prevent transmission of HBV from HCW to the patients

As mentioned before, the first regulations to prevent transmission from HCW to patients came from USA.[17, 18] Similar recommendations[21] followed in the UK after the British investigations were reported.[19] Earlier a Consensus Conference held by the Health Canada Laboratory Center in 1996 proposed a ban on an HBeAg infected HCW continuing with EPIP.[22] This move was opposed by both the Canadian medical and dental associations, thus delaying the health policy on this issue.[23] A notice was issued by the Canadian health department in 1998.[23] Soon there were further recommendations which held that HBsAg and HBeAg positive HCW should be prevented from carrying out exposure-prone invasive procedures.[22]

To prevent HCW from getting infected in the first place, it was recommended that all the HCW should be vaccinated to acquire >10 mIU/ml of anti-HBs titers in the serum. Others have suggested that the HBsAg screening should begin at the point of entry in medical schools, followed by vaccination of the susceptible and counseling of positive students so that they do not choose disciplines that make them perform EPIP.

Legal issues

Before discussing the legal aspects, it may be worth mentioning that the heath-care providers are obliged to protect patients from any harm that might result from diagnostic and treatment modalities. They also have a duty to be responsible to their fellow colleagues, their hospitals, institutions, and the society. The actual implementation of these obligations brings to the fore several complex issues because of self-interest of different groups involved. It is, however, morally appropriate that an infected HCW should disclose infection status before exposing patients to the risks of infection and should also inform the hospital so as to permit the authorities to take appropriate action.

What is the legal position? In the USA,[24] two federal statutes, the Rehabilitation Act of 1973 and the Americans with Disabilities Act of 1990 provide anti-discrimination protection to employees with disabilities, provided the employee, despite his handicap, is able to perform basic duties for which he was hired. The employer is expected to display reasonable accommodation while permitting him to work. In 1987, however, the US Supreme Court ruled that the employment of an infective person carried significant risk and that employer was obliged to continue that employee in position provided he is satisfied that he presented no significant risk to others.[24] Significant risk was defined as the product of four factors: nature, duration, severity, and probability of transmission of infection. This judgment imposed that while continuing to provide employment, the hospital authorities have to examine in detail the individual HCW's case so as to ensure safety to patients, emphasize improved infection control, and allow restriction or reassignments of duties only if the employee rejects reasonable restrictions.

Health care provider in the USA has also to abide by the regulations of the Occupational Safety and Health Administration standards.[25] These refer to the need to conduct applied research to analyze risk and to carry out protective and educational programs, all of which are costly. If these standards are not followed, the hospital is liable to face legal action from the patients. Infected HCWs are therefore not expected to perform EPIP unless they have sought counsel from an expert review panel regarding what procedures they can perform without risk to the patients. Before they perform these procedures, the HCW are expected to notify about their infection status to the prospective patients and obtain their informed consent.

Currently, USA since 1991,[17] UK since 1993,[21] and Canada since 1998[23] are the only three countries that have government agencies regulations on transmission of blood-borne and intra-operative infections from HCW to patients. The United Kingdom has additionally regulations with the National Health Service that empowers the employer to test the HBV status of HCW at the time of offering employment and even for nursing and medical students at entry into their courses and deny them employment or admissions. It is expected that such regulations may eventually be adopted by other countries too.[26]

The Indian scene

Commensurate with a higher HBsAg prevalence rate[27] of up to 10% in Indian HCW, there is a possibility that the HCW performing EPIP could be transmitting infections to their patients at a higher rate than in the western countries. However, paucity of published work poses difficulty in realistic assessment of the situation prevailing in our hospitals.[28] There is an urgent need to carefully investigate patients who get infected following EPIP in our hospitals and trace these infections to their source. Undoubtedly, any such investigations or regulatory measures that might follow are likely to meet resistance from the HCW, of whom surgeons, form the major group. Such investigations need support from the hospital administrators, who may not be enthusiastic about investigating their staff. Alternatively, we may adopt the same steps that have been taken by advanced countries without generating data on the presumption that frequency of HBV transmission from the HCW-to-patient in our hospitals is much higher than in the western countries.

The issue of an HBV infected HCW requires a wide debate among the experts in our country and eventually an awareness campaign to educate HCWs, administrators, medical students, and nursing students. Since medical insurance is round the corner in the country, we can expect brisk activity of data generation and appropriate preventive steps in this direction in the near future. It stands to common sense and logic, however, that we ought to anyway have the following hospital regulations in place sooner than later: (i) HBsAg survey for all the HCW, (ii) HBeAg/HBV-DNA testing of all HBsAg positive HCW, (iii) counseling and education of all potentially infective HCW, (iv) prevention of infective HCW from performing EPIP, and (v) instituting policy regarding disclosing the infective status of the HCW to their patients.

What then is in store for an HBV infected Indian HCW in the future? Those currently merrily performing EPIP are likely to be uneasy since debates like those mentioned in this article are bound to attract the attention of the media and the public. Eventually, the following complex situations may arise: (i) identification of more HCW as carrying a risk to their patients, (ii) attempts by administration to move HCW to 'safer', possibly administrative duties or offering them early retirement benefits, (iii) attempts to resist such relocations by individuals or employees' associations through industrial actions and lawsuits, (iv) demands by administrators for informed consent from patients to be operated by infected HCW after detailed explanation of the risks of transmission of infection, and (v) litigations and demand for payment of compensation from patients detected to be infected for the first time after surgery. The last named situation demands a more thorough preoperative work-up for blood-borne or intraoperatively transmissible infections. An important fall out surely will be a higher hospital cost for patients.

What are the problems that will await the Indian hospitals? Issues that will be debated in future are the compensation to the HCW infected while working in the hospital and the retirement plans to be offered to them. To avoid these problems, hospitals need to have regulations in place that make it mandatory (a) to assess the baseline infection status at the time of employment, (b) to monitor periodically their infective status, (c) to have preventive policies like vaccination, disinfection and sterilization, use of universal precautions, etc., and (d) to issue timely warnings to an errant HCW. The HCW working in hospitals ignoring these aspects are likely to demand a high compensation from the hospitals accusing them for being responsible for their infections and health consequences and for being laid off specialized professional duties. Hospitals may have difficulty in deciding the exact quantum of compensation and the type of retirement benefits that can be offered to such an HCW. If all these hospital regulations are not in place at the time of original employment of an HCW, running hospitals may well prove a difficult problem with litigations and unwelcome court judgments after prolonged legal proceedings that are the order of the day in the Indian legal scene.

REFERENCES

1. Denes AE, Smith JL, Maynard JE, Doto IL, Berquist KR, Finkel AJ. Hepatitis B infection in physicians. Results of a nationwide seroepidemiologic survey. *JAMA* 1978; 239:210-2.
2. Segal HE, Llewellyn CH, Irwin G, Bancroft WH, Boe GP, Balaban DJ. Hepatitis B antigen and antibody in the US Army: Prevalence in health care personnel. *Am J Public Health* 1976;66:667-71.
3. Favero MS, Boylard EA. Microbiologic considerations. Disinfection and sterilization strategies and the potential for airborne transmission of blood-borne pathogens. *Surg Clin N Am* 1995;75:1071-89.
4. Robinson CG, Gladstone JL, Goodman S, Shulman BD. Outbreak of viral hepatitis in a municipal hospital. *Arch Intern Med* 1968;122:318-21.
5. Jovanovich JF, Saravolatz LD, Arking LM. The risk of hepatitis B among select employee groups in an urban hospital. *JAMA* 1983;250:1893-4.
6. Dienstag JL, Ryan DM. Occupational exposure to hepatitis B virus in hospital personnel: Infection or immunization? *Am J Epidemiol* 1982;115:26-39.
7. Hadler SC, Doto I, Maynard JE, Smith J, Clark B, Mosley J, Eickhoff T, et al. Occupational risk of hepatitis B in hospital workers. *Infect Control* 1985;6:24-31.
8. Wood RC, MacDonald KL, White KE, Hedberg CW, Hanson M, Osterholm MT. Risk factors for lack of detectable antibody following hepatitis B vaccination of Minnesota health care workers. *JAMA* 1993;270:2935-9.
9. Grady GF, Lee VA, Prince AM, Gitnick GL, Fawaz KAI. Hepatitis B immune globulin for accidental exposures among medical personnel: Final report of a multicenter controlled trial. *J Infect Dis* 1978; 138:625-38.
10. Centers for Disease Control: Universal precautions for preventing transmission of human immunodeficiency virus, hepatitis virus, and blood-borne pathogens in health-care settings. *MMWR* 1988;37: 377-88.
11. Lewis TL, Alter MJ, Chalmers TC, Holland PV, Purcell RH, Alling DW. A comparison of the frequency of hepatitis B antigen and antibody in hospital and non-hospital personnel. *N Engl J Med* 1973;289: 647-51.
12. Bell DM, Shapiro CN, Culver DL, Martone WJ, Curran JW, Hughes JM. Risk of hepatitis B and human immunodeficiency virus transmission to a patient from an infected surgeon due to percutaneous injury during an invasive procedure: estimates based on a model. *Infect Agents Dis* 1992;1:263-9.

13. Rimland LM, Parkin WE, Miller GB, Schrack WB. Hepatitis B outbreak traced to an oral surgeon. *N Engl J Med* 1977;296:953-8.
14. Snydman DR, Hindman SH, Wineland MD, Bryan JA, Maynard JE. Nosocomial viral hepatitis B: a cluster among staff with subsequent transmission to patients. *Ann Intern Med* 1976;85:573-7.
15. Centers for Disease Control: Recommendations for prevention of HIV transmission in health care settings. *MMWR* 1987;36(suppl 2S):16SA.
16. Chamberland ME, Ciesielski CA, Howard RJ, Fry DE, Bell DM. Occupational risk of infection with human immunodeficiency virus. *Surg Clin N Am* 1995;75:1057-70.
17. Centers for Disease Control: Recommendations for preventing transmission of human immunodeficiency virus and hepatitis B during exposure-prone invasive procedures. *MMWR* 1991; Morb Mortal Wkly Rep 40(No. RR-8):1-9.
18. Bell DM, Shapiro CN, Ciesielski CA, Chamberland ME. Preventing blood-borne pathogen transmission from health care workers to patients. The CDC perspective. *Surg Clin N Am* 1995;75:1189-1203.
19. The Incident Investigation Teams and others. Transmission of hepatitis B to patients from four infected surgeons without hepatitis B e antigen. *N Engl J Med* 1997;336:178-84.
20. Caspari G, Gerlich WH. Mandatory hepatitis B virus testing for doctors. *Lancet* 1998;352:991.
21. United Kingdom Health Departments: Protecting health care workers and patients from hepatitis B: Recommendations of the Advisory Group on Hepatitis. London, Her Majesty's Stationery Office, 1993.
22. Proceedings of the Consensus Conference on Infected Health Care Workers – risks for transmission of blood-borne pathogens. *Canad Commun Dis Rep* 1998:24(suppl 4).
23. Mandatory HBV-testing for Canada's doctors. *Lancet* 1998;352:466.
24. Rhodes RS, Telford GL, Hierholzer WJ, Barnes M. Blood-borne pathogen transmission from health care worker to patients. Legal issues and provider perspectives. *Surg Clin N Am* 1995;75:1205-17.
25. Department of Labor, Occupational Safety and Health administration: Occupational exposure to blood-borne pathogens: Final rule. *Federal Register* 1991;56:64175-81.
26. Chiarello LA, Cardo DM. Preventing transmission of hepatitis B virus from surgeons to patients. *Infect Control Hosp Epidemiol* 2002;23:301-2.
27. Kant L. *ICMR Bulletin* 1995.
28. Singal AK, Singal A, Shukla DK. Prevention and management of hepatitis B in India: results of a natural survey. *Indian J Gastroenterol* 2002;210(suppl 1):A15 (abstract).

Section V
Hepatitis B vaccination

33

Standardization and efficacy of hepatitis B vaccines in India

Surinder Singh, Rajesh Bhatia

Historically vaccines have been shown to be the most cost-effective approach to prevent, control, and eradicate communicable diseases. Safe and immunogenic vaccines are now available against hepatitis B, and it is possible to effectively prevent this serious infection. Hepatitis B vaccine also protects against hepatitis D virus, which being a defective virus is dependent on hepatitis B virus (HBV) for replication. World Health Organization (WHO) has recommended to include the hepatitis B vaccine in the national expanded program of immunization (EPI),[1] and this has been endorsed by the Indian Academy of Paediatrics[2] and the Indian Association for the Study of the Liver (INASL).[3] Presently, two types of vaccines are in use, i.e., the first generation, plasma derived heat inactivated HBV vaccines, and the second generation, genetically engineered or recombinant HBV vaccines. The classical approach of producing an attenuated or inactivated vaccine is not possible because HBV cannot be propagated in tissue culture. High production costs and the resultant high price of these vaccines is a major limiting factor in their use in the EPI. Live recombinant vaccines in vectors such as *Baculovirus* or bacteria or use of naked nucleic acid vaccines are the newer methodologies that are being studied.

PLASMA DERIVED VACCINES

The plasma derived vaccines consist predominantly of purified 22 nm particles of the S antigen of HBV that are derived from the plasma of healthy individuals with chronic HBV infection and inactivated with heat or formalin. Some vaccines also include varying amounts of pre-S1 or pre-S2 antigens. The effectiveness and safety of these vaccines has been demonstrated in adults and in neonates born to HBsAg positive mothers.[4] The inherent drawbacks of this vaccine include: limited availability of the serum as a source of the antigen for producing vaccine, elaborate purification and virion inactivation procedures, and ever lurking concern about contamination with other human pathogens associated with blood.[5]

RECOMBINANT DNA VACCINES

The genetically engineered hepatitis B vaccines are prepared by recombinant DNA technology by expressing hepatitis B surface antigen in the prokaryotic cells (*Escherichia coli* and *Bacillus subtilis*) or in eukaryotic system such as mammalian cells, and yeast cells *(Saccharomyces cerevisiae, Pichia pastoris,* or *Hansenula polymorpha)*. Eukaryotic systems are candidates of choice because they have a better capability of expressing and assembling recombinant HBsAg in its native configuration. The development and production of a recombinant vaccine in an expression system and its quality assurance goes through a number of steps (Fig. 1).

The yeast cell derived vaccines presently available in India contain only the protein S of the hepatitis B virus and not the additional pre-S1 and pre-S2 sequences of the S protein. Some studies have shown that pre-S containing vaccines tended to produce a more rapid immuno-

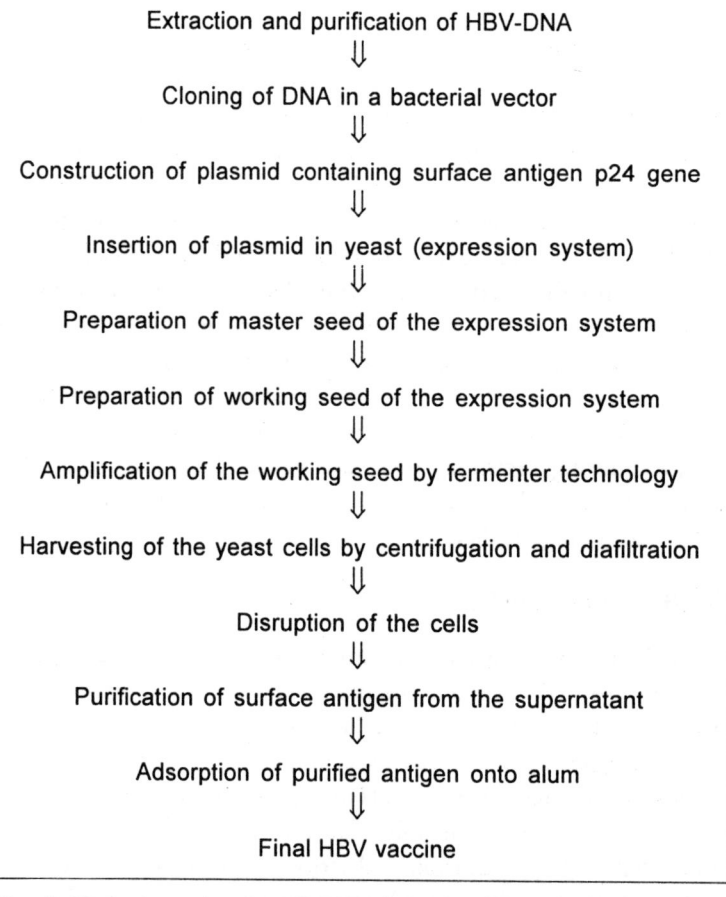

Fig. 1. Flow chart showing manufacturing process of rDNA vaccine

genic response.[5] The development of vaccines that comprise more than one antigenic viral protein, i.e., antigens encoded by the S, pre-S1, and pre-S2 genes of the hepatitis B virus envelope, is underway.[6] The hepatitis B vaccines containing the pre-S gene product may also help in the control of escape mutant of hepatitis B and mutations to the "a" determinant of HBsAg which enable the hepatitis virus to resist neutralization by specific immunoglobulin (HBIg) or vaccine induced anti-HBs.

Quality assurance of rDNA hepatitis B vaccines

There is a system of pre-release certification of vaccines in our country involving various agencies (Fig. 2). This national regulatory mechanism comprises:

(a) Drugs Controller General of India, who is the Chief Licensing Authority for vaccines, and
(b) National Institute of Biologicals (NIB) which is being set up by the Government of India as an apex institution to monitor the quality of biologicals including vaccines before they are released for EPI/non-EPI programs and for marketing. Till such time National Institute of Biologicals becomes fully functional, the quality control of various vaccines including hepatitis B vaccines is being done by the Central Drugs Laboratory, Kasauli, HP.

Assessing the potency of hepatitis B vaccines is the most critical quality control parameter. Potency is estimated by either mouse immunogenicity test or a suitably validated *in vitro* HBsAg control assays, i.e., ELISA or RIA using a reference preparation in parallel. The reference preparation material can be developed either in-house or obtained from the WHO.

Every new vaccine to be introduced in the market must demonstrate its immunogenicity and safety in healthy subjects. This is to ensure that the intended vaccine can consistently produce predictable rise in antibody titers and can offer protection to the human beings. Although

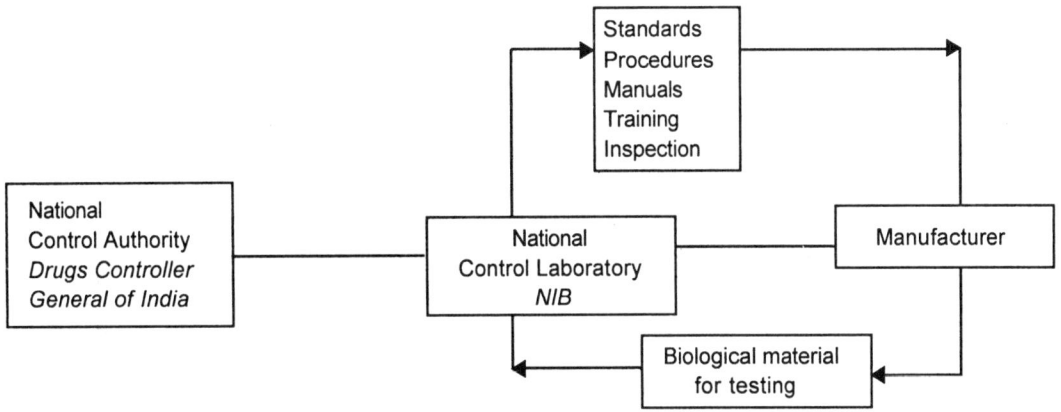

Fig. 2. National regulatory mechanism of release of vaccines

both the plasma derived and the recombinant vaccines are equally effective in preventing HBV transmission, the latter has the advantages of unlimited supply, no blood products being involved, and a shorter production cycle. In most parts of developed world the recombinant vaccines have gradually replaced the plasma derived HBV vaccines and the same is happening in India.

Vaccine dosage and administration

Hepatitis B vaccine is available as a one ml suspension containing 20 µg of protein (adult dose) or as a 0.5 ml suspension containing 10 µg protein (pediatric dose), adsorbed onto aluminium hydroxide adjuvant and thiomersal is included as a preservative. This vaccine should be administered by intramuscular (IM) injection in the deltoid region in adults and children, and in the anterolateral thigh in infants. Gluteal administration may result in sub optimal result. The vaccine should not be given intravenously or intradermally. Intradermal administration is associated with an inferior immunological response compared with IM administration.[7,8] However, subcutaneous administration should be used in patients with severe bleeding tendencies such as haemophilia, to reduce the risk of haematoma.

Two schedules are recommended for vaccination with hepatitis B vaccines; 0, 1 and 6 months which is the standard schedule; 0, 1, 2 and 12 months which is the immunization schedule used when rapid protection is required. These schedules give maximum flexibility and optimum protection in different circumstances. However, after completion of 3 doses of hepatitis B vaccine, seroprotection rates and/or anti-HBs geometric mean titers have been reported to be significantly higher in those receiving the standard schedule.[9,10] This vaccine is not available in a freeze dried form. It must not be used if it is frozen inadvertently. Inoculation of such preparation can lead to granuloma formation and may result in vaccine failure.

Efficacy studies

The immunogenicity of hepatitis B vaccines is generally evaluated according to three parameters: the sero-conversion rate, seroprotection rate and peak geometric mean titers (GMT) of antibody to hepatitis-B surface antigen (anti-HBs). Seroprotection is defined as the development of the anti-HBs titers ≥ 10 mIU/ml after the vaccination schedule. This antibody concentration has been accepted as conferring protection against clinically significant infection by the US Advisory Committee on Immunization Practices (ACIP), and the WHO.[11] In the United Kingdom the limit of 100 mIU/ml is considered necessary for protection, particularly in high-risk individuals.[12-14] It has been demonstrated that the best indication of response towards hepatitis B vaccination is the measurement of antibodies to HBsAg in the serum obtained 1–3 months after the last dose.

The hepatitis B vaccine is highly immunogenic. The sero-conversion and seroprotection rates are found to be more than 96% after three doses. In some cases there is a virtual 100% seroconversion and seroprotection following 3 doses and there appears to be a dose-dependent effect on the antibody concentrations.[11,15] The antibody response of the neonates and the children receiving 10 µg dose of the vaccine have been found to be slightly higher than the response in the adults receiving 20 µg dose.[16] The clinical data of hepatitis B vaccines available in India is given in Table 1.[17-29a] The hepatitis B vaccines, which are being produced indigenously, are yeast derived and different manufacturers are using different yeasts as expression systems, i.e., *Saccharomyces cerevisiae*, *Pichia pastoris* or *Hansenula polymorpha* depending upon the technology available. These indigenously produced recombinant hepatitis B vaccines contain only the protein-S of the hepatitis B virus. Both the published and unpublished reports of field studies done in India on these rDNA vaccines indicate excellent seroconversion and seroprotection (>95%) in almost all the vaccines. These vaccines have been

Table 1. Clinical trials of recombinant vaccines available in India in healthy adults, children and neonates

Manufacturer/ Importer (brand name)	No. of vaccines	Age (yrs)	Vaccine dose (µg)	Immunization schedule (months)	Time of sampling for anti-HBs (months)	Seroprotection rates in % anti-HBs titres (mIU/ml)	Geometric mean titers (mIU/ml)
Bharat Biotech Intl. Ltd., Hyderabad[17] (Revac-B)	60	5-10	10	0,1,2	3	100	17000
Shantha Biotechnics Pvt. Ltd., Hyderabad[18,19] (Shanvac-B)	81 55	18-40 18-40	20 20	0,1,2 0,1,2	3 3	100 96.4	2246 419
Panacea Biotec Ltd., Delhi[20-23] (Enivac-B)	60 61 102 110	18-24 17-50 40-65 14-35	20 20 20 20	0,1,6 0,1,6 0,1,6 0,1,6	7 4 7 7	100 100* 85.30 100	1456 NM 136.10 NM
SmithKline Beecham, Belgium[24-29a] (Engerix-B)	241 507 392 81 205 223 42	20-50 16-40 39-70 0-10 <10 2-6 22-60	20 vs 10 20 vs 10 20 vs 10 10 10 10 vs 2.5 20	0,1,6 0,1,6 0,1,6 0,1,6 0,1,6 0,1,6 0,1,6	7 7 8 7 7 7 7	98.3 vs 93.1 99.6 vs 99.2 91 vs 85 98 99.9 98.4 vs 98.3 95	15018 vs 1110 22601 vs 3569 837 vs 340 7640 9500 8062 vs 3732 NM

NM : Not mentioned
* Only sero-conversion data mentioned.

demonstrated to be safe, potent, and efficacious. The choice of the vaccine to be used depends upon the cost and the discretion of the clinician. The seroprotective levels of anti-HBs have been reported to persist for at least 10–12 years in most of the immunized children and adults.[30] The greatest reduction in anti-HBs titers occurs during the first year after immunization, and the rate of decline appears to depend upon the peak anti-HBs response attained after completion of a full immunization course.[30] The individuals with higher anti-HBs titers maintain seroprotective level of anti-HBs for a longer period as compared to individuals with lower anti-HBs titers.

Low-responders and non-responders

Although, the immune response after three doses hepatitis B vaccine course is generally good, there is a small proportion of population which does not respond adequately to immunization with currently used vaccination schedule.[31] About 5–10% of adults are low responders, i.e., they develop anti-HBs titers ranging from 10–99 mIU/ml only. Host-related factors such as obesity, smoking, age, male gender, and genetic factors have been recognized to be significant factors responsible for non-or low-response to vaccination.[32,33] However, non-responsiveness to hepatitis B vaccines can be overcome in almost all the cases by an appropriate vaccination schedule.[21,34]

Safety and reactogenicity

The adverse events associated with hepatitis B vaccines are generally mild and transient. Of the adverse events reported, mild soreness lasting for 1–2 days and induration at the injection site are the most frequent local reactions; fatigue and headache were the most common systemic symptoms. Other less common symptoms include influenza-like symptoms, vomiting, dizziness, pruritus, arthralgia, myalgia, diarrhoea, urticaria, paraesthesia, and somnolence.[35,36] Serious adverse events have been reported rarely in patients immunized with hepatitis-B vaccine and no causal relationship has been established between the development of chronic illness including multiple sclerosis, rheumatoid arthritis or other immune-mediated or neurological disorders and the administration of hepatitis B vaccine.[37-42]

FUTURE NEEDS

Hepatitis B vaccines have proved to be an effective tool to tackle the problem of HBV infection. Moreover, they have a significant potential to reduce the incidence of hepatocellular carcinoma. Indigenously produced recombinant hepatitis B vaccines are safe, generally well tolerated, and highly immunogenic as seen from the various clinical trials and their use under field conditions. However, these vaccines are very costly and are beyond the reach of an average human being in India. The cost of the vaccine is the main factor hampering the introduction of hepatitis B vaccine in the EPI. The Indian biotech industry needs to develop technology which can help to bring down the cost of these vaccines to the same as that of EPI vaccines. There is also a need to develop hepatitis B vaccines that comprise more than one antigenic viral protein, as studies have shown that pre-S containing vaccines tend to produce a more rapid immunogenic response.[43] Mathematical models forecast that immunity after hepatitis B vaccination may last more than 20 years or even life-long, however, long-term follow-up is necessary to determine the exact persistence of protective immunity against HBV infection.

REFERENCES

1. Centres for Disease Control. Protection against viral hepatitis. Recommendations of the Immunization Practices Advisory Committee (ACIP). *MMWR* 1990;39:1-26.
2. Indian Academy of Pediatrics's immunization timetable in pediatrics. *Indian Pediatr* 1995;32:1329.
3. Sarin SK. Summary and recommendations of single theme conferences on hepatitis B and C: Indian Association for Study of the Liver (INASL). *J Gastroenterol Hepatol* 2002;17:S197-203.
4. Panda SK, Ramesh R, Rao Kanury VS, Gupta A, Zuckerman AJ, Nayak NC. Comparative evaluation of the immunogenicity of yeast derived (recombinant and plasma-derived hepatitis B vaccine in infants. *J Med Virol* 1991;35:297-302.
5. Lee PI, Lee CY. Practical considerations in converting from plasma-derived to recombinant hepatitis B vaccines. *Biodrugs* 1998;10:11-25.
6. Iwarson S. New approaches to hepatitis A and B vaccines. *APMIS* 1995;103:321-6.
7. Struve J, Aronsson B, Frenning B, Granath F, Von Sydown, Weiland O. Intramuscular versus intradermal administration of a recombinant hepatitis B vaccine: a comparison of response rates and analysis of factors influencing the antibody response. *Scand J Infect Dis* 1992;24:423-9.
8. Hollinger FB. Factors influencing the immune response to hepatitis B vaccine, booster dose guidelines, and vaccine protocol recommendations. *Am J Med* 1989;87(suppl 3A):536-40.
9. Marsano LS, Greenberg RN, Kirkpatrick RB, Zetterrman RK, Christiansen A, Smith DJ, De Medina MD. Comparison of a rapid hepatitis B immunization schedule to the standard schedule for adults. *Am J Gastronterol* 1996;91:111-5.
10. Hess G, Hingst V, Cseke J, Bock HL, Clemens R. Influence of vaccination schedules and host factors on antibody response following hepatitis B vaccination. *Eur J Clin Microbiol Infect Dis* 1992;11:334-40.
11. Assad S, Francis A. Over a decade of experience with a yeast recombinant hepatitis B vaccine. *Vaccine* 2000;18:57-67.
12. Lunn JA. Hepatitis B vaccination. *Br Med J* 1993;307:732.
13. Halsey NA, Duclos P, Van Damme P, Margolis H. Hepatitis B vaccine and central nervous system demyelinating diseases. *Pediatr Inf Dis J* 1999;18:23-4.
14. Morgan D, Ed. A code of practice for implementation of the UK hepatitis B immunization guidelines for the protection of patients and staff. London: *BMA*, 1995 (edited for British Medical Assoc. Board of Science and Education).
15. Gunn TR, Woodfield DG. The persistence of anti-hepatitis B surface antibodies to three years of age: is a hepatitis B vaccine booster required? *Z Med J* 1993;106:499-501.
16. Wood RC, MacDonald K, White KE, Hedberg CW, Hanson M, Osterholm MT. Risk factors for lack of detectable antibody following hepatitis B vaccination of Minnesota health care workers. *JAMA* 1993;270:2935-9.
17. Lakshmi G, Reddy RP, Kumar KK, Bhawani NV, Dayanand M. Study of the safety, immunogenicity

and sero-conversions of a Hepatitis B vaccine in malnourished children of India. *Vaccine* 2000;18: 2009-14.
18. Abraham P, Mistry FP, Bapat MR, Sharma G, Reddy GR, Prasad KS, Ramanna V. Evaluation of a new recombinant DNA hepatitis B vaccine (Shanvac B). *Vaccine* 1999;17:1125-9.
19. Joshi N, Kumar A, Sreenivas DV, Palan S, Kumar N. Safety and immunogenicity of indigenous recombinant hepatitis B vaccine (Shanvac-B) in comparison with commercially available vaccine. *Indian J Gastroenterol* 2000;19:71-3.
20. Kaur H, Mani A. Seroprotection following Enivac HB, a recombinant hepatitis B vaccine. *Indian J Gastroenterol* 2000;19:41.
21. Kar P, Jandwani, P, Khurana V, Kumar V, Gupta RK, Sama S, Wadhawan S. Sero-conversion with rDNA hepatitis B vaccine of Cuban Origin. *Indian J Gastroenterol* 1997;16:161.
22. Das K, Kar P, Singh S, Kumar V, Sharma BK. HLA phenotype and response to a single booster dose in non-responders to hepatitis B vaccination among age group more than forty years in north Indians. *J Gastroenterol Hepatol* 2000;15(suppl):B32.
23. Jain A, Mathur US, Jandwani P, Gupta RK, Kumar V, Kar P. A multicentric evaluation of recombinant DNA hepatitis B vaccine of Cuban origin. *Trop Gastroenterol* 2000;21:14-7.
24. Renzulli G, Gottardell L, Canazza S, Hansen E. Immunogenicity of two hepatitis B vaccines produced by means of recombinant DNA technique. In 35th Congresso Nazionale de Igiene. Montecatini Termi, Italy. October 21-24, 1992; pp. 116-9.
25. Chairamonte M, Majori S, Ngatchu T, Moschen ME, Baldo V, Renzulli G, Simoncello I, et al. Two different dosages of yeast derived recombinant hepatitis B vaccines, a comparison of immunogenicity. *Vaccine* 1996;14:135-7.
26. Treadwell TL, Keeffe EB, Lake J, Read A, Friedman LS, Goldman lS, Howell CD, et al. Immunogenicity of two recombinant hepatitis B vaccines in older individuals. *Am J Med* 1993;95:584-8.
27. Moyes C. Milne A. Immunogenicity of a recombinant yeast derived hepatitis B vaccine (Engerix-B) in children. *NZ Med J* 1988;101:162-4.
28. Catania G, Di Ciommo V, Concato C. Vaccination against hepatitis B virus in children and adolescents in a pediatric hospital. *Recenti Prog Med* 1996;87:271-4.
29. Goldfarb J, Medendorp SV, Nagamori K, Buscarino C, Krause D. Comparison study of the immunogenicity and safety of 5 and 10 µg dosages of a recombinant hepatitis B vaccine in healthy children. *Pediatr Infect Dis* 1996;15:768-71.
29a. Broor SL, Singal AK. Efficacy and safety of Engerix B in Indian subjects. Data on file (unpublished) SKB Pharmaceuticals, 1989.
30. Gesemann M. Scheierman N. Quantification of hepatitis B vaccine-induced antibodies as a predictor of anti-HBs persistence. *Vaccine* 1995;13:443-7.
31. Grob PJ. *Unresolved issues in hepatitis B immunization. In:* Hollinger FB, Ed. Viral hepatitis and liver disease. Baltimore: Williams & Wilkins, 1990; pp. 856-60.
32. Leroux Roels G. Nonresponsiveness to hepatitis B vaccine. *Hepatocite Int Hepatitis Update* 1993;10: 17-8.
33. Desombere I. Willems A, Leroux-Roels G. Response to hepatitis B vaccine: multiple HLA genes are involved. *Tissue Antigens* 1998;51:593-604.
34. Bock HL, Clemens R, Sanger R, Vadheim M. Low and non-responders do respond after additional hepatitis B vaccine doses. Triennial International Symposium on Viral Hepatitis and Liver Disease. Rome, Italy, 1996.
35. Andre FE. Overview of a 5-year clinical experience with a yeast-derived hepatitis B vaccine. *Vaccine* 1990;8(suppl):S74-8.
36. Singh S, Sharma DR. Tolerability of a recombinant DNA hepatitis B vaccine-results of post-marketing surveillance. *J Commun Dis* 1999;31:53-5.

37. Kakar A, Sethi PK. Gullian Barre syndrome associated with hepatitis B vaccination. *Indian J Pediatr* 1997;64:710-2.
38. Expanded program on Immunization (EPI): lack of evidence that hepatitis B vaccine causes multiple sclerosis. *Weekly Epidemiological Record* 1997;72:149-52.
39. Hepatitis B vaccine: What you may have heard and what you should know (fact sheet). Hepatitis Branch, National Center for Infectious Diseases; National Immunization Program: Centers for Disease Control and Prevention (CDC): 1998;30.
40. Geier MR, Geier DA. Hepatitis B vaccination safety. *Ann Pharmacother* 2002;36:370-4.
41. Geier DA, Geier MR. Hepatitis B vaccination and arthritic adverse reactions: analysis of the Vaccine Adverse Events Reporting System (VAERS) database. *Clin Exp Rheumatol* 2002;10:119.
42. McPhillips H, Marcuse EK. Vaccine safety. *Curr Probl Pediatr* 2001;31:91-121.
43. Guaan XJ, Guan XJ, Wu YZ, Jia ZC, Shi TD, Tang Y. Construction and characterization of an experimental ISCOMS-based hepatitis B polypeptide. *Vaccine* 2002;8:294-7.

Hepatitis B: who should be vaccinated?

Philip Abraham

The epidemiology of hepatitis B virus (HBV) infection varies with the geographic and socio-economic patterns. India is in intermediate-endemicity zone, with a reported HBsAg prevalence rate of 3–5%.[1-3] Whereas in high-endemicity regions newborns of infected mothers are at maximum risk for acquiring HBV infection (vertical transmission), in intermediate-endemicity areas the populations at high-risk include children in the early years of life, medical and paramedical personnel exposed to blood and blood products, individuals with multiple sexual partners, those who need to receive multiple blood transfusions, intravenous drug abusers, family members, and contacts of infected patients (horizontal transmission).

PREVENTION STRATEGIES

Universal barrier precautions, use of disposable instruments, adequate sterilization of reusable equipment, and blood-banking discipline go a long way in preventing the spread of the hepatitis B infection. However, the only fail-safe way to prevent this dreaded disease is hepatitis B vaccination.

VACCINATION OPTIONS FOR INDIA

The question that arises when undertaking a vaccination program on a wide scale is whether it should be extended to the entire population, only to those at high-risk, or to all the newborns. The last option is undertaken with the aim of long-term benefit to the population. To initiate a program for long-term benefit requires commitment; first, the benefits are not immediate and second, the immediate consequences of hepatitis B infection are only sometimes fatal and are not very morbid, and so are not sensational. However, a program of newborn vaccination has been shown to give dramatic benefits over a decade or so in other countries with similar endemicity.[4,5]

Vaccination of total population

Vaccinating an entire population is unrealistic. The cost in India, based on the current commercial price of approximately Rs. 200 per dose for the recombinant vaccine, would be a staggering Rs. 600 billion or so. A more selective and rational approach to vaccination is therefore required. It should be clear that determining an appropriate approach is relevant only to a program sponsored through public funds. An individual's decision to get vaccinated at his own cost, irrespective of the level of risk, should always be accepted. The present practice of conducting public camps where this vaccine is administered at subsidized cost by non-governmental agencies may also be seen in this light.

Vaccination of high-risk population

In the United States, a low-endemicity country, a strategy to vaccinate only high-risk individuals was followed when the vaccine was first introduced.[6] Intermediate-endemicity countries like India were advised by the WHO to follow a similar policy. Retrospective analysis, however, showed that this strategy was a failure; there was no decline in the incidence of HBV infection in the US till the late 1980s. In fact, there was a rise in the incidence among certain groups (77% increase among parenteral drug abusers).[6]

The major problems with this strategy were the difficulty in identifying and approaching all members of high-risk groups, many of whom did not wish to avail of health care facilities. Inadequate motivation was another problem, less than 50% of high-risk health care workers, even in the US, availed of complete vaccination despite full information about the disease and the inherent risk.[6] Our own experience with vaccination showed high default rate, especially among doctors, despite the vaccine being made available at no cost to them.[7] Similar experience has been reported from other centers in the country, both in the public and private sectors.[8] Although vaccinating the high-risk groups is still prudent for those groups, to make a large-scale impact, the target base has to be widened.

Based on cost-benefit calculations, the other approaches considered included vaccination of newborns, adolescents (all or only high-risk), and high-risk adults, in different combinations. The current recommendation from the Immunization Practices Advisory Committee (ACIP), US Department of Health and Human Services, is universal immunization of infants, and all the high-risk adolescents and adults.[9] Could a similar policy be adopted in India?

Vaccination of newborns or infants

Universal immunization of infants has been calculated to be cost-effective in our country; in fact, in the long-term, it has been calculated to be less expensive than a policy of screening mothers for HBV markers and vaccinating only at risk newborns.[10] Apart from the cost saving, it must be remembered that the major route of transmission in intermediate-endemicity countries is horizontal, and infants are more likely to acquire the infection in early life rather than at birth.

The HBeAg positivity rate among HBsAg positive Indian women was only 12% in one study.[11] This information is important because immunization of babies born to HBeAg-positive mothers is only 50–75% effective in preventing transmission of HBV, whereas it is 95–100% effective in preventing infection in children born to HBeAg–negative mothers. The advantages of universal infant vaccination are manifold. Parents are likely to accept a vaccine against hepatitis B, especially if it could be delivered in combination with the other vaccines. In addition to decreasing the prevalence of infection, this strategy reduces the risk of horizontal transmission, thus conferring 'herd immunity'.

While it is theoretically possible that hepatitis B infection could be eradicated by universal childhood immunization, there are several biological and practical issues that make this difficult. First, a small proportion of infections occur *in utero* (from HBsAg positive mothers) and cannot be prevented by active or passive immunization at birth. Second, both combined passive/active immunization and active immunization alone fail to prevent transmission completely between HBeAg-positive mothers and their newborns, irrespective of the doses and schedules used. In general, active/passive immunization can be expected to reduce transmission from chronically infected HBeAg-positive mothers by more than 90%. Third, programs that rely upon interventions shortly after birth, or within the first days of life, are difficult to implement at least in rural areas, where the health system is not geared to deliver the vaccine.

Since the benefit from vaccinating newborns will be seen only after a few decades, there is a need for continuing immunization of high-risk adolescents and adults, the population at more immediate risk of infection. Adolescents are specifically considered because of their imminent exposure to the world of risk. Vaccinating all the newborns and persons below 16 years of age was considered in Israel, another country with intermediate endemicity (HBsAg prevalence rate of 2%). This approach was shown to yield a benefit-to-cost ratio of 1.9:1 for health services only; inclusion of indirect benefits increased the ratio to 2.8:1. This plan was, however, shelved because of the high initial investment required, which was calculated as US$ 18 million (in 1990).[12] A subsequent decision to vaccinate only newborns was still shown to yield a benefit ratio of 1.5:1.[13] Direct extrapolation of these results to our country may be difficult as health care costs are possibly less and so the benefit-to-cost ratio would be lower. This brings down the available option to targeting only high-risk adolescents and adults in addition to vaccinating all newborns.

WHO IS "HIGH-RISK"?

Health care workers

Exposure to HBV infection is an occupational hazard for health care workers and public safety workers who are exposed to blood in the work place.[9] Surgeons, pathologists, gastroenterologists, operating room staff, blood bank, laboratory technicians, staff working in hemodialysis centers, emergency staff, and dentists and dental assistants represent the highest risk groups. In one study, the prevalence of HBsAg among doctors, nurses, and technicians was found to be 8%, 10%, and 12%, respectively, much higher than in the general population and among office workers and ancillary staff (lift operators, floor supervisors, watchmen, etc.) working in the hospital, who had a prevalence of only 1%.[14]

Thus, workers who perform tasks involving contact with blood or body fluids should be vaccinated, and vaccination should be completed during training in schools of medicine, dentistry, nursing, laboratory technology, and other allied health professions, i.e., before trainees have their first contact with blood. Workers whose exposure to blood is extremely infrequent may not be included in the high-risk vaccination program.

Recipients of blood products or hemodialysis

Vaccination for patients receiving blood products is mandatory especially in India, where a large number of blood banks do not screen for HBV or use methods which are not sensitive.[15, 16] It should be initiated as soon as the diagnosis of a disease requiring blood products or multiple blood transfusions is made, e.g., hemophilia, aplastic anemia, leukemia, hemoglobinopathies, and patients awaiting major surgery. Pre-vaccination screening may be worthwhile if a patient has received multiple transfusions earlier.

Both patients and staff of hemodialysis centers are susceptible. In India, approximately 25% of patients undergoing hemodialysis contract hepatitis B (our unpublished data) or are chronically infected with HBV.[17] Transmission of patient-to-patient and from patient-to-staff in dialysis centers may result from dialyser malfunctions, sharing of contaminated equipment, accidental tissue penetrations with contaminated needles, possible airborne spread, and environmental contamination. Unfortunately, in patients with chronic renal failure on maintenance hemodialysis, the rate of development of anti-HBs after standard doses of vaccine is disappointing.[18, 19] Hence, twice the usual dose of hepatitis B vaccine has been recommended.[9] Vaccination in patients with chronic renal disease appears to be more effective if initiated before the onset of hemodialysis.[20] Family members of these patients are also at high-risk; hence, routine vaccination should be advised for them also.

Inmates and staff of institutions for mentally handicapped

Exposure to blood, saliva, skin lesions, and other infective body fluids imposes an increased risk of infection in this category. Thus, patients on first entry into such institutions should be vaccinated. Personnel, including training and teaching staff, directly involved in patient care over a period of time in such institutions should be given the benefit of vaccination.

Homosexual men and individuals with multiple sexual partners

All susceptible patients presenting to sexually-transmitted disease clinics, those with homosexual habits, promiscuous heterosexuals, and prostitutes should be vaccinated as early as possible, after these sexual practices begin.

Parenteral drug abusers

The incidence of infection is very high in this group due to sharing of contaminated needles; vaccination should ideally begin as soon as drug abuse begins, a goal that possibly cannot be achieved.

Contacts and sexual partners of HBV patients

All individuals in close contact with HBsAg positive subjects over a period of time are at increased risk of acquiring HBV, sexual partners being at the highest risk. Thus, vaccination is recommended for all household and sexual contacts of a person identified to be having chronic HBV infection. The risk is highest amongst spouses, followed by parents, offspring, and siblings.[21] Casual contacts of HBsAg positive subjects in whom exposure occurs in classroom or working place do not appear to be at increased risk, and vaccination for them is not recommended.[9]

Family contacts of patients with acute hepatitis B, other than infants less than one year of age, may not require prophylaxis for hepatitis B unless they have had identifiable exposure to blood and body fluids of the index patient. Post-exposure vaccination of spouses of patients with acute hepatitis B failed to provide protection,[22] and hepatitis B immune globulin (HBIg) has been shown to be 75% effective in preventing infections among them.[23] The ACIP recommendation in this situation is to administer a single dose of HBIg (0.06 ml/kg) and vaccination should be initiated if it can be started within 14 days of the last sexual contact. If the persons are not from a high-risk group for whom vaccine is routinely recommended, only a single dose of HBIg need to be given. Repeat test of HBsAg can be done after 3 months, with no vaccination required if it is negative.

Following inadvertent percutaneous or mucosal exposure to HBsAg-positive (or possibly positive) blood, unvaccinated persons should be immediately vaccinated. Administration of HBIg is recommended by the ACIP if the source is known to be HBsAg-positive. If the person has been previously vaccinated, with the response to vaccination unknown, a test for anti-HBs should be done and booster dose of vaccine administered if the titer is inadequate.

Others

Long-term prisoners are at increased risk of acquiring HBV, mainly by homosexual activity and parenteral drug abuse; they should thus be vaccinated. Alcoholics are at increased risk of acquiring HBV; also, the response to vaccination in this population is subnormal. Double-dose vaccination has been tried with variable success. Staff of custodial institutions and rescue services also should be vaccinated.

Is screening necessary before vaccination?

Another aspect that needs to be considered is whether to screen for HBV markers prior to vaccination. This will depend on the cost of screening and of the vaccine, and the likely yield from screening.

Let us consider this in health care workers in our country, where the prevalence of HBsAg is 5–10% while that of anti-HBs is nearly 15%,[7,14] a total of 25% who may not require vaccination (presuming titers are protective). If a cohort of 10,000 high-risk individuals is to be vaccinated without screening, the cost will be Rs. 6 million (at Rs. 200 a dose, excluding administrative costs). If the same cohort is to be screened before vaccination, the cost of testing will be approximately Rs. 6 million (cost per test of HBsAg and anti-HBs, or of anti-HBc alone, Rs. 600), which will have to be added to the cost of vaccinating susceptible individuals (75%), i.e., Rs. 4.5 million. Thus, this approach will be costlier than vaccinating individuals without screening. These calculations will obviously not hold true if the prevalence of markers in the cohort is higher or the cost of screening and vaccine is considerably lower.[24] It should be remembered that the positivity of viral markers depends on the duration a health-care worker has been in the profession. For a mass vaccination policy, an approach of no prior screening may therefore be followed. However, at an individual level, this raises two problems. First, the vaccinated person will be under the false notion of being safe and protected. Second, this opens the possibility of a misdiagnosis of vaccine failure.

MUTANT VIRUSES

Finally, a few important considerations about mutant viruses need to be addressed. Immune pressure exerted by immunoprophylaxis at birth may select for a mutant virus. Mutations in the 'a' determinant have been detected in almost 22% of vaccinated children as compared to the finding of precore mutant in almost half the unvaccinated children who developed infection.[25] However, mutation in the 'a' determinant was not an important cause of failure to prevent maternal-infant transmission of HBV by active post-exposure hepatitis B immunization in China.[26]

The identification of hepatitis B antibody escape mutants may have important implications for vaccine efficacy. Antibodies to the surface antigen are present in the sera of immunized subjects, but the mutant virus is not neutralized by this antibody and can replicate as a competent virus. The causes for concern are the failure to detect HBsAg, which may lead to HBV transmission through donated blood[27] and second, the mutated HBV may infect previously immunized subjects.[28] Newer vaccines may be needed with immunogenicity against mutants, though the number of subjects who would benefit from this exercise would be small.

REFERENCES

1. Elavia AJ, Banker DD. Prevalence of hepatitis B surface antigen and its subtypes in high-risk group subjects and voluntary blood donors in Bombay. *Ind J Med Res* 1991;93:280-5.
2. Tandon BN, Acharya SK, Tandon A. Epidemiology of hepatitis B virus infection in India. *Gut* 1996;38(suppl 2):S56-9.
3. Satoskar A, Ray V. Prevalence of hepatitis B surface antigen (HBsAg) in blood donors from Bombay. *Trop Geogr Med* 1992;44:119-21.
4. Goh KT. Prevention and control of hepatitis B virus infection in Singapore. *Ann Acad Med Singapore* 1997;26:671-81.
5. Chunsuttiwat S, Biggs BA, Maynard J, Thamapalo S, Laoboripat S, Bovoronsin S, Charavasari U, et al. Integration of hepatitis B vaccination into the expanded program on immunization in Chonburi and Chiangmai provinces, Thailand. *Vaccine* 1997;15:769-74.
6. Bloom BS, Hillman AL, Fendrick AM, Schewartz JS. A reappraisal of hepatitis B virus vaccination strategies using cost-effectiveness analysis. *Ann Intern Med* 1993;118:298-306.
7. Rajadhyaksha KP, Haridas V, Plumber ST, Pipalia DH, Kamat RS, Abraham P, Naik SR. Efficacy of low-dose intradermal hepatitis B vaccine. *Indian J Gastroenterol* 1988;7:111.
8. Desai HG, Trikannad S, Thakkar R, Dhunjibhoy KR, Karnik SR. Intradermal route for prophylaxis against hepatitis B: loss of potency in relation to time. *Indian J Gastroenterol* 1988;7:109-10.
9. Recommendations of the Immunization Practices Advisory Committee (ACIP). Hepatitis B virus: a comprehensive strategy for eliminating transmission in the United States through universal childhood vaccination. *MMWR* 1991;40:1-25.
10. Aggarwal R, Naik SR. Prevention of hepatitis B infection. The appropriate strategy for India. *Natl Med J India* 1994;7:216-20.
11. Prakash C, Sharma RS, Bhatia R, Verghese T, Datta KK. Prevalence in north India of hepatitis B carrier state amongst pregnant women. *Southeast Asian J Trop Med Public Health* 1998;29:80-4.
12. Ginsberg GM, Berger S, Shouval D. Cost benefit analysis of a nationwide inoculation programme against viral hepatitis B in an area of intermediate endemicity. *Bull WHO* 1992;70:757-67.
13. Ginsberg GM, Shouval D. Cost-benefit analysis of a nationwide neonatal inoculation programme against hepatitis B in an area of intermediate endemicity. *J Epidemiol Community Health* 1992;46:587-94.
14. Elavia AJ, Banker DO. Hepatitis B virus infection in hospital personnel. *Natl Med J India* 1992;5:265-8.
15. Desai DC. Post transfusion hepatitis — now HCV, how many more? *J Assoc Phys India* 1993;41:190-1.
16. Kapoor D, Saxena R, Sood B, Sarin SK. Blood transfusion practices in India: results of a national survey. *Indian J Gastroenterol* 2000;19:64-7.
17. Gunasekaran V, Kirubakaran MG, Jhony KV, Sahstry JC, John TJ. Hepatitis B viral infection in a renal unit in India. *Ind J Med Res* 1979;70:1-4.
18. Stevens CE, Szmuness W, Goodman AI, Weseley SA, Fotino M. Hepatitis B vaccine: immune responses in hemodialysis patients. *Lancet* 1980;ii:1211-3.
19. Stevens CA, Alter HJ, Taylor PE, Zang EA, Harlay EJ, Szmuness W. Hepatitis B vaccine in patients receiving hemodialysis: immunogenicity and efficacy. *N Engl J Med* 1984;311:496-501.
20. Seaworth B, Drucker J, Starling J, Drucher R, Stevens C, Hamilton J. Hepatitis B vaccines in patients with chronic renal failure before dialysis. *J Infect Dis* 1988;157:332-7.
21. Dhorje SP, Pavri KM, Prasad SR, Sehgal A, Phule DM. Horizontal transmission of hepatitis B virus infection in household contacts, Pune. *Ind J Med Virol* 1985;16:183-9.
22. Koff RS. *Viral hepatitis*. In: Schiff L, Schiff ER, Eds. Diseases of Liver. JB Lippincott, Philadelphia 1993; pp. 492-577.
23. Redeker AG, Mosley JW, Gocke DJ, Mckae AP, Pollack W. Hepatitis B immune globulin as a prophylactic measure for spouses exposed to acute type B hepatitis. *N Engl J Med* 1975;293:1055-9.

24. Blostein J, Clark PA. Cost-effectiveness of pre-immunization hepatitis B screening in high-risk adolescents. *Public Health Rep* 2001;116:165-8.
25. Lee PI, Chang LY, Lee CY, Huang LM, Chang MH. Detection of hepatitis B surface gene mutation in carrier children with or without immunoprophylaxis at birth. *J Infect Dis* 1997;176:427-30.
26. He JW, Lu Q, Zhu QR, Duan SC, Wen YM. Mutations in the 'a' determinant of hepatitis B surface antigen among Chinese infants receiving active post-exposure hepatitis B immunization. *Vaccine* 1998;16:170-3.
27. Daw BC, Yates P, Galea G, Munro H, Buchanan I, Ferguson K. Hepatitis B vaccines may be mistaken for confirmed hepatitis B surface antigen–positive blood donors. *Vox Sang* 2002;82:15-7.
28. Scwarzwald H, Kline NE. False positive hepatitis B surface antigen test caused by hepatitis B vaccine. *Pediatr Infect Dis J* 2001;20:1049-54.

35

Hepatitis B vaccination: are boosters needed?

Premashish Kar, Surinder S Rana

In an attempt to reduce the burden of hepatitis B virus (HBV) infection, the WHO in 1991, recommended that hepatitis B vaccine be integrated into the national immunization programs in all countries.[1] The protective efficacy of the primary course of vaccination is well established but there is no consensus on the need for booster vaccination. There are two schools of thought regarding the need for booster vaccination, one for and the other against. The group which does not recommend booster vaccination bases its opinion on two facts:

(a) Good *in vivo* anamnestic response that follows immunization with HBV vaccine, and
(b) Persistent protective memory, particularly B-cell mediated even with waning or absent antibody responses.

The other group recommends booster vaccination when anti-HBs titers fall below 10 mIU/ml (protective level), citing the fact that delay between infection and stimulation of memory lymphocytes might permit the virus to invade hepatocytes and cause the disease.

HEPATITIS B VACCINE INDUCED IMMUNITY

The strength of immune response after administration of HBsAg has been assessed by measuring antibody to HBsAg (anti-HBs) with commercial kits. A level above 10 mIU/ml is generally taken to be protective,[2] but the potential for low anti-HBs levels to mask significant infection has led some countries to adopt a higher reference level (e.g., 100 mIU/ml in the UK).[3] The persistence of anti-HBs is closely related to the peak anti-HBs response of the vaccine. There is a rapid decline in the antibody levels in the first 12 months after the third dose and a more gradual decline over time.[4-7a] Among adult vaccinees, anti-HBs levels decline to <10 mIU/ml in 7 to 50% by about 5 years after vaccination and in 30 to 60% by 9–11 years[7] (Table 1). A recent data from India,[12] however, has shown that in the Indian population, anti-HBs levels decline more rapidly.

Table 1. Long-term protection among adults who responded (peak anti-HBs titer ≥ 10 mIU/ml) to a primary hepatitis B vaccination schedule

Group	No. of subjects	Length of follow-up (Yrs.)	% of patients showing anti-HBs loss	Number of late infections All*	Chronic
Health care workers[8]	144	11	31	0	0
Homosexual men[9]	127	11	61	0	0
Medical students[10]	100	5	19	1	0
Health care workers[11]	143	5	7	4	0
Health care workers[12]	18	8	81	1	0

Anamnestic antibody response

Clonal proliferation after primary exposure to HBsAg gives rise to a population of memory B lymphocytes and on subsequent exposure to specific antigen, these can proliferate differentiate and produce anti-HBs within days. Various studies have shown that there is a time lag of about 4 days between exposure to HBsAg and initiation of significant antibody production in subjects who responded well to their initial vaccination series.[5] There is no data documenting the exact duration of the replicative cycle of hepatitis B virus in human beings. A recent data on *in vitro* infection of cultured human hepatocytes with HBV revealed that HBcAg was observed intranuclearly as soon as 3 days after inoculation.[6]

On theoretical grounds, the 3 day delay in regaining protective antibody levels after a booster would allow infection of liver cells, thus making revaccination mandatory. Despite this risk, we do not know of any published case where a vaccinated person who has had a transient benign breakthrough infection (i.e., positive for anti-HBc but negative for HBsAg) has gone on to develop chronic liver disease as a direct result of HBV infection.

Despite accepting immunological memory as a mechanism of protection against infection, many of the researchers advocate a cautious approach to administration of booster doses according to an assessment of vaccine induced antibody. This approach is based on the following three major concerns.

(a) Most of the data indicating long-term strong immunological memory have been performed on vaccinees given plasma derived rather than the recombinant vaccine. Antigen content of both vaccines is the HBsAg protein. However, HBsAg of the plasma derived and recombinant vaccine is not exactly similar from the point of its physicochemical properties. Because of the existing differences, it is still important to determine whether the recombinant antigen is immunogenic for as long a time as demonstrated by the plasma derived vaccine.

(b) The time of antibody disappearance ranges widely among subjects.

(c) Although there is virtual absence of development of chronicity after a breakthrough HBV infection in subjects who respond to the vaccine, case reports of anti-HBcAg conversions have been reported. This is an indication of an infection, although subclinical, with a potentially oncogenic virus. Thus, because of this conflicting data, no consensus has emerged on the need for booster vaccination for HBV (Table 2).

Table 2. Global recommendations on the need for boosters of hepatitis B vaccine for health care workers

Vaccination Policy	Country		
	Netherland	UK	USA
Vaccination schedules (months)	0,1,6	0,1,6 or 0,1,2,12	0,1,6
Post-vaccination anti-HBs testing	Yes	Yes	Yes
Booster vaccination (in relation to anti-HBs titers in mIU/ml)	No, if >100 Yes, if 10–100	Yes, single booster after 5 yr. only	No for adults whose immune status is normal

With the above background, there are three options for ensuring protection against HBV infection and/or disease:

(i) Reliance on immunological memory rather than booster doses to protect against clinically significant breakthrough infections. But there is no cheap and convenient method to assess immunological memory and the exact duration of immunological memory is also not known.

(ii) Provision of regular booster vaccinations to all vaccinated people without assessing anti-HBs status.

(iii) Testing anti-HBs one month after the primary vaccination and administering booster before the minimum protective anti-HBs level is reached.

The duration of immunological memory is still under investigation. Hence, it remains contentious for whom and after how much time should booster vaccination be recommended? Unnecessary hepatitis B booster vaccinations are wasteful. Boosters should be used only if there is a time when vaccinees become susceptible to significant breakthrough infection. Data from the west have shown persistant of immunological memory for as long as 12 years after a course of primary vaccination.[7] Similar reports have appeared from India also. In one such study from India,[12] it has been shown that immunological memory after vaccination against hepatitis B lasts for at least 10 years.

Till the role and duration of immunological memory is clearly elucidated, following recommendations regarding booster dose of HBV vaccine may be adopted.

Children and adolescents

Immunological memory has been shown to be robust in infants. One study in area of low HBV infection (i.e., low chance of natural boosters) demonstrated that vaccine induced immunological memory persists for at least 12 years in children vaccinated as infants.[7, 7a] To date, there is no evidence to support the use of boosters in children.

Health care workers and others at occupational risk

As this cohort is at a very high-risk of acquiring HBV infection, it is recommended that a cautious approach should be followed and anti-HBs levels should be maintained at >10 mIU/ml. As already mentioned, the time of disappearance of protective antibody varies widely among subjects.[13] Therefore, the opinions concerning when to schedule revaccination differ widely. The International group recommended[2] that anti-HBs levels should be tested in every vaccinee 1–3 months after the last dose to be sure to achieve anti-HBs titers >10 mIU/ml. It has been shown that in the Indian population, anti-HBs levels decline rapidly.

Immune compromised patients

Patients with impaired immune function such as those with chronic renal failure and those who are HIV positive, tend to have lower peak anti-HBs levels. Primary and secondary humoral responses are also slower. Hence routine booster vaccination is recommended in such patients to maintain anti-HBs >10 mIU/ml. Since antibody is likely to persist for less time in immunocompromised patients than immunocompetent individuals, post-vaccination testing every 6–12 months is advisable.

General population

A cost effective and safe strategy will be to give a booster dose to all without preliminary testing for anti-HBs levels. The time when the booster dose should be given will depend upon large population based studies which will determine the time when the proportion of individuals adequately protected in the population falls below an acceptable level.

The cautious approach mentioned earlier is supported by concerns that appear more theoretic and duration of immunological memory is shown to be at least more than 10 years.[14, 15] Therefore, it seems that there is no need for boosters for at least 10–13 years after initial vaccination. Ongoing studies should provide information on the need for booster doses during the second decade after vaccination.

The old debate on the need for booster vaccination in the HBV vaccination schedule still continues. As there is no consensus on this subject, no universally acceptable guidelines are available. Based upon the experimental evidence available at present, it is recommended that at least high-risk groups should be given booster dose of the vaccine.[16] The need for giving booster dose to general population can be answered only after large population based studies are undertaken to determine the exact duration of immunological memory.

REFERENCES

1. World Health Organization, WHO expanded programme on immunization. *Report of 14th Global Advisory group* (Antalya, Turkey, Oct. 14-18, 1991). Geneva: WHO; 1991: WHO/EPI/GEN/92-1.
2. International group. Immunization against hepatitis B. *Lancet* 1988;I:875-6.
3. Salisbury DM, Begg NT, Eds. *Immunization against infectious disease*. London: HM Stationary Office, 1996;95-108.
4. Jilg W, Schmidt M, Deinhardt F. Four year experience with a recombinant hepatitis B vaccine. *Infection* 1989;17:70-6.
5. Jilg W, Schmidt M, DeinHardt F. Immune response to hepatitis B revaccination. *J Med Virol* 1988; 24:377-84.
6. Rijntjes PJM. The in vitro infection of human hepatocytes with hepatitis B virus. Thesis 1987. University of Nijmegen, The Netherlands: ISBN: 90-9001929-4.
7. West DJ, Watson B, Lichtman J, Hisley TM, Hedberg K. Persistence of Immunological memory for twelve years in children given hepatitis B vaccine in infancy. *Pediatr Infect Dis J* 1994;13:745-7.
7a. Seto D, West DJ, Ioli VA. Persistence of antibody and immunologic memory in children immunized with hepatitis B vaccine at birth. *Pediatr Infect Dis J* 2002;21:793-5.
8. Mahoney FJ, Stewart K, HVH, Coleman P, Alter MJ. Progress toward the elimination of hepatitis B virus transmission among health care workers in the United States. *Arch Intern Med* 1997;157: 2601-5.
9. Stevens CE, Toy PT, Taylor PE, Leet, Yip HY. Prospects for control of hepatitis B virus infection: implications of childhood vaccination and long-term protection. *Pediatrics* 1992;90:(suppl):170-3.
10. Goh KT, Oon CJ, Heng BH, Lim BK. Long-term immunogenicity and efficacy of a reduced dose of plasma derived hepatitis B vaccine in young adults. *Bull WHO* 1995;73:523-7.
11. Courouce AM, Laplanche A, Benhamou E, Jungers P. Long-term efficacy of hepatitis B vaccination in healthy young adults. *Alan R Liss* 1988, New York N.Y.
12. Chadha MS, Arankalle VA. Ten year serological follow-up of hepatitis B vaccine recipients. *Indian J Gastroenterol* 2000;19:168-71.
13. Williams JL, Christensen CJ, Mcmahon BJ, Bulkow LR, Cagle HH, Mayes JS, Zanis CL, et al. Evaluation of the response to a booster dose of hepatitis B vaccine in previously immunized health care workers. *Vaccine* 2001;19:4081-5.
14. Mahoney FJ. Update on diagnosis, management and prevention of hepatitis B infection. *Clin Microbiol Rev* 1999;12:351-6.
15. Watson B, West DJ, Chilkatowsky A, Piercy S, Ioli VA. Persistence of immunologic memory for 13 years in recipients of a recombinant hepatitis B vaccine. *Vaccine* 2001;283:110-20.
16. Consensus statements: Indian Association for Study of Liver. *Indian J Gastroenterol* 2000;20(suppl 3): C54-66.

36

Post-vaccination screening: for whom and why?

Virender Chauhan, Yogesh K Chawla

Hepatitis B vaccine is highly effective and more than 95% of subjects develop antibodies against HBsAg.[1] Because of very high sero-conversion rates in immunocompetent individuals, post-vaccination testing usually is not necessary. Protective levels of antibodies persist in the majority of responders (68% at 4 years).[2] Even if antibody titers decline and anti-HBs levels become no longer detectable, this does not necessarily mean loss of protection. These subjects usually show an anamnestic response when re-exposed to HBV and *in vitro* studies of B-cells from these individuals have demonstrated immunologic memory.[2] Therefore, routine testing of vaccinated individuals and routine booster vaccinations are not recommended.[2]

However, there are no clear guidelines presently for the post-hepatitis B vaccination screening except in select circumstances like immunocompromised individuals, health care workers, and infants born to HBeAg positive mothers. Revaccination of such high-risk individuals who fail to show an adequate response may be needed with or without other immuno-adjuvants like granulocyte macrophage colony stimulating factor (GMCSF) and interleukin–2.[3]

INFANTS BORN TO HBV POSITIVE MOTHERS

Failed post-natal immuno-prophylaxis for hepatitis B in infants born to HBsAg positive mothers has also been reported.[4] In certain instances, failure could be attributed to factors that predispose to peri-natal infections such as prematurity,[5] prolonged labor,[6] delay or omission in HBIg administration and failure to achieve full vaccination.[7] However, HBV infection has been reported in full-term infants who were delivered by obstetric intervention and given full prophylaxis. Past studies have associated such 'breakthrough' infections with intrauterine infection,[8] high-level maternal viremia[9] and infection by vaccine escape HBV mutants.[10] Recently, allelic base changes in maternal HBV C158, A328, G365, and A479 have also reported to be associated with a higher transmission rate in infants.[11] Whether these subgroups of patients should be subjected to post-HBV vaccination screening needs to be investigated further. In spite of these situations, a 10-year long-term follow-up study did not show development of chronic HBV infection in 118 infants, born to HBeAg positive mothers, who were vaccinated at birth.[12]

HIV INDIVIDUALS

Presently, hepatitis B vaccination is essential in HIV infected patients[13] as it is associated with higher progression rate of HBV infections to chronicity and lower rate of serum HBsAg loss. It has been shown that these individuals have decreased anti-HBs response after a standard vaccination schedule (3 doses, 20 micrograms).[13,14] Preliminary results show that doubling the number of hepatitis B vaccinations (six) in HIV-infected patients might significantly improve anti-HBs response rate; however, close monitoring of anti-HBs is necessary because of its short-lived persistence.[13] So, this subgroup of patients may also merit post-HBV vaccination screening.

HEMODIALYSIS PATIENTS

Immunocompromised patients, including those receiving hemodialysis have a reduced chance of mounting protective immune response after vaccination.[2] Studies from different centers have reported sero-conversion rates of 23–33% after three doses of vaccine at 0, 1, and 2 months, which after the fourth booster dose increased to 40–60%. In spite of the use of hepatitis B vaccine in chronic renal failure patients, the risk of developing fresh infections is still higher (7.04%) than in the general population (0.9–2.2%).[15] Additional and higher doses of vaccine increase the response rate.[2,16] The initial immune response to hepatitis B vaccine is an important determinant of duration of immunity and the risk of infection is inversely related to maximal anti-HBs response.[17,18] It was previously thought that protection against HBV occurred with anti-HBs titer >10 mIU/ml. In contrast, now it has been shown[16] that those with anti-HBs titers lesser than 100 mIU/ml, 3 months after the vaccination are susceptible to HBV infection and effective protection requires an anti-HBs titer > 100 mIU/ml. Similarly, it has also been shown that in dialysis patients who received HBV vaccine, 92% of those with anti-HBs titers between 10 mIU/ml to 100 mIU/ml had lost their anti-HBs after one year of follow-up compared to only 3.3% of the cases who had anti-HBs titer of over 100 mIU/ml.[16,19] These findings suggest that in chronic renal failure patients on dialysis, a post-vaccination anti-HBs titer of over 100 mIU/ml is required for effective protection.[19]

PATIENTS WITH MALNUTRITION AND ASSOCIATED HCV INFECTION

Malnutrition has been shown to negatively influence the response to hepatitis B vaccine in hemodialysis patients.[20] It has also been shown that the antibody response to HBV vaccine in chronic renal failure patients who are anti-HCV-positive showed a poorer response as demonstrated by a post-vaccination antibody titer of >100 mIU/ml than those who were anti-HCV negative (23% vs. 63%).[19]

A high-dose, short-interval HBV vaccination schedule may produce an effective and early antibody response in chronic hepatitis C patients. In one of the recent studies,[21] 109 out of 152 (72%) patients of chronic hepatitis C seroconverted (anti-HBs >10 mIU/ml) in comparison to 24 of 26 (92%) of controls (p<0.05). The response was significantly lower in cirrhotics in comparison to non-cirrhotics (54% vs. 80%, p<0.001).

SMOKERS

Smoking has been shown to result in increased cytotoxic/suppressor and decreased inducer/helper T-cell numbers, as well as lower immunoglobulin titers[22] and these may be the mechanisms of action for non-response to hepatitis B vaccination. In one of the studies,[23] it was recommended that high-risk health care workers who are smokers and who are above 50 years of age and with weight height index of 29 in males and[3] 42 in females, should have anti-HBs titers determined.[23]

HEALTH CARE WORKERS

Hepatitis B vaccination response has been reported to be poor in Costa Rican health care workers. They reported an adequate anti-HBs response of >100 mIU/ml in only 64% of health care workers compared to an excellent response in healthy university students.[24] Post-vaccination testing of health care workers is done in many institutions and has been recommended in some countries. Those who have not responded can be offered additional doses of the vaccine and appropriately counseled if they do not respond.

The Centres for Disease Control and Prevention (CDC) recommends that health care workers who receive three doses of HBV vaccine, should be followed by assessment of the anti-HBs titers to document response in high-risk health care workers.[25] Determining this titer increases the cost of a vaccine course by $9.27 in the US. If it is possible to predict high rate of response, then the determination of the post-vaccination anti-HBs titers and its cost can be avoided. In one of the studies, Alimonos et al[23] showed that the anti-HBs response can be predicted in health care workers by looking at the gender, smoking status, and the weight-height index (WHI). Female non-smokers with age of less than 50 years and WHI less than 42 had a 98.2% probability of response. Male non-smokers less than 50 years and WHI less than 29 also had a 94.7% probability of response. They suggested that assessment of anti-HBs titers might be unnecessary in these groups. They also applied economic analysis to the cost of determining the anti-HBs titers following three doses of HBV vaccine versus not determining the titers but giving post-exposure prophylaxis for hepatitis B and they found the later policy to be cheaper.[23]

GENETIC FACTORS AND AGE

In addition to smoking status and WHI, genetic factors may also modulate the immune response to vaccination.[26, 27] Craven et al[26] found that among the 17 non-responders and 3 hypo-responders, 9 (45%) had HLA DR7 and 8 (40%) had HLA DR3, compared with an expected rate of 23% in general population. At least one of the two extended haplotypes (B44, DR7, FC31 or B8, DR3, SC01) were detected in 6 of the 9 who did not respond to vaccination compared to 2 of 11 who responded to second course of vaccine.

Patients over 50 years of age and those with HLA B8 also exhibit a decreased antibody response to hepatitis B vaccine.[28, 29] But whether these individuals should be subjected to screening for anti-HBs antibodies after vaccination has not been clearly defined in available literature, and can be areas of further studies.[30]

REFERENCES

1. Szmuness W, Stevens C, Harley EJ, Zang EA, Alter HJ, Taylor PE, Devera A, et al. Hepatitis B vaccine in medical staff of hemodialysis units: Efficacy and sub-type cross-protection. *N Engl J Med* 1982;307:1481-6.
2. Wright TL, Terrault NA, Ganem D. *Hepatitis B virus*. In: Richman DD, Whitley RJ, Hayden FG, Eds. Clinical Virology: New York, Churchill Livingstone, 1996; pp. 663-82.
3. Meuer SC, Dumann H, Meyer Zum Buschenfelde K, Kohler H. Low-dose interleukin–2 induces systemic responses against HBsAg in immunodeficient responders to hepatitis B vaccination. *Lancet* 1989;1:15-8.
4. Agui SL, Andrew NJ, Underhill GS, Heptonstall J, Teo CG, et al. Failed post-natal immuno-prophylaxis for hepatitis B: characteristics of maternal hepatitis B virus as risk factors. *Clin Infect Dis* 1998;27:100-6.
5. Mullida MJ, Stietim ER. Neonatal hepatitis B infection: Clinical and immunological considerations. *J Perinatol* 1994;14:2-9.
6. Lin HH, Chang MH, Chen DS, Sung JL, Hong KH, Young YC, Young KH, et al. Early predictor of efficacy of immunoprophylaxis against perinatal hepatitis B transmission: analysis of prophylaxis failure. *Vaccine* 1991;9:457-60.
7. Smith CP, Parle M, Morris DJ. Implementation of government recommendations for immunizing infants at risk of hepatitis B. *Br Med J* 1994;309:1339.
8. Stevens CE, Taylor PE, Tong MJ. *Prevention of perinatal hepatitis B virus infection with HBIg and hepatitis B vaccine*. In: Zucherman AJ, Ed. Viral hepatitis and liver diseases: New York, Alan R Liss 1988; pp. 982-9.
9. Del Canho R, Grosheide PM, Schalm SW, de Vries RRP, Heitjink RA. Failure of neonatal hepatitis B vaccination: the role of HBV-DNA levels in hepatitis B carrier mothers and HLA antigens in neonates. *J Hepatol* 1994;20:483-6.
10. Oon CJ, Lim GK, Ye Z, Goh KT, Tan KL, Yo SL, Hopes E, et al. Molecular epidemiology of hepatitis B virus vaccine variants in Singapore. *Vaccine* 1995;13:699-702.
11. Naoumov NY, Thomas MG, Mason AL, Chokshi S, Bodicky CJ, Farzaneh F, Williams R, et al. Genomic variations in hepatitis B core gene: a possible factor influencing response to interferon-alpha treatment. *Gastroenterology* 1995;108:505.
12. Huang LM, Chang BL, Lee CY, Lee PI, Chi WK, Chang MH. Long-term response to hepatitis B vaccination and response to booster in children born to mothers with HBeAg. *Hepatology* 1999;29: 954-9.
13. Rey D, Krantz V, Partisani M, Schmitt MP, Meyer P, Libbrecht E, Wendling MJ, et al. Increasing the

number of hepatitis B vaccine injections augments anti-HBs response rate in HIV infected patients. Effect on HIV-1 viral load. *Vaccine* 2000;18:1161-5.
14. Collier AC, Corey L, Murply VL, Handsfield HH, et al. Antibody to human immuno-deficiency virus (HIV) and sub-optimal response to hepatitis B vaccination. *Ann Intern Med* 1988;109: 101.
15. Choudhry N, Ramesh B, Saraswat S, Naik SR. Effectiveness of mandatory transmissible diseases screening in Indian blood donors. *Ind J Med Res* 1995;101:229-32.
16. Shusterman, N, Singer I. Infectious hepatitis in dialysis patients. *Am J Kidney Dis* 1987;9:447-55.
17. Hadler SC, Francis D, Maynard IE, Thompson SE, Judson FN, Echenberg DF, Ostrow DG, et al. Long-term immunogenicity and efficacy of hepatitis B vaccine in homosexual men. *N Engl J Med* 1986;315:209-14.
18. Hollinger F. Factors influencing immune response to hepatitis B vaccine. Booster dose guidelines and vaccine protocol recommendations. *Am J Med* 1989;87:S336-40.
19. Navarro JF, Fernandez CN. Antibody level after hepatitis B vaccination. *Nephrol Dial Transplant* 1997;12:2207.
20. Fernandez E, Betrice MA, Gomer R. Response to hepatitis B virus vaccine in haemodialysis patients. Influence of malnutrition and its importance as a risk factor for morbidity and mortality. *Nephrol Dial Transplant* 1996:11;1559-63.
21. Idilman R, De MN, Colantoni A, Nadir A, Van T. The effect of high-dose and short interval HBV vaccination in individuals with chronic hepatitis C. *Am J Gastroenterol* 2002;97:435-9.
22. Johnson JD, Houchens DP, Kuwe WM, Craig DK, Fisher GL, et al. Effects of mainstream and environmental tobacco smoke on immune system in animals and humans: a review. *Clin Rev Toxicol* 1990;20:369-95.
23. Alimonos K, Nafziger AN, Murray J, Bertino JS Jr. Prediction of response to Hepatitis B vaccine in health care workers: Whose titers of antibody to hepatitis B surface antigen should be determined after a three dose series, and what are the implications in terms of cost- ectiveness? *Clin Infec Dis* 1998;26:566-71.
24. Taylor L, Garcia Z, Herrera G, Luftig RB, Visona KB, et al. Low response to hepatitis B vaccine in Costa Rican health care workers. *Hepatology* 1998;27:637.
25. Centres for Disease Control. Hepatitis Virus; a comprehensive strategy for eliminating transmission in the United States through universal childhood vaccination. Recommendations of the immunization Practices advisory committee (ACIP). *MMWR* 1991;40(RR-13):1-25.
26. Craven DE, Awdeh ZL, Kunches LM, Yunis EJ, Dienstag JL, Werner BG, Polk F, et al. Nonresponsiveness to hepatitis B vaccine in health care workers. *Ann Intern Med* 1986;105:356-60.
27. Durupinar B, Okten G. HLA tissue types in non-responders to hepatitis B vaccine. *Indian J Pediatr* 1996;63:369-73.
28. *MMWR*. Hepatitis surveillance Report no. 52 Atlanta. Center for Disease Control, Public health services 1989.
29. *MMWR*. Protection against viral hepatitis. Recommendations of the immunization practices advisory committee (ACIP) 1990;39:1.
30. Rendi-Wagner P, Weidermann G, Stemberger H, Kollaritsch H. New vaccination strategies for low- and non-responders to hepatitis B vaccine. *Wien Klin Wochenschr* 2002;114:175-80.

Hepatitis B vaccination policy for health care workers

Hiralal G Desai, Ashwani K Singal

PREVENTION OF HEPATITIS B VIRUS INFECTION AMONG HEALTH CARE WORKERS

Hepatitis B virus (HBV) infection is a well recognized occupational risk for health care workers. The risk of infection has been demonstrated to be primarily related to the degree of contact with blood at the workplace. In serological studies conducted in the United States during the 1970s, health care workers were demonstrated to have a prevalence of HBV infection up to 10 times higher compared to the general population. Due to the high-risk of hepatitis B among health care workers, routine pre-exposure vaccination of health care workers against hepatitis B and the use of universal precautions to prevent exposure to blood and other potentially infectious body fluids have been recommended since the early 1980s. Regulations recently issued by the Occupational Safety and Health Administration (OSHA) should increase compliance with these recommendations and further decrease the risk of HBV transmission in the workplace.

Who is a health care worker?

Any person who is involved in the implementation of the health care program is a health care worker, including the administrative staff. However, in general, health workers are those who are directly involved in patient's management, both in therapeutic and diagnostic aspects as well as at the hospital or community level. These mainly include doctors, nurses, laboratory technicians, and other paramedical workers such as maids, ward boys, and cleaning staff. All these groups are at high-risk of acquiring HBV infection. However, the risk is not the same for all of them. So they can be categorized in three different groups, viz., high-risk, medium-risk, and low-risk, depending upon the nature of their work and the potential for exposure. The high-risk group includes physicians, surgeons, anesthetists, dialysis staff, laboratory technicians (dealing with the blood), blood bank staff, dentists, pediatricians, gynecologists, nurses working in ICUs and operation theaters, etc. Medium-risk group includes physicians (family practitioners, psychiatrists, etc.), nurses, sanitary staff, etc. The rest are in the low-risk group.

Risk factors for health care workers

During the last few decades, the sero-prevalence studies in the health care workers have defined the risk factors for acquiring HBV infection. It was also shown that, though, there is a risk of HBV transmission to the patients from infected health care workers, it is minimal when compared with the risk of health care workers getting infection from the patients. Studies from the US have shown that prevalence of HBV markers increases with duration in the profession reaching as high as 30% amongst those who have worked for 20 years or more as compared to 5% in comparable age group in the general population. Risk of HBV infection also increases with the nature of work, being highest in the laboratory technicians. Important risk factors for acquiring HBV infection are listed in Table 1.[1]

The most important determinant for risk in the work place is the frequency of exposure to blood and blood derived fluids and the frequency of needle stick accidents. Another important risk factor is the rate of HBsAg positivity in the patient population. Health personnel working with patients with higher HBsAg prevalence rate are at higher risk compared to those working with patients having low prevalence rate of HBsAg.[2] In sero-prevalence studies of patients consecutively admitted to hospitals in the United States, 0.9–1.5% were found to be HBsAg positive.[3] The prevalence of HBV infection among patients has been found to vary by geographic location and by the degree of specialization of the hospital; the highest prevalence was found in urban, tertiary care hospitals.[4,5] Only a small fraction (<20%) of subjects with chronic hepatitis B infection admitted to hospitals had a history of liver disease.[3] This finding provides the rationale for using universal precautions to prevent exposure to blood or body fluids in hospitals and for vaccination of all health care workers who have exposure to blood, since health care workers may treat five HBsAg positive persons for each one they recognize. It has been shown that health care workers in developed countries working in urban hospitals or tertiary care centers are at higher risk because of greater exposure to blood and other facilities like hemodialysis, etc. This may also be true for the developing countries. Persons working in rural hospitals or PHCs in these countries may also have substantial risk of acquiring infection due to other factors like sanitation, inadequate sterilizing facilities, re-use of the instruments, socio-economic status of the population, etc. However, no hard data are available in this regard. Asymptomatic HBsAg positive individuals are an important source of infection amongst health care workers. Since all patients who get treated in hospitals are not screened for HBsAg and are not clinically suspected to have HBV infection, the usual barrier precautions are not taken while handling their blood samples or doing procedures.

Modes of Transmission

Blood contains the highest HBV titers of all body fluids and is the most important vehicle for

Table 1. Risk factors for acquiring HBV infection

Frequency of exposure
contact with blood or blood derived fluids
accidents with needle / sharp instruments
Type and location of hospital
metropolitan vs. rural
tertiary care vs. primary care
hemodialysis vs. no hemodialysis
Patient group
homosexual men
parenteral drug abusers
Asian or African born persons
institutional, developmentally disabled
immunocompromised patients
Work area in hospital

transmission in the health care setting. Following are the principle modes of HBV transmission in the health care setting: (a) direct percutaneous inoculation of blood or body fluids containing HBV via needle stick or other injuries from sharp instruments, (b) direct inoculation of blood or body fluids containing HBV onto mucous membranes, cutaneous scratches, abrasions, burns, or other lesions, and (c) indirect inoculation of HBV from environmental surfaces contaminated with blood or body fluids onto mucous membranes, cutaneous scratches, abrasions, burns, or other lesions.

HBV transmission from needle-sticks and other sharp instrument injuries

Injuries from needles containing HBV infected blood are one of the most efficient means of HBV transmission in the health care setting. The average volume of blood inoculum during a needle-stick injury with a 22 gauge needle is approximately 1 microliter,[6] a sufficient quantity to contain up to 100 infectious doses of HBV.[7]

The reported frequency of needle-stick and other sharp instrument injuries in hospitals ranged from 7.5–16 per 100 employees per year.[8-10] Higher injury rates were reported among nursing, housekeeping, and laboratory personnel compared to rates reported among physicians, students, and x-ray technicians. The risk of developing clinical hepatitis from a needle depends on the 'e' antigen status of the patient (Table 2).[11]

Table 2. Risk of hepatitis B after needle-stick injury

	Clinical hepatitis (%)	Serological positivity (%)
HBeAg +ve blood	22 – 31	37 – 62
HBeAg –ve blood	1 – 6	23 – 37

HBV transmission from other direct blood or body fluid exposures

While overt percutaneous injuries are one of the most efficient modes of HBV transmission, only about 10% of the health care workers could recall a specific percutaneous injury; however 29–38% could recall caring for an HBsAg positive patient within 6 months prior to the onset of illness.[12-14] Transmission via the respiratory tract or through the gastrointestinal tract, although theoretically possible, is not seen in the practical situation.

HBV transmission from environmental surfaces

HBV has been shown to survive in dried blood at room temperature on environmental surfaces for at least one week.[15] Hence indirect inoculation of HBV can occur via inanimate objects. The potential for HBV transmission through contact with environmental surfaces has been demonstrated in investigations of HBV outbreaks among patients and staff of hemodialysis units.[16-18] Contact with HBV contaminated blood from the surface of dialysis machines and instruments and transfer of HBV on the hands of medical personnel to patients was suspected to be the primary mode of transmission in these outbreaks. With the extensive use of infection control procedures, the annual incidence of HBV infection among staff in dialysis centers decreased more than 25-fold from 2.6% during 1976 to 0.1% during 1989.[19]

Sero-prevalence of HBV infection among health care workers

Estimates of the annual risk of HBV infection among selected health care worker groups ranges from 0.5–6% in various studies.[20,21] The prevalence of HBV infection has been found to vary considerably among persons in the same profession including dentists (4–30%),[22,23] physicians (9–35%),[24,25] nurses (3–32%), and laboratory personnel (3-26%).[26,27] Prevalence estimates have also been found to be different in various work areas in the hospital. This variation appears to be related to differences in the frequency of blood contact. There also appears to be an increased risk of infection associated with a longer duration of time in medical practice[20,21] and for persons recently entering medical practice.[28] Although health care workers continue to have a substantial risk of acquiring HBV infection, there is evidence that the risk is declining, presumably as a result of hepatitis B vaccination.[29]

Indian scenario

Limited information is available on the incidence or prevalence of HBV infection in health care workers from India. A few isolated studies from different parts of the country (Table 3) suggest that health care workers are at very high-risk for HBV infection.[30-33] Epidemiological and environmental set up also supports this, which includes medium HBsAg prevalence rate (3–35%), poor facilities in hospitals, inadequate sterlization, non-availability of disposable items, absence of screening facility for HBsAg, socio-economic background, etc.

Table 3. Frequency of HBsAg positivity in health care workers in India[30-34]

Center	Method	No. tested	HBsAg +ve (%)
Pre–1995			
Madras	CIEP	224	8.0
	RPHA	127	16.5
Bombay	RIA	114	7.9
	ELISA	863	10.0
	ELISA	606	6.6
Delhi	ELISA	83	10.9
	ELISA	184	8.2
Shimla	ELISA	250	16.0
	RPHA	200	8.0
Ahmednagar	RPHA	188	2.1
Trivandrum	CIEP	150	0.6
Chandigarh	ELISA	202	4.0
Pune	ELISA	510	2.16
Post–1995			
Shimla	ELISA	400	5.0
Mumbai	ELISA	166	3.33
Delhi	ELISA	86 (pre-clinical)	2.3
		68 (clinical)	1.4*

CIEP – Counter Immuno electro phoresis; RPHA – Reverse passive hemagglutination
RIA – Radio immuno assay; ELISA – Enzyme linked immunosorbent assay
* Although the HBsAg positivity was less in the clinical group, the overall positivity for HBV markers was more likely in the clinical group compared to the pre-clinical group, e.g., anti-HBc positivity 55% vs. 10.4, and anti-HBs positivity 69% vs. 18%.

Strategies for control of HBV transmission in the health care workers

Prevention of HBV infection is the only cost-effective approach, as the specific treatment (interferon, lamivudine) of chronic HBV infection is costly, prolonged, and with unsatisfactory response (<40%), along with significant side-effects of parenteral interferon. Prevention of HBV infection is possible by various measures (Table 4). The most effective way is to use active and passive immunization.[34]

The strategy to control HBV infection in a country will depend on the HBsAg positivity, the incidence of HBeAg in HBsAg positive subjects, the main route of transmission (vertical or

Table 4. Prevention of HBV infection in health care workers

General / universal measures
Blood and body fluid precautions
Barrier techniques
Proper disposal of infected instruments and materials
Patient screening and isolation
Medical history
Serological testing
Post-exposure prophylaxis
Hepatitis B immunoglobulin (HBIg)
Hepatitis B vaccine
Pre-exposure prophylaxis
Hepatitis B vaccine

horizontal), the age of exposure, the cost–benefit ratio of immunoprophylaxis, and the availability of resources. World Health Organization (WHO) initially recommended all infant immunization in high and intermediate endemicity countries and immunization of high-risk only in low endemicity countries.[35] Subsequently, WHO recommended infant immunization in all countries. Till infant immunization is practiced for at least a few decades, all countries should offer active immunization to high-risk groups. Here we shall be dealing with prevention of HBV infection in the health care workers.

Use of hepatitis B vaccine

Vaccination of health care workers who are regularly exposed to blood is the most effective means of preventing HBV infection in the health care setting.

Whose responsibility? Health care workers should be administered the hepatitis B vaccine at the earliest, preferably in the first few days of joining. Whether the cost should be borne by the government or the municipality or the institute or the staff member himself has been debated for long. In a survey of hospitals in the United States conducted during 1990 by OSHA, 91% of hospitals had hepatitis B vaccination programs for their employees; of these, 64% paid for the cost of vaccination for employees involved in direct patient care and laboratory work (high-risk employees) (OSHA, personal communication). Those health care workers who are maximally exposed to blood and who cannot afford the cost of vaccine should be provided vaccine from institute's funds.

Which vaccine? Plasma derived vaccine (PV) prepared from human plasma is cheap, safe, and immunogenic but is not used because of unreasonable fear of possible transmission of infections. The recombinant vaccines (RV) are mostly in use. Over the years, the cost of the vaccine is significantly reduced now as the vaccine is manufactured in India. Both PV and RV have only one antigen and hence newer vaccines (HEPAGENE) with pre-S1, pre-S2, S are manufactured which have significantly quicker and higher sero-conversion.[36, 37]

Route Intra-dermal route with 0.1 ml or 2 µg of Engerix B achieves 90% sero-conversion but with a lower anti-HBs titer; the cost is markedly reduced.[38, 39] In institutes with limited resources, intra-dermal route may be used for HCWs. Experienced technicians or nurses are required to administer intra-dermal injection.

Pre-vaccination screening All decisions regarding pre-vaccination screening are based on cost–benefit ratio. Pre-vaccination screening is not necessary when vaccination is offered to all medical, dental, nursing students on joining the hospital. To decide vaccination of elderly (>40 years) HCWs, pre-vaccination screening will be cost-effective. Pre-vaccination screening is usually not cost–effective for groups with a low expected prevalence of HBV serological markers (<20%), such as health care professionals in training or during their early carrier years. If a decision is made to do pre-vaccination screening, only one antibody test is generally needed (anti-HBs or anti-HBc).[40]

Non-responsiveness While sero-conversion occurs in about 95% of healthy young (<40 years) HCWs; non-responsiveness significantly increases in those over the age of 50 years (5–30%).[41] Double dose on each deltoid or a newer vaccine (HEPAGENE) may be tried in non-responders.[37] A few will respond to either method but most will persist as non-responders.

Post-vaccination screening Post-vaccination testing for anti-HBs is not compulsory in subjects below the age of 40 years but is required in elderly. Periodic anti-HBs testing after 5 years to monitor for protective anti-HBs level (>10 mIU/ml) is not required as most experts believe that booster dose is not needed even in those with undetectable levels (relying on immunological memory).[42-46]

Escape mutants Single amino acid substitution from glycine (G) to arginine (A) occurs at position 145 of 'a' determinant of all subtypes of HBsAg. Such a mutation is likely to occur in two situations: (a) active and passive immunization, and (b) HBIg use in liver transplant to prevent reinfection of transplanted liver. However, the appearance of a mutant is rare but may occasionally complicate vaccination strategy.

Declination of vaccine Even HCWs who are frequently in contact with blood, acceptance of vaccine is about 75 per cent. Acceptance by HCW is much less in those who occasionally come in contact with blood or body fluids. The declination of vaccine is expected to be much lower over the next few years. Concern about the safety and efficacy of hepatitis B vaccine and lack of perceived risk were the major reasons cited for not being vaccinated in studies of vaccine acceptance among hospital employees.[47, 48]

Use of infection control practices

As some health care workers will not develop an adequate antibody response to vaccine, and few shall not accept the vaccine, use of other infection control practices are needed to prevent transmission of HBV in the health care setting. The most important of these infection control practices is the use of "universal precautions".[49] Universal precautions emphasize that all patients should be assumed to be infectious for HBV and other blood-borne pathogens and that precautions should be taken to prevent exposure to all blood and blood derived body fluids. These precautions include use of gloves, gowns, masks, and protective eyewear. Measures that can be taken to prevent needle-stick and other sharp instrument injuries include avoidance of recapping needles before disposal, use of impervious containers for the disposal of needles, use of self-sheathing needles for blood drawing and intravenous lines, use of gloves that are puncture resistant, and use of laser cutting devices as substitutes for scalpels. Measures to control mucous membrane exposure to HBV include avoidance of practices such as mouth pipetting, eating, and smoking in the work area. Environmental control measures are also important, including appropriate use of hand washing[50] and rigorous maintenance of a work environment that is free of blood contamination.[51]

Routine screening for HBsAg before intervention is also recommended as one of the ways to effectively reduce the transmission of HBV. Initially it was recommended only in dialysis units,[52] but of late, more and more data are emerging to recommend it before elective surgeries.[53]

OSHA regulations

In 1991, in response to the requests from various unions representing health care workers, OSHA developed regulations to protect workers from occupational exposures to blood-borne hazards.[54, 55] These regulations became law in December 1991 and require all employers to provide the following:

(a) Hepatitis B vaccine free of charge to all employees who have occupational exposure to blood or other potentially infectious materials,

(b) personal protective clothing and equipment when there is a potential for exposure to blood or blood derived body fluids,

(c) engineering and work practice controls including facilities for hand washing, provisions for immediate disposal of needles after use without recapping, and prohibition of eating, drinking, or smoking in areas where there is a potential for occupational exposure,

(d) appropriate housekeeping procedures, including cleaning and disinfection of equipment and environmental surfaces after contact with blood or other potentially infectious material, and appropriate disposal of infectious waste and laundry,

(e) medical follow-up of exposure incidents, including use of HBIg, when appropriate, and

(f) training of health care workers regarding the measures they can take to prevent exposure to HBV in the workplace.

REFERENCES

1. Hadler SC. Hepatitis B virus infection and health care workers. *Vaccine* 1990;8:24-8.
2. Pattison CP, Maynard JE, Berquist DR, Webster HM. Epidemiology of hepatitis B in hospital personnel. *Am J Epidemiol* 1975;101:59-64.
3. Mahoney JP, Richman AV, Teague PO. Admission screening for hepatitis B surface antigen in a university hospital. *South Med J* 1978;71:624-8.
4. Denes AE, Smith JL, Maynard JE, Doto IL, Berquist KR, Finkel AJ. Hepatitis B infection in physicians: results of nationwide seroepidemiologic survey. *JAMA* 1978;239:210-2.
5. Osterholm MT, Graylade SM. Clinical viral hepatitis B among Minnesota hospital personnel: results of a ten year statewide survey. *JAMA* 1985;254:3207-12.
6. Napoli VM, McGowan JE. How much blood is in a needle-stick? *J Infect Dis* 1987;155:828.
7. Shikata T, Karasawa T, Abe K, Uzawa T, Suzuki H, Oda T, Imai H, et al. Hepatitis B e antigen and infectivity of hepatitis B virus. *J Infect Dis* 1977;136:571-6.
8. Jacobson JT, Burke JP, Conti MT. Injuries of hospital employees from needles and sharp objects. *Infect Control* 1983;4;100-2.
9. McCormick RD, Maki DG. Epidemiology of needle-stick injuries in hospital personnel. *Am J Med* 1981;70:928-32.
10. Dandoy SE, Kirkman-Liff BL, Krakowski FM. Hepatitis B exposure incidents in community hospitals. *Am J Public Health* 1984;74:804-7.
11. Seeff LB, Wright EC, Zimmerman HJ, Alter HJ. Type B hepatitis after needle-stick exposure: prevention with hepatitis B immune globulin. Final report of the Veterans Administration Cooperative Study. *Ann Intern Med* 1978;88:285-93.
12. Chaudhuri AKR, Follett EAC. Hepatitis B virus infection in medical and health care personnel. *Br Med J* 1982;284:1408.
13. Callender ME, White YS, Williams R. Hepatitis B virus infection in medical and health care personnel. *Br Med J* 1982;284:324-6.
14. Public health Laboratory Service. Acute hepatitis B. *Br Med J* 1975;3:603.
15. Bond WW, Favero MS, Peterson NJ, Gravelle CR, Ebert JW, Maynard JE. Survival of hepatitis B virus after drying and storage for one week. *Lancet* 1981;1:550-1.
16. Hennekens CH. Hemodialysis associated hepatitis: an outbreak among hospital personnel. *JAMA* 1973;225:407-8.
17. Garibaldi RA, Forrest JN, Bryan JA, Hanson BF, Dismukes WE. Hemodialysis associated hepatitis. *JAMA* 1973;225:384-9.
18. Snydman DR, Bryan JA, Macon EJ, Gregg MB. Hemodialysis associated hepatitis: report of an epidemic with further evidence on mechanism of transmission. *Am J Epidemiol* 1976;104:563-70.
19. Alter MJ, Favero MS, Moyer LA, Bland LA. National surveillance of dialysis associated disease in the United States. *ASAIO Trans* 1991;37:97-109.
20. Segal HE, Llewellyn CH, Irwin G, Bancroft WH, Boe GP, Balaban DJ. Hepatitis B antigen and antibody in the US army: prevalence in health care personnel. *Am J Public Health* 1976;66:667-71.
21. Snydman DR, Munoz A, Werner BG, Polk BF, Craven DE, Platt R, Crumpacker C, et al. A multivariate analysis of risk factors for hepatitis B virus infection among hospital employees screened for vaccination. *Am J Epidemiol* 1984;120:684-93.

22. Smith JL, Maynard JE, Berquist KR, Doto IL, Webster HM, Sheller MJ. Comparative risk of hepatitis B among physicians and dentists. *J Infect Dis* 1978;133:705-6.
23. Krugman S, Friedman H, Lattimer C. Hepatitis A and B: serologic survey of various population groups. *Am J Med Sci* 1978;275:249-55.
24. Hollinger FB, Grander JW, Nickel FR, Suarez MS. Hepatitis B prevalence within a dental student population. *JADA* 1977;94:521-7.
25. Levy BS, Harris JC, Smith JL, Washburn JW, Mature J, Davis A, Crosson TJ, et al. Hepatitis B in ward and clinical laboratory employees of a general hospital. *Am J Epidemiol* 1977;106:330-5.
26. Dienstag JL, Ryan DM. Occupational exposure to hepatitis B virus in hospital personnel: infection or immunization? *Am J Epidemiol* 1982;115:26-9.
27. Hirshowitz BI, Dasher CA, Whitt FJ, Cole GW. Hepatitis B antigen and antibody and tests of liver function: a prospective study of 310 hospital laboratory workers. *Am J Clin Path* 1980;73:63-8.
28. Hadler SC, Doto IL, Maynard JE, Smith J, Clark B, Mosley J, Eickoff T, et al. Occupational risk of hepatitis B infection in hospital workers. *Infect Control* 1985;6:24-31.
29. Alter MJ, Hadler SC, Margolis HS, Alexander WJ, Hu PY, Miller JK, Moyer LA, et al. The changing epidemiology of hepatitis B in the United States: need for alternative vaccination strategies. *JAMA* 1990;263:1218-22.
30. Joshi YK. *Prevalence of hepatitis B in health care workers.* In: Sarin SK, Singal AK. Eds. Hepatitis B in India: Problems and Prevention. CBS Publishers & Distributors, New Delhi, 1996;pp. 33-8.
31. Ganju SA, Goel A. Prevalence of HBV and HCV infection among health care workers (HCW). *J Commun Dis* 2000;32:228-30.
32. Mohite JB, Urhekar AD. Prevalence of HBsAg positivity in staff and patients at MGM medical college and hospital, navi-mumbai. *Indian J Med Sci* 1999;53:434-8.
33. Khanna V, Kar P, Mansharamani N, Jain V, Kanodia A. Differences in hepatitis B markers between clinical and pre-clinical health care personnel. *Trop Gastroenterol* 1997;18:69-71.
34. Desai HG. Prevention and control of hepatitis B virus in India. *Nat Med J Ind* 1988;1:233-6.
35. Desai HG. WHO recommendation for hepatitis B immunization. *Indian J Gastroenterol* 1986;5:291.
36. Dhawan PS, Gill HH, Shah S, Rajan R, Trikanad VS, Desai HG. Immunogenicity of hepatitis B vaccine with pre-S1, pre-S2, and S antigens. *Natl Med J India* 1996;9:201.
37. McDermott AB, Cohen SB, Zuckerman JN, Madrigal JA. Hepatitis B third generation vaccines: improved response and conventional vaccine non-response – evidence for genetic basis in humans. *J Viral Hepat* 1998;(suppl 2):9-11.
38. Desai HG, Trikanand S, Thakkar R, Dhunjibhoy KR, Karnik SR. Intradermal route for prophylaxis against hepatitis B: loss of potency in relation to time. *Indian J Gastroenterol* 1988;7:109-10.
39. Cardell K, Fryden A, Normann B. Intradermal hepatitis B vaccination in health care workers. Response rate and experiences from vaccination in clinical practice. *Scand J Infect Dis* 1999;31:197-200.
40. Centers for Disease Control, Hepatitis B virus: a comprehensive strategy for eliminating transmission in the United States through universal childhood vaccination. Recommendations of the Immunization Practices Advisory Committee (ACIP). *MMWR* 1991;40:1-25.
41. Barash C, Conn MI, DiMarino AJ Jr., Marzano J, Allen ML. Serologic hepatitis B immunity in vaccinated health care workers. *Arch Intern Med* 1999;159:1481-3.
42. Marinho RT, Moura MC, Pedro M, Ramalho FJ, Velosa JF. Hepatitis B vaccination in hospital personnel and medical students. *J Clin Gastroenterol* 1999;28:317-22.
43. Mahoney FJ, Stewart K, Hu H, Coleman P, Alter MJ. Progress toward the elimination of hepatitis B virus transmission among health care workers in the United States. *Arch Intern Med* 1997;157:2601-5.

44. Peces R, Laures AS. Persistence of immunologic memory in long-term hemodialysis patients and health care workers given hepatitis B vaccine: role of a booster dose on antibody response. *Nephron* 2001;89:172-6.
45. Williams JL, Christensen CJ, McMohan BJ, Bulkow LR, Cagle HH, Mayers JS, Zanis CL. Evaluation of the response to a booster dose of hepatitis B vaccine in previously immunized health care workers. *Vaccine* 2001;19:3936-9.
46. Bonnani P, Bonacorsi G. Vaccination against hepatitis B in health care workers. *Vaccine* 2001;19: 2389-94.
47. Crossley KB, Gerding DN, Petzel RA. Acceptance of hepatitis B vaccine by hospital personnel. *Infect Control* 1985;6:147-9.
48. Fulton JP, Bodenheimer HC, Kramer PD. Acceptance of hepatitis B vaccine among hospital workers: A follow-up. *Am J Public Health* 1986;76:1339-40.
49. Centers for Disease Control, Update: Universal precautions for prevention of transmission of human immunodeficiency virus, hepatitis B virus, and other blood borne pathogens in health care setting. *MMWR* 1988;37:377-82, 387-8.
50. Garner JS, Favero MS. Guideline for washing and hospital environmental control, 1985. Atlanta: Public Health Service, Centers for Disease Control, 1985. *HHS publication* no. 1985; 99.
51. Favero MS. Sterlization, disinfection, and antisepsis in the hospital. *Manual of Clinical Microbiology*, 4th Ed., American Society for Microbiology, Washington, DC, 1985;pp. 129-37.
52. Favero MS, Alter MJ, Bland LA. *Dialysis associated infections and their control*. In: Bennett JV, Brachman PS, Eds. Hospital Infections: Little, Rown and Co., Boston, MA, 1992;pp. 375-403.
53. Recommendations: Indian Association for Study of Liver (INASL). Hepatitis B in India–Prevention and Management. *Indian J Gastroenterol* 2000;20(suppl 3):C67
54. Occupational Safety and Health Administration. Occupational exposure to blood-borne pathogens; final rule. *Fed Reg* 1991;56:64005-182.
55. Sagoe-Moses C, Pearson RD, Perry J, Jagger J. Risks to health care workers in developing countries. *N Engl J Med* 2001;345:538-41.

38

Hepatitis B vaccination in patients with chronic renal failure

Devender S Rana, Dinesh Khullar, Ashwani Gupta, Anil K Bhalla, Ashwani K Singal

Hepatitis B virus (HBV) infection in patients with chronic renal failure (CRF) or end-stage renal disease (ESRD) is an important cause of mortality and morbidity. It is further promoted by the characteristic immunological dysfunction that develops in renal failure and interferes with the patient's ability to eliminate the virus. The prevalence of HBV in the dialysis population in India is reported to range between 3.4% and 42%.[1] The acute course of the infection is often anicteric and peak transaminases concentration is significantly less than in patients with normal renal function. Up to 60% of patients on dialysis with HBV infection develop chronic hepatitis with persistence of HBsAg and infectivity.

The general health care of patients with chronic renal failure (CRF) or end-stage renal disease (ESRD) is often provided by nephrologists. Since anemia is a very common feature of renal disease at times requiring blood transfusions, these patients are at an increased risk of acquiring blood-borne diseases like hepatitis B. Moreover, once they progress to a stage requiring hemodialysis, they are again at an increased risk of procedure related acquisition the viral disease. One of the major risk factors, that, render dialysis patients prone to acquire hepatitis B, is the high prevalence of the infection in this population. Patients with chronic hepatitis B are infective for patients and the staff. Hemodialysis patients are treated in centers and they need regular vascular puncture. This increases the risk of transmission of blood from one patient to another.[2] One of the principal means for prevention of HBV infection in this population is the administration of hepatitis B vaccine. Giving hepatitis B vaccine to patients with CRF and ESRD is one of the main components of management of these patients by the nephrologist.

HEPATITIS B VACCINATION IN PATIENTS WITH CRF

In the early years of hemodialysis in the Western Europe and the USA, hepatitis B caused endemic outbreaks in dialysis centres and was one of the major risks for both patients and dialysis staff.[3]

This is still true in many regions of the world with low hygienic standards and without access to vaccination. Patients with CRF have a reduced response to vaccination because of the general suppression of the immune system associated with uremia. Compared to vaccination in normal subjects, dialysis patients have lower antibody titers and an inability to maintain adequate antibody titers over time.[4] The sero-conversion rate following hepatitis B vaccination in patients with chronic renal failure has been in the range of 10–82% in various studies. Not only the titers are low, they also appear late and wane early.[5-8] The relative antibody response to a vaccine also appears to correlate with the degree of renal failure, but not with the specific mode of dialysis. In patients with ESRD on regular dialysis, the adequacy of dialysis has a bearing on the response to the vaccine.[9]

Despite the evidence of decreased efficacy, there has been a large impact on the HBV prevalence in these patients. In 1990, 6.1% of dialysis patients in the registry of the European Dialysis and Transplantation Association were positive for HBsAg. This number is already a reflection of the effect of prophylactic measures because in 1978, 28.8% had been positive in France and 12.8% in Germany.[10] The reduction in the incidence of hepatitis B has mainly been because of the greater awareness about the disease, use of universal precautions and more effective vaccination. Therefore, current recommendations are to vaccinate patients with CRF or ESRD.[11, 12] This gains more importance in the light of the fact that hepatitis B-related chronic liver disease is an important cause of morbidity and mortality when these patients undergo kidney transplantation. Support for this recommendation is provided by a case control study which found that hemodialysis patients vaccinated against hepatitis B had a 70% lower risk of infection compared with non-vaccinated patients.[13]

Mechanisms of non- or hypo-response

Non-response to the hepatitis B vaccine in uremics and patients on hemodialysis has been extensively investigated in the last two decades. A generalized state of immunodeficiency has been demonstrated in patients with CRF that sets in early in the course of illness and affects almost all the components of the immune system including the antigen processing cells, various T-cell subsets, T-cell B-cell cooperation, B-cell function, cytokine production, and the complement cascade (Table 1).[14]

The mechanisms underlying the defective responses in phagocytic cells, lymphocytes, and antigen processing are likely due to either failure to adequately eliminate suppressive compounds by the defective kidneys or to improper metabolic processing of the factors by the damaged renal parenchyma. That some of the defects are reversed by transplantation and not dialysis suggests that renal parenchymal metabolic activities may be involved, although it is also possible that functioning glomerular cells are capable of filtering substances that mem-

Table 1. Mechanisms of non- or hypo-response to hepatitis B vaccine in patients with chronic renal failure

Genetic pre-disposition
Defects in IL-2 and IL-2R expression
Antigen presentation defect
B-cell dysfunction
Defects in the complement system

branes are not currently capable of eliminating.[15] Despite the multitude of major defects in humoral, cellular, and inflammatory processes, uremic patients who are cared for today, although they remain at higher risk of serious infectious complications, can and do maintain a good quality of life, with most remaining free of major infections for years and decades.

Dosage and timing of vaccination

It has been shown that the sero-conversion rates are superior with 4-dose schedule compared with 3-dose schedule and using 40 µg dose in comparison to 20 µg dose.[16-18] Similar results were obtained by a well conducted study from India by Agarwal et al.[19] Two schedules of vaccination; 0, 1, 2 (group A, $n = 75$) and 0, 1, 2, 6 (group B, $n = 42$), were studied in patients with mild (creatinine levels 1.5–3.0 mg%), moderate (creatinine levels 3.0–6.0 mg%), and severe (creatinine levels > 6.0 mg%) chronic renal failure. The sero-conversion rates in group A were 87.5%, 66.6%, and 35.7% in mild, moderate, and severe CRF respectively, while same results in group B were 100%, 77%, and 36.36% respectively. The authors concluded that patients of CRF should be vaccinated at a very early stage of the disease using 40 µg of vaccine. Four-dose schedule of 0, 1, 2, 6 months gives better results than the three- dose schedule in patients with early CRF.

Duration of protection and the need for boosters

The duration of protection in patients with CRF and on hemodialysis is also short.[20, 21] This was elegantly shown in a recent study from Spain,[22] wherein 76 hemodialysis patients (60 after primary vaccination and 16 with natural immunity) and 46 health care workers (32 after primary vaccination and 14 with natural immunity) were followed up for 10 years to evaluate the persistence of immunity. Ten years after vaccination, the analysis showed a lower sero-conversion rate (38 vs. 75%, $p < 0.001$) in HD patients as compared with health care workers. To assess the immunological memory, they administered a booster dose of the vaccine 3–12 years (mean 6.7±0.6 years) after primary vaccination in a selected group of 37 HD patients who presented a decline of their antibodies or were non-responders. Anamnestic response could be shown in 100% of the health care workers while only 51% of HD patients could mount such a response. The authors concluded that patients undergoing HD not only have lower rates of immunization to hepatitis B than healthy adults, but also that these are frequently transient. Booster doses after a primary course of vaccine are effective in about half of HD patients who presented a decline of their antibodies or were non-responders but whether they are necessary is unclear. What has not been analysed in this study is the occurrence of breakthrough infections. If this is shown to be increased significantly in patients with HD, compared to healthy adults, there becomes a strong point for the use of booster dose in patients with CRF and patients on HD. It is recommended to do serial monitoring of anti-HBs levels in these patients, and use the booster dose of 40μg if the titers fall below 10 mIU/ml.[12]

Intra-dermal vs. intra-muscular administration

Intra-dermal administration of hepatitis B vaccine achieves better sero-conversion in patients on dialysis compared to intra-muscular route. This has been shown in many studies using twice weekly intra-dermal administration[23] of 5 μg of vaccine every 2 weeks up to a peak anti-HBs titer of 1000 mIU/ml.[24,25] The advantages of the intra-dermal vaccination are that it induces a better immunity compared to intra-muscular route, is efficacious in patients failing on intra-muscular route, and need for lower total dose of the vaccine. However, the routine use of this route in clinical practice is limited as it is reported to have a short lasting immunity, has a poor compliance because of the need for frequent and larger number of injections, and being more expensive and less cost-effective compared to intra-muscular route.

Overcoming non- or hypo-responsiveness

As the response rate to hepatitis B vaccination in patients with CRF are low, it is advisable and recommended to do post-vaccination screening for anti-HBs protective (>10 mIU/ml) titers. If after 4 doses of 40 μg each, given at 0, 1, 2, 6 months, the anti-HBs levels (done 1 month after the last dose) are not in the protective range, these are labelled as non-responders. There are many options available to overcome such non-responsiveness such as increasing the dose of the vaccine, increasing the number of doses, using the intra-dermal route, use of erythropoietin,[23] and use of immune stimulants, e.g., granulocyte macrophage stimulating factor (GM-CSF). There was initial optimism towards the role of interleukin-2 and erythropoietin in improving the response rate to the vaccine but the same could not be confirmed in subsequent studies. Out of all these options, the last option of the use of GM-CSF has been most commonly used and has drawn the attraction of the clinicians. The use of this adjuvant has been shown to increase the response to the vaccine from all over.

More recently, however, there have been promising reports regarding the efficacy of granulocyte macrophage colony stimulating factor (GM-CSF) as an adjuvant to hepatitis B vaccination for improving sero-conversion rate in maintenance HD patients. In one such study, Anandh et al[26] randomly assigned twelve chronic HD patients to receive either hepatitis B vaccination alone or hepatitis B vaccination 24 hours after one dose of GM-CSF for primary immunization.

Sero-protective antibody titers appeared in only 33% patients who did not receive GM-CSF as compared to 83% patients who received the adjuvant. In the same study, a second group of 16 chronic HD patients, who had not sero-converted after a standard two dose hepatitis B vaccination were randomly assigned either to a booster dose of hepatitis B vaccine alone or a booster dose given 24 hours after one dose of GM-CSF. There was sero-conversion in 87.5% patients who had received GM-CSF as compared to only 25% of those who did not receive the same. The sero-protective antibody titers even when they appeared in patients who received hepatitis B vaccine alone were significantly lower when compared to patients who had received GM-CSF as an adjuvant. In another study, Kapoor et al (Table 2) also showed similar results in 15 patients.[27] These patients at the time of indication of dialysis were stratified to receive either 40 µg of hepatitis B vaccine at 0, 1, 2 and 6 months (group A, $n = 9$) or 3 µg/kg GM-CSF on day 1 followed by the vaccination schedule as described above (group B, $n = 6$). Titres of anti-HBs were quantified at 1, 2, 6 and 7 months from the first dose of vaccine. Protective antibody titres developed in 44% (4/9) of the patients in group A compared to 100% (6/6) in group B. Moreover, 50% of responders in group A developed protective levels after the 4th dose of vaccine while 67% of responders in group B were protective after only the 2nd dose of vaccine ($P = 0.046$). These findings suggest that administration of one dose of GM-CSF as adjuvant therapy, prior to primary or booster dose hepatitis B vaccination may significantly increase sero-conversion rate and sero-protective antibody titers in chronic HD patients. Newer agents are being developed to improve the vaccination results in these patients, e.g. erythropoietin, levamisole,[29] etc.

Table 2. Summary of trials of effect of GM-CSF on hepatitis B vaccination in hemodialysis patients

Reference no.	anti-HBs > 10 mIU/ml	
	Group A* (%)	Group B** (%)
26	33 (6)	83 (6)
27	44 (8)	100 (6)
28	25 (8)	87.5 (8)

* Hepatitis B vaccine at 0, 1, 2 and 6 months **GMCSF + hepatitis B vaccine at 0, 1, 2 and 6 months
figures in parathenses indicate number of patients studied

RECOMMENDATIONS

The following recommendations for vaccination against hepatitis B in patients with CRF are proposed.[12]

(a) Patients of renal disease should be screened for HBsAg. Patients with past history of jaundice should additionally be screened for anti-HBs.

(b) Patients with mild to moderate renal failure and negative for HBsAg and without any protective titers of antibodies (if tested) should be given four doses of hepatitis B vaccine as per the following schedule.

Dose	40 µg
Route and site	Intramuscular over deltoid muscle
1st dose	0 day
2nd dose	30th day (1 month)
3rd dose	60th day (2 months)
4th dose	180 (6 months)

(c) Patients should be tested for development of antibodies after 4 to 6 weeks of the last dose. If antibody titers are less than 10 mIU/ml, patient should be given GM-CSF (150 to 300 mg subcutaneously) followed 24 hours later by an intramuscular booster dose of 40 µg of hepatitis B vaccine.

(d) Patients with ESRD about to be initiated on dialysis, who have not been vaccinated against hepatitis B and not having protective antibody titers should be given GM-CSF as an adjuvant before the first dose of immunization schedule.

(e) Patients negative for HBsAg and without protective titers of antibody against HBsAg should be screened monthly for HBsAg, and if found positive, should be isolated from HBsAg negative patients.

(f) Patients having protective titers of antibody should be screened for antibodies once in 6 to 12 months and if the titers are declining, should be given a booster dose of 40 µg of vaccine.

REFERENCES

1. Saha D, Agarwal SK. Hepatitis and HIV infection during hemodialysis. *J Indian Med Assoc* 2001;99:194-9, 203, 213.
2. Jalava T, Ranki M, Bengtstrom M, Pohjanpelto P, Kallio A. A rapid and quantitative solution hybridization method for detection of HBV-DNA in serum. *J Virol Methods* 1992;36:171-80.
3. London WT, Difiglia M, Sutnick AI, Blumberg BS. An epidemic of hepatitis in a chronic hemodialysis unit. *N Engl J Med* 1969;281:571.
4. Rodby RA, Trenholme GM. Vaccination of the dialysis patient. *Semin Dial* 1991;4:102.
5. Schwebke J, Mujais S. Vaccination in hemodialysis patients. *Int J Artif Organs* 1989;12:481-4.

6. Stevens CE, Alter JH, Taylor PE, et al. Hepatitis B vaccine in patients receiving hemodialysis. Immunogenecity and efficacy. *N Engl J Med* 1984;311:496.
7. Buti M, Viladomiu L, Jardi R, et al. Long-term immunogenicity and efficacy of hepatitis B vaccine in hemodialysis patients. *Am J Nephrol* 1992;12:144-7.
8. Crosnier J, Jungers P, Couroce AM. Randomized placebo-controlled trial of hepatitis B vaccine in French hemodialysis units: II, Hemodialysis patients. *Lancet* 1981;1:779-80.
9. Dacko C, Holley JL. The influence of nutritional status, dialysis adequacy and residual function on the response to hepatitis B vaccination in peritoneal dialysis patients. *Adv Perit Dial* 1996;12:315-7.
10. Ribot S, Rothstein M, Goldblat M, Grasso M. Duration of hepatitis B surface antigenemia in hemodialysis patients. *Arch Intern Med* 1979;139:178-80.
11. Moyer LA, Alter MJ, Fovero MS. Hemodialysis associated hepatitis B: revised recommendations for serologic screening. *Semin Dial* 1990;3:201.
12. Consensus statements. Indian Association for Study of Liver. Hepatitis B in India-Prevention and management. *Indian J Gastroenterol* 2000;20(suppl.3):C54-66.
13. Miller ER, Atter MJ, Tokars JI. Protective effect of hepatitis B vaccine in chronic hemodialysis patients. *Am J Kidney Dis* 1999;33:356-60.
14. Saraswat VA. *Hepatitis B vaccination: special groups*. In: Sarin SK, Singal AK. Eds. Hepatitis B in India – Problems and Prevention: CBS Publishers & Distributors: New Delhi. 1996;pp. 162-74.
15. Pesanti EL. Immunologic defects and vaccination in patients with chronic renal failure. *Infect Dis Clin North Am* 2001;15:813-22.
16. Bruguera M, Rodicio JL, Alcazar JM. Effects of different dose levels and vaccination schedules on immune response to a recombinant DNA hepatitis B vaccine in hemodialysis patients. *Vaccine* 1990;88: S47-9.
17. Guan R, Tay HH, Choong LL. Hepatitis B vaccination in chronic renal failure patients undergoing hemodialysis: the immunogenecity of an increased dose of a recombinant DNA hepatitis B vaccine. *Ann Acad Med Singapore* 1990;19:793-7.
18. Marangi AL, Giordano R, Montanaro A, et al. Hepatitis B virus infection in chronic uremia: long-term follow-up of a two step integrated protocol of vaccination. *Am J kidney Dis* 1994;25:537-42.
19. Agarwal SK, Irshad M, Dash SC. Comparison of two schedules of hepatitis B vaccination in patients with mild, moderate and severe renal failure. *J Assoc Phys Ind* 2000;48:266-7.
20. Pillion G, Chiesa M, Maisin A. Immunogenicity of hepatitis B vaccine (HEVAC-B) in children with advanced renal failure. *Pediatr Nephrol* 1990;4:627-9.
21. Dukes CS, Street AC, Starling JF, Hamilton JD. Hepatitis B vaccination and booster in pre-dialysis patients: a 4 year analysis. *Vaccine* 1993;11:229-32.
22. Peces R, Laures AS. Persistence of immunologic memory in long-term hemodialysis patients and health care workers given hepatitis B vaccine: role of a booster dose on antibody response. *Nephron* 2001;89:172-6.
23. Anandh U, Thomas PP, Shastry JC, Jacob CK. A randomized controlled trial of intra-dermal hepatitis B vaccination and augmentation of response with erythropoietin. *J Assoc Phys Ind* 2000;48: 1061-3.
24. Vlassopoulos D, Arvanitis D, Lilis D, Hatjiyannakos D, Louizou K, Hadjiconstantinou V. Complete success of intra-dermal vaccination against hepatitis B in advanced chronic renal failure and hemodialysis patients. *Ren Fail* 1997;19:455-60.
25. Charset AF, McDougall J, Goldstein MB. A randomized comparison of intra-dermal and intra-muscular vaccination against hepatitis B virus in incident chronic hemodialysis patients. *Am J Kidney Dis* 2000;36:976-82.

26. Anandh U, Bastani B, Ballal S. Granulocyte macrophage colony stimulating factor as an adjuvant to hepatitis B vaccination in maintenance hemodialysis patients. *Am J Nephrol* 2000;20:53-6.
27. Kapoor D, Aggarwal SR, Singh NP, Thakur V, Sarin SK. Granulocyte macrophage colony stimulating factor enhances the efficacy of hepatitis B virus vaccine in previously unvaccinated hemodialysis patients. *J Viral Hepat* 1999;6:405-9.
28. Sudhagar K, Chandrasekar S, Rao MS, Ravichandran R. Effect of granulocyte macrophage colony stimulating factor on hepatitis B vaccination in hemodialysis patients. *J Assoc Phys Ind* 1999;47:602-4.
29. Kayatas M. Levamisole treatment enhances protective antibody response to hepatitis B vaccination in hemodialysis patients. *Artif Organs* 2002;26:492-6.

39

Vaccination against hepatitis A and B in patients with chronic liver disease

Vivek A Saraswat, Sanjay K Somani

Viral hepatitis continues to be a major public health problem around the world. Over the last two decades, effective vaccines have been developed against hepatitis A and B. The medical community is still in the process of evolving optimal strategies and determining cost–benefit equations for utilizing these vaccines to eradicate hepatitis A virus (HAV) and hepatitis B virus (HBV) infections. Patients with chronic liver diseases (CLD) due to a variety of causes including alcohol or chronic HBV and hepatitis C virus (HCV) infection constitute a subgroup that is especially vulnerable to superinfection by these viruses, since they are likely to develop severe, often life-threatening illness after such infections. Routine immunization of patients with chronic liver diseases against HAV has been recommended by the Advisory Committee for Immunization Practices (ACIP) in the USA. Is it time now to recommend routine vaccination against HAV for patients with CLD due to HBV, HCV, alcohol or other etiologies and against HBV for patients with non-hepatitis B-related CLD (non-B CLD)patients in India also? Several issues need to be dealt with before this question can be answered satisfactorily. Before offering vaccination against HAV, it is necessary to review the following: (a) likelihood of HAV infection occurring in an adult in India, (b) the course of acute HAV infection in CLD, (c) the efficacy of HAV vaccine in CLD, and (d) the cost–benefit equation of universal immunization of all patients with CLD versus a policy of selective immunization after screening for anti-HAV antibodies, etc. Similarly, before considering vaccination against HBV in patients with non-B CLD, it is necessary to review the role of HBV in progression of non-B CLD, the efficacy of HBV vaccines in CLD, the optimum vaccination schedules and other related issues.

VACCINATION AGAINST HAV IN PATIENTS WITH CLD

Hepatitis A in the world

Hepatitis A continues to be a major health problem, with an estimated burden of about 1.4

million cases per annum worldwide concentrated mainly in Asia, Africa and eastern Europe. The epidemiology of HAV infection is changing around the globe. The general paradigm has been a shift to the right in the age-related sero-prevalence graph with improving standards of environmental sanitation and personal hygiene that have accompanied improvement in socio-economic status. This shift began after World War II in Japan, North America and northern and western Europe and has now reached all except the most elderly segments of the population in these areas.[1-3] In USA, sero-prevalence for HAV was 10% below 10 years, 15% in 11–20 years, 18% in 31–40 years and 45% in 41–50 years age groups, rising to 70% in 51–70 years group.[4] This shift has also been noted in the developing world over the last 1–2 decades. In Taiwan, prevalence of anti-HAV dropped to 11.7% in 11–14 years age-group in 1984 compared to 72.5% in 1975-76.[5] In Malaysia, between 1985 and 1994, sero-prevalence fell from 43% to 15% in people below 10 years of age and from 64% to 28% in the 11–20 years age group.[6] Similar changes have been reported from Singapore.[7] Correlation between socio-economic status and HAV sero-prevalence, which was low in high socio-economic groups, has been reported from Thailand.[8]

Hepatitis A in India

The general impression is that India is a region highly endemic for hepatitis A and that infection and immunity are acquired almost universally in early childhood. However, published data of HAV sero-prevalence in India are rather scanty. A study from Pune found that HAV infected a majority of children by the age of 3, virtually all by the age of 10–15 and that age-specific sero-prevalence had shown no change between 1982 and 1992.[9] Data from Chandigarh revealed that 96% of school-going children from lower socio-economic groups and 85% from higher socio-economic groups had acquired antibodies against HAV.[10] In Vellore,[11] virtually all children studied before 1990, had antibodies to HAV by 10 years of age. In 1996, 78% of a large cohort ($n = 670$) were found to have detectable anti-HAV antibodies in Mumbai.[12] By 5 years of age, 62% were seropositive, with the figure rising to 77% by 10 years of age, and, 83% by 15 years of age. Except for an unexplained dip to 67% in the age group of 16–20, the seropositivity remained unchanged up to 40 years of age rising to 95.8% after that. However, interestingly, when compared with low socio-economic groups, seropositivity was found to be significantly lower in the high socio-economic group. This was seen in the group below 40 years of age as a whole, as well as in almost all age groups compared, while it was similar above 40 years of age. This supports the impression that, in higher socio-economic groups, perhaps due to improved hygiene and sanitation, a shift to the right is appearing as exposure to HAV decreases in younger age groups of this stratum. Age-group specific sero-prevalence of HAV was reported recently from Hyderabad[13] in a small sample of 90 subjects. Though the number in each age-group was small, sero-prevalence rose rapidly from 14.2% below the age of 5 years of age to 31% by 10 years of age and 75% by 15 years of age. The prevalence in children below 12 years was lower than in adults (31.8% and 94.4%; $p<0.001$).[13] Though socio-economic status of the cohort was not reported, these data suggest that there may be a change in the pattern of HAV infection in some parts of India, with fewer infections occurring in children, while older age-groups exhibit high levels of seropositivity, probably from previous exposure. Thus, at least some segments of the Indian population may be undergoing the demographic transition from high to low prevalence for HAV. Data on the sero-prevalence of HAV infection among cirrhotics from India are very scarce. Anti-HAV antibodies were detected in only 5.3% of a series of 94 consecutive patients with liver cirrhosis seen at a north Indian hospital, suggesting that a very large proportion of the cirrhotic population is at risk of acute hepatitis A. However, more data from other centers are needed to corroborate this observation.[14] In India, HAV does not appear to be a major cause of serious liver disease. Investigators from north India found that HAV caused fulminant hepatitis in 1.7%[15] and sporadic acute hepatitis in 5% of cases.[16]

HAV superinfection in HBV-related chronic liver disease

Hepatitis A is usually an anicteric, uncomplicated and mild illness in children. However, in adults, it often has severe symptoms, with high levels of transaminases and serum bilirubin, and is frequently complicated by severe cholestasis, resulting in more loss of time from work. Fulminant and subacute liver failure also occur more commonly in adults.[17, 18] Thus, paradoxically, while improving hygiene and sanitation decreases childhood HAV infections, the burden of symptomatic illness in adults is often increased.

Initial reports suggested, that the outcome of acute hepatitis A was not modified by the coexistence of pre-existing chronic HBV infection.[19-24] During an outbreak of 143 cases of acute hepatitis A in the age group of 5–30 years in Taiwan,[19] the clinical and biochemical course in 28 (20%) patients with chronic HBV infection was no different than in those without HBV infection. However, it is well known that hepatitis A is milder in younger age groups and younger patients with chronic HBV infection are more likely to be healthy subjects rather than affected with chronic liver disease. Small studies from Munich[20] ($n = 30$) and Athens[21] ($n = 10$), as well as a few case reports of 1 to 3 patients[22-24] found that hepatitis A in chronic HBsAg positive subjects was a mild disease that did not differ from hepatitis A in patients without chronic HBV infection.

However, not all reports presented such an optimistic outlook. Fulminant hepatic failure developed following acute hepatitis A in a patient with chronic hepatitis.[25] Experience from large outbreaks of hepatitis A and in large populations followed over long periods suggests that acute hepatitis can have a grave outcome in the presence of HBV-related CLD. The 1988 Shanghai hepatitis A epidemic[26] resulted in 3,10,746 cases of acute hepatitis A with a total of 47 deaths. Deaths were due to fulminant hepatitis A in 25, hepatitis A superimposed on chronic HBV infection in 15 and miscellaneous diseases in 7 patients. Case fatality rate in acute hepatitis A superimposed on chronic HBV infection was 5.6 fold higher than without chronic HBV infection (0.05% vs. 0.009%).[26] The increased mortality of HAV superinfection in chronic HBV infection was hypothesized to be the result of enhanced T-cell-mediated destruction of HBV-infected hepatocytes during acute HAV infection.[27] In the United States, 381 deaths occurred among 1,15,551 cases of acute hepatitis A reported to CDC, Atlanta, between 1983 and 1988, of which 27 (7%) occurred in 231 patients with chronic HBV infection and 108 (28%) deaths occurred in patients with non-B, non-alcoholic cirrhosis. The case fatality rate in acute hepatitis A superimposed on chronic HBV infection was 11.7% compared with 0.2% in those without HBV infection.[28] Thus, it appears that underlying liver disease predisposes to a more severe outcome from HAV infection.

A study from Japan differentiated between subjects with chronic HBV infection and those with chronic liver disease.[29] It was found that, among 29 patients with acute hepatitis A superimposed on chronic HBV infection, severe clinical course (deep jaundice, prothrombin time <50% in 7; death in 2) was seen in those who had severe chronic hepatitis (2), cirrhosis (4) or massive hepatic necrosis (3) on liver biopsy. Biopsies done in 8 others with chronic HBV infection who had a benign uncomplicated course, revealed only acute hepatitis (5) or mild chronic hepatitis (3). The remaining patients, who were not biopsied, were healthy chronic HBsAg positive subjects and experienced a mild course, similar to that seen in patients without chronic HBV infection. It appeared, in this review, that hepatitis A was severe mainly in patients with hepatitis B (HB)-related CLD, while in chronic HBsAg positive subjects, it was similar to hepatitis A in the absence of HBV infection.

In contrast, a study from Thailand[30] found that hepatitis A was equally severe in healthy chronic HBsAg positive subjects and those with CLD. Acute hepatitis A in 20 asymptomatic hepatitis B surface antigen (HBsAg) positive subjects and 12 patients with chronic liver disease (CLD; due to HBV in 8, HCV in 4), was compared with the course of HAV infection in 100 patients without any other disease. While all patients with isolated HAV infection recovered fully, fulminant or submassive hepatitis occurred in 11 (55%) HBsAg positive subjects and 4 (33%) with HBV or HCV related CLD. Nine of 15 patients with severe hepatitis died (5/11 HBsAg positive subjects, all 4 with CLD), mortality being similar among chronic HBsAg positive subjects and CLD patients 25% vs. 33%; p = 0.15).[30] Although baseline serum alanine aminotransferase (ALT) was comparable between the groups, liver histology in the HBsAg positive subjects was not reported.

It appears that the outcome of hepatitis A in patients with chronic HBV infection depends on the extent of pre-existent liver damage and degree of compromise of liver function. Healthy HBsAg positive subjects with normal transaminases and normal liver histology fare no worse than individuals without prior liver disease; however, in the presence of chronic hepatitis or liver cirrhosis, the risk of a severe or fatal illness is high.

HAV superinfection in other chronic liver diseases

A few reports suggest that hepatitis A in patients with other forms of liver diseases also has an adverse outcome. In the United States, of 381 deaths occurring among 1,15,551 cases of acute hepatitis A reported between 1983 and 1988, 108 (28%) deaths occurred in patients with non-B, non-alcoholic cirrhosis.[28] Death due to fulminant hepatitis A occurred in 4 patients with alcoholic liver disease (hepatitis 1, cirrhosis 2, cirrhosis with hepatitis 1) reported from Los Angeles.[31]

Vento[32] followed 432 patients with chronic hepatitis C for 7 years. Fulminant hepatic failure (FHF) developed in 7 (41%) of 17 patients with chronic HCV infection developing acute hepatitis A compared with 3 of 415 (0.7%; p< 0.03) without HAV infection over this period.[32] None of the HCV patients had liver cirrhosis. This suggests that severe, life-threatening acute liver damage may develop following HAV superinfection in HCV-related chronic hepatitis, even in the absence of cirrhosis.

Vaccination against HAV is effective in CLD

Lee evaluated the safety and immunogenicity of an inactivated hepatitis A vaccine in 56 patients with chronic hepatitis B and 4 with chronic hepatitis C.[33] A two-dose schedule, given at 0 and 6 months, produced 100% sero-conversion. All individuals remained sero-positive for 12 months, the majority maintaining high levels of antibody during a 5-year follow-up period. Though the inactivated hepatitis A vaccine was found to be well tolerated and immunogenic in patients with CLD, the immune response generated was inferior to that observed in healthy individuals, indicating the need for a higher dose and the two-dose schedule to ensure adequate protection.[33] In another study comparing two doses of an inactivated hepatitis A vaccine in patients with CLD and healthy subjects, Keeffe[34] found that the vaccine was well tolerated and induced a satisfactory immune response in patients with chronic hepatitis B; 97.7% of patients with chronic hepatitis B and 98.2% healthy adults had seroconverted at 7 months.[34] Among children, anti-HAV response was found to be lower in vaccine recipients positive for hepatitis B surface antigen (11/16, 68.8%) compared with those negative for HBsAg (95/101, 94.1%; p <0.01) when tested 15 days after the priming dose.[35] There are very few data about the efficacy and sero-conversion rates after HAV vaccination in patients with alcoholic liver disease, a group found to seroconvert poorly after HBV vaccination.

Liver failure significantly reduced the antibody response to hepatitis A vaccine and liver transplant recipients were unable to respond to it. Dumot[36] vaccinated 16 end-stage liver disease patients and 8 liver transplant recipients. Median antibody titer, undetectable in liver transplant recipients, was higher in liver failure patients (34.7 mIU/ml; p <0.001) but lower than the level seen in healthy individuals or even those patients with early CLD. Although small, this study suggested that immunization against HAV should be considered early for susceptible patients with chronic liver disease because the development of liver failure may blunt the immune response to the vaccine and it might be ineffective after immunosuppresion.

Based on these and other data, the Advisory Committee on Immunization Practices (ACIP) recommended in December 1996 that all patients with chronic liver disease should be immunized against HAV infection.[37] In the consensus statement on the role of hepatitis A vaccination in patients with chronic liver disease,[38] it was concluded that improved sanitation and hygiene in the developing world have led to a decline in immunity against HAV. As a result, growing number of adults are now susceptible to infection, with those who have not been vaccinated against hepatitis B virus (HBV) being at risk for dual infection and potentially more severe illness. It was recommended that patients with CLD should be targeted for hepatitis A vaccination as soon as CLD is diagnosed.[38]

Vaccination against HAV for chronic liver disease patients in India

From the forgoing review, it is clear that adults with chronic liver disease due to HBV, HCV or alcohol are at a high-risk for the development of fatal or serious complications after hepatitis A. It also appears that vaccination against HAV is effective in patients with HBV and HCV related CLD, especially if undertaken before the development of end-stage liver disease or liver transplantation. Data about its efficacy in alcoholic liver disease are lacking. However, available reports suggest that HAV is a rare cause of acute hepatitis or fulminant hepatic failure in India. Hepatitis A causing deterioration in patients with CLD has not been widely reported from India. The prevalence of pre-existing anti-HAV antibodies, especially among adults, is in excess of 75%, though almost no information is available among those with CLD. Sero-prevalence may be declining in age groups below 40 years in higher socio-economic groups; however, only a few good studies have been undertaken to establish this point. Very limited work has been published regarding the efficacy of the commonly used HAV vaccines in the Indian population. Particularly, there are reports confirming efficacy of the HAV vaccine in Indian patients with chronic liver disease. Firm recommendations in favour of universal immunization against HAV of adult Indian CLD patients must await the availability of more data about frequency and levels of anti-HAV antibodies, frequency of HAV-related worsening in stable patients with CLD, and the efficacy and optimum dosage schedules of current vaccines. Until then, clinicians will have to exercise their clinical judgement in recommending vaccination to individuals on the basis of their perceived risk assessed on the basis of factors such as higher socio-economic status and whether they belong to the identified high-risk groups in the population. A strategy of screening before vaccination, with selective immunization for those lacking protective levels of antibodies should be considered and may be better suited to the needs of a population with high background levels of anti-HAV antibodies. Until large-scale studies documenting the efficacy and optimum vaccination schedule for Indian cirrhotics are available, antibody testing and monitoring should be undertaken among those offered vaccination against HAV to ensure continued protection. Universal immunization against HAV as a part of the National Immunization Program will be the long-term solution of the problem of HAV infection among all population groups. However, no such proposal has hitherto been floated for India.

VACCINATION AGAINST HEPATITIS B IN PATIENTS WITH NON-B CLD

HBV infection in the world

Hepatitis B is one of the most common infectious diseases in the world. It has been estimated that 350 million people world-wide have chronic hepatitis B virus infection. More than 75% of these carriers live in over 40 countries of the Western Pacific and South East Asia, which are the largest and most populous of the six World Health Organization regions.[39] The global prevalence of chronic HBV infection is high ($\geq 8\%$) in sub-Saharan Africa, east Asia and the western Pacific, intermediate (2–7%) in southern and eastern Europe and India and low ($\leq 2\%$) in western Europe, northern America and Australia. The predominant routes of transmission vary according to the prevalence of the HBV infection. In high-prevalence areas, transmission is mainly perinatal whereas in low-prevalence areas, sexual contact amongst high-risk adults is the predominant route. Between one-third and one-fourth of people with chronic HBV infection are expected to develop progressive liver disease including cirrhosis and primary liver cancer.[40]

Impact of immunization for HBV

All infants and/or adolescents are routinely vaccinated in over 100 countries which have included hepatitis B (HB) immunization in their national immunization programs. Many more countries are planning to launch this program in the next two years. Ten to 15 years follow-up data are now being reported from population based studies of HB immunization from around the world, showing a reduction in chronic HBsAg positivity rates from high ($\geq 8\%$) to low ($\leq 2\%$) prevalence in immunized cohorts.[41]

HBV in India

The average estimated HBsAg positivity rate in India is 4%, with a pool of approximately 43 million infected subjects. Professional blood donors constitute a major high-risk group for HBV infection in India, with hepatitis B surface antigen positivity rates of 14–36%.[42] Blood transfusions represent the most important route of HBV transmission among adults. However, most of India's infected pool is established in early childhood, predominantly by horizontal spread due to crowded living conditions and poor hygiene. HBV is reckoned to be the etiological agent in 42% and 45%, respectively, of adults with acute and subacute liver failure which are common complications of viral hepatitis in India. HBV is reported to be responsible for 70% of chronic hepatitis and 80% of liver cirrhosis patients in India. About 60% of patients with hepatocellular carcinoma are positive for HBV markers.[43]

HBV and HCV infection and progression of alcoholic liver disease

The role of HBV and HCV infection in the progression of alcoholic liver disease remains the subject of debate. Many studies from different parts of the world report a high frequency of

HBV and HCV infection among alcoholics.[44-47] It appears that alcoholism and HBV infection exert synergistic effects on liver injury. Alcoholism, HBV and HCV seem to interact and each amplifies liver injury due to the others.[46-48] Alcoholics with HBV infection have been reported to have accelerated liver injury and HCC, as well as decreased survival compared with alcoholics who are not HBV infected.[49]

Alcoholics are considered a high-risk group for HBV infection in eastern Europe. At least one marker of HBV infection was present in 50% and anti-HCV was detected in 24% of 144 unselected patients attending an outpatient clinic for alcoholics in Poland, significantly higher than in a matched control population.[44] Among 129 Alaskan natives, HBV markers were present in 34.4% of alcoholics and in only 11.7% of controls ($p = 0.012$).[45]

In Brazil, both HBsAg (1.9%) and anti-HBc (28.3%) were more frequent ($p<0.001$) among 365 alcoholics with or without cirrhosis than among controls (0.4%, 4.0% respectively). The frequency of HBsAg in alcoholics without cirrhosis was similar to controls, whereas it was significantly higher among those who progressed to cirrhosis, suggesting that HBV may be implicated in the progression to cirrhosis in some alcoholic individuals.[46]

A study from Taiwan[47] comparing 123 alcoholic patients with liver disease with 44 alcoholics without liver disease found HBsAg in 30.1% of the former compared with 11.4% of the latter ($p<0.05$). HBsAg was detected in 40.7% with cirrhosis and HCC, in 30.7% with cirrhosis alone and in 29.4% with other liver diseases. Similar findings were noted in those with HCV infection. Serum ALT level was higher in those with alcohol and virus when compared with those without HBV or HCV. Thus, patients with more advanced alcoholic liver disease were more likely to be infected by HBV, suggesting a role for the virus in the progression of liver disease.

A case-control analysis in central Harlem, New York, underlined the role of hepatitis viruses in the development of chronic liver disease among alcoholics.[48] Patients with both alcoholism and either HBV (odds ratio [OR] 6.3;95% CI 0.5–33.4) or HCV infection (OR 2.9;CI 1.3-6.2) were at an increased risk for CLD whereas risk was similar to controls in patients with only one of these three factors.

While alcoholics have been reported to have a high frequency of exposure to HBV, as suggested by the presence of anti-HBc and/or anti-HBs, the frequency of replicating infection, contributing to the progression of liver disease, remains uncertain. In order to clarify this issue, Nalpas[50] looked for HBV-DNA as well as other markers of HBV infection in the serum of 146 chronic alcoholics, with normal liver function (group I), 67 with alcoholic liver disease without cirrhosis (group II) and 31 with alcoholic cirrhosis (group III). HBV markers were present in 37% of the whole group, though serum HBV-DNA was detected only in total of 17 patients (11.6%): 6 (12.5%) in group I, 7 (10.4%) in group II and 4 (12.9%) in group III, compared to none in 100 healthy controls ($p<0.01$). Among the HBV-DNA positive patients, HBsAg was detected in 3, anti-HBc and/or anti-HBs in the absence of HBsAg in 5, while no HBV marker was found in 9 patients. Eight of the 68 patients studied were also positive for HBV-DNA in the liver.[50] Thus, this study found that although HBV infection occurred in over one-third of alcoholics, HBV-DNA was present in only about 12% and may have played a role in the development or progression of liver disease in only half of these, since in the others HBV-DNA was present in the absence of other HBV markers, suggesting cleared or inactive infection.

Outcome of acute hepatitis superimposed on CLD

The development of acute viral hepatitis, due to any virus (HAV, HBV, HCV), often results in severe liver disease or death in patients with established liver cirrhosis, including alcoholic cirrhosis. Four patients with alcoholic liver disease developing acute hepatitis A died after a fulminant illness.[31] Two of the 4 patients with alcoholic liver disease developing acute hepatitis B in another report also died after a fulminant course.[51] Acute non-A, non-B (probable HCV) transfusion-associated hepatitis developed in 6 patients receiving factor IX concentrates; 3 of 4 with underlying cirrhosis died after a fulminant course.[52] Liver failure (hepatic coma and/or ascites) developed in 12 of 20 (60%) patients with alcoholic cirrhosis developing acute, probably transfusion associated hepatitis, due to HBV in 2 and NANBV (? HCV) in 18. Four (20%) died after a fulminant illness.[53] Thus, these reports clearly show that development of acute hepatitis of any etiology can have devastating consequences for patients with underlying liver cirrhosis, particularly decompensated cirrhosis of any etiology.

Vaccination against HBV in alcoholic liver disease patients

Several workers have reported that sero-conversion rates after HBV vaccination in alcoholic liver disease ranges from 43–70%[54-58] compared with over 90% in nonalcoholic subjects. With advanced liver disease, sero-conversion rate drops even further.[59, 60] Factors responsible for poor sero-conversion are not well understood. It remains unclear whether this inadequate antibody response to vaccination is the result of age, alcoholism, cirrhosis, malnutrition or poor general health and whether it is unique for the HBV vaccine or is seen with other vaccines used in alcoholics and other types of CLD. Some reports suggest that age may influence sero-conversion rates among alcoholics. McMahon[45] did not find poor sero-conversion among younger alcoholics. Standard 3-dose HBV vaccination was given to 72 subjects (32 alcoholics, 40 controls) in Alaska. Among 62 who seroconverted, those below the age of 45 showed no difference in the mean anti-HBs titers between alcoholics and controls. Alcoholics over the age of 45, had lower anti-HBs titers than age-matched controls, though the difference was insignificant. Reduced rates of conversion after the age of 55 have been reported by others also.[60] Nalpas[58] found that mean anti-HBs titer was significantly lower during follow-up among those alcoholics who had seroconverted after vaccination against HBV but resumed drinking, suggesting a direct effect of alcohol on the response. Advanced liver disease is known to reduce sero-conversion for HAV as well as HBV vaccination. Only

47% of 132 patients with end-stage liver disease, including 7 alcoholics, referred for liver transplantation seroconverted after a 3-dose course of recombinant HBV vaccine.[60]

Degos[54] used 3 or 4 doses of a recombinant vaccine in alcoholic patients with or without cirrhosis. Among 32 cirrhotics, 20 received three injections of hepatitis B vaccine at monthly intervals and 12 received the fourth dose one month later. Anti-HBs titer at 6 months did not differ between the 3- and 4-injection groups. Only 2 patients were good responders (peak anti-HBs >300 mIU/ml), 14 had a low response (<30 mIU/ml) and 16 (50%) had no detectable anti-HBs response. Alcoholics without cirrhosis were given 4 injections and all had detectable anti-HBs but peak antibody response (mean 97.7 ± 4 mIU/ml) was not very satisfactory. There were no obvious differences in the response to the vaccine on the basis of age, sex or continuation of alcohol intake.[54]

Mendenhall[55] found sero-conversion among only 18% of alcoholics with clinical liver disease after 3 doses of HBV vaccine, compared to 70% among alcoholics without overt liver disease and 89% among nonalcoholic controls. The levels of anti-HBs were also significantly lower among those with overt liver disease as compared to the other two groups. Maruyama[56] could detect an anti-HBs response in only 8 out of 15 alcoholics given standard, 3-dose vaccination against hepatitis B. Villaneuva[57] found that sero-conversion occurred in only 60% of alcoholics compared to 83% in nonalcoholic subjects and anti-HBs levels were significantly lower among alcoholics. Using a rapid, high-dose schedule did not improve sero-conversion rates or anti-HBs titers among the alcoholics.

Modifications in the HBV vaccination strategy for alcoholics, in an effort to improve sero-conversion rates and antibody titers, have included concentrating on alcoholics without cirrhosis, using high-dose, 4-injection schedules and booster doses at 1 year.[61,62] One hundred alcoholic subjects, including 10 with clinical or pathologic evidence of cirrhosis, received either standard (20 micrograms at 0, 1 and 6 months) or high-dose (40 micrograms at 0, 1, 2, and 6 months) recombinant hepatitis B vaccine (Engerix-B).[61] Thirty-six of 48 (75%) patients seroconverted in the high-dose group compared with 24 of 52 (46%) in the standard dose group ($p<0.005$). Mean anti-HBs titer in the high-dose group was greater than in the standard dose group (76.4 vs. 39.4 mIU/ml, $p<0.01$), though in both groups, it was lower than the usual response in non-alcoholics. Logistic regression demonstrated a significant effect on sero-conversion for the vaccine dose ($p <0.005$) and serum albumin ($p = 0.05$) but not for other variables such as race, age, drinking during the study, serum creatinine, arm muscle circumference and cirrhosis.[61]

A prospective randomized trial compared serovaccination with standard hepatitis B vaccination in patients with alcoholic cirrhosis.[62] In the vaccination group, 3 doses of GenHevac B vaccine at 0, 1, 6 months were followed by a 4th, 1 dose at 9 months while the serovaccination group received the same vaccination schedule followed by an injection of hepatitis B immunoglobulins (HBIg 500 IU). After 12 months, seroconversion rates were 69% and

67% in the two groups. Thus, serovaccination did not increase immunogenicity of hepatitis B vaccination in patients with alcoholic cirrhosis and cannot be recommended.[62]

Nalpas[58] assessed the efficacy of a 1-year booster dose in 28 alcoholics with minimal liver disease who had received primary immunization with a 3-dose course of HBV vaccine. Seroconversion rate rose from 43% after primary vaccination to 82% after the booster. Anti-HBs titers were measured 1 month and 2 years after the booster dose. Those with a 1-month post-booster anti-HBs titer above 1000 mIU/ml still had high anti-HBs levels(>100 mIU/ml) at 2 years whereas 80% of these with 1–month post-booster levels below 1000 mIU/ml had low levels (<100mIU/ml) or below protective levels (<10 mIU/ml) of anti-HBs at 2 years. They suggested that alcoholics should routinely receive a booster dose at 1 year and that those with low 1 month post-booster levels should be tested at regular intervals, so that further doses can be given as required.

Vaccination against HBV for HCV-related CLD patients

Chronic hepatitis C results in liver disease, cirrhosis, and hepatocellular carcinoma. Its prevalence is estimated to be 70–92% among intravenous drug users, who are also at high-risk of acquiring parenteral or sexually transmitted hepatitis B infection. Other than intravenous drug abusers, other groups of patients infected with HCV (hemophiliacs, thalassemics and others receiving frequent blood transfusions, dialysis and transplant recipients, etc.) also form high-risk groups for HBV infection. Since infection with hepatitis B virus may accelerate liver damage due to underlying hepatitis C and liver damage due to the two viruses may be synergistic, it appears logical to offer vaccination against HBV to patients with chronic HCV infection.

A group of 126 consecutive patients with chronic HCV infection (intravenous drug abuse 88, exposure to blood or blood products 22, no identifiable risk factor 16) was studied prospectively.[63] Seventy-five were negative for all serum markers of hepatitis B infection at inclusion and were therefore still at risk. Only 10 of 126 patients received vaccination against hepatitis B after counselling by physicians or to meet visa requirements for travel abroad. Forty-one per cent (51/126) developed serologic markers of hepatitis B infection during follow-up, confirming that patients with chronic hepatitis C were at risk for HBV infection and are likely to benefit from vaccination against HBV. This study suggested that opportunities for vaccination against HBV were being missed. Vaccination might not have been offered due to failure to recognize that patients with hepatitis C are at risk for hepatitis B as well as failure to appreciate that intravenous drug users have inconsistent contact with health care professionals.[63]

Investigating the profile of dual infections with both hepatitis B and C viruses, workers in Saudi Arabia[64] found that liver cirrhosis was more common in patients with dual infection than in controls infected with HCV alone (95% vs. 48.5%, $p<0.01$). Patients with dual infection often had decompensated liver disease, with more of them classified as Child-Pugh grade C compared to controls. Similarly, hepatocellular carcinoma was more common in patients with dual infection than in controls (63% vs. 15%, p<0.01).[64]

Both HBV and HCV are blood-borne viruses; however, HBV is transmitted efficiently by both percutaneous and mucosal exposures while HCV is transmitted predominantly by percutaneous exposure. Because the relative importance of various modes of transmission of these viruses differs in different parts of the world, the choice of specific prevention and control strategies depends primarily on the epidemiology of infection in a particular country. Comprehensive hepatitis B prevention strategies should include (a) prevention of perinatal HBV transmission, (b) hepatitis B vaccination at critical ages to interrupt transmission, and (c) prevention of nosocomial HBV transmission.[65,66]

Vaccination against HBV for non-B related CLD patients

Although the need for immunizing alcoholics and those with other forms of liver cirrhosis against HBV infection is beyond question, several problems with HBV vaccination for patients with alcoholic liver disease have yet to be resolved. Sero-conversion rates are low in alcoholics in general and especially so in those with liver cirrhosis, precisely the group at highest risk from intercurrent hepatitis B infection.[67] Sero-conversion is rare after progression to end-stage liver disease and after liver transplantation. Anti-HBs levels attained after vaccination are low and wane rapidly. The optimum dose, schedule, need for boosters and for monitoring anti-HBs levels have yet to be established. Data about efficacy of vaccination against HBV in HCV related CLD or in other forms of cirrhosis are even more scanty. Hitherto, vaccination against HBV for patients with alcoholic or other forms of liver cirrhosis has not been recommended by the ACIP, FDA, or any other regulatory authority. Presently, vaccination against HBV should be offered on a case-by-case basis, after evaluating risk and benefit in the individual patient. Since a standard schedule has not yet been prescribed for these patients, the onus for monitoring antibody response and finding a schedule adapted to the individual patient, to maintain protective antibody levels in responders, will rest on the clinician recommending vaccination.

REFERENCES

1. Shapiro CN, Coleman PJ, McQuillan GM, Alter HJ, Margolis HS. Epidemiology of hepatitis A: seroepidemiology and risk groups in the USA. *Vaccine* 1992;10(suppl 1):59-62.
2. Frosner GG, Papaevangelou G, Butler R, Iwarson S, Lindholm A, Conrouce-Pauty A, Haas H, et al. Antibody against hepatitis A in seven European countries. I. Comparison of prevalence data in different age groups. *Am J Epidemiol* 1979;110:63-9.
3. Gust ID. Epidemiological patterns of hepatitis A in different parts of the world. *Vaccine* 1992;10 (suppl 1):56-8.
4. Lemon SM, Shapiro CN. The value of immunization against hepatitis *Infect Agents Dis* 1994;1:38-49.
5. Hsu HY, Chang MH, Chen DS, Lee CY, Sung JL. Changing seroepidemiology of hepatitis A infection in Taiwan. *J Med Virol* 1985;17:297-301.

6. Malik VA, Baharin R. Changing prevalence of hepatitis A in Malaysia. Presented at 4th Western Pacific Congress on Chemotherapy and Infectious Diseases, Dec 1994, Manila, Phillipines.
7. Committee on Epidemic Diseases. Epidemiology of hepatitis A virus infection in Singapore. *Epidemiol News Bull* 1992;18:63-4.
8. Pruksananoda P, Kothiphan J, Dejvorraasuthi S, Pissasarakti B, Akarwong K. Sero-prevalence of hepatitis A antibody in high socio-economic Thai population residing in Bangkok, Thailand. Presented at 7th ASEAN Pediatric Federation Conference, Nov 1994, Bangkok
9. Arankalle VA, Tsarev SA, Chadha MS, Alling DW, Emerson SU, Banerjee K, Purcell RH. Age-specific prevalence of antibodies to hepatitis A and E viruses in Pune, India, 1982 and 1992. *J Infect Dis* 1995;171:447-50.
10. Thapa BR, Singh K, Singh V, Broor S, Nain CK. Patterns of hepatitis A and B markers in cases of acute sporadic hepatitis in healthy school children from northwest India. *J Trop Pediatr* 1995;41:328-9.
11. John TJ, Chandy GM. What priority for prevention of hepatitis A in India? *Indian J Gastroenterol* 1998;17:2-3.
12. Dhawan PS, Shah SS, Alvares JF, Kher A, Shankaran, Kandoth PW, Sheth PN, et al. Sero-prevalence of hepatitis A virus "in Mumbai and immunogenicity and safety of hepatitis A vaccine. *Indian J Gastroenterol* 1998;17:16-8.
13. Joshi N, Nagarjun Kumar, Kumar A. Age related sero-prevalence of antibodies to hepatitis A virus in Hyderabad, India. *Trop Gastroenterol* 2000;21:63-5.
14. Das K, Kar P, Gupta RK. Chronic liver disease: what is the risk of decompensation by hepatitis A superinfection? *Indian J Gastroenterol* 1999;18(suppl 2):A42.
15. Acharya SK, Dasrathy S, Kumar TL, Sushma S, Prasanna KS, Tandon A, Sreenivas V, et al. Fulminant hepatitis in a tropical population: clinical course, cause and early prediction of outcome. *Hepatology* 1996;23:1448-55.
16. Datta R, Panda SK, Tandon BN. Acute sporadic non-A, non-B viral hepatitis of adults in India-epidemiological and immunological studies. *J Gastroenterol Hapatol* 1987;2:333-45.
17. Boughton C, Hawkes B, Ferguson V. Viral hepatitis A and B. *Med J Aust* 1980;1:177-80.
18. Hadler SC, McFarland L. Hepatitis A in day care centers: epidemiology and prevention. *Rev Infect Dis* 1986;8:548-57.
19. Yang CY, Chu CM, Liaw YF, Au C, Sheen IS, Lin DY, Chang-Chen CS, et al. A clinical study on acute hepatitis A: with special reference to its occurrence in HBsAg carriers. *L Formos Med Assocn* 1983;82: 1128-32.
20. Zachoval R, Roggendorf M, Deinhardt F. Hepatitis A infection in chronic carriers of hepatitis B virus. *Hepatology* 1983;3:528-31.
21. Tassopoulos N, Papaevangelou G, Roumeliotou-Karayannis A, Kalafatas P, Engle R, Gerin J, Purcell RH. Double infection with hepatitis A and B viruses. *Liver* l985;5:348-53.
22. Conteas C, Kao H, Rakela J, Weliky B. Acute type A hepatitis in three patients with chronic HBV infection. *Dig Dis Sci* 1983;28:684-6.
23. Viola LA, Barrinson JG, Coleman JC, Murray-Lyon IM. The clinical course of acute type A hepatitis in chronic HBsAg carriers: A report of 3 cases. *Postgrad Med J* 1982;58:80-1.
24. Davis GL, Hoofnagle JH, Waggoner JG. Acute type A hepatitis during chronic hepatitis B infection: Association of depressed hepatitis B virus replication with appearance of endogenous alpha interferon. *J Med Virol* 1984;14:141-7.
25. Wang JY, Lee SD, Tsai YT, Lo KJ, Chiang BN. Fulminant hepatitis A in chronic HBV carrier. *Dig Dis Sci* 1986;31:109-11.
26. Yao G. *Clinical spectrum and natural history of viral hepatitis A in a 1988 Shanghai epidemic.* In: Hollinger FB, Lemon SM, Margolis H, Eds. Viral hepatitis and liver disease: Baltimore, Williams & Wilkins, 1991:pp.76-8.

27. Cooksley WG. What did we learn from the Shanghai hepatitis A epidemic? *J Viral Hepat* 2000; (suppl 1):1-3.
28. Hadler SC. *Global impact of hepatitis A virus infection: changing patterns. In:* Hollinger FB, Lemon SM, Margolis H, Eds. Viral hepatitis and liver disease: Baltimore, Williams & Wilkins, 1991;pp.14-20.
29. Fukumoto Y, Okita K, Konishi T, et al. *Hepatitis A infection in chronic carriers of hepatitis B virus. In:* Sung JL, Chen DS, Eds. Viral hepatitis and hepatocellular carcinoma: Amsterdam, Excerpta Medica, 1990: pp.43-8.
30. Pramoolsinsap C, Poovorawan Y, Hirsch P, Busagorn N, Attamasirikul K. Acute hepatitis A superinfection in HBV carriers or chronic liver disease related to HBV or HCV. *Ann Trop Med Parasitol* 1999;93:745-51.
31. Akriviadis EA, Redeker AG. Fulminant hepatitis A in intravenous drug users with chronic liver disease. *Ann Intern Med* 1989;110:838-9.
32. Vento S, Garofano T, Renzine C, Cainceli F, Casali F, Ghironzi G, Ferraro T, et al. Fulminant hepatitis A associated with hepatitis A superinfection in patients with chronic hepatitis C. *N Engl J Med* 1998;338:286-90.
33. Lee S. Hepatitis A vaccination in patients with chronic liver disease in Taiwan. *J Viral Hepat* 2000; (suppl 1):19-21.
34. Keeffe EB, Iwarson S, McMahon BJ, Lindsay KL, Koff RS, Manns M, Baumgarten R, et al. Safety and immunogenicity of hepatitis A vaccine in patients with chronic liver disease. *Hepatology* 1998;27:881-6.
35. Lee SD, Chan CY, Yu MI, Wang YJ, Lo KJ, Safary A. Single-dose inactivated hepatitis A vaccination schedule for susceptible youngsters. *Am J Gastroenterol* 1996;91:1360-2.
36. Dumot JA, Barnes DS, Younossi Z, Gordon SM, Avery RK, Domen RE, Henderson JM, et al. Immunogenicity of hepatitis A vaccine in decompensated liver disease. *Am J Gastroenterol* 1999;94: 1601-4.
37. Center for Disease Control and Prevention. Prevention of hepatitis A through active or passive immunization recommendations of the Advisory Committee on Immunization Practices (ACIP). *MMWR* 1996;45:1-30.
38. Cooksley WG. Consensus statement on the role of hepatitis A vaccination in patients with chronic liver Disease. *J Viral Hepat* 2000;(suppl 1):29-30.
39. Gust ID. Epidemiology of hepatitis B infection in the Western Pacific and South East Asia. *Gut* 1996;38(suppl 1):S18-23.
40. Maddrey WC. Hepatitis B: an important public health issue. *J Med Virol* 2000;61:362-6.
41. Kane MA. Expanded Program on Immunization, World Health Organization, Geneva, Switzerland. *Vaccine* 1998;16(Suppl):S104-8.
42. Sood B, Saxena R. *What is safe blood? In:* Sarin SK, Singal AK, Eds. Hepatitis B in India: Problems and Prevention. CBS Publishers and Distributors, New Delhi. 1996; pp.86-104.
43. Tandon BN, Acharya SK, Tandon A. Epidemiology of hepatitis B virus infection in India. *Gut* 1996;38(suppl 2):S56-9.
44. Laskus T, Radkowski M, Lupa E, Horban A, Cianciara J, Slusarczyk J. Prevalence of markers of hepatitis viruses in out-patient alcoholics. *J Hepatol* 1992;15:174-8.
45. McMahon BJ, Wainwright K, Bulkow L, Parkinson AJ, Lindenbaum M, Helmiak C. Response to hepatitis B vaccine in Alaska natives with chronic alcoholism compared with nonalcoholic control subjects. *Am J Med* 1990;88:460-84.
46. de Oliveira LC, Buso AG, de Oliveira AT, Arantes CA, Borges LV, Valente SR. Prevalence of hepatitis B and hepatitis C markers in alcoholics with and without clinically evident hepatic cirrhosis. *Rev Inst Med Trop Sao Paulo* 1999;41:69-73.
47. Chang TT, Lin CY, Chow NH, Hsu PI, Yang CC, Lin XZ, Shin JS, et al. Hepatitis B and C virus

infection among chronic alcoholic patients with liver disease in Taiwan. *J Formos Med Assoc* 1994;93: 128-33.
48. Frieden TR, Ozick L, McCord C, Nainan OV, Workman S, Comer G, Lee TP, et al. Chronic liver disease in central Harlem: the role of alcohol and viral hepatitis. *Hepatology* 1999;29:883-8.
49. Ohnishi K, Lida S, Iwwama S, Goto N, Nomura F, Takashi M, Mishima A, et al. The effect of chronic habitual alcohol intake on the development of liver cirrhosis and hepatocellular carcinoma: relation to hepatitis B surface antigen carriage. *Cancer* 1982;49:672-7.
50. Nalpas B, Berthelot P, Thiers V, Duhamel G, Courouce AM, Tiollais P, Brechot C. Hepatitis B virus multiplication in the absence of usual serological markers. A study of 146 chronic alcoholics. *J Hepatol* 1985;1:89-97.
51. Theodossi A, Wilkinson SP, Portmann B, White Y, Eddleston AL, Williams R, Zuckerman AJ. De novo acute and activation of hepatitis B virus in established cirrhosis. *Br Med J* 1979;ii:893-5.
52. Wyke RJ, Tsiquaye KN, Thornton A, White Y, Portmann B, Dags PK, Zuckerman AJ, et al. Transmission of non-A, non-B hepatitis to chimpanzees after fatal complications in patients with chronic liver disease. *Lancet* 1979;1:520-4.
53. Feller A, Uchida I, Rakela J. Acute viral hepatitis superimposed on alcoholic liver cirrhosis: clinical and histopathologic features. *Liver* 1985;5:239-46.
54. Degos F, Duhamel G, Brechot C, Nalpas B, Courouce AM, Tron F, Berthelot P. Hepatitis B vaccination in chronic alcoholics. *J Hepatol* 1986;2:402-9.
55. Mendenhall C, Roselle GA, Lybecker LA, Marshall LE, Grossman CJ, Myre SA, Weesner RE, et al. Hepatitis B vaccination: response with and without liver injury. *Dig Dis Sci* 1988;33:263-9.
56. Maruyama N, Sata M, Ishii K, Atono Y, Ono K, Matuda T, Suzuki H, et al. Hepatitis B vaccination in alcoholics. *Kansenshogaku Zasshi* 1989;63: 27-34.
57. Villaneuva C, Enriquez J, Just J, Teixido M, Mendez C, Rodrigo O. Vaccination against hepatitis B virus in alcoholics. *Med Clin (Barc)* 1991;96:211-4.
58. Nalpas B, Thepot V, Driss F, Pol S, Courouce AM, Saliou P, Berthelot P. Secondary immune response to hepatitis B virus vaccine in alcoholics. *Alcohol Clin Exp Res* 1993;17:295-8.
59. Clemente-Ricote G, Perez-Roldan F, Banares-Canizares R, Vicario JL, Santos-Castro L, Perez Marin C, Callaja Kempin J, et al. The response to hepatitis B vaccine prior to orthotopic liver transplantation. *Rev Esp Enferm Dig* 1995;87:516-20.
60. Van Thiel DH, Gavaler JS. Response to HBV vaccination in patients with severe liver disease. Absence of an HLA effect. *Dig Dis Sci* 1992;37:1447-50.
61. Rosman AS, Basu P, Galvin K, Lieber CS. Efficacy of a high and accelerated dose of hepatitis B vaccine in alcoholic patients: a randomized clinical trial. *Am J Med* 1997;103:217-22.
62. Bronowicki JP, Weber-Larivaille F, Gut JP, Doffoel M, Vetter D. Comparison of immunogenicity of vaccination and serovaccination against hepatitis B virus in patients with alcoholic cirrhosis. *Gastroenterol Clin Bio J* 1997;21:848-53.
63. Wong V, Wreghitt TG, Alexander GJ. Prospective study of hepatitis B vaccination in patients with chronic hepatitis C. *Br Med J* 1996;312:1336-7.
64. Mohamed A el S, al Karawi MA, Mesa GA. Dual infection with hepatitis C and B viruses: clinical and histologic study in Saudi patients. *Hepatogastroenterology* 1997;44:1404-6.
65. Mast EE, Alter MJ, Margolis HS. Strategies to prevent and control hepatitis B and C virus infections: a global perspective. *Vaccine* 1999;17:1730-3.
66. Idilman R, De MN, Colantoni A, Nadic A, Van T. The effect of high-dose and short interval HBV vaccination in individuals with chronic hepatitis C. *Am J Gastroenterol* 2002;97:435-9.
67. Argudas MR, Mcguire BM, Fallon MB. Implementation of vaccination in patients with cirrhosis. *Dig Dis Sci* 2002;47:384-7.

40

Post-exposure prophylaxis of hepatitis B virus infection

Premashish Kar, Surinder S Rana

Viral hepatitis is a serious health problem in India. It is estimated that approximately 4 million people in India suffer every year from acute viral hepatitis. Hepatitis B virus (HBV) infection accounts for about 40% of all cases of sporadic hepatitis in adults and about 18% in children. HBV infection occurring after an accidental exposure like needle-stick poses a serious hazard for medical personnel. Since there is no specific treatment available, prevention of HBV infection is of utmost importance.

The discovery of hepatitis B surface antigen (HBsAg) in 1965 made a much needed serological marker available, that improved the surveillance procedure and improved physical methods to prevent spread of the disease.[1] It also led to the development of new biological products that have proved to be effective agents for passive and active immunization against hepatitis B. In the past three decades, there have been remarkable advances in the knowledge of hepatitis B and its prevention.

PASSIVE IMMUNOPROPHYLAXIS

The concept of successful passive immunization against viral hepatitis dates back to 1945, when studies demonstrated the efficacy of immunoglobulin (Ig) in preventing the spread of viral hepatitis, presumably type A in origin.[2-4] During the following three decades, numerous additional studies confirmed that Ig was protective against hepatitis A.[5-7]

This led to initiation of studies, evaluating the role of Ig in hepatitis B. From a study conducted in late 1960, it became apparent that Ig with detectable anti-HBs, had the capability of reducing the frequency of endemically acquired hepatitis B.[8] Shortly thereafter, a special Ig preparation was developed by collecting plasma exclusively from donors, who were anti-HBs positive, so that the final globulin preparation contained extremely high anti-HBs titers.[9] This hyperimmune Ig was subsequently referred to as hepatitis B immunoglobulin (HBIg) and was evaluated extensively for both pre-exposure and post-exposure prophylaxis.[10] Since HBIg contains much higher levels of HBV specific antibody, it was found to be much more effective in providing immediate protection.

HBIg should be given as soon as possible, preferably within 6 hours and upto 48 hours after exposure. The antibody (anti-HBs) can be detected in the serum within 3 days of administration of HBIg and it lasts up to 3 months.

POST-EXPOSURE PROPHYLAXIS

There are three different circumstances in which post-exposure prophylaxis is useful:

(a) Sexual contact,
(b) accidental needle-stick exposure, and
(c) perinatal exposure from HBsAg positive mother.

Of the studies involving HBIg for sexual contact, a single injection of HBIg has shown protection against both clinical disease and subclinical infection, proving the efficacy of HBIg.[11] Studies conducted for evaluating the role of HBIg for accidental needle-stick exposure showed that two injections of HBIg given one month apart did prevent transmission of the disease in about 80% of cases.[10,12] The likelihood of infection following a prick amounts to only 50%, suggesting that percutaneous transfer of HBV particles sufficient to induce infection is not an invariable result of needle-stick accident. The likelihood of hepatitis B transmission is far greater, if the blood to which exposure has occurred, is positive for both HBsAg and HBeAg. Studies carried out to evaluate the role of HBIg in preventing perinatal exposure from HBsAg positive mothers, have shown efficacy of 71% provided HBIg is administered within 24 hr. of birth.[13,14]

Role of hepatitis B vaccine

Though HBIg has proved to be effective in preventing post-exposure transmission, it has limited applicability because HBIg (a) is only partially effective, (b) has a short half-life, and so it does not give any long-term protection in high-risk situations and also does not prevent reinfection, and (c) interferes with long-lasting immunity by inhibiting active immunization.

However, with the advent of hepatitis B vaccine, a solution to these problems appeared. In order to circumvent the problem of delayed immune response to hepatitis B vaccine alone, a study was undertaken to evaluate the effect of combination of HBIg with hepatitis B vaccine.[15,16] This combined regimen not only is capable of inducing an early and prolonged antibody response, but is also highly effective in preventing sustained and recurrent HBV infection. Further, HBIg-induced passive immunization did not inhibit vaccine-induced active response.

RECOMMENDATIONS FOR POST-EXPOSURE PROPHYLAXIS[17,18]

The type of exposure that are believed to warrant immnoprophylaxis include perinatal, percutaneous, and perhaps sexual contact.

Neonates of HBsAg positive mothers

The risk of transmission of HBV infection to the newborn depends upon the gestational age. If the mother develops acute hepatitis due to HBV in the first or the second trimester, the risk of transmission is very low but if mother develops acute hepatitis in the third trimester, the risk is very high.[19] It has been shown that the risk of transmission of HBV infection depends upon the HBe/anti-HBe status of the mother.[20] If the mother is HBeAg positive, 85% of the newborns will acquire the infection, whereas if mother is anti-HBe positive, the new borns usually do not acquire infection, although 6% develop acute or fulminant hepatitis at 2–3 months of age.[21]

The risk of acquiring HBV infection by the newborn can be graded into 3 categories, depending upon the presence of serological markers of HBV infection in the mother.

HBeAg +ve   –   high-risk
HBsAg +ve   –   relatively high-risk
HBsAg –ve   –   low-risk

It has been proven that HBIg is effective in decreasing the rate of chronic hepatitis in newborns but not completely.[22] Therefore, it is recommended that newborns born to HBsAg positive mothers be immunized at birth along with the administration of HBIg. The immunoglobulin along with the vaccine should be given shortly after birth. The second and third dose of the vaccine is recommended to be given at 1 and 6 months of age respectively.

The protocol followed is to give HBIg immediately at birth followed by additional injections at 3 and 6 months of age. But many studies on combined immunoprophylaxis have suggested that either or both of HBIg injections at 3 and 6 months of age can be deleted.[23-26] This conclusion is based upon the observation, that hepatitis B vaccine is highly immunogenic in the newborns. However, according to Esteban et al,[26] immune response to the vaccine is not immediate. Hence, more than 50% of infants do not develop protective antibodies at 3 months after birth. This delay in vaccine responsiveness will be even greater in low birth weight or pre-term infants. This is more so in our country where malnutrition and low birth weight are common problems. Hence, we advocate continuation of the old protocol where HBIg is given at birth and then repeated at 3 and 6 months of age.

There have been few studies which have reported that vaccination alone is effective in reducing the risk of neonatal HBV infection.[27,28] However, various long-term studies have proven that vaccination is less effective than combined treatment in the prevention of HBV infection.[23] The other question which needs to be addressed is the effect of HBIg on the immune response to the vaccine. Beasley et al,[24] Wong et al[23] and Mazel et al[25] reported that simultaneous administration of HBIg had no effect on the immune response to the HBV vaccine. Contrary to this, Esteban et al[26] reported that simultaneous administration of HBIg and vaccine impaired the immune response to vaccine. But majority of studies have suggested that simultaneous administration of HBIg and HBV vaccine have no effect on the immune response to vaccine and thus combined immunoprophylaxis can be given. Esteban et al[26] suggested that in low-risk hepatitis B areas, hepatitis B vaccine alone should be used for prophylaxis instead of simultaneous administration of HBIg and hepatitis B vaccine. They demonstrated that passive, active and combined immunoprophylaxis were equally effective in preventing the development of chronic HBV infection in the newborns of HBsAg positive mothers from low-risk hepatitis B areas. This was due to small number of HBeAg positive mothers in the three groups, which is a common finding in areas of low prevalence for HBV infection. However, in our country where HBV is a public health problem, combined immunoprophylaxis should be adopted to prevent the perinatal transmission of HBV infection (Fig. 1).

Needle-stick exposure

After the exposure of the health care workers to HBV either through accidental needle-stick or mucosal contamination to body secretions, early administration of HBIg is recommended for the prevention of HBV infection. Considering the expense of the product, the following protocol has been suggested.

Known HBsAg positive source

Immediate intramuscular administration of HBIg (0.06 ml/kg), along with the HBV vaccine within 7 days is recommended. Following this, the recipient sample is tested for anti-HBs. No further treatment is required if anti-HBs exceeds 10 mIU/ml. In such cases, a single booster

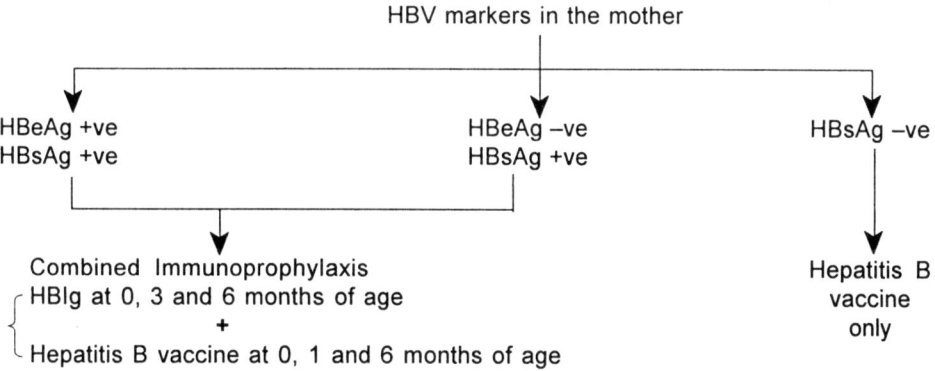

Fig. 1. Algorithm for prevention of perinatal transmission of hepatitis B virus

dose of vaccine is all that is needed. If anti-HBs is absent or less than 10 mIU/ml, anti-HBc testing is conducted. If this is also negative, two more doses of the vaccine at 1 and 6 months should be administered.

Known source but unknown HBsAg status

If the source is a recognized high-risk individual like a homosexual man, drug abuser, a patient on dialysis; the donor and the recipient blood sample should be obtained immediately and a dose of HBIg (0.06 ml/kg) should be administered as soon as possible. If donor is HBsAg negative, discontinue therapy. If donor is HBsAg positive, the protocol mentioned earlier should be followed. If the source is low-risk, prophylaxis is optional.

Source and HBsAg status unknown

The same protocol is recommended as that suggested for a high-risk source exposure. The recommendation pertaining to post-exposure prophylaxis following needle-stick exposure are outlined in Fig. 2.

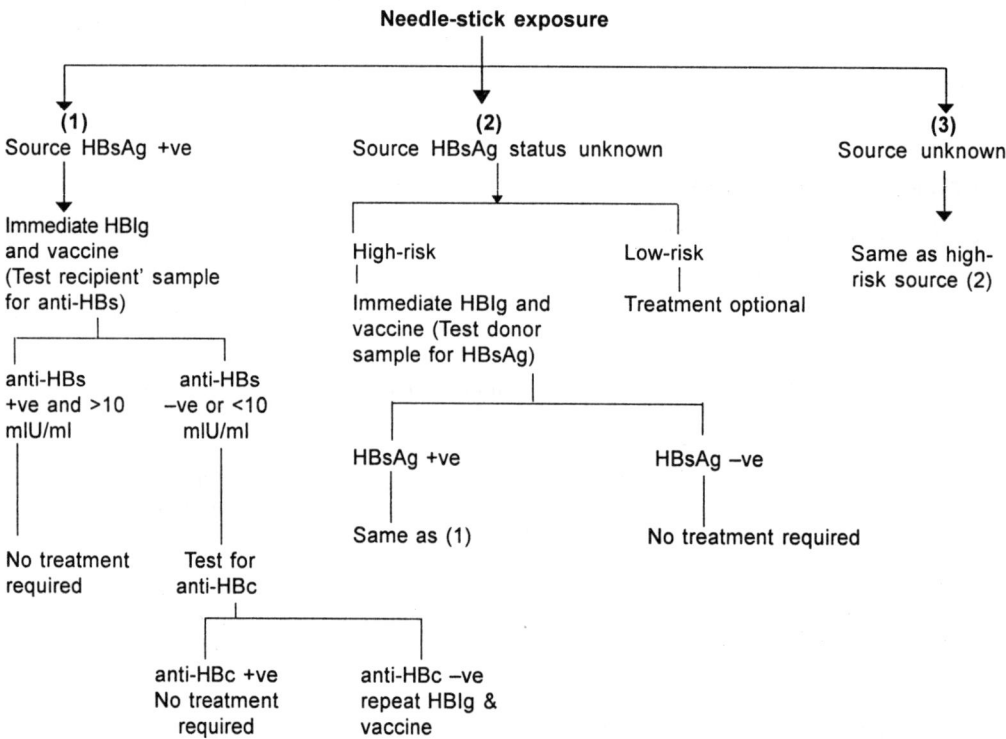

Fig. 2. Algorithm for prophylaxis after needle-stick exposure from patients

REFERENCES

1. Blumberg BS, Alter HJ, Visnich S. A "new" antigen in leukemia sera. *JAMA* 1965;191:541-6.23
2. Stokes J, Jr., Neefe JR. The prevention and attenuation of infectious hepatitis by gamma globulin. *JAMA* 1945;127:144-5.
3. Gellis SS, Stokes J Jr., Brother GM, Gilmore, HR, Hall WM, Beyer E, Morrissey RA. The use of human immune serum globulin (gamma globulin) in infectious (epidemic) hepatitis in the Mediterranean theater of operations. I. Studies on prophylaxis in two epidemics of infectious hepatitis. *JAMA* 1945;128:1062-3.
4. Havens WP Jr., Paul JR. Prevention of infectious hepatitis with gamma globulin. *JAMA* 1945;129:270-2.
5. Brooks BF, Hisa DY, Gellis SS. Family outbreaks of infectious hepatitis: prophylactic use of gamma globulin. *N Engl J Med* 1953;249:58-60.
6. Hisa DY, Lonsway M, Gellis SS. Gamma globulin in the prevention of infectious hepatitis: studies on the use of small doses in family outbreak. *N Engl J Med* 1954;250:417-9.
7. Cline AI, Mosley JW, Scovel FG. Viral hepatitis among American missionaries abroad. A preliminary study. *JAMA* 1967;199:551-3.
8. Prophylactic gamma globulin for prevention of endemic hepatitis: effects of US gamma globulin upon the incidence of viral hepatitis and other infectious diseases in US soldiers abroad. *Arch Intern Med* 1971;128:723-38.
9. Prince AM, Szmuness W, Woods KR, Grady GF. Antibody against serum hepatitis antigen. Prevalence and potential use as immune serum globulin in prevention of serum-hepatitis infections. *N Engl J Med* 1971;285:933-8.
10. Krugman S, Giles JP, Hammond J. Viral hepatitis, type B (MS-2 strain) prevention with specific hepatitis B immune serum globulin. *JAMA* 1971;218:1665-70.
11. Redeker AG, Mosley JW, Gocke DJ, Mckee PA, Pollack W. Hepatitis B immune globulin as a prophylactic measure for spouses exposed to acute type B hepatitis. *N Engl J Med* 1975;293:1055-9.
12. Seeff LB, Wright EC, Zimmerman HJ, McCollum RW, VA Cooperative Study Group. VA cooperative study of post-transfusion hepatitis, 1969-1974: incidence and characteristics of hepatitis and responsible risk factors. *Am J Med Sci* 1975;270:355-62.
13. Beasley RP, Hwang LY, Lin CC, Stevens CE, Wang KY, Sun TS, Hsieh FJ, et al. Hepatitis B immune globulin (HBIg) efficacy in the interruption of perinatal transmission of hepatitis B virus carrier state. Initial report of a randomized double blind placebo-controlled trial. *Lancet* 1981;ii:388-93.
14. Beasley RP, Hwang LY, Stevens CE, Lin CC, Hseih FJ, Wang KY, Sun TS, et al. Efficacy of hepatitis B immune globulin for prevention of perinatal transmission of the hepatitis B virus carrier state: Final report of a randomized double-blind placebo-controlled trial. *Hepatology* 1983;3:135-41.
15. Szmuness W, Stevens CE, Oleszko WR, Goodman A. Passive-active immunization against hepatitis B: immunogenicity studies in adult Americans. *Lancet* 1981;i:575-7.
16. Zachoval R, Deinhardt F, Fronser H, Szmuness W, Wang KY. *Active and passive-active immunization against hepatitis B. In:* Szmuness W, Alter HJ, Maynard JE, Eds. Viral hepatitis. Philadelphia: Franklin Institute Press, 1982:pp.757.
17. Immune globulin for protection against viral hepatitis. Recommendations of the Immunization Practices Advisory Committee (ACIP). *MMWR* 1981;30:423.
18. Inactivated hepatitis B virus vaccine. Recommendations of the immunization Practice Advisory Committee. *Ann Intern Med* 1982;97:379.
19. Schweitzer IL, Dunn AE, Peters RL, Spears RL. Viral hepatitis B in neonates and infants. *Am J Med* 1973;55:762-71.

20. Okada K, Kamiyama I, Inomata M, Imai M, Miyakawa Y. e antigen and anti-e in the serum of asymptomatic carrier mothers as indicators of positive and negative transmission of hepatitis B virus to their infants. *N Engl J Med* 1976;294:746-9.
21. Shiraki K, Yoshihara N, Sakurai M, Eto T, Kawana T. Acute hepatitis B in infants born to carrier mother with antibody to hepatitis B 'e' antigen. *J Pediatr* 1980;97:768-70.
22. Beasley RP, Hwang LY, Lin CC, Stevens CE, Wang KY, Sun TS, Hseih FJ, et al. Hepatitis B immunoglobulin (HBIg) efficacy in the interruption of perinatal transmission of hepatitis B carrier state. Initial report of a randomized double-blind placebo-controlled trial. *Lancet* 1981;ii:388-93.
23. Wong VC, Ip HM, Reesink HW, Lelie PN, Reerink-Bronges EE, Yeung CY, Ma HK. Prevention of the HBsAg carrier state in new born infants of mothers who are chronic carriers of HBsAg and HBeAg by administration of hepatitis-B vaccine and hepatitis-B immunoglobulin. Double-blind randomized placebo-controlled study. *Lancet* 1984;i:921-6.
24. Beasley RP, Hwang LY, Lee GC, Lan CC, Roan CH, Huang FY, Chen CL. Prevention of perinatally transmitted hepatitis B virus infections with hepatitis B immunoglobulin and hepatitis B vaccine. *Lancet* 1983;ii:1099-1102.
25. Mazel JA, Schalm SW, de Gast BC, Nujiten AS, Heijink RA, Botman MJ, Banffer JR, et al. Passive active immunization of neonates of HBsAg positive carrier mothers: preliminary observations. *Br Med J* 1984;288:513-5.
26. Esteban JI, Genesca J, Esteban R, Hemandez JM, Seijo G, Buti M, Muniz R, et al. Immunoprophylaxis of perinatal transmission of the hepatitis B virus: efficacy of hepatitis B immune globulin and hepatitis B vaccine in a low-prevalence area. *J Med Virol* 1986;18:381-91.
27. Poovorawan Y, Sanpavat S, Chumdermpadetsuk S, Safary A. Long-term hepatitis B vaccine in infants born to hepatitis B e antigen positive mothers. *Arch Dis Child Fetal Neonatal Ed.* 1997;77:F47-51.
28. Lolekha B, Warachit B, Hiruny achote A, Bowon Kiratikachorn P, West DJ, Poerschke G. Protective efficacy of hepatitis B vaccine without HBIg in infants of HBeAg-positive carrier mothers in Thailand. *Vaccine* 2002;20:3739-43.

41

Ideal schedule for vaccinating children against hepatitis B in India

Anju Agarwal, Ashok K Patwari

Immunization of children in India against hepatitis B assumes immense importance because of estimated 43 million subjects with chronic infection of hepatitis B virus (HBV) constituting about 10% of the pool of HBV infected subjects in the world. India falls in the intermediate prevalence zone, i.e., 2–7% of the population are infected with the virus.[1] No effective treatment is available for the disease and prevention through vaccination is very important.

In 1990, World Health Organization (WHO) recommended the hepatitis B vaccine to be included in the Expanded Program of Immunization (EPI). This has been endorsed by the Indian Academy of Pediatrics, however, it is still to be included in the EPI in India.[2,3] In order to formulate an ideal immunization schedule for vaccinating children against hepatitis B, it is prudent to consider common modes of transmission, cost of vaccine, and suitability of administration.

WHO SHOULD BE VACCINATED AND WHEN?

Most important mode of transmission of hepatitis B in children is perinatal. Other modes of transmission are through blood and blood products, sexual and through unsafe injection practices.[1,4] The chronic HBV infection rate is 90% if the infection is acquired at birth compared to 8–10% in those who acquire the infection after five years of age. About two-thirds of the chronic HBV infection is established by two years of age.[5] Hence, any vaccination schedule should target infants at birth for maximum benefit.

Initially a policy of selective immunization after screening the mothers for HBsAg was implemented in many countries but it did not bring down the chronic HBV infection rate and was not cost-effective.[6] Screening of high-risk groups is not cost-effective. It was difficult to identify the high-risk groups and many such patients do not avail of the health facilities. Hence a strategy of universal immunization of infants and selective high-risk groups without prior screening has been adopted and shown to be cost-effective.

In India, this policy has been calculated to be cost-effective and should be adopted. This would prevent vertical transmission and also confer life-long immunological memory which prevents future possibility of horizontal transmission. This will lead to ultimate eradication of the virus over a period of time.

Hence, a rationale approach in India would be to vaccinate all newborns at birth, family contacts of patients with liver disease, thalassemics, hemodialysis patients, hemophiliacs, and health care workers at point of entry to health services.

WHO, American Academy of Pediatrics and almost all health agencies have recommended that the first dose of the vaccine should be given at birth, as early as possible, and preferably not after 48 hours. A study from Taiwan has demonstrated that vaccination started at 7 days after birth gave almost 24% less protection compared to early vaccination (within 48 hours).[7]

VACCINE

Two types of vaccines are commercially available; the plasma derived and the recombinant DNA vaccine. Both the vaccines have equal efficacy, immunogenicity and safety. With the decreasing supply of high-risk plasma in the world, the supply of plasma derived vaccine is decreasing. Now various companies are indigenously manufacturing recombinant DNA hepatitis B vaccine. The cost of vaccine has been drastically brought down due to technological advances and these hepatitis B vaccines have been demonstrated to be efficacious in the Indian population.[8-10]

Dose of vaccine

The 10 µg or 0.5 ml, intramuscularly, is the standard dose of the vaccine till 10 years of age and 20 µg or 1.0 ml intramuscularly, after 10 years of age. A dose of 40 µg is recommended for patients undergoing dialysis and in immunocompromized adults.[11]

Route of administration

Intramuscular injection should be given over the anterolateral part of thigh or over the deltoid region. Immunogenicity is decreased if vaccine is given over the gluteal region.[11] Intradermal route does not produce adequate immune response.

Stability of vaccine

Vaccine should be stored at 2–8°C and has a shelf-life of 2 years at this temperature. Though it is reported to remain efficacious for a week at 45°C and for a month at 37°C, it is preferable to maintain the cold chain.

Adverse reactions

About 1–6% of the recipients report pain at the injection site and fever after vaccination. Rarely, some children have urticaria and anaphylaxis.[12]

Vaccination schedule

As already discussed, the first dose of the vaccine should be given within 48 hours of birth for the vaccination schedule to be effective in decreasing mortality and morbidity due to hepatitis B. An ideal vaccination schedule would be of 0, 1, 6 months with the first dose given within 48 hours of birth. An alternative schedule of 0, 1, 2, 12 months is followed if rapid protection is required as in cases of infants born to HBsAg positive mothers or in cases with accidental exposure to hepatitis B. Though the antibody levels are higher at third month if 0, 1, 2, 12 schedule is followed, the overall antibody levels are higher if 0, 1, 6 month schedule is followed.[13]

PROBLEMS IN INCLUDING THE VACCINE IN EPI IN INDIA

In India, 80% of the deliveries take place at home and hence accessibility of infants at birth is difficult. With the increasing awareness and education of parents regarding the need of vaccination at birth, the implementation of ideal vaccination program is possible. In fact, with the implementation of rural child health program and other programs targeted to have 100% deliveries attended by trained dais, it is possible to access the infants at birth. For this to happen, we should have a positive attitude and include the vaccine in the Universal Immunization Program (UIP). Countries with poor perinatal services have tried to link hepatitis B immunization with DPT vaccination. This strategy has decreased the chronic HBV infection rate but failed to prevent all cases of vertical transmission. In India, studies have been carried out with 3 doses of hepatitis B vaccine given with DPT vaccine at 6, 10, 14 weeks and demonstrated an adequate sero-conversion.[14, 15] Implications of such a schedule as far as protective efficacy and prevention of perinatal transmission is concerned, requires further evaluation.[16] In south east Asian countries where vaccination has been implemented at birth, a definite decrease in the chronic HBV infection rate has been documented, though only up to 40% of infants receive vaccine at birth.[17] Even school-based vaccination program has been shown to be cost-effective.[18] Hence hepatitis B needs to be included in the Universal Immunization Program of India even if all infants are not accessible at birth.[19-21] Efforts to access infants at birth should continue through the existing national programs.

Cost is another factor which deters the government to include it in the UIP but it has been documented to be cost effective in studies in our country[1] and abroad. Hence it should be included in UIP with the first dose at birth and second and third doses to be clubbed with other EPI vaccines.

NEED FOR BOOSTERS

Hepatitis B vaccines have been demonstrated to be efficacious for at least 10–15 years following vaccination.[11,22] Anti-HBs concentration of 10 mIU/ml has been taken as a protective level but there is no definite correlation between the antibody level and the protective efficacy. At present, booster dose is not recommended routinely. However, further studies are needed in this direction. In patients on hemodialysis and in immunocompromised patients, the dose of the vaccine should be repeated when antibody levels fall below 10 mIU/ml.[11]

PREVENTION OF PERINATAL HBV INFECTION

With prompt hepatitis B vaccination within 12 hours of birth, one month later, and at 6 months, the protection rates achieved are 90–95%.

If 0.5 ml of hepatitis B immunoglobulin (HBIg) is given simultaneously at a separate site, the protective efficacy increases to 95–98%. Ideally, HBIg should be given to all infants born to HBsAg positive mothers at birth or within 7 days (if HBsAg status is known) after birth of the child. Four dose rapid schedule of hepatitis B vaccination should be followed if hepatitis B immunoglobulin is not available.[12]

FUTURE DIRECTIONS

Future studies should address the question of need for boosters, development of combination vaccines and methods to improve the immunogenicity of the vaccine. New recombinant vaccines containing both pre-S and S-antigen produced in yeast or in stably transferred mammalian lines are being developed.[19]

REFERENCES

1. Aggarwal R, Naik SR. *Cost efficacy estimation of inclusion of hepatitis B vaccine in Expanded Programme of Immunization.* In: Sarin SK, Singal AK, Eds. Hepatitis B in India: Problems and Prevention. CBS Publishers & Distributors, New Delhi, 1996; pp. 206-16.
2. Center of Disease Control. Protection against viral hepatitis. Recommendation of the Immunization Practices Advisory Committee (ACIP). *MMWR* 1990;39:5-7.
3. IAP's immunization time table in Pediatrics. *Indian Pediatr* 1995;32:1329-33.
4. Chowdhury A, Santra A, Choudhary S, Ghosh A, Banerjee P, Mazumdar DN. Prevalence of hepatitis B injection in general population; a rural community based study. *Trop Gastroentrol* 1999;20:75-7.
5. Universal Hepatitis B immunization. Committee on Infectious Diseases. *Pediatrics* 1992;89:795-8.
6. Alter SK, Halder SC, Margolia HS. The changing epidemiology of hepatitis B in United States need for alternative vaccination strategies. *JAMA* 1990;263:1218-22.
7. Mittal SK, Kumar N. Optimizing Hepatitis B vaccine use in India. *Pediatr Today* 1998;1:35-40.
8. Lakshmi G, Reddy RP, Kumar KK, Bhavani NV, Dayanand M. Study of safety, immunogenicity and sero-conversion of hepatitis B vaccine in malnourished children of India. *Vaccine* 2000;18:2009-14.

9. Joshi N, Kumar A, Sreenivas DV, Palan S, Nagarjuna YR. Safety and immunogenicity of indigenous recombinant hepatitis B vaccine (Shanvac B) in comparison with commercially available vaccine. *Indian J Gastroentrol* 2000;19:71-3.
10. Jain A, Mathur US, Jandwani P, Gupta RK, Kumar V, Kar P. A multicenteric evaluation of recombinant Hepatitis B vaccine of Cuban origin. *Trop Gastroentrol* 2000;21:14-7.
11. *Hepatitis B. In*: Peter G, Ed. 1997 Red Book: Report of Committee of Infectious Diseases: 24th ed. Elk Grove Village IL: American Academy of Pediatrics 1997;pp. 427-59.
12. Sachdev HPS. Immunization dialogue Hepatitis B vaccine. *Indian Pediatr* 1995;32:715-8.
13. Safary A. *Hepatitis B vaccination : now and in future. In*: Sarin SK, Singal AK, Eds. Hepatitis B in India: Problems and Prevention. CBS Publishers & Distributors, New Delhi 1996;pp. 132-51.
14. Gomber S, Sharma R, Ramachandran VG, Talwar V, Singh B. Immunogenicity of hepatitis B vaccine incorporated into expanded programme of immunization schedule. *Indian Pediatr* 2000;17:411-3.
15. Mittal SK, Rao S, Kumar S, Aggarwal V, Prakash C, Thirupuram S. Simultaneous administration of hepatitis B vaccine with other EPI vaccines. *Indian J Pediatr* 1994;6:183-8.
16. Mathew A. First dose of hepatitis B vaccine in infacts. *Indian Pediatr* 2002; 39:981-2.
17. Wilson N, Ruff TA, Ranat BJ, Leydon J, Locarnini S. The effectiveness of the infant hepatitis B immunization programme in Fiji, Kiribati, Tonga and Vanuata. *Vaccine* 2000;18:3059-66.
18. Wilson T. Economic evaluation of a metropolitan-wide, school based hepatitis B vaccination program. *Public Health Nurse* 2000;17:323-7.
19. Dasgupta R, Priya R. The sustainability of hepatitis B immunization within the Universal Immunization Program in India. *Health Policy Plan* 2002;17:99-105.
20. Mittal SK. Desirability and feasibility of hepatitis B vaccine in EPI. *Indian J Pediatr* 2001;68(suppl): S61-5.
21. Sokhey J, Jain DC, Harit AK, Dhariwal AC. Moderate immunization coverage levels in East Delhi: Implications for disease control programs and introduction of new vaccines. *J Trop Pediatr* 2001;47: 199-203.
22. Gill HH. *Hepatitis B vaccine: Current and New. In*: Sarin SK, Singal AK, Eds. Hepatitis B in India: Problems and Prevention. CBS Publishers & Distributors, New Delhi 1999;pp. 206-16.

42

Economic burden of hepatitis B in India

Kishore Chaudhary, Shiv K Sarin

Hepatitis B infection is an important global cause of mortality and morbidity, being responsible for over 250,000 deaths annually out of estimated over 300 million persons infected with HBV.[1] Although India falls in the intermediate prevalence zone (2 to 7%) of HBV infection; the magnitude of the problem acquires a huge dimension due to its population size. The country has above 40 million subjects suffering from chronic HBV infection and 4 million patients with chronic liver disease.[2] HBV infection may result in a broad range of clinical presentations, varying from clinically asymptomatic stage to chronic hepatitis, cirrhosis, and hepatocellular carcinoma. The natural history of chronic viral hepatitis is complex and the morbidity is affected by many interactive factors, like age, gender, ethnic group, viral co-infection, mutations, and alcohol consumption.[3-5] This implies that the cost incurred by the patients in getting the treatment would also be variable depending upon the presence of the symptoms, availability of diagnostic and therapeutic facilities around their place of residence and the socio-economic status of the patient.

ESTIMATION OF THE COST

The cost of therapy can be divided into two major subgroups, i.e., direct and indirect costs. The direct cost may be related to medical or non-medical expenses. Direct medical cost includes expenditure on consultation with physicians, investigations, drugs (adjuvant as well as specific), procedures (diagnostic or therapeutic) and hospitalization. Direct non-medical cost includes money spent on travel to hospital or diagnostic facility, additional expenses on boarding and lodging to get the treatment. Indirect cost includes loss of wages incurred for getting the treatment or disability or reduced efficiency, and loss to the society due to premature death. These expenses or losses may be incurred by the patients or their relatives/friends. In many countries like India, the health services are often subsidized by the government or non-governmental organizations (NGOs). Therefore, in any economic analysis, their contribution should also be taken into account.

Limited information is available on cost of treatment of hepatitis B. These studies have tended to assess the cost of management of the HBV-related chronic liver disease with newer specific therapies, like interferon or lamivudine. Dusheiko et al[6] using a transitional probability model of estimation of progression of liver disease over a 30-year period, studied cohorts of hypothetical patients with either chronic hepatitis B or C. They compared the treated cohort (with interferon-alpha) with the untreated cohort and reported excess benefits over cost in cohort of patients treated with interferon-alpha. However, this study was full of assumptions, e.g., hypothetical cohort of patients, transitional probability model for progression of disease, etc. Miller et al[7] reported that lamivudine will deliver economic value in the treatment of chronic hepatitis B but again this was based on interviews with hepatologists and other physicians and not on hard data collected from the patients. The expenditure assessment in these studies either excluded the direct non-medical expenditure or assigned a fixed sum for each patient. The cost of direct medical expenditure was often based on subjective assessment by physicians or on the rates of packages offered by the hospitals.

HEALTH SERVICES IN INDIA

Health care to people in India is available through state run health services, private fee-for-service approach, health insurance schemes for specific groups, public sector run health insurance schemes, and through services provided by NGO. Although, the state run hospitals and dispensaries do not generally charge for their facilities, they invariably are not in a position to provide the entire care for management of the diseases. Thus, patients do have to spend themselves, the quantum of which differs depending upon the facilities available at the contacted health care center for the disease being treated.

About two-thirds of registered hospitals in India are private, but account for less than 40% of available beds. Indian health services are largely financed by out-of-pocket household-level payments, with small contributions by state and central government contributions through direct service provision. Per capita expenditure by government run insurance schemes, namely, CGHS and ESI was Rs. 260 and Rs. 338.4 per capita during the year 1995-96. The per capita premium under the public sector run health insurance–Mediclaim varied from Rs. 152 to 751 during the same year (Garg C.C. Implications of current experience of health insurance in India. Paper presented during the National seminar on health insurance, organized by Ministry of Health & Family Welfare, New Delhi, 16th & 17th November 1999).

ASSESSMENT OF ECONOMIC BURDEN OF HBV vs. VACCINATION COSTS IN INDIA

For the purpose of assessing the cost of management of HBV-related diseases, it would be easiest to use the data from health service records. However, in view of the chronic nature of the illness and variations in the availability of facilities at different centres (and thus, out-of-pocket expenditure by patients), it would not be correct to consider the average cost of health care as representative of the average cost of treatment of HBV-related diseases. It may be possible to collect some information on expenditure on selected HBV-related diseases incurred by government run health insurance schemes like CGHS or ESIC (total beneficiaries less than 40 million), but the expenditure would not be representative of the entire country. The available data from any of the health service records can at the maximum provide rough estimates of direct medical expenditure incurred by the government. It would not provide any information on the direct medical care cost borne by the patients, the direct non-medical costs and indirect costs of HBV-related diseases. Thus, existing health care records are not likely to provide a true picture on the subject.

The current management scenario for HBV-related diseases suggests that prevention of the infection would be the most practical strategy for its control. The endeavour in the current study is to assess the cost of treating patients with hepatitis B and to compare with the cost of possible strategies for vaccination against HBV in India. The existing scientific literature regarding cost of management of HBV-related diseases was reviewed and its adequacy was assessed for generalization of the results to the country. Population estimates were available from the population projections made by the Registrar General of India,[8] for the years 1996 to 2016. These projections are based on the 1991 census of India and estimated birth and death rates for various years. The limitations of the available study on the cost estimates were also assessed.

India has seen a lot of change on cost of vaccine against hepatitis B virus. Availability of an indigenously manufactured vaccine in 1998 saw a nearly three-fold reduction in its cost. The current cost of these vaccines varies between Rs. 180 and 288 per ml in a multidose vial, which is the expected packaging used in a national program on immunization. The program may provide three doses of 0.5 ml each for children. As the cost of commodities also depends on the turnover of the product, this cost is still likely to reduce if it is introduced under the country's expanded program of immunization (EPI). Estimates on expected cost after nationwide use vary between Rs. 20 and Rs. 80 per dose. It is felt that a 50% reduction in the cost after nationwide use may be a practical proposition.

Only one study has reported cost of management of HBV-related diseases on pilot basis.[9] The study developed a model for assessing the social cost of HBV-related illnesses by correcting some of the identified lacunae in the earlier reported studies. The study interviewed HBV infected persons and patients of chronic liver disease due to HBV, to collect data on expenditure related to their disease under various heads, namely, consultation, investigations, therapy, hospitalization, extra expenditure on food, lodging, transport charges, loss of income, and any expenditure by relatives or friends. Chronic HBV infection was defined as a person positive for HBsAg for more than 6 months. Any expenditure on conditions not related to hepatitis was excluded. Average expenditure by a case with HBV infection during preceding six months was Rs. 4,122 (range 20 to 28,600) with investigations accounting for about 57% of the expenditure (Table 1). A patient of chronic liver disease spent an average

Table 1. Mean and range of expenditure (rupees) incurred by subjects with chronic HBV infection and patients of chronic liver disease during the last 6 months

Expenditure Head	Subjects with chronic HBV infection (n=23)		Patients of chronic liver disease (n=43)	
	Mean expenditure (Rs.)	Range of expenditure (Rs.)	Mean expenditure (Rs.)	Range of expenditure (Rs.)
Consultation	191	0-1,550	106	0-1,000
Investigations	2,345	0-19,000	3,376	0-30,415
Drugs	498	0-2,500	13,099	0-70,600
Admission charges	304	0-6,000	944	0-20,000
Extra food	142	0-1,000	1,529	0-10,000
Lodging	0	0	381	0-6,000
Transport	438	0-2,500	1,599	0-8,000
Relatives' loss/ expenditure	135	0-2,500	466	0-9,000
Loss of income	69	0-1,000	2,059	0-42,000
Total expenditure	4,122	36,050	23,559	1,97,015

Source: Ref. no. 9

of Rs. 23,561 during last six months (range Rs. 60 to 1,11,395/-). Major expenditure heads included drugs (56%), investigations, loss of income, transport, extra money on food, etc. Multivariate regression analysis revealed a significant model with hospitalization, residence outside Delhi, and higher family income, significantly resulting in higher expenditure. The pilot data indicated an enormous expenditure by patients of HBV-related diseases. This study, however, did not estimate the cost incurred by the treating institution and the cost due to premature death of the patients.

Table 2 presents the data on the cost of management of all possible patients with HBV-related diseases for the year 2000, after applying 10% discounting to correct the effect of inflation (which is approximately the current inflation rate in India). The cost to the country

Table 2. Cost of HBV infection and chronic liver disease in India (rupees)

	HBV infection	Chronic liver disease
Annual mean expenditure, 1999	8,243	47,121
No. of patients in India	4 crore	40 lac
Cost for India, 1999	32,972 crore	18,848 crore
	51,820 crore	
Cost for India, 2000	57,002 crore	

1 crore = Rs. 10,000,000/-   1 lac = Rs. 100,000/-

due to hepatitis B virus infection and chronic liver disease in the year 2000, amounts to 57,002 crores.

The cost to the country on account of HBV vaccination is given in Table 3. The cost of immunizing the entire population in a single year would amount to Rs. 46,576 crore at current prices. The cost considers immunization of children under 12 years with 0.5 ml of vaccine and older persons with 1 ml of vaccine per dose. The immunization of children less than 5 years of age would cost Rs. 2,978 crore at the current cost, which may reduce to half if the entire country is covered. The cheapest approach would be the strategy of immunizing only the newborns, which would cost Rs. 652 crore at the current prices and Rs. 326 crore at the expected reduced prices, in the event of HBV vaccination getting included under the EPI program.

Table 3. Cost of vaccination against HBV in India, 2000 (rupees)

Vaccination strategy	Cost at current vaccine prices (@Rs. 90 / per dose)	Cost at reduced vaccine prices (@Rs. 45 / per dose)
Entire population (1.002 b)	46,576 crore*	23,288 crore*
Under 5 years (110.298 m)	2,978 crore	1,489 crore
Newborns (24.148 m)	652 crore	326 crore

1 crore = 10,000,000   b = billion, m = million
Cost per dose for persons >12 years = Rs. 180

The study estimates the annual cost to India due to hepatitis B virus related diseases. The expenditure incurred by the patients with HBV infection and chronic liver diseases had been reported in an earlier pilot subject by the authors.[9] The expenditure related to the direct medical as well as direct non-medical expenditure and loss of wages incurred by the patients had been reported in that study. The data was discounted to convert it to prices in the year 2000, in order to adjust for the effect of inflation. The cost to the country due to HBV related diseases amounts to a substantial Rs. 57,002 crore in the year 2000.

Generalization of the data from a pilot study on cost of management of HBV related diseases to the entire country, has limitations. The study conducted in a tertiary hospital may not have the patients in proportion to their distribution in the country. However, the study collected data only on direct costs and partial indirect cost in the form of lost wages. The cost due to premature death due to the disease is expected to be substantial. A study by one of the authors (KC) on cost of management of tobacco related cancers indicates that cost to the society due to premature death caused by such chronic diseases is substantial.[10] The expenditure incurred by the host institution was also not estimated. Many services in government and non-governmental hospitals in India are free or highly subsidized and thus this expenditure by the society is also likely to be substantial. Therefore, the current estimates are not likely to be an abstract figure but should present a reality.

In the background of the substantial expenditure incurred by the patients of HBV related diseases, the expenditure on vaccination against HBV has also been estimated. Cost with various strategies for immunization has been assessed keeping in mind the current cost as well as anticipated reduction in the event of the HBV vaccination finding a place in the regimen of Indian Expanded Program on Immunization.[11,12] One may ideally like to immunize the entire population against the disease. However, the whopping cost of Rs. 46,576 crore at the current vaccine prices, would make it impractical. It may be useful to note that the total state and central government spending on public health care services in India is only US$ 2-3 per capita per year.[13] Even if one considers the expenditure at the upper end of US$ 3 (or Rs. 135 at the current rate of exchange), the entire annual expenditure would amount to approximately Rs. 13,500 crore. The cost of immunization of the entire population under five years of age may be a better option, but given the entire gamut of diseases to be covered by health services, it may not be a workable proposition. The expenditure of covering all the newborns with HBV vaccination seems to be the most acceptable option with an annual expenditure of Rs. 652 crores at the current vaccine prices. Vaccine manufacturers do indicate a reduction in price if there is a substantial market, as would occur in the event of the HBV vaccination being accepted under EPI. The present study considers a reduction of vaccine prices by half, although price reduction to one-third level may also be possible.

With less optimistic price reduction (by half) the estimated cost of 100% immunization coverage of the newborns in the country in the year 2000 would be Rs. 326 crore. The recurring cost in the future years is expected to be of the similar magnitude in view of the anticipated reduction of birth rate. As per the projected population estimates, the cost of vaccination of all newborns for the years 2006, 2011 and 2016 is likely to be Rs. 339 crore, 356 crore and 367 crore, respectively (at year 2000 price level). Therefore, the strategy of covering only newborns with an eye on price reduction of vaccine seems to be a feasible option for prevention of the substantial HBV related disease in our country.

REFERENCES

1. Maynard JE. Hepatitis B: global importance and need for control. *Vaccine* 1990;8(suppl):S18-20.
2. Thyagarajan SP, Jayaram S, Mohanavalli B. *Prevalence of HBV in the general population of India. In:* Sarin SK, Singal AK, Eds. Hepatitis B in India: Problems and Prevention. CBS Publishers & Distributors, New Delhi 1996; pp.5-16.
3. Lok AS, Lai CL. Acute exacerbations in Chinese patients with chronic hepatitis B virus (HBV) infection. Incidence, predisposing factors and aetiology. *J Hepatol* 1990;10:29-34.
4. Chu CM, Sheen IS, Lin SM, Liaw YF. Sex difference in chronic hepatitis B virus infection: studies of serum HBeAg and alanine aminotransferase levels in 10,431 asymptomatic Chinese HBsAg carriers. *Clin Infect Dis* 1993;16:709-13.

5. Hsieh CC, TZ Onou A, Zavitsanos X, Kaklamani E, Lan SJ, Trichopoulos D. Age at first establishment of chronic hepatitis B virus infection and hepatocellular carcinoma risk: a birth order study. *Am J Epidemiol* 1992;136:1115-21.
6. Dusheiko GM, Roberts JA. Treatment of chronic type B and C hepatitis with interferon-alpha: An economic appraisal. *Hepatology* 1995;22:1863-73.
7. Miller DW, Reckford XL. An economic evaluation of lamivudine for the treatment of chronic hepatitis B in China. *Research report to Glaxo Wellcome.*
8. Registrar General. *Population projections for India and States: 1996-2016.* Registrar General, India, Ministry of Home Affairs, Government of India, August 1996.
9. Chaudhry K, Gupta R, Murthy NS, Ojha RS, Sarin SK. A novel approach to economic appraisal of management of hepatitis B virus related liver disease–A pilot study.
10. Chaudhry K, Rath GK. *Estimation of cost of management of tobacco related cancers–Report of an ICMR task force study.* Indian Council of Medical Research, New Delhi, 1999.
11. Sachdev P, Sehgal A, Puliyel J. Under estimation of cost of hepatitis B vaccination in India. *Indian J Gastroenterol* 2001;20:205-6.
12. Singal AK, Kaur V. Prevalence of HBsAg in population referred to a hospital in North Delhi. *Indian J Gastroenterol* 2000;19(suppl 3):C75-6.
13. Naylor CD, Jha P, Woods J, Shariff A. *A Fine Balance–Some Options for private and public health care in Urban India.* The World Bank, Washington DC, 1999.

43

Hepatitis B vaccine failure

Yong Poovorawan, Pantipa Chatchatee, Voranush Chongsrisawat

Hepatitis B virus (HBV) infection constitutes a major public health problem on a global scale. This is particularly so in Southeast Asia where vertical transmission plays a significant role in the spread of HBV.

Hepatitis B vaccine has proven to be highly effective in preventing the HBV infection. Moreover, this is also the first vaccine shown to be able to effectively prevent the occurrence of cancer, in this context hepatocellular carcinoma.[1] Hence, universal administration of hepatitis B vaccine to neonates constitutes the sole means of efficiently reducing the occurrence of HBV infection and this in turn might eventually lead to the eradication of this disease. However, there have been reports of cases of non-responders as well as vaccine failures upon receipt of the complete course of inoculations.[2,3] We have reviewed the prevalence and pathogenetic mechanisms observed among cases of non-response and vaccine failure.

NON-RESPONDERS

Approximately 5 to 10% of individuals receiving standard hepatitis B vaccination fail to produce protective antibody levels (above 10 mIU/ml).[4,5] This lack of response has been attributed to genetic factors and various defects in the immune reaction. These include: defects in antigen uptake, processing and presentation,[6, 6a] T-cell dependent suppression of antibody production, defects of T-cell response as well as T-cell repertoire,[7, 7a] and failure of T-cells to assist B-cells in producing anti-HBs.[8, 9]

Based on the evidence available, non-responsiveness may be related to genetic factors in that the HLA-linked immune response may also control the response to HBsAg. For example in mice, antibody response has been demonstrated to be major histocompatibility complex (MHC) controlled in that certain strains are non-responders, some show intermediate response, while others demonstrate good response.[10, 11, 12] The ability to respond is inherited as a dominant and lack of response as a recessive trait.

In humans, numerous studies have shown the association between certain HLA haplotypes and poor antibody response. Those HLA haplotypes found associated with non-response are summarized in Table 1. As for non-responsiveness, the exact mode of inheritance has as yet not been clearly defined, since the results available at present differ between different research groups. A study conducted in Japan suggested non-responsiveness to be associated with the particular HLA haplotypes HLA-Bw54; DR4; DRw53, respectively, and to be inherited as a dominant trait.[13] Studies performed among Caucasian populations revealed non-responsiveness to be associated with haplotypes HLA-DR3 and -DR7, as well as with the extended haplotypes [HLA-B8;SC01;DR3] and [HLA-B44; FC31;DR7]. With the latter two haplotypes, a certain overrepresentation of the homozygous has been observed suggesting non-responsiveness to be a recessive trait.[14]

Table 1. HLA types associated with non-responsiveness to hepatitis B vaccination

HLA types	Study
DR7	Walker et al[15]
DR7	Durupinar et al[16]
B44;DR7;FC31 B8;DR3;SC01 DRB1*0701;DQB1*0202	Craven et al[14] McDermott et al[17]
DQB1*0604;DQA1*0102; DRB1*1302	Largö-Warensjö et al[18]
BW54;DR4;DRw53;DQw4	Watanabe et al[13]

* indicated molecular HLA typing

Following are the immunological mechanisms proposed to induce non-responsiveness to hepatitis B vaccine.

Defects in antigen uptake, processing and presentation

This defect which might be due to defects of antigen presenting cells resulting in failure to produce peptide fragments of HBsAg. Those HBsAg fragments are supposed to interact with MHC class II molecules. Any given peptide to tightly fit into the peptide binding groove of MHC class II may depend on the quality of certain MHC haplotypes, a hypothesis supported by non-responsiveness demonstrated to be associated with particular haplotypes. Positive response has also been speculated to be evoked by a dominant immune response gene located within the MHC and, hence non-responsiveness to result from either defects or total lack of this gene.[19] Conversely, several data do not support the hypothesis of defective antigen presenting cells. For example, HBsAg specific T-cell lines cocultured with HBsAg and unfractionated peripheral blood mononuclear cells (PBMC) derived from non-responders proliferated *in vitro*, suggesting the antigen presenting cells in non-responders not to be defective and thus arguing against the above hypothesis.[20]

Presence of HBsAg-specific suppressor T-cells

This hypothesis has been suggested subsequent to the results obtained from various studies performed in Japan showing lack of response to be mediated by HBsAg specific suppressor T-cells.[13, 21, 22] Removing CD8+ cells from non-responders' peripheral blood *in vitro* resulted in proliferative response along with the antibody production upon exposure to HBsAg. Conversely, data obtained from the study conducted among Caucasian populations have failed to confirm the role of suppressor T-cells as a potential basis for non-responsiveness.[23] Peripheral blood cells derived from non-responders were not found to proliferate upon exposure to recombinant HBsAg *in vitro*, even if the cell preparation employed had been deprived of suppressor T-cells, suggesting a defect in T-cell response rather than the presence of specific suppressor T-cells as the mechanism responsible for non-responsiveness. The discrepancies emerging from those two studies might have been caused by the ethnic differences between the populations investigated.

Defects in T-cell response

CD4+ cells derived from the peripheral blood of non-responders showed a lack of proliferative response to recombinant HBsAg *in vitro*, whereas cells originating from responders proliferated vigorously. This failure to proliferate upon exposure to HBsAg remained unaltered upon removal of CD8+ cells.[23] Another experiment employed pairs of HLA-matched individuals, a responder and a non-responder to HBsAg, respectively. Isolated T-cells derived from responders proliferated when cocultured with PBMC–derived adherent cells originating from non-responders whereas non-responder T-cells could not be induced to proliferate upon exposure to HBsAg presented by adherent cells isolated from responders. These data suggest non-responsiveness to be caused by either a defect in HBsAg specific T-helper cells or more generally by a defect in the T-cell repertoire.

Insufficient or devoid T-cell assistance

HBsAg is one of the few exogenous antigens which can be presented to MHC class I molecules. Antigen-specific B-cells have been demonstrated to deliver HBsAg to class-I restricted cytotoxic lymphocytes which in turn destroy the B-lymphocytes.[9] This might be speculated to represent one of the mechanisms potentially responsible for the suppression of antibody response, be that among non-responders to hepatitis B vaccine or among those progressing towards the stage of chronic HBV infection.

OVERCOMING NON-RESPONSIVENESS

Since non-responders constitute a small but significant proportion of individuals immunized with hepatitis B vaccine, several attempts have been made to solve this problem. A novel recombinant vaccine containing S, pre-S1 and pre-S2 antigenic components (Hepagene, Medeva plc, London, UK) has been found to be highly immunogenic and capable of stimulating strong cellular as well as humoral immune responses.[17,24,25] Also, administration of novel adjuvants displaying the potential to induce a balanced Th-1 and Th-2 response has been proposed. In a non-responder strain of mice, application of the cationic lipid 3-[N-(N', N'-dimethylaminoethane) carbamoyl] cholesterol (DC-Chol) has been shown to vanquish the lack of response to HBsAg.[26] Nucleic acid immunization performed in mice has been proven to vanquish non-responsiveness at the cytotoxic T-cell level and likewise, to augment the level of anti-HBs upon immunization.[27] Along with the improved insight into the mechanisms underlying non-responsiveness, the prospects for us to accomplish this problem in the near future will also increase.

INTRA-UTERINE HBV INFECTION

Apart from viral escape mutants, three additional possible causes of HB vaccine failure have been proposed.[28,28a] First, due to intra-uterine infection, the child might have been rendered immunologically tolerant to HBV antigens. Second, early administration of hepatitis B immunoglobulin (HBIg) could have prevented viremia to develop in the child. Third, based on the child's genetic make-up the vaccine might have elicited a weak response, thus permitting horizontal infection. In neonates born to HBV positive mothers, the rate of intra-uterine HBV transmission has been reported to range between 10 and 16%.[29] Table 2 shows the

Table 2. Prevalence of intrauterine hepatitis B virus infection among high-risk neonates

Country	Number of mothers	Number of intrauterine infections n (%)
China	27 HBsAg+	12 (44) HBV-DNA+ in fetal liver[28]
		5 (19) HBsAg, HBcAg, or anti-HBc IgM+
	48 HBsAg+	4 (8) in fetus[30]
	122 HBsAg+	8 (6) HBsAg+ in serum at birth[31]
Taiwan and Japan	32 HBeAg+	5 (16)[32] (3 HBsAg+ in cord blood, 2 HBsAg+ at 1 mo)
Turkey	158 HBsAg+	34 (22) (28 PCR+ in PBMC 9 PCR+ in serum at birth)[33]
Singapore	345 HBeAg+	25 (7) HBV-DNA+ in serum[2]
Thailand	13 HBsAg+ and 19 HBsAg+ and HBeAg+	0 (0) (in neonatal PBMC)[34]
	55 HBsAg+ and HBeAg+	4 (7) HBsAg+ in venous[35] blood at birth

*PCR – polymerase chain reaction, PBMC – peripheral blood mononuclear cells

prevalence of intra-uterine HBV infection among high-risk neonates as reported from various locations ranging from the Middle East to the Far East. The mechanism involved in intra-uterine HBV infection have been investigated by Lin et al who reported babies of HBeAg positive mothers displaying signs and symptoms of either impending abortion and/or pre-term labor to be infected *in utero*.[32] This observation suggests transplacental leakage of maternal blood induced by uterine contractions during pregnancy to be a likely route of intra-uterine HBV infection. Administration of HBIg to babies within the first week after pre-term delivery successfully prevented perinatal HBV transmission. This study also demonstrated intra-uterine HBV infection that neither corelates with maternal hepatic dysfunction, nor with the concentration of HBsAg, HBeAg or HBV-DNA in the maternal serum.

On the other hand, Lazizi et al have shown transplacental passage of the HBV to be correlated with the presence of viral DNA in maternal peripheral blood mononuclear cells (PBMC).[33] Twenty-three out of 24 babies born to mothers harboring HBV-DNA in their PBMC were found to be HBV-DNA positive. Based on the observation that viral genomes detectable by spot hybridization amounted to a mere 3 out of the 28 PCR positive newborn sera, it was concluded that HBV was transmitted at a low titer. Of the 14 babies, not having responded by three months of age, nine without receiving a booster sero-converted to anti-HBs at month 15, having completely cleared the virus. In these late responders, the C gene was undetectable in PBMC at birth, whereas 4 of 5 persistent non-responders retained the complete HBV genome in their PBMC as shown by PCR employing primers specific for the S, C, and X-gene sequences, respectively. From these results the authors concluded the duration of non-responsiveness to the hepatitis B vaccine apparently to be correlated with the load of virus at birth. Thus, in the course of progressing viral infection, passage through PBMC might represent one step prior to the virus entering the hepatocytes and consequently, immunoprophylaxis administered at birth might prevent hepatocytes from getting infected.

As for the mechanism of intra-uterine transmission of HBV, Xu et al have suggested two possible routes of transmission, i.e., hematogenous due to damage of placental vessels and cellular due to trans-placental transfer of HBV.[36] The study conducted by this group of researchers on HBsAg positive mothers demonstrated HBsAg positivity to be 100% in decidual cells, 59.38% in trophoblasts, 65.50% in the villous mesenchyme, and 39.38% in villous capillary endothelial cells (VCEC). The HBsAg positivity in VCEC in particular was found to be significantly corelated with intra-uterine infection. Retrospective analysis of the outcome of pregnancy among HBsAg-positive women with invasive tests performed for pre-natal diagnosis was conducted to determine if amniocentesis constitutes an increased risk of intra-uterine HBV transmission.[37] Amniocentesis had been performed on 17 HBsAg positive women (2 were both HBsAg and HBeAg positive). Their babies received HBIg immediately after birth and hepatitis B vaccine within the first year of life. All infants were HBsAg negative and proceeded to develop an active immune response to the vaccine, suggesting that amniocentesis represents a low-risk for intra-uterine HBV transmission. However, definite conclusions cannot be drawn for HBeAg positive women. Identical results as to the effect of amniocentesis on intra-uterine HBV transmission have been reported by Ko et al.[38] The HBsAg positive rates determined in the cord blood of infants born to HBsAg positive mothers with and without amniocentesis amounted to 2.9 and 3.1%, respectively. The failure rates of immunoprophylaxis of neonates born to HBsAg positive mothers observed in the group that had undergone amniocentesis compared with infants immunized in the National Hepatitis B Prevention Program (serving as controls), were similar (9.4% vs. 11%).

A study performed on intra-uterine HBV infection in induced abortions has shown HBV-DNA to be detectable not only in fetal liver, but also in spleen, pancreas, kidney and placenta.[39] Approximately 40% of fetuses infected with HBV *in utero* express viral antigens, possibly due to the immaturity of fetal tissues. Another study performed in fetuses employing serology, immunohistochemistry in the liver tissue and molecular hybridization using P-labeled HBV-DNA as a probe showed the rate of intra-uterine HBV infection to amount to 20.0% (7/35), 5.9% (1/17), and 44.4% (12/27), respectively.[40] Some babies with intra-uterine HBV infection failed to produce either HBsAg or anti-HBc. Alexander and Eddleston proposed that maternal anti-HBc suppresses fetal viral antigen expression and viral replication, thus preventing fetal immune response to HBV-associated antigens.[41] HBIg administered after birth delays the onset of viral replication until the immune system is sufficiently mature to clear the virus. Damiani et al[42] evaluated the HBV markers in maternal and fetal blood and tissues in relation with the vaccine response. HBsAg, anti-HBc, and anti-HBe were found to be 42.8%, 100%, and 50%, respectively, in amniotic fluid extracted by trans-abdominal amniocentesis. In contrast, the percentage of the same markers detectable in funicular blood samples obtained immediately after delivery amounted to 50% for HBsAg and 100% for anti-HBc and anti-HBe. Passive–active immunization elicited a protective response in all the neonates, irrespective of their antigen status during intra-uterine life.

A study performed on high-risk neonates focused on the effect of hepatitis B immunoglobulin (HBIg) administered before delivery on the prevention of intra-uterine HBV transmission.[29] Each subject in the HBIg group received 200 IU of HBIg intramuscularly at months 3, 2 and 1 prior to delivery, whereas the control group did not receive HBIg. The results showed the rates of intra-uterine transmission in both the groups to have decreased from 14.7% to 5.7%. Recently, a preliminary report has been published on the efficacy of lamivudine, a potent inhibitor of HBV replication applied to prevent perinatal transmission.[43] Three women with HBV titers above 1.2×10^9 genome equivalents/ml received lamivudine during the final 4 weeks of pregnancy. Standard passive–active immunization was administered to their infants, who subsequently were found to have seroconverted to anti-HBs and who remained negative for HBV-DNA during the 12-month follow-up period.

The potential of intra-uterine HBV infection, though slight, ought not to be neglected. The underlying mechanism(s) and future strategies aimed at preventing intra-uterine HBV transmission merit further study.

VACCINE ESCAPE MUTANTS

Hepatitis B virus, though a DNA virus, employs an intracellular pre-genomic RNA intermediate for replication of its genome. As known with retroviruses, reverse transcriptase required to transcribe this RNA intermediate lacks proofreading capacity and hence, incurs a higher number of mutations than commonly found among DNA viruses. Thus, the viral genome undergoes an estimated mutation rate of 2×10^4 substitutions per site per year.[44] The variations observed within the HBs gene can be as follows.

Subtype related variations

Variations within the S-gene lead to the emergence of subdeterminants, e.g., *adr, adw, ayr, ayw*. Amino acid position 122 discriminates between subdeterminants *d* and *y*, more specifically, lysine at this position indicates subtype *d*, whereas arginine is characteristic for subtype y. Lysine at amino acid position 160 distinguishes subtype *w* from subtype *r* which harbors arginine, instead. Yet, there have been reports on some additional minor alterations affecting positions 126, 127, 134, 141 and 143 which can serve to discriminate between subtypes.[45] Those substitutions show a geographical distribution and hence are important for epidemiological studies.

Escape mutants

Escape mutants of HBV usually occur in the major hydrophilic region (amino acid positions 100-160) of HBs protein which represents the antibody binding site employed by the host's immune response as well as in laboratory tests. These mutations which usually coexist with anti-HBs might evolve as a reaction to immunoprophylaxis and have a major impact in that they may impair laboratory diagnosis as well as immunoprophylaxis by HBIg, vaccine, or both combined.[2,3,46-48]

The "*a*" determinant harbors the major B-cell epitopes and constitutes the antigenic determinant located between amino acid positions 124 and 147 common to all subtypes.[49] It comprises two cysteine loops, with the first one located at amino acid positions 121-138 and the second one starting between positions 139 and 147/149, and projecting outward from the viral surface. This region represents the most important recognition site for diagnosis, as well as a crucial target for the immune system to confer protection against the major HBV subtypes (*adr, adw, ayr, ayw*).[45] There have been numerous reports on mutations within the "*a*" determinant detected among subjects with chronic HBV infection displaying anti-HBs,[48] liver transplant patients receiving HBIg therapy,[50,51] and failure of immunoprophylaxis in neonates. Significant alterations most frequently reported are those occurring within the second loop at positions 144 (D144A) and 145 (G145R) as shown in Fig. 1.[2,52-54] Numerous studies aimed at investigating the molecular basis of the impact of "*a*" determinant on vaccine failure among neonates receiving hepatitis B prophylaxis have shown the frequency of infection with surface

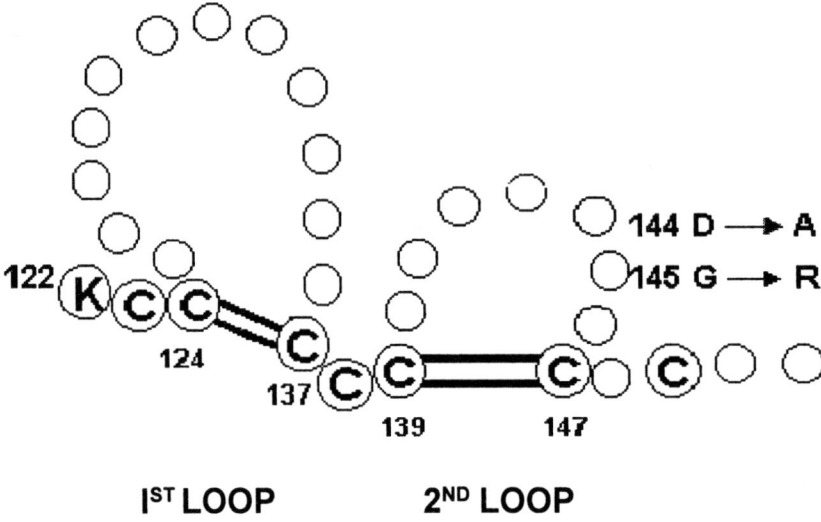

Fig. 1. Schematic diagram of common escape mutants shows substitution of aspartate (D) for alanine (A) and arginine (R) for glycine (G) at aa 144 and 145, respectively in the "a" determinant of HBsAg

gene mutants to be far lower than with the wild type. The HBs gene mutations detectable in children chronically infected with HBV following immunoprophylaxis are shown in Table 3. However, in the course of serosurveys, HBV escape mutants have also been detected among individuals who had developed chronic infection subsequent to natural infection, devoid of

Table 3. Escape mutants of HBs gene among the infants with hepatitis B vaccine failure

Countries	Hepatitis B vaccine failure			
	Vaccine failure (number)	Escape mutant (number)	%	Reference
Taiwan	27	6	22	Lee et al[55]
	33	12	36	Hsu et al[56]
Thailand	11	2	18	Poovorawan et al[3]
	13	4	30	Theamboonlers et al[57]
England and Wales	17	2	11	Ngui et al[47]
Singapore	41	16	39	Oon et al[2]
Japan	46	12	26	Miyake et al[46]

any immune pressure (Table 4). The occurrence of escape mutants discernible among vaccinated as opposed to naturally infected children was not strikingly higher. These findings suggest natural immunity prevailing among humans and hence, the potential selection of variant types as a consequence of vaccination.

Table 4. Mutants of "a" determinant of hepatitis B surface antigen in vaccinated and non-vaccinated children during the serosurvey

Country	Mutants of "a" determinant of HBsAg						Reference
	Vaccinated children			Non-vaccinated children			
	Total	mutants	%	Total	mutants	%	
Taiwan	33	12	36	153	15	9	Hsu et al[56]
	27	6	22	21	0	0	Lee et al[55]
Thailand	13	4	30	36	7	19	Theamboonlers et al[57]

The majority of children infected with escape mutant strains remained asymptomatic, showing normal growth and development. Similarly, there was no evidence of the mutant strain(s) being horizontally transmitted to other vaccinated children.[58] Recently, there has been a report on murine monoclonal antibodies displaying adequate reactivity with all mutant HBs antigens, including G145R.[59] Furthermore, two licensed recombinant hepatitis B vaccines derived from wild type HBV and solely containing HBs protein completely protected chimpanzees from infection with the frequently found vaccine escape mutant strain (Gly 145 Arg).[60] To conclude, escape mutants do occur, though rather infrequently, and there has been evidence as to the licensed vaccine's protective efficacy against all the strains described, including the most prevalent mutant strain (G145R). Hence, to incorporate the mutant gene into a newly formulated hepatitis B vaccine does not appear imperative at present.

Role of vaccine storage

Hepatitis B vaccine should be stored at 2 to 8°C. Freezing dissociates the antigen from the alum and interferes with the immunogenicity of the vaccine. Heating of the vaccine at 45°C for 1 week or 37°C for 1 month did not alter immunogenicity of the vaccine.[61] The vaccine was still effective even after storage for 1 to 2 months at an average temperature of 25°C.[62]

ACKNOWLEDGMENTS

The authors would like to express their gratitude towards the entire staff of the Viral Hepatitis Research Unit, Department of Pediatrics, Faculty of Medicine, Chulalongkorn University Hospital, for their tireless effort in collecting the multitude of data required. They also like to thank the Thailand Research Fund, Senior Research Scholar and Molecular Research Project, Faculty of Medicine, Chulalongkorn University, for supporting their group, and Ms. Petra Hirsch in editing the manuscript.

REFERENCES

1. Chang MH, Chen CJ, Lai MS, Hsu HM, Wu TC, Kong MS, Liang DC, et al. Universal hepatitis B vaccination in Taiwan and the incidence of hepatocellullar carcinoma in children. Taiwan childhood hepatoma study group. *N Engl J Med* 1997;336:1855-9.
2. Oon CJ, Lim GK, Ye Z, Goh KT, Tan KL, Yo SL, Hopes E, et al. Molecular epidemiology of hepatitis B virus vaccine variants in Singapore. *Vaccine* 1995;13:699-702.
3. Poovorawan Y, Themboonlers A, Chongsrisawat V, Sanpavat S. Molecular analysis of the a determinant of HBsAg in children of HBeAg-positive mothers upon failure of post-exposure prophylaxis. *Int J Infect Dis* 1998;216-20.
4. Szmuness W, Stevens CE, Harley EJ, Zang EA, Oleszko WR, William DC, Sadovsk YR, et al. Hepatitis B vaccine: demonstration of efficacy in a controlled clinical trial in a high-risk population in the United States. *N Engl J Med* 1980;303:833-41.
5. Dienstag, JL, Werner BG, Polk BF. Hepatitis B vaccine in health care personnel: safety, immunogenicity, and indicators of efficacy. *Ann Intern Med* 1984;101:34-40.
6. Nouri-Aria KT, Magrin S, Alexander GJ, Anderson MG, Williams R, Eddlestion AL. Abnormal T-cell activation in chronic hepatitis B infection: a consequence of monocyte dysfunction? *Immunology* 1988;64:733-8.
6a. Swennen B, Van Damme P, Vellinga A, Coppieters Y, Depoorter AM. Analysis of factors influencing vaccine uptake: perspectives from Belgium. *Vaccine* 2001;20:S5-7.
7. Salazar M, Deulofeut H, Granja C, Deulofeut R, Yunis DE, Marcus-Bagley D, Awdeh Z, et al. Normal HBsAg presentation and T-cell defect in the immune response of non-responders. *Immunogenetics* 1995;41:366-74.
7a. Bauer T, Weinberger K, Jilg W. Variants of two major T-cell epitopes within the hepatitis B surface antigen are not recognized by specific T helper cells of vaccinated individuals. *Hepatology* 2002;35:455-65.
8. Vingerhoets J, Vanham G, Kestens L, Penne G, Leroux-Roels G, Gigase P. Deficient T-cell responses in non-responders to hepatitis B vaccination: absence of Th-1 cytokine production. *Immunol Lett* 1994;39:163-8.
9. Barnaba V, Franco A, Alberti A, Benvenuto, Balsano F. Selective killing of hepatitis B envelope antigen-specific B-cells by class I-restricted, exogenous antigen-specific T-lymphocytes. *Nature* 1990;345:258-60.
10. Milich DR, Chisari FV. Genetic regulation of the immune response to the hepatitis B surface antigen (HBsAg). I. H-2-restriction of the murine humoral immune response to the a and d determinants of HBsAg. *J Immunol* 1982;129:320-5.
11. Milich DR, Leroux-Roels GG, Chisari FV. Genetic regulation of the immune response to the hepatitis B surface antigen (HBsAg) II. Qualitative characteristics of the humoral immune response to the a, d, and y determinants of HBsAg. *J Immunol* 1983;130:1395-400.
12. Milich DR, Leroux-Roels GG, Louie RE, Chisari FV. Genetic regulation of the immune response to hepatitis B surface antigen (HBsAg) IV. Distinct H-2-linked Ir genes control antibody responses to different HBsAg determinant on the same molecule and map to the I-A and I-C subregions. *J Exp Med* 1984;159:41-56.
13. Watanabe H, Okumura M, Hirayama K, Sasazuki T. HLA-Bw54-DR4-DRw53-DQw4 haplotype controls non-responsiveness to hepatitis B surface antigen via CD8–positive suppressor T-cells. *Tissue Antigens* 1990;36:69-74.
14. Craven DE, Awdeh ZL, Kunches LM, Punis EJ, Dienstag JL, Werner BG, Poek BF, et al. Non-responsiveness to hepatitis B vaccine in health care workers results of revaccination and genetic typings. *Ann Intern Med* 1986;105:356-60.

15. Walker M, Szmuness W, Stevens CE, Rubinstein P. Genetics of anti-HBs responsiveness. I HLA DR 7 and non-responsiveness to hepatitis vaccination. *Transfusion* 1981;21:601.
16. Durupinar B, Okten G. HLA tissue types in non-responders to hepatitis B vaccine. *Indian J Pediatr* 1996;3:369-73.
17. McDermott AB, Madrigal JA, Sabin CA, Zuckerman JN, Cohen SBA. The influence of host factors and immunogenetics on lymphocyte responses to hepagene vaccination. *Vaccine* 1999;17:1329-37.
18. Lango-Warensjo A, Cardell K, Lindblom B. Haplotypes comprising subtypes of the DQB1 *06 allele direct the antibody response after immunization with hepatitis B surface antigen. *Tissue antigens* 1998;52: 374-80.
19. Alper CA, Kruskall MS, Marcus-Bagley D, Craven DE, Katz AJ, Brink SJ, Dienstag JL, et al. Genetic prediction of non-response to hepatitis B vaccine. *N Engl J Med* 1989;321:708-12.
20. Desombere I, Hauser P, Rossau R, Paradijs J, Roels GL. Non-responders to hepatitis B vaccine can present envelope particles to T-lymphocytes. *J Immunol* 1995;520-9.
21. Hatae K, Kimura A, Okubo R, Watanabe H, Erlich HA, Ueda K, Nishimura Y, et al. Genetic control of non-responsiveness to hepatitis B virus vaccine by an extended HLA haplotype. *Eur J Immunol* 1992;22:1899-905.
22. Watanabe H, Matsushita S, Kamikawaji N, Hirayama K, Okumura M, Sasazuki T. Immune suppression gene on HLA-Bw54Dr4-Drw53 haplotype controls non-responsiveness to hepatitis B surface antigen via CD8-positive suppressor T-cells. *Tissue Antigens* 1988;22:9-17.
23. Egea E, Iglesias A, Zalazar M, Watanabe H, Erlich HA, Ueda K, Nishimura Y, et al. The cellular basis for lack of antibody response to hepatitis B vaccine in humans. *J Exp Med* 1991;173:531-8.
24. Pride MW, Bailey CR, Muchmore E, Thanavala Y. Evaluation of B and T-cell responses in chimpanzees immunized with hepagene a hepatitis B vaccine containing pre-S1, pre-S2 and S-gene products. *Vaccine* 1998;16:543-50.
25. McDermott AB, Cohen SBA, Zuckerman JN, Madrigal JA. Human leukocyte antigens influence the immune response to a pre-S/S hepatitis B vaccine. *Vaccine* 1999;17:330-9.
26. Brunel F, Darbouret A, Ronco J. Cationic lipid DC-Chol induces an improved and balanced immunity able to overcome the unresponsiveness to the hepatitis B. *Vaccine* 1999;17:2192-2203.
27. Schirmbeck R, Bohm W, Ado K, Chisari FV, Reimann J. Nucleic acid vaccination primes hepatitis B virus surface antigen-specific cytotoxic T lymphocytes in non-responder mice. *J Virol* 1995;5929-34.
28. Tang SX, Yu GL. Intra-uterine infection with hepatitis B virus. *Lancet* 1990;3;335:302.
28a. Leroux-Roels G, Cao T, Deknibber A, Meuleman P, Roobrouck A, Farhoudi A, Vanlandschoot P, et al. Prevention of hepatitis B infections: vaccination and its limitations. *Acta Clin Belg* 2001;56:209-19.
29. Zhu Q, Lu Q, Gu X, Xu H, Duan S. A preliminary study on interruption of HBV transmission in uterus. *Chin Med J* 1997;110:145-7.
30. Li L, Sheng MH, Tong SP, Chen HZ, Wen YM. Transplacental transmission of hepatitis B virus. *Lancet* 1986;2:872.
31. Liu ZH, Men K, Xu D. A follow-up study on correlated factors for intra-uterine infection of hepatitis B virus. *Chung Hua Yu Fang I Hsueh Tsa Chih* 1997;31:263-5.
32. Lin HH, Lee TY, Chen DS, Sung JL, Ohto H, Etoh T, Kawanna T, et al. Transplacental leakage of HBeAg-positive maternal blood as the most likely route in causing intra-uterine infection with hepatitis B virus. *J Pediatr* 1987;111:877-81.
33. Lazizi Y, Badur S, Perk Y, Ilter O, Pillot J. Selective unresponsiveness to HBsAg vaccine in newborns related with an in utero passage of hepatitis B virus DNA. *Vaccine* 1997;10:1095-100.
34. Poovorawan Y, Chongsrisawat V, Theamboonlers A, Vimolkej L, Yano M. Is there evidence for intra-uterine HBV infection in newborns of hepatitis B carrier mothers? *Southeast Asian J Trop Med Public Health* 1997;28:365-9.

35. Poovorawan Y, Sanpavat S, Pongpunlert W, Chumdermpadetsuk S, Sentrakul P, Safary A. Protective efficacy of a recombinant DNA hepatitis B vaccine in neonates of HBe antigen positive mothers. *JAMA* 1989;261:3278-81.
36. Xu D, Yan Y, Xu J. A molecular epidemiologic study on the mechanism of intra-uterine transmission of hepatitis B virus. *Chung Hua Liu Hsing Ping Hsueh Tsa Chih* 1998;19:131-3.
37. Grosheide PM, Quartero HW, Schalm SW, Heijtink RA, Christiaens GC. Early invasive prenatal diagnosis in HBsAg-positive women. *Prenat Diagn* 1994;14:553-8.
38. Ko TM, Tseng LH, Chang MH, Chen DS, Heih FJ, Chuang SM, Lee TY, et al. Amniocentesis in mothers who are hepatitis B virus carriers does not expose the infant to an increased risk of hepatitis B virus infection. *Arch Gynecol Obstet* 1994;255:25-30.
39. Tang S. Study on the mechanisms and influential factors of intra-uterine infection of hepatitis B virus. *Chung Hua Liu Hsing Ping Hsueh Tsa Chih* 1991;12:325-6.
40. Tang S. Study on the HBV intra-uterine infection and its rate. *Chung Hua Liu Hsing Ping Hsueh Tsa Chih* 1990;11:328-30.
41. Alexander GJ, Eddleston AL. Does maternal antibody to core antigen prevent recognition of transplacental transmission of hepatitis B virus infection? *Lancet* 1986;1:296-7.
42. Damiani S, Attanasio P, Maneschi F, Speciale P, La Ferla A, Navetta A, Tripi S, et al. Maternal-fetal transmission of infection with hepatitis B virus: evaluation of viral markers in maternal and fetal biological materials and relation with the vaccine response. *Ann Ostet Ginecol Med Perinat* 1989;110:217-25.
43. van Nunen AB, de Man RA, Heijtink RA, Niesters HG, Schalm SW. Lamivudine in the last 4 weeks of pregnancy to prevent perinatal transmission in highly viremic chronic hepatitis B patients. *J Hepatol* 2000;32:1040-1.
44. Howard CR. The structure of hepatitis B envelope and molecular variants of hepatitis B virus. *J Viral Hepat* 1995;2:165-70
45. Magnius LO, Norder H. Subtypes, genotypes and molecular epidemiology of the hepatitis B virus as reflected by sequence variability of the S-gene. *Intervirology* 1995;38:24-34.
46. Miyake Y, Oda T, Li R, Sugiyama K. A comparison of amino acid sequences of hepatitis B virus S-gene in 46 children presenting various clinical features for immunoprophylaxis. *Tohoku J Exp Med* 1996;180:233-47.
47. Ngui SL, Connell SO, Eglin RP, Heptonstall J, Teo CG. Low detection rate and maternal provenance of hepatitis B virus s-gene mutants in cases of failed postnatal immunoprophylaxis in England and Wales. *J Infect Dis* 1997;176:1360-5.
48. Yamamoto K, Horikita M, Tsuda F, Itoh K, Akahane Y, Yotsumoto S, Okamoto H, et al. Naturally occurring escape mutants of hepatitis B virus with various mutations in the S-gene in carriers seropositive for antibody to hepatitis B surface antigen. *J Virol* 1994;2671-6.
49. Stirk HJ, Thornton JM, Howard CR. A topological model for hepatitis B surface antigen. *Intervirology* 1992;33:148-58.
50. Protzer-Knolle U, Naumann U, Bartenschlager R, Berg T, Hopf U, Beuschen felde KH, Neuhaus P, et al. Hepatitis B virus with antigenically altered hepatitis B surface antigen is selected by high-dose hepatitis B immune globulin after liver transplantation. *Hepatology* 1998;27:254-63.
51. Carman WF, Trautwein C, Van Deursen FJ, Colman K, Dornan E, McIntyre G, Waters J, et al. Hepatitis B virus envelope variation after transplantation with and without hepatitis B immune globulin prophylaxis. *Hepatology* 1996;24:489-93.
52. Okamoto H, Yano K, Nozaki Y. Mutations within the S-gene of hepatitis B virus transmitted from mothers to babies immunized with hepatitis B immune globulin and vaccine. *Pediatr Res* 1992;32:264-8.

53. Fujji H, Moriyama K, Sakamoto N, Kondo T, Yasuda K, Hiraizumi Y, Yamazaki M, et al. Gly145 To arg substitution in HBs antigen of immune escape mutant of hepatitis B virus. *Biochem Biophys Res Commun* 1992;184:1152-7.
54. Hsu HY, Chang MH, Ni YH, Lin HH, Wang SM, Chen DS. Surface gene mutants of hepatitis B virus in infants who develop acute of chronic infections despite immunoprophylaxis. *Hepatology* 1997;26:786-91.
55. Lee PI, Chang LY, Lee CY, Huang LM, Chang MH. Detection of hepatitis B surface gene mutation in carrier children with or without immunoprophylaxis at birth. *J Infect Dis* 1997;176:427-30.
56. Hsu HY, Chang MH, Liaw SH, Ni YH, Chen HL. Changes of hepatitis B surface antigen variants in carrier children before and after universal vaccination in Taiwan. *Hepatology* 1999;30:1312-7.
57. Theamboonlers A, Chongsrisawat V, Jantaradsamee P, Poovorawan Y. Variants within the "a" determinant of HBs gene in children and adolescents with and without hepatitis B vaccination as part of Thailand's Expanded Program of Immunization (EPI). *Tohuku J Exp Med* 2000;193:197-205.
58. Oon CJ, Tan KL, Harrison T, Zuckerman A. Natural history of hepatitis B surface antigen mutants in children. *Lancet* 1996;348:1524.
59. Cooreman MP, Van Roosmalen MH, te Morsche R, Sunmen CM, de Ven EM, Jansen JB, Tytgat GN, et al. Characterization of the reactivity pattern of murine monoclonal antibodies against wild-type hepatitis B surface antigen to G 145 R and other naturally occurring "a" loop escape mutations. *Hepatology* 1999;30:1287-92.
60. Ogata N, Cote PJ, Zanetti AR, Miller RH, Shapiro M, Garin J, Purcell RH, et al. Licensed recombinant hepatitis B vaccines protect chimpanzees against infection with the prototype surface gene mutant of hepatitis B virus. *Hepatology* 1999;30:779-86.
61. Van Damme P, Cramm M, Safary A, Vandepapeliere P, Meheus A. Heat stability of a recombinant DNA hepatitis B vaccine. *Vaccine* 1992;10:366-7.
62. Xu ZY, Cao HL, Liu CB, et al. *Control of hepatitis B in China. In* : Rizzetto M, Purcell PH, Gerin JL, Berme G, Eds. Viral Hepatitis and Liver Disease : Turin, Edizioni Minerva Medica, 1997;pp. 689-90.

Section VI

Treatment of chronic hepatitis B

44

Treatment of chronic hepatitis B: current trends and Indian perspectives

Shiv K Sarin, Rakesh Kumar, Manoj K Sharma

The spectrum of clinical manifestations of hepatitis B virus (HBV) infection varies in both acute and chronic disease. During the acute phase, manifestations range from subclinical hepatitis to anicteric hepatitis, icteric hepatitis, and fulminant hepatitis. Ninety-five percent of the adults with acute hepatitis B are known to clear the viral infection spontaneously. Hence, there is little rationale at present to recommend antiviral therapy in uncomplicated acute hepatitis B. In patients with complications of acute hepatitis, the use of antiviral therapy is being evaluated.

Chronic HBV infection is defined as the presence of HBsAg in serum for 6 months or longer after the initial detection. The prevalence of chronic HBV infection is high in China, Southeast Asia, among Eskimos. India falls in the intermediate prevalence region[1]. Chronic HBV infection could lead to a wide spectrum of manifestations, from an asymptomatic infection to chronic hepatitis, cirrhosis, and hepatocellular carcinoma. Most patients with chronic hepatitis B are asymptomatic, and a fair number have only nonspecific symptoms such as fatigue. Signs and symptoms of clinical liver disease are more often found in older patients[2] and those with more advanced histologic disease.[3]

FACTORS INFLUENCING SURVIVAL

Patients with a prolonged replication phase of HBV have a poor prognosis. In a study of 98 patients with HBsAg positive compensated cirrhosis,[4] the five-year survival rate in HBeAg positive was lower than anti-HBe positive patients (72 versus 97 percent). Clearance of HBeAg was associated with a 2.2-fold decrease in death rate. In another series of 366 European compensated cirrhotic patients, the five-year survival rates were 77 and 88 percent in patients who were HBeAg positive and negative, respectively.[5] The worse prognosis in patients with a prolonged replicative phase may be related to a longer duration of necroinflammation. Recurrent episodes of hepatitis may, either directly or indirectly through immune-mediated injury, increase the risk of fibrosis, cirrhosis, and perhaps carcinogenesis. Other independent factors associated with poor survival are older age, hypoalbuminemia, thrombocytopenia, splenomegaly, and hyperbilirubinemia.

Even among patients with decompensated cirrhosis, suppression of HBV replication and HBsAg clearance can result in improvement in liver disease. The annual rates of development of HCC range from 2% per year in Italy[6] to 4.1% per year in Japan.[7] In compensated cirrhosis type B, figures range from 2.2% to 2.8% per year in Taiwan[4, 8] and 2.7% per year in Japan. In the Western world, an annual rate of 1.5% per year was reported.[9]

PATIENT EVALUATION FOR THERAPY
Initial evaluation

The evaluation of a patient with chronic HBV infection should include a thorough history and physical examination. Efforts should be made to determine the mode of acquisition of infection. Risk factors for co-infection, alcohol use, family history of HBV infection and liver cancer should be looked for. Investigations should include assessment for overt or latent liver disease (using imaging modalities such as an ultrasound or a CT scan), evidence of portal hypertension (imaging studies, UGI endoscopy), markers of HBV replication (HBeAg), and tests for co-infection with HCV, HDV and HIV in those at risk.

HBV-DNA Assay

There is limited role of doing HBV-DNA by PCR in the treatment of a patient with chronic HBV infection. Mere presence of a low level of viremia does not constitute an indication for treating chronic HBV infection. A quantitative test for the viral load is needed. An arbitrary value of >10^5 copies/mL has been chosen as a criterion for treating chronic hepatitis B at a recent NIH conference.[10] Besides being expensive, there are some difficulties with this definition. First, the assays for HBV-DNA quantification are not well standardized. Second, some patients with chronic hepatitis B have fluctuating HBV-DNA levels that may at times fall below 10^5 copies/mL. Third, the threshold HBV-DNA level that is associated with progressive liver disease is unknown.

In general, if a patient is HBeAg positive and has raised ALT levels, there is no need for doing any HBV-DNA test, except for study protocols. Only in patients who are HBeAg negative, there is a need to do DNA estimation to confirm that the rise in ALT in a given patient is due to viral replication and consequent injury.

Liver Biopsy

The liver biopsy helps to assess the severity of liver injury and to exclude other causes of liver disease. Histologic findings may help in predicting prognosis.[3] An international panel of experts has recommended that the histologic diagnosis of chronic hepatitis should include the etiology, grade of necroinflammatory activity, and stage/extent of fibrosis.[11] Liver histology helps in assessing response to therapy as it improves significantly in patients who have sustained response to antiviral therapy or spontaneous HBeAg sero-conversion. Liver biopsies can be used for immunohistochemical staining for HBsAg and hepatitis B core antigen.

Patient Selection

The ideal patient to consider for therapy is HBsAg and HBeAg positive for a minimum of six months with elevated, but stable transaminases, histological evidence of chronic hepatitis and without cirrhosis.[12]

Patients with cirrhosis, HBeAg negative patients, neonatally infected individuals, and patients with co-infection especially with delta virus are difficult to treat and require special protocols.

The need for treatment in HBV can be broadly decided according to an algorithmic approach suggested in a Consensus Conference of the Indian Association for the Study of the Liver held in 1998 (Fig. 1).[13]

DRUG THERAPY FOR CHRONIC HEPATITIS B

Several drugs having antiviral properties are available for the treatment of chronic HBV. The two common drugs are Interferon (IFN) and lamivudine.

Selection of patients for IFN therapy

Interferons are cytokines with immunomodulatory, antiproliferative and antiviral properties. Interferon alpha (IFN-α) and interferon beta (IFN-β) have potent antiviral properties, while interferon gamma (IFN-γ) has more marked immunoregulatory properties.

Predictors of response to IFN therapy

Since interferon therapy is effective only in a proportion of patients and is associated with significant side effects, identification of predictive factors for a favorable response is needed. These factors include low pretreatment HBV-DNA level, elevated transaminases (>2 × normal), short duration of disease, significant inflammation on liver biopsy, HBeAg positive, adult acquired infection, immunocompetent state, female gender and no contraindication to therapy.

None of these variables, however, can predict with certainty the likelihood of success with interferon therapy in an individual patient. Many patients lacking these criteria do respond to treatment and hence these characteristics cannot be used to exclude patients from receiving treatment.

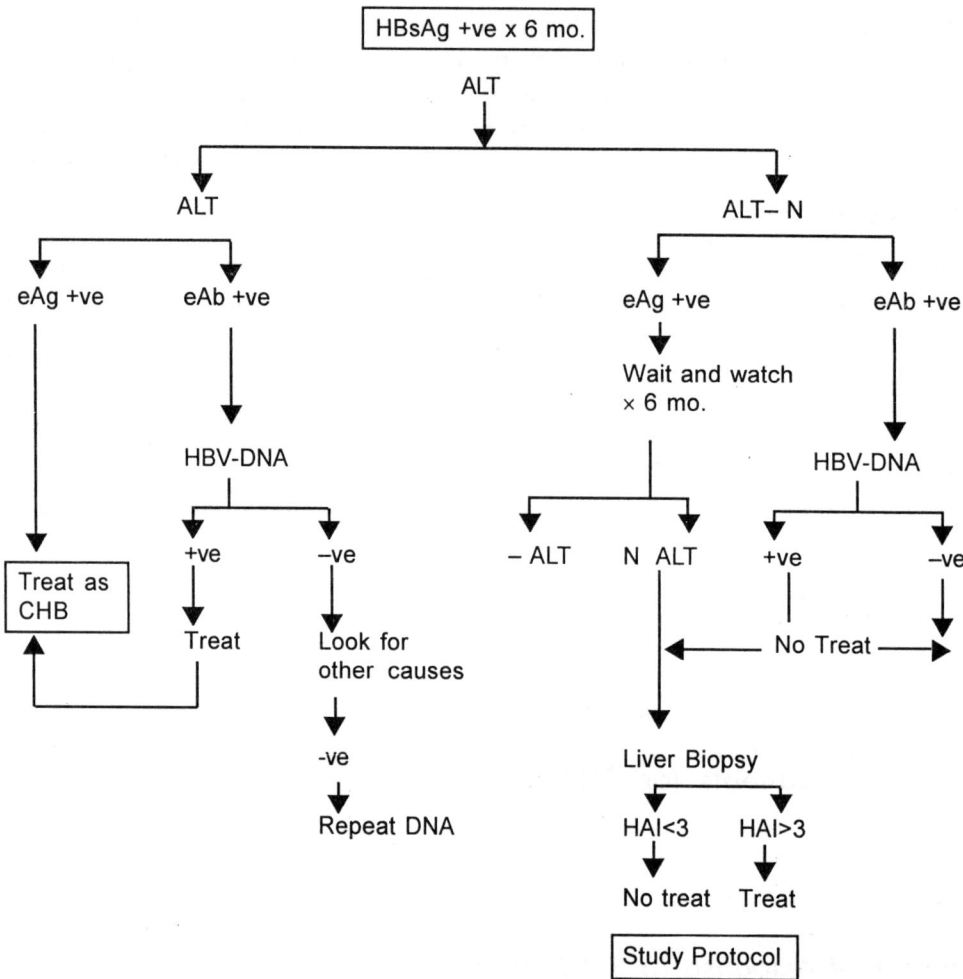

Fig. 1. Evaluation and management of patients with chronic HBV infection

HBV genotypes are recently being evaluated to define response to therapy. The precore mutation is more common with genotype D (more prevalent in the Mediterranean region and India) and is rare in patients with genotype A (more common genotype in the Unites States and Western Europe and India).

Patients in the immune tolerant phase of chronic hepatitis B infection, with circulating HBeAg and HBV-DNA but normal or near normal (<2 times) ALT levels, have very low response rates to interferon. HBeAg-positive patients with high serum HBV-DNA but normal ALT levels should be monitored at three-to-six month intervals.

Patients with extrahepatic manifestations of chronic hepatitis B infection, such as polyarteritis nodosa and various glomerular diseases, may also respond to interferon therapy.

Contraindications to interferon Therapy

Patients with concomitant HCC, pregnancy, co-morbid conditions such as significant coronary artery disease, renal failure, psychiatric disorders, brittle diabetes, seizures should not receive interferon therapy. A neutrophil count below $1,500 \times 10^3/L$ or a platelet count below $70 \times 10^5/L$ is a contraindication to therapy. An ANA titre above 1/160 and a history suggestive of autoimmune disease contraindicates IFN treatment.

Patients receiving treatment should be monitored clinically and with laboratory studies including liver function tests (alanine aminotransferase [ALT], albumin and total leucocyte count and platelets) every 1 to 2 weeks during treatment. Additionally, HBsAg, HBeAg, and HBV-DNA should be measured at initiation, completion, and 6 months after treatment. Preceding seroconversion, patients may have a "flare" of serum aminotransferases. It may take months to years after completing treatment for HBeAg and HBsAg to become negative.[14]

The dose of interferon should be reduced or terminated if the patient shows evidence of decompensation of liver disease (decreased albumin or increased bilirubin), significant bone marrow depression, severe depression, or intolerable side effects. Between 10% and 40% of patients require dose reduction and 5% to 10% discontinue therapy early. Approximately 2% of patients develop severe side effects, including bacterial infection, autoimmune disease, severe depression, suicide, seizure, acute cardiac or renal failure, and pneumonitis.

Selection of patients for lamivudine therapy

Only chronic hepatitis B patients with active HBV replication who are HBeAg-positive and/or have quantifiable HBV-DNA with raised serum ALT are suitable candidates for lamivudine therapy. Lamivudine is also effective in IFN non-responders. Non-response to interferon does not appear to influence the treatment response to lamivudine.[15]

Lamivudine has also been safely administered to liver transplant recipients to prevent or to treat recurrent hepatitis B following transplantations.[16, 17] However, lamivudine-resistant YMDD mutants emerge more frequently and earlier in immunosuppressed transplant recipients, compared with immunocompetent patients.

Prophylactic use of lamivudine in chronic hepatitis B patients receiving chemotherapy or immune suppression has been suggested.[18, 19]

Predictors of response to lamivudine

Pretreatment ALT level is an important predictor of response.[20-24] According to a pooled analysis of 406 patients who received 100 mg of lamivudine daily for one year, the rates of HBeAg sero-conversion correlated directly with pretreatment ALT levels and were detected in 2%, 9%, 21%, and 47% of patients with normal ALT level, one–twofold, two–fivefold and more than fivefold ALT elevations, respectively.[25] The corresponding figures in the placebo groups were 0%, 5%, 11%, and 14%, respectively.

Adverse effects

Oral lamivudine therapy is relatively safe and has no adverse effect on the bone-marrow. Potentially serious, but uncommon adverse effects reported in patients receiving lamivudine include pancreatitis and lactic acidosis.[26, 27] Lamivudine is predominantly excreted by the kidney and the dose should be reduced in patients with renal insufficiency.

ANTIVIRAL THERAPY

The short-term goal of the antiviral therapy is to achieve loss of infectivity (sero-conversion/loss of HBV-DNA), biochemical (normalization of ALT) and histological remission (reduction in inflammation). The long-term goal is to eradicate HBV infection, remission of the liver disease (which will prevent progression to cirrhosis and HCC) with or without reversal of fibrosis and prolongation of survival.

Definition of Response

At a recent NIH workshop on the management of hepatitis B, it was proposed that responses to antiviral therapy of chronic hepatitis B should be categorized as biochemical (BR), virological (VR) or histological (HR) and as, on-therapy or sustained off-therapy (Table 1).[10]

Table 1. Definition of different categories of response to antiviral therapy

Biochemical (BR)	Decrease in serum ALT to within normal range
Virological (VR)	Decrease in serum HBV-DNA to undetectable levels in unamplified assays (10^5 copies / mL), and loss of HBeAg in patients who were initially HBeAg positive
Histological (HR)	Decrease in histological activity index by at least 2 points compared with pre-treatment liver biopsy
Complete Response (CR)	Fullfil criteria of biochemical and virological response and loss of HBsAg
Time of assessment	
On-Therapy	During therapy
	• Maintained – persist throughout the course of treatment
	• End of treatment- At the end of a defined course of therapy
	After discontinuation of therapy
	• Sustained (SR-6) – 6 mo. after discontinuation of therapy
Off-Therapy	• Sustained (SR-12) – 12 mo. after discontinuation of therapy

Aims of Treatment

Initial goals are to suppress HBV replication and to induce remission of liver disease. The ultimate goals are to eliminate HBV, prevent disease progression to cirrhosis or hepatocellular carcinoma (HCC) and to improve patient survival (Table 2).[28]

Table 2. Goals of antiviral treatment of chronic HBV infection

Sustained suppression of HBV replication
HBV-DNA undetectable in serum
HBeAg to anti-HBe sero-conversion
HBsAg to anti-HBs sero-conversion
Remission of liver disease
Normalization in serum ALT levels
Decreased necroinflammation in liver
Improved clinical outcome
Decreased risk of developing cirrhosis, liver failure and HCC
Increased survival

TREATMENT OF HBeAg POSITIVE CHRONIC HEPATITIS B (e+ CHB)

Interferon Therapy

IFN has antiviral, antiproliferative, and immunomodulatory effects, all of which may be important in HBV therapy. IFN increases cytotoxic T-cell immune response and also prevents viral entry and uncoating, as well as mRNA translation and assembly. IFN-α has been shown to inhibit viral RNA pregenome packing into core particles and also enhance the expression of HBsAg and HBcAg on the hepatocytes.

IFN therapy can achieve a beneficial response (defined as sero-conversion from HBeAg to anti-HBe) in 30 to 40 percent of patients, when administered as subcutaneous injections in doses of 5 million units (MU) daily or 10 MU three times a week for 16 weeks. There is also evidence that IFN-α may be beneficial in patients with extrahepatic manifestations of chronic HBV infection.

Patterns of Response

A treatment response is defined as normalization of liver enzymes, loss of HBV-DNA by hybridization assay, and loss of HBeAg with or without conversion to anti-HBe positivity. This is assessed at the end of therapy (ETR) given for 4–6 months. A sustained response (SR) is defined as HBeAg loss, anti-HBe +ve and HBV-DNA [<10^5 copies/ml] with normalization of ALT six months after stopping treatment.[29]

IFN therapy leads to a gradual decline in ALT levels and a fall in serum HBV-DNA. This may or may not lead to viral clearance. On the other hand, in responder patients, an increase in transaminases, often up to 10 times normal, between week 7 and 12 of therapy can be seen. This "flare" in hepatitis is usually associated with a dramatic decline in HBV-DNA followed by loss of HBeAg and development of anti-HBe. This is called sero-conversion and response.

Months to years later, up to 70% of the patients may also clear HBsAg. This is termed as "cure". HBV-DNA is undetectable in the serum by an ultra-sensitive PCR assay, but detectable in the liver tissue. Liver biopsies of these patients show markedly less hepatic inflammation, but mild activity often persists.

Forty percent of patients with ALT between 100 and 200 IU/L and 50% with ALT>200 IU/L will normalize serum ALT on treatment. Sixty-seven percent of patients with ALT between 100 and 200 IU/L and close to 100% of those with ALT >200 will develop undetectable HBV-DNA on treatment.[30] Thirty-seven percent of patients will develop a sustained loss of HBV-DNA, 33% a sustained loss of HBeAg, and 8% will lose HBsAg over time. IFN therapy is associated with flares (at least twofold increase over baseline) in serum ALT concentrations in 30 to 50 percent of patients. This response is thought to reflect immune-mediated lysis of infected hepatocytes. IFN may need to be discontinued or the dose reduced if the flare is severe and accompanied by symptoms or a substantial rise in the serum bilirubin concentration and or hepatic decompensation.

A meta-analysis of available trials (15 RCTs) involving 837 adult patients who received IFN-α in doses of 5–10 MU daily, 3 times weekly for 4–6 months indicates loss of HBeAg in 33% of treated patients compared with 12% of controls. Loss of HBsAg was seen in 8% of interferon treated patients compared with only 1.8% in control group. Loss of HBV-DNA and normalization of ALT was more common in the treated group.[31]

Despite wide spread experience, there is limited published data from India on the use of IFN in patients with chronic hepatitis B. Sarin et al in 1996 studied 41 patients who were randomized to receive either 3 million units alpha-interferon on alternate days for 4 months (n=20) or no therapy (n=21). All patients completed the trial without any serious adverse effects. The HBeAg and HBV-DNA clearance was 50% and 57% respectively with sero-conversion in 37%. The HBsAg clearance was 15% at the end of one year of follow-up. The HAI as assessed by Knodell's score, significantly decreased in treated patients compared to controls. The response was better in patients with chronic hepatitis and patients with high ALT levels than in cirrhotics and those with lower ALT levels.[32]

Mazumder et al studied 24 patients with histological evidence of chronic hepatitis with or without cirrhosis and persistent elevation of serum aminotransferases and persistent positivity for HBsAg and HBeAg for more than 6 months. Fourteen patients were treated with interferon-alpha-2b 3 million units thrice a week for 16 weeks; Ten patients who could not afford the drug served as control. At the end of 1 year, HBeAg clearance occurred in 9 (64%) in IFN group and in one in the control group (p<0.01). HBsAg clearance occurred in only one patient in the treatment group during a follow-up of 2.4 (range 1-4) years. Patients having high ALT (>100 IU/L) levels at the beginning of the treatment had significantly higher HBeAg clearance rate (7 of 7) than patients with low ALT levels (2 of 7; p<0.05).[33]

Relapse after IFN therapy is rare. In one long-term study, only 3 of 23 (13%) patients relapsed and became HBeAg positive again. Most of these relapses occurred within one year of therapy.

In those who fail to respond to IFN-α therapy, the options are to observe, enroll in a trial of retreatment with IFN-α,[34] treat with lamivudine or other anti-virals.

Successful sero-conversion to anti-HBe and HBV-DNA negative states results in decreased decompensated liver disease and mortality for Western patients.[35-37]

Pegylated interferon is now being studied for the treatment of chronic hepatitis B.

Cooksley et al[38] looked at a 24-week course of pegylated interferon-alpha-2a and compared it with regular interferon-α-2a. Twelve percent of patients who received short-acting interferon, compared with 27% of patients who were treated with 90 or 180 μg per week of pegylated interferon, achieved a sustained response.

Duration of Therapy

The optimal duration of IFN therapy for chronic hepatitis B is not clear. A multicenter trial from Europe demonstrated benefit of continuing therapy in patients in whom HBeAg had not cleared by 16 weeks but who had low levels of HBV-DNA (<10 pg/ml).[39] There is very little data on longer courses of treatment in patients with HBeAg positive chronic hepatitis B. Scully et al found that the response was similar in patients who received 12 versus 24 weeks of IFN-α.[40] Janssen et al[39] reported that among patients who have not cleared HBeAg after 16 weeks of INF-α, those randomized to continue treatment until 32 weeks had significantly higher rates of HBeAg clearance compared to those who stopped treatment.

The durability of response to IFN therapy varies in Asian and North American or European patients. Nearly 95–100% of responders remain HBeAg negative during 5–10 years of follow-up and 30–86% of the responders even lose HBsAg as shown in studies from Europe and North America.[35, 37] While Asian studies showed lower rate of durable response and rare loss of HBsAg, the rate of HBeAg loss was in similar proportion of treated and untreated patients.[41, 42]

Interferon-alfa therapy for chronic hepatitis B in children

Only a few studies have been carried out in this population. The safety and efficacy has not been as carefully evaluated in children. However, they appear to tolerate interferon better than adults.

A recent trial at several centers in Canada, Europe and the United States examined the use of interferon-alpha in children between the ages of 1 and 17 years with chronic hepatitis B. Seventy patients received 24 weeks of interferon-alpha-2b (6 million units per square meter three times a week) and 74 were observed. Serum HBeAg and viral DNA became negative in 26% of treated and 11% of observed children (P < 0.05). Hepatitis B surface antigen became negative (most likely indicative of viral clearance and cure) in 10% of treated children and 1% of controls.[43]

Lebensztejn et al[44] looked at the sustained response to short-acting interferon-alfa given to 71 children with chronic hepatitis B. Thirty-two of 71 (45%) developed a sustained response to 3 million units of IFN-α given 3 times per week for 20 weeks. All patients had negative HBV-DNA assays and maintained their sero-conversion to anti-HBe. Fifteen trials were analyzed in a meta-analysis involving 240 children treated with doses 3–10 MU/m² given 3 times/week for 12–48 weeks. Loss of HBeAg was seen in 23% in treated group compared to 11% in control; while HBsAg loss was 1.5% in treated patients and none in control.[45] The response of IFN therapy in children however, has been variably reported with higher response in European children compared to the Asian Chinese. They are known to respond poorly to IFN even with steroid priming.

We studied recombinant interferon therapy in 22 children with CHB infection, HBeAg positive and HBV-DNA positive, 16 (73%) with chronic hepatitis and the remaining with cirrhosis. Loss of HBeAg and HBV-DNA was seen in 9 (41%), 3 of 9 (33.3%) in vertically transmitted group and 6 of 13 (46%) in horizontally transmitted group. Sero-conversion to anti-HBe was seen in 4 (18%) patients. IFN was well tolerated with no serious side-effects.[46]

Lamivudine Therapy

Lamivudine is the pyrimidine nucleotide analogue, the negative enantiomer of 3- thiacytidine. It is well absorbed orally and has potent antiviral action against HBV, both *in vivo* and *in vitro*. The drug has the advantages of better tolerability, safety, and oral administration. Almost all patients initially become HBV-DNA-negative on treatment.

Four long-term studies have shown an increased rate of HBeAg sero-conversion with lamivudine therapy.[21, 23, 47, 48] At one year, 32% loss of HBeAg and a 17% sero-conversion rate has been reported. Results are similar in Asians and whites, with the highest response rates seen in patients with increased serum ALT levels. In one study of long-term therapy in Asian patients, the HBeAg conversion rate was 47% after 4 years of continued lamivudine treatment.[47] Patients with ALT > 5 times normal, clear HBeAg in about 64% of cases at 1 year of treatment, compared with 34% in the control group. Treatment beyond one year is controversial.

Response to therapy results in suppression of viral replication and a reduction in hepatic necroinflammatory activity. Improvement in fibrosis occurs in patients with cirrhosis and bridging fibrosis.

Lamivudine resistance

Resistance to lamivudine on treatment develops due to selection of resistant mutants of HBV. These mutants have characteristic changes of the amino acid substitution over the conserved YMDD-motif of the RNA-dependent DNA polymerase.[49] The methionine (M) at codon 552 is either replaced by an isoleucine (M552I) or by a valine (M552V). The M552V mutation is frequently accompanied by another mutation, a leucine 528-to-methionine (L528M) substitution. YMDD variants do not replicate as effectively as wild-type HBV *in vitro* and this is most likely due to the lower affinity of the viral polymerase for its nucleotide substrates.[49, 50] *In vitro* studies have demonstrated that these mutations confer up to 10,000-fold resistance and hence increase in dose of lamivudine does not help.[49]

Prevalence of YMDD variants

The YMDD variants usually occur after the first six months of lamivudine therapy and their frequency increases with longer duration of treatment. In Asian studies, the frequency of YMDD variants at 1 year is 14–32%, at 2 year 38%, at 3 year 49% and 66% at 4 year of treatment.[15, 25, 49, 51]

Reappearance of wild-type virus after cessation of lamivudine therapy is common. After 3-4 months of discontinuation of lamivudine treatment, a reduction in the prevalence of YMDD variants occurs from 27–32% to 21–29%.[21, 48, 52] In one study, reemergence of wild-type HBV that appear as the dominant strain occurred by the end of 12–16 week of a lamivudine-free period.

Virological consequences of YMDD variants

The development of YMDD mutants is usually associated with breakthrough infection, but their long-term clinical significance is not known. Median pretreatment values of serum ALT and HBV-DNA were higher in patients who subsequently developed YMDD variants. However, lamivudine can suppress HBV-DNA, with most patients becoming HBV-DNA negative during treatment, suggesting that there may be a continued suppressive effect of lamivudine on the wild-type virus and replication deficient nature of mutant. With continued therapy, the median serum ALT and HBV-DNA levels remained below the pretreatment values and below the median values at the end of two years.

HBeAg sero-conversion occurred even after the development of YMDD mutant in 22% patients who continued lamivudine treatment.[51] Stopping therapy in patients with such variants results in a reversion to wild type HBV and is associated with an increase in levels of HBV-DNA and ALT.[49] It is currently recommended that patients who develop YMDD mutants may remain on lamivudine, if they are experiencing a clinical benefit.[24]

Biochemical consequence of YMDD variants

Lamivudine generally results in normalization of serum ALT levels, regardless of whether YMDD variants are detected during therapy. In Asian patients, marked transient ALT elevations usually occur during emergence of YMDD variants.[53] This flare of serum ALT elevation is suggested to be attributable to hepatic decompensation or significant liver damage caused by the mutant virus. Nevertheless, 62% of patients with hepatitis flares have been found to subsequently attain HBeAg sero-conversion,[53] similar to that of spontaneous HBeAg seroconversion in patients with wild-type HBV. Compared to those treated with placebo, patients who continue to receive lamivudine despite breakthrough infection have continued suppression of HBV-DNA, significant histologic improvement, and sustained normalization of serum ALT.[54,55]

Histologic findings of patients treated for 2 years with lamivudine show improvement despite the presence of YMDD variants.[56]

Duration of therapy

The exact duration of lamivudine therapy is an unresolved issue. Patients who do not lose HBeAg often relapse with increase in HBV-DNA and ALT to pretreatment value on stopping treatment with occasional flare of ALT above the base line values (17%) and rarely becoming severely symptomatic.[57]

In those who clear HBeAg and remain negative for next 3 months with or without anti-HBe, the loss is sustained in 86% and 25% of the patients also lose HBsAg.[57] The rate of sustained loss was lower in Asian patients (73%).[25]

Relapse rates as high as 50% after loss of HBeAg have been reported from Korea. The practice guideline of AASLD recommends lamivudine therapy for one year in HBeAg +ve patients or till the loss of HBeAg. The recommendation is primarily to prevent the development of YMDD mutants. If however, they have already emerged, lamivudine should be continued and if available, adefovir should be added wherever required as rescue therapy.

Combination Therapy

Combination therapy with lamivudine and IFN-α has not been consistently proven superior to monotherapy with either IFN or lamivudine. In one multicenter trial combined IFN and lamivudine therapy had higher HBeAg sero-conversion rate (29%) versus those receiving lamivudine (19%) or IFN (18%) monotherapy but it was not significant.[21]

TREATMENT OF HBeAg NEGATIVE CHRONIC HBV (e-CHB)

A fair proportion of patients with chronic HBV infection despite becoming HBeAg negative, continue to have replicative HBV and on-going hepatic inflammation. The HBeAg negativity is usually attributed to a mutation in the precore region (G1896A). Chronic hepatitis B due to the e negative variant (e-CHB) could have a more aggressive course with persistent or intermittent HBV replication and liver disease activity. Since such patients have a relatively high annual rate of development of cirrhosis and hepatocellular carcinoma, an effective antiviral regimen for them is needed.[58,59]

The aim of therapy in e-CHB is to achieve normalization of ALT, sustained loss of quantifiable HBV-DNA (<10^5 copies/ml) and histological improvement.

Interferon Therapy

Interferon alpha has been shown in e-CHB to be less effective. Despite 60–90% ETR, majority of the patients relapse.[60, 61] In a recent meta-analysis of 4 RCTs,[60, 61] with 86 IFN treated and 84 untreated patients, the SR was 10–47% after 12 months of cessation of treatment vs. 0% in the untreated controls.[60, 61] A 24-month course of IFN in dose of 6 MU thrice weekly was found to achieve a combined biochemical and virological response in 38% of 21 patients as compared to 10% of untreated controls (Table 3).[62] In a study of 216

Table 3. Comparison of the efficacy of interferon in e-CHB various trials

Author (year)	Type of study	IFN dose	Duration of Rx (months)	Follow-up duration (months)	No. of patients		End of treatment response (%)		Sustained response (%)	
					Rx	Ctr	Rx	Ctr	Rx	Ctr
Brunetto (1989)	RCT	9 mu 3x weekly	16–18 week	nr	12	12	66	0	25	0
Hadziyannis (1990)	RCT	3 mu 3x weekly	14–16	12	25	25	59	0	47	0
Fattovich (1992)	RCT	5 mu 3x weekly	6	12	30	30	57	10	40	0
Pastore (1992)	RCT	5 mu/m² 3x weekly	6	24	10	8	90	37	10	0
Brunetto (1995)	NRT	6–18 mu 3x weekly	4–6	2–7 years	53	–	60	–	9.4	–
Lampertico (1997)	RCT	6 mu 3x weekly	24	24	21	21	38	10	28	0
Kako (1998)	NRT	702 mu*	6	24	24	–	58	25	–	–
Guptan (1998)	NRT	3 mu 3x weekly	4	–	18	–	72	–	–	–
Alberti (1998)	RCT	5 mu 3x weekly	6	3–6 months	–	–	57	33	–	–
Lin[62] (2001)	NRT	6–10 mu 3x weekly	6–12	32 months	30	28	57	18	30	7
Brunetto (2002)	NRT	4–12 mu 3x weekly	9	21 months	103	195	68.5	–	21	–

RCT–Randomized controlled trial, NRT–non randomized trial, Ctr–control group, Rx–treatment group, *total dosage of interferon

patients from Greece, using 3 and 5 MU, the SR rate was 11.5% and 22% with a 6 or 12 month course respectively.[63] The duration of therapy was found by multivariate analysis, to be inversely related to the relapse rate. A proportion of the long-term responders also become HBsAg negative (range, 15–32%).[64] Recently, Brunetto et al,[65] reported a SR of 21% and two-thirds of the patients with SR lost HBsAg and half of them even developed anti-HBs. These workers also demonstrated that IFN-α treatment slowed down the disease progression by 2.5 fold in comparison to untreated patients. Liver disease improved in 16% of IFN treated vs. 1.6% of untreated controls.

From India, Guptan et al[66] showed that approximately 15% of Indian patients with hepatitis B virus related chronic liver disease have infection with precore mutant form. Interferon-alpha 2b was given at 3 MU on alternate days for 4 months. Thirteen of 18 (72.2%) patients responded to treatment (response was defined as loss of HBV-DNA by dot blot hybridization). However, 7 of 13 (54%) relapsed and became HBV-DNA positive during a mean follow-up period of 14±6 months. This study showed that interferon therapy is beneficial only to a limited extent in HBV precore mutant related chronic liver disease. It is ineffective in eliminating the mutant HBV infection, which explains the high relapse rate.[27,66] In Western trials also, despite 60–90% end-of-treatment response in e-CHB, majority of patients relapse. In a recent study of 103 patients treated with 4–12 MU IFN-α for 9 months, thrice weekly, the end-of-treatment response was 68.5%, but the sustained response was only in 21%.[67]

The end-point of therapy in patients of e-CHB is little unclear at present. Approximately 20–25% patients of e-CHB who are long-term responders will lose their HBsAg. However, this cannot be used as a therapeutic target, as HBsAg loss occurs rather late and infrequently. Since HBeAg is undetectable in e-CHB, the HBV-DNA levels should be the targets of therapeutic response. However, HBV-DNA assay by molecular hybridization may be negative in patients with biochemical remission,[64] but positive by PCR in both e-CHB and e+CHB, despite sustained biochemical response or HBeAg clearance.[63,68] Persistence of low level viremia in the face of sustained biochemical remission has little clinical significance.[69] In fact, therapy with IFN has been found to significantly reduce the development of liver decompensation and or HCC development, only in the subset of patients with sustained biochemical response.[68] Hence, besides HBV-DNA negativity or low level viremia, sustained biochemical response should be an end-point. Finally, it should be emphasized that e-CHB patients should be followed-up for at least 2 years following therapy, as only 2% patients relapse within six months and 25% between 6 to 12 months, and 20% between 12 to 24 months after discontinuation of interferon therapy.[70] Relapse may sometimes be associated with quite severe hepatitic flare with ALT values exceeding the levels seen in acute hepatitis and occasionally even with the development of liver decompensation.[69] Re-treatment with IFN-α may have the same or even better efficacy compared with that of IFN-α therapy in naïve patients.[70]

Recently, mutations in basal core promoter region (BCP) were demonstrated to influence IFN response. Yeun et al studied 96 IFN treated patients. Sum of mutations in the BCP correlated with response to IFN. Responder patients carried more mutations in BCP area than non-responders who otherwise had comparable histology and HBV-DNA levels. They had more nucleotide exchanges in the nucleotide region 1753 to 1766 compared to non-responders.[71]

Lamivudine Therapy

A randomized trial of lamivudine therapy for 52 weeks in e-CHB patients showed HBV-DNA loss in 63% patients at the end-of-treatment compared to 6% in the placebo group (Table 4).[72] However, the SR rate to lamivudine therapy is now known to be around 13–15%.[73, 74] It has been observed that continuing lamivudine treatment beyond one year is associated with progressively reduced virological and biochemical remission. Hadziyannis et al[74] have shown the response rate at 1, 2 and 3 year of 50%, 46%, 33% respectively. This progressive decrease in response rate with lamivudine treatment has been alleged to be due to the emergence of YMDD mutant stains.

Table 4. Efficacy of lamivudine in e-CHB compared in different studies

Author (year)	Type of study	Total patients	Duration of treatment	Dosage (mg)	ETR Lam	ETR Placebo	SVR Lam	SVR Placebo	YMDD, mutant (%)
Tassopoulis (1999)	RCT	60	52 weeks	100	63	6	nr	nr	27
Santantonio (2000)	NRT	15	52 weeks	100	74	–	13	–	13
Hadziyannis (2000)	NRT	25	26±7 months	150	41.6	–	nr	–	50
Lok (2000)	NRT	29	21±7 (months)	100/150	–	–	–	–	56
Kazim (1998)	NRT	22	36 (months)**	100	33	–	–	–	50

RCT–Randomized controlled trial, NRT–non randomized trial, Lam–Lamivudine, nr–not reported, *at 24 months of treatment, **at 36 months of treatment

In addition, it has been found that the core-promotor mutations are most likely to be associated with the selection of lamivudine resistance mutants.[75] The level of ALT flare during the viral breakthrough may reach that of acute hepatitis range. On stopping lamivudine, severe exacerbation of liver disease due to re-emergence of wild type strains has been reported.[76] It is therefore recommended that lamivudine therapy should be restricted to only 12 months to prevent development of drug resistant mutants.

Resistant mutants have been reported in patients treated for HBeAg-negative chronic hepatitis

B.[77] The cumulative rate of detection of lamivudine resistant mutations after 1 and 2 years were 10% and 56%, respectively.

Combination Therapy

Combination therapy of IFN with lamivudine, is being actively studied.[78] In a pilot study by Tatulli et al,[79] the ETR was as high as 93%, however, the SR remained at 14%. None of the patients developed viral breakthrough during treatment. A combined regimen with 3g gancyclovir with 4.5 mu IFN thrice weekly for 6 months was tried and compared with IFN alone. The SR was only 15%.[80] Similarly, combination with ribavarin in a pilot study showed response of 21% only.[81]

Treatment of Non-responders to Interferon

These patients constitute a difficult group to treat. There is limited information available on the management of these patients.

In one study, combination therapy was not found to be superior in patients who had failed IFN monotherapy.[48]

In a recent trial,[82] a combination of interferon and granulocyte macrophage colony stimulating factor was compared with a combination of interferon and lamivudine. Both the treatments were given for a period of 6 months. Forty percent and 28% of patients respectively responded to the combination therapy. There is need for larger clinical trials in these patients to develop proper therapeutic protocols.

Decompensated Cirrhosis

Interferon

Interferon therapy is not recommended in these patients as there is a significant risk of aggravating the hepatic decompensation. Even low dose IFN is associated with major complications such as bacterial infections and gastrointestinal bleeding.

Lamivudine

Lamivudine has been reported to increase albumin levels, decrease bilirubin levels, decrease Child-Pugh scores, prolong survival, and possibly delay the need for liver transplantation in these patients. In the Quebec study, up to 80% of 35 patients with decompensated HBV-related cirrhosis (10 Child-Pugh class B and 25 Child-Pugh class C) treated for 6 months or more with lamivudine improved biochemically and clinically with a reduction of Child-Pugh score of at least 2 points. Improvement was time-dependent and most obvious after 9±12 months of treatment. In this study, the majority of patients who died from complications of liver disease did so within the first 6 months of treatment, marking this period as a likely critical interval for determining the likelihood of long-term survival during lamivudine treatment.[83] Yao et al. studied 13 patients with HBV-related decompensated cirrhosis (9 HBeAg-positive and 4 HBeAg-negative) with detectable viremia, and showed that lamivudine was effective in improving severe hepatic decompensation with a mean follow-up of 17.5 months. Child-Pugh score improved in 69%. HBV-DNA became and remained negative in serum among most patients, and nearly half of HBeAg-positive patients lost HBeAg during follow-up although without sustained sero-conversion to anti-HBe.[84] A study conducted at our center by Kapoor et al included 18 patients with HBV-related decompensated cirrhosis (10 HBeAg positive and 8 HBeAg-negative) with detectable viremia (bDNA assay; sensitivity 2.5 pg/mL). Lamivudine was found effective in suppressing HBV-DNA (100% of patients by 8 weeks of therapy) and in inducing anti-HBe sero-conversion (30% of patients). Furthermore, lamivudine therapy improved biochemical and clinical outcome, characterized by reduction of ALT levels (from 111 to 58 IU/L, $P < 0.01$), improvement of Child-Pugh score, and significant reduction in liver-related morbidity and hospitalizations before and after lamivudine therapy.[85]

Lamivudine treatment is well tolerated in patients with decompensated cirrhosis, and effectively suppresses serum HBV-DNA.[83-85] In patients who were treated for at least 6 months with lamivudine, it was found that all of those with Child-Pugh class B status improved, and that 14 of the 15 with Child-Pugh class C status became class B or A.[83]

The three parameters which predict the likelihood of early death in patients receiving lamivudine for decompensated chronic hepatitis B include pretreatment elevated serum bilirubin, elevated creatinine levels and detectable hepatitis B virus DNA. These parameters help to identify patients requiring urgent liver transplantation despite antiviral therapy.[86]

Famciclovir

This drug also lowers significantly the HBV viral counts and ALT in patients previously not treated with it, in those who did not respond to interferon, and in patients who have received transplants; however, it is probably not as potent as lamivudine.[87, 88] Mutations can occur with famciclovir, especially in the DNA polymerase gene, which can limit the ability of famciclovir to suppress HBV. Some, but not all, of the mutations in HBV when exposed to famciclovir are the same as with lamivudine.[89] Sequential treatment with lamivudine after famciclovir appears to be efficacious until lamivudine-associated mutations form. Generally, famciclovir is well tolerated with only minimal clinically significant side effects. Overall, famciclovir appears to be less potent and has a more transient effect than lamivudine. It is currently less preferred compared to other antiviral agents.

Adefovir dipivoxil

Adefovir has just been approved by FDA for the treatment of wild-type and lamivudine-resistant chronic hepatitis B.

Adefovir dipivoxil is an orally bioavailable prodrug of adefovir, a phosphonate nucleotide analog of adenosine monophosphate which possesses potent *in vitro* activity against hepadnaviruses. The active intracellular moiety, adefovir diphosphate, acts as an inhibitor via chain-termination of HBV replication mediated by hepatitis B virus (HBV) DNA polymerases.

Adefovir dipivoxil 10 mg has been shown to have significant clinical and antiviral activity in a broad spectrum of patients with chronic hepatitis B. This includes both HBeAg positive and anti-HBe positive, DNA positive (presumed precore mutant) patients with compensated liver disease, patients with lamivudine-resistant HBV, patients in post-OLT period with compensated and decompensated liver disease, and patients co-infected with HIV. In studies 437 and 438, the effects of adefovir dipivoxil 10 mg on other markers of chronic hepatitis B, including virologic, biochemical and serologic markers confirmed its efficacy.[90, 91] Statistically significant reductions in serum HBV-DNA and ALT levels were seen compared to placebo after 48 weeks of treatment. Adefovir dipivoxil 10 mg enhances HBeAg sero-conversion and HBeAg loss compared to placebo.

In both the placebo-controlled studies, histological benefit was also observed. In patients with HBeAg positive chronic hepatitis B, 53% of patients receiving adefovir dipivoxil 10 mg showed histological improvement compared with 25% of patients who received placebo.[90] A similar treatment difference was seen in study 438 in patients with anti-HBe positive chronic hepatitis B. Sixty-four percent of patients in the adefovir dipivoxil 10 mg group showed histological improvement compared with 33% in the placebo group.

Adefovir has *in vitro* and *in vivo* activity against lamivudine resistant YMDD variants. In post-liver transplantation patients, treatment with adefovir dipivoxil 10 mg rapidly and significantly reduced serum HBV-DNA levels in patients with lamivudine-resistant HBV. The response was consistent regardless of the pattern of lamivudine-resistant HBV mutations present at baseline.[92] In patients with advanced liver disease, the clinical benefits of adefovir dipivoxil therapy were also manifested as improvements in Child-Pugh-Turcotte score. An overall survival benefit was also seen.

Another benefit of adefovir is in patients co-infected with HIV. Significant reductions in serum HBV-DNA levels were accompanied by reductions in ALT levels. In this study, biopsies were performed and histological improvements were again demonstrated.[93]

Adefovir appears to be effective and no resistance has been reported up to 136 weeks of treatment.[91] Adefovir can cause renal insufficiency and is contraindicated in patients with chronic renal failure.

Entecavir

This is another nucleoside analog under study for the treatment of chronic hepatitis B.[94, 95] It is a potent inhibitor of HBV-DNA polymerase and is also active against wild-type virus and lamivudine-resistant YMDD mutations.

Other treatments

Future strategies may use adefovir and lamivudine in combination to treat patients in this setting. Trials are currently in progress using pegylated interferon in combination with lamivudine. The preliminary results of these studies appear promising. Other nucleoside analogues under study for the treatment of chronic hepatitis B include emtricitabine and tenofovir. A phase 2 dose-ranging study of Val-LdC, an L-nucleoside agent with activity against hepatitis B, showed patients treated for 28 days achieved a 3.6-$\log_{10}$ drop in HBV viral loads. Information on other potentially useful agents such as IL-12, ganciclovir, and thymosin is limited.

Other potential therapies for chronic HBV infection

Several other lines of investigation are being taken in the approach to treatment of chronic HBV infection. As with other viral agents, vaccination with antigenic epitopes are being investigated. Antisense oligonucleotides and ribozymes have some theoretical potential and are being studied. Recently, an inhibitor of the endoplasmic reticulum, a-glucosidase, which prevents proper folding and transport of the hepadnavirus glycoproteins, has been reported to be successful in the woodchuck hepatitis model. Human studies are planned.

CONCLUSIONS

More effective therapy is needed for the treatment of patients with chronic hepatitis B. Current therapies produce a complete cure (loss of HBsAg) in only 8–10% of patients. The goals of treatment at present are therefore restricted only to produce HBeAg sero-conversion. This usually results in a significant improvement in liver histology and may slow or prevent the development of cirrhosis. Currently, candidates for treatment include patients with aminotransferases >2 × normal, chronic hepatitis on liver biopsy, HBV-DNA levels >100,000 by hybridization assay, and HBeAg positivity. Like for HIV, we probably need to use a cocktail of antiviral drugs with the hope of reducing resistance and improving response rates. The consideration of cost, development of mutations and possible discovery of better antiviral therapy such as second generation nucleoside analogs in future would modify the treatment regimens in different parts of the world.

REFERENCES

1. Margolis HS, Alter MJ, Hadler SC. Hepatitis B: evolving epidemiology and implications for control. *Semin Liver Dis* 1991;11:84-92.
2. Koff RS. Management of the hepatitis B surface antigen (HBsAg) carrier. *Semin Liver Dis* 1981;1(1): 33-43.
3. Weissberg JI, Andres LL, Smith CI, et al. Survival in chronic hepatitis B. An analysis of 379 patients. *Ann Intern Med* 1984;101:613.
4. Liaw YF, Lin DY, Chen TJ, Chu CM. Natural course after the development of cirrhosis in patients with chronic type B hepatitis: A prospective study. *Liver* 1989;9:235.

5. Realdi G, Fattovich G, Hadziyannis S, et al. Survival and prognostic factors in 366 patients with compensated cirrhosis type B: A multicenter study. *J Hepatol* 1994; 21:656.
6. Colombo M, de Franchis R, Del Ninno E, Sangiovanni A, De Fazio C, Tommasini M, Donato MF, et al. Hepatocellular carcinoma in Italian patients with cirrhosis. *N Engl J Med* 1991;325:675-80.
7. Tsukuma H, Hiyama T, Tanaka S, Nakao M, Yabuuchi T, Kitamura T, Nakanishi K, et al. Risk factors for hepatocellular carcinoma among patients with chronic liver disease. *N Engl J Med* 1993;328: 1797-801.
8. Beasley RP. Hepatitis B virus. The major etiology of hepatocellular carcinoma. *Cancer* 1988;61: 1942-56.
9. Fattovich G, Giustina G, Schalm SW, Hadziyannis S, Sanchez-Tapias J, Almasio P, Christensen E, et al. Occurrence of hepatocellular carcinoma and decompensation in western European patients with cirrhosis type B. *Hepatology* 1995;21:77-82.
10. Lok AS, Heathcote EJ, Hoofnagle JH. Management of Hepatitis B 2000, Summary of a Workshop. *Gastroenterology* 2001;120:1828.
11. Desmet VJ, Gerber M, Hoofnagle JH, Manns M, Scheuer PJ. Classification of chronic hepatitis: diagnosis, grading and staging. *Hepatology* 1994;19:1513-20.
12. Brook MG, Karayiannis P, Thomas HC. Which patients with chronic hepatitis B virus infection will respond to a-interferon therapy? A statistical analysis of predictive factors. *Hepatology* 1989;10:761-3.
13. Indian Association For Study of the Liver (INASL). Changing terminology of hepatitis B and C carriers: Consensus statement. *Indian J Gastroenterol* 1999;28(suppl 1):515-20.
14. Lau DT, Everhart J, Kleiner DE, Park Y, Vergalla J, Schmid P, Hoofnagle JH. Long-term follow-up of patients with chronic hepatitis B treated with interferon-alfa. *Gastroenterology* 1997;113:1660-67.
15. Lai CL, Chien RN, Leung NW, Chang TT, Guan R, Tai DI, Ng KY, et al. A one-year trial of lamivudine for chronic hepatitis B. Asia Hepatitis Lamivudine Study Group. *N Engl J Med* 1998; 339:61-8.
16. Perrillo R, Rakela J, Dienstag J, Levy G, Martin P, Wright T, Caldwell S, et al. Multicenter study of lamivudine therapy for hepatitis B after liver transplantation. *Hepatology* 1999;29:1581-6.
17. Nery JR, Weppler D, Rodriguez M, Ruiz P, Schiff ER, Tzakis AG. Efficacy of lamivudine in controlling hepatitis B virus recurrence after liver transplantation. *Transplantation* 1998;65:1615-21.
18. Al-Taie OH, Mork H, Gassel AM, Wilhelm M, Weissbrich B, Scheurlen M. Prevention of hepatitis B flare-up during chemotherapy using lamivudine: case report and review of the literature. *Ann Hematol* 1999;78:247-9.
19. Ahmed A, Keeffe EB. Lamivudine therapy for chemotherapy-induced reactivation of hepatitis B virus infection. *Am J Gastroenterol* 1999;94:249-51.
20. Schiff E, Cianciara J, Kowdley K, et al. Durability of HBeAg sero-conversion after lamivudine monotherapy in controlled phase II and III trials. *Hepatology* 1998;28:163A.
21. Schalm S, Heathcote J, Cianciare J. Lamivudine and alpha-interferon combination treatment of patients with chronic hepatitis B infection: a randomized trial. *Gut* 2000;46:562-8.
22. Lai CL, Yuen MF, Cheng CC, et al. An open comparative study of lamivudine and famciclovir in the treatment of chronic hepatitis B infection. *Hepatology* 1998;28:318A.
23. Dienstag JL, Schiff ER, Wright TL, et al. Lamivudine as initial treatment for chronic hepatitis B in the United States. *N Engl J Med* 1999;341:1256-63.
24. Chien RN, Liaw YF, Atkins M, Asian Hepatitis Lamivudine Trial Group. Pretherapy alanine aminotransferase level as a determinant for hepatitis B e antigen sero-conversion during lamivudine therapy in patients with chronic hepatitis B. *Hepatology* 1999;30:770-4.
25. Liaw YF, Leung NW, Chang TT, Guan R, Tai DI, Ng KY, Chien RN, et al. Effects of extended lamivudine therapy in Asian patients with chronic hepatitis B. Asia Hepatitis Lamivudine Study Group. *Gastroenterology* 2000;119:172-80.

26. Ben-Ari Z, Shmueli D, Mor E, Shapira Z, Tur-Kaspa R. Beneficial effect of lamivudine in recurrent hepatitis B after liver transplantation. *Transplantation* 1997;63:393-6.
27. Lok AS, Heathcote EJ, Hoofnagle JH. Management of hepatitis B 2000, summary of a workshop. *Gastroenterology* 2001;120:1828-53.
28. Pramoolsinsup C. Management of viral Hepatitis B. *J Gastroentrol Hepatology* 2002;17(suppl)S125-45.
29. Core Working Party for Asia Pacific Consensus on Hepatitis B and C. Consensus Statements on the prevention and management of hepatitis B and C in the Asia Pacific region. *J Gastroenterol Hepatol* 2000;15:825-41.
30. Perrillo R. Hepatitis B: Treatment, AASLD State-of-the-Art Lecture. *Digestive Disease Week* 2002; May 19-22.
31. Wong DKH, Cheung AM, O'Rourke K, Naylor CD, Detsky AS, Heathcote J. Effect of alpha interferon treatment in patients with hepatitis B e antigen-positive chronic hepatitis B *Ann Intern Med* 1993;119:312-23.
32. Sarin SK, Guptan RC, Thakur V, Malhotra V, Banerjee K, Khandekar P. Efficacy of low-dose alpha-interferon therapy in HBV-related chronic liver disease in Asian Indians: a randomized controlled trial. *J Hepatol* 1996;24:391-6.
33. Mazumder DG, Chaudhuri S, Konar A, Santra A, Pal B, Sarkar S. Response to low-dose interferon in chronic liver disease due to hepatitis B virus infection. *Ind. J Gastroenterol* 1998;17:97-9.
34. Carreno V, Marcellin P, Hadziyannis S, Salmeron J, Diago M, Kitis GE, Vafiadis I, et al. Retreatment of chronic hepatitis B e antigen-positive patients with recombinant interferon-alpha-2a. The European Concerted Action on Viral Hepatitis (EUROHEP). *Hepatology* 1999;30:277-82.
35. Lau DT, Everhart J, Kleiner DE, Park Y, Vergalla J, Schmid P, Hoofnagle JH. Long-term follow-up of patients with chronic hepatitis B treated with interferon alfa. *Gastroenterology* 1997;113:1660-67.
36. Fattovich G, Giustina G, Sanchez-Tapias J, Quero C, Mas A, Olivotto PG, Solinas A, et al. Delayed clearance of serum HBsAg in compensated cirrhosis B: Relation to interferon-alpha therapy and disease prognosis. European Concerted Action on Viral Hepatitis (EUROHEP). *Am J Gastroenterol* 1998;93:896-900.
37. Niederau C, Heintges T, Lange S, Goldmann G, Niederau CM, Mohr L, Haussinger D. Long-term follow-up of HBeAg-positive patients treated with interferon alfa for chronic hepatitis B. *N Engl J Med* 1996;334:1422-7.
38. Cooksley GE, et al. 40 KDA Peginterferon alpha 2a (Pegasys): Efficacy and safety results from a phase II, randomized, actively controlled, multicenter trial in the treatment of HBeAg positive chronic hepatitis B. *Hepatology.* 2001;34:349:710A.
39. Janssen HL, Gerken G, Carreno V, Marcellin P, Naumov NV, Craxi A, Ring-Larsen H, et al. Interferon alfa for chronic hepatitis B infection : increased efficacy of prolonged treatment. The European Concerted Action on Viral Hepatitis (EUROHEP). *Hepatology* 1999;30:238-43.
40. Scully LJ, Shein R, Karayiannis P, McDonald JA, Thomas HC. Lymphoblastoid interferon therapy of chronic HBV infection. A comparison of 12 vs. 24 weeks of thrice weekly treatment. *J Hepatol* 1987;5:51-8.
41. Lok ASF, Chung H-T, Liu VWS, Ma OCK. Long-term follow-up of chronic hepatitis B patients treated with interferon alfa. *Gastroenterology* 1993;105:1833-8.
42. Lin SM, Sheen IS, Chien RN, Chu CM, Liaw YF. Long-term beneficial effect of interferon therapy in patients with chronic hepatitis B virus infection. *Hepatology* 1999;29:971-5.
43. Sokal EM, Conjeevaram HS, Roberts EA, Alvarez F, Bern EM, Goyens P, Rosenthal P, et al. Interferon alfa therapy for chronic hepatitis B in children: a multinational randomized controlled trial. *Gastroenterology* 1998;114:988-95.
44. Lebensztejn DM, Kaczmarski M, Sinkiewicz J, et al. Long-term evaluation of children with chronic

hepatitis B after HBeAg/Anti-HBe sero-conversion caused by interferon-alpha treatment. *Gastroenterology* 2002;122:A-303.
45. Torre D, Tambini R. Interferon-alpha therapy for chronic hepatitis B in children: a meta-analysis. *Clin Infect Dis* 1996:23:131-7.
46. Guptan RC, Thakur V, Malhotra V, Sarin SK. Recombinant Interferon Therapy In Indian Children with HBV-related Chronic Liver Disease. *Indian Pediatrics* 2002;39:462-7.
47. Lai C-L, Chien R-N, Leung NWY, Chang T-T, Guan R, Tai D-I, Ng K-Y, et al. Asia Hepatitis lamivudine Group. A one year trial of lamivudine for chronic hepatitis B. *N Engl J Med* 1998;339: 61-8.
48. Schiff ER, Karaylcin S, Grimm I, Perillo R, Dienstag J, Husa P, Schalm, et al. A placebo controlled study of lamivudine and interferon-alpha-2b in previously failed interferon therapy. *Hepatology* 1998;28:388A.
49. Allen MI, Deslauriers M, Andrews CW, Tipples GA, Walters KA, Tyrrell DL, Brown N, et al. Identification and characterization of mutations in hepatitis B virus resistant to lamivudine. *Hepatology* 1998;27:1670-7.
50. Ono SK, Kato N, Shiratori Y, Kato J, Goto T, Schinazi RF, Carrilho FJ, et al. The polymerase L528M mutation cooperates with nucleotide binding site mutations increasing, hepatitis B virus replication and drug resistance. *J Clin Invest* 2001;107:449-55.
51. Leung NWY, Lai CL, Chang TT, Guan R, Lee CM, Ng KY, Lim SG, et al. Extended lamivudine treatment in patients with chronic hepatitis B enhances hepatitis B e antigen sero-conversion rates: results after 3 years of therapy. *Hepatology* 2001;33:1527-32.
52. Dienstag JL, Schiff ER, Mitchell M, Casey DE Jr, Gitlin N, Lissoos T, Gelb LD, et al. Extended lamivudine retreatment for chronic hepatitis B. Maintenance of viral suppression after discontinuation of therapy. *Hepatology* 1999;30:1082-7.
53. Liaw YF, Chien RN, Yeh CT, Tsai SL, Chu CM. Acute exacerbation and hepatitis B virus clearance after emergence of YMDD motif mutation during lamivudine therapy. *Hepatology* 1999;30:567-72.
54. Schiff ER, Heathcote J, Dienstag JL, et al. Improvements in liver histology and cirrhosis with extended lamivudine therapy. *Hepatology* 2000;32:296A.
55. Atkins M, Hunt CM, Brown N, et al. Clinical significance of YMDD mutant hepatitis B virus (HBV) in a large cohort of lamivudine-treated hepatitis B patients. *Hepatology* 1998;28:319A.
56. Leung N, Wu PC, Tsang S, et al. Continued histological improvement in Chinese patients with chronic hepatitis B with 2 years lamivudine. *Hepatology* 1998;28:489A.
57. Schiff E, Cianciara J, Karayalacin S, et al., The international lamivudine investigator group. Durable HBeAg and HBsAg sero-conversion after lamivudine for chronic hepatitis B. *J Hepatol* 2000;32(suppl):99.
58. Hadziyannis SJ. Hepatitis HBeAg negative chronic hepatitis B from clinical recognition to pathogenesis and treatment. *Viral Hepat Rev* 1995;1:7-36.
59. Sarin SK, Satapathy SK, Chauhan R. Hepatitis B e-antigen negative chronic hepatitis B. *J Gastroenterol Hepatol* 2002;17:S311-21.
60. Brunetto MR, Oliveri F, Rocca G, Criscuolo D, Chiaberge E, Capalbo M, David E, et al. Natural course and response to interferon of chronic hepatitis B accompanied by antibody to hepatitis B e antigen. *Hepatology* 1989;10:198-202.
61. Pastore G, Santantonio T, Millela M, et al. Anti HBeAg positive chronic hepatitis B with HBV-DNA in the serum: response to a 6 month course of lymphoblastoid interferon. *J Hepatol* 1992;14:2215.
62. Lampertico P, Del Ninno E, Manzin A, Donato MF, Rumi MG, Lunghi G, Morabito A, et al. A randomized, controlled trial of a 24-month course of interferon-alpha-2b in patients with chronic hepatitis B who had hepatitis B virus DNA without hepatitis B e antigen in serum. *Hepatology* 1997;26:1621-5.
63. Manesis EK, Hadziyannis SJ. Interferon alpha treatment and retreatment of hepatitis B e antigen – negative chronic hepatitis B. *Gastroenterology* 2001;121:101-9.

64. Lin CC, Wu JC, Chang TT, Huang YH, Wang YJ, Tsay SH, Chow NH, et al. Long-term evaluation of recombinant interferon alpha 2b in the treatment of patients with hepatitis B e antigen –negative chronic hepatitis B in Taiwan. *J Viral Hepat* 2001;8:438-46.
65. Brunetto MR, Oliveri F, Coco B, Leandro G, Colombatto P, Gorin JM, Bonino F. Outcome of anti-HBe positive chronic hepatitis B in alpha-interferon treated and untreated patients: a long-term cohort study. *J Hepatol* 2002;36:263-70.
66. Guptan RC, Thakur V, Malhotra V, Sarin SK. Low dose recombinant interferon therapy in anti-HBe positive chronic hepatitis B in Asian Indians. *J Gastroenterol Hepatol* 1998;13:675-9.
67. Alberti A, Fattovich G, Pontisso P, Brollo L, Belussi F, Ruol A. Interferon treatment of anti-HBe positive and HBV-DNA positive chronic hepatitis B. *Chemioterapia* 1998;(suppl):15-19.
68. Papatheodoridis GV, Hadziyannis SJ. Diagnosis and management of precore mutant chronic hepatitis B. *J Viral Hepat* 2001;8:311-21.
69. Papatheodoridis GV, Manesis EK, Hadziyannis SJ. Long-term outcome of interferon a in treated and untreated patients with HBeAg negative chronic hepatitis B. ?? 2001;39:306-13.
70. Papatheodoridis GV, Manesis EK, Hadziyannis SJ. Long-term follow-up after initial response to interferon therapy in patients with HBeAg negative chronic hepatitis B. *Hepatology* 2000;32(suppl):378A.
71. Yeun MF, Hui CK, et al. Long-term follow-up of interferon-alpha treatment in Chinese patients with chronic hepatitis B infection: The effect on hepatitis B antigen sero-conversion and development of cirrhosis related complications. *Hepatology* 2002;34:139-45.
72. Tassopoulos NC, Volpes R, Pastore G, Heathcote J, Buti M, Goldin RD, Hawley S, et al. Efficacy of lamivudine in patients with hepatitis B e antigen-negative/hepatitis B virus DNA-positive (precore mutant) chronic hepatitis B. Lamivudine Precore Mutant Study Group. *Hepatology* 1999;29:889-96.
73. Santantonio T, Mazzola M, Iacovazzi T, Miglietta A, Guastadisegni A, Pastore G. Long-term follow-up of patients with anti-HBe/HBV-DNA–positive chronic hepatitis B treated for 12 months with lamivudine. *J Hepatol* 2000;32:300-6.
74. Hadziyannis SJ, Papatheodoridis GV, Dimou E, Laras A, Papaioannou C. Efficacy of long-term lamivudine monotherapy in patients with hepatitis B e antigen-negative chronic hepatitis B. *Hepatology* 2000;32:847-51.
75. Lok AS, Hussain H, Carsano, et al. Evolution of hepatitis B virus polymerase gene mutation in hepatitis B e antigen negative patients receiving lamivudine therapy. *Hepatology* 2000;32:1145-53.
76. Honkoop P, de Man RA, Niesters HGM, Zondervan PE, Schalm SW. Acute exacerbation of chronic hepatitis virus infection after withdrawal of lamivudine therapy. *Hepatology* 2000;32:635-9.
77. Wakil SM, Kazim SN. Khan LA, Raisuddin S, Parvez MK, Guptan RC, Thakur V, Hasnain SE, Sarin SK. Prevalence and profile of lamivudine induced mutation in the polymerase and surface genes of hepatitis B virus among Indian population. *J Med Virol* 2002;68:311-8.
78. Schalm SW, De Man RA, Janssen HLA. Combination and newer therapies for chronic hepatitis B. *J Gastroenterol Hepatol* 2002;17:S338-41.
79. Tatulli I, Francavilla R, Rizzo GL, Vinciguerra V, Ierardi E, Amoruso A, Panella C, Francavilla A. Lamivudine and alpha-interferon in combination long-term for precore mutant chronic hepatitis B. *J Hepatol* 2001;35:805-10.
80. Hadziyannis S, Alexopoulou A, Papakonstantinou A, Petraki K, Manesis E. Interferon treatment with or without oral ganciclovir in HBeAg–negative chronic hepatitis B: a randomized study. *J Viral Hepat* 2000;7:235-40.
81. Cotonat T, Quiroga JA, Lopez-Alcorocho JM, Clouet R, Pardo M, Manzarbeitia F, Carreno V. Pilot study of combination therapy with ribavirin and interferon-alfa for the retreatment of chronic hepatitis B e antibody–positive patients. *Hepatology* 2000;31:502-6.
82. Guptan RC, Thakur V, Kazim SN, Sarin SK. Efficacy of granulocyte-merophage colony-stimulating

factor or lamivudine combination with recombinant interferon in non-responders to interferon in hepatitis B virus-related chronice liver disease patients. *J Gastroenterol Hepatol* 2002;17:765-71.

83. Villeneuve JP, Condreay LD, Willems B, Pomier-Layrargues G, Fenyves D, Bilodeau M, Leduc R, et al. Lamivudine treatment for decompensated cirrhosis resulting from chronic hepatitis B. *Hepatology* 2000;31:207-10.

84. Yao FY, Bass NM. Lamivudine treatment in patients with severely decompensated cirrhosis due to replicating hepatitis B infection. *J Hepatol* 2000;33:301-7.

85. Kapoor D, Guptan RC, Wakil SM, Kazim SN, Kaul R, Agarwal SR, Raisuddin S, Hasnain SE, Sarin SK. Beneficial effects of lamivudine in hepatitis B virus-related decompensated cirrhosis. *J Hepatol* 2000;33:308-12.

86. Fontana RJ, Hann HW, Perrillo RP, Vierling JM, Wright T, Rakela J, Anschuetz G, et al. Determinants of early mortality in patients with decompensated chronic hepatitis B treated with antiviral therapy. *Gastroenterology* 2002;123:719-27.

87. Han SH, Kinkhabwala M, Martin P, Holt C, Murray N, Seu P, Rudich S, et al. Resolution of recurrent hepatitis B in two liver transplant recipients treated with famciclovir. *Am J Gastroenterol* 1998;93:2245-7.

88. Kruger M, Tillmann HL, Trautwein C, Bode U, Oldhafer K, Maschek H, Boker, et al. Famciclovir treatment of hepatitis B virus recurrence after liver transplantation: A pilot study. *Liver Transpl Surg* 1996;2:253-62.

89. Bartholomew MM, Jansen RW, Jeffers LJ, Reddy KR, Johnson LC, Bunzendahl H, Condreay LD, et al. Hepatitis B virus resistance to lamivudine given for recurrent infection after orthotopic liver transplantation. *Lancet* 1997;349:20-2.

90. Marcellin P, Gee Lim S, Tong MJ, Sievert W, Schiffmann M, Jeffers, et al. A double-blind, randomized, placebo-controlled study of adefovir dipivoxil for the treatment of patients with HBeAg + chronic hepatitis B infection : 48 week Results. *Hepatology* 2001;34:340A.

91. Yung H, Westland CE, Ho V, Miller M, et al. Resistance monitoring in chronic hepatitis B patients exposed to adefovir dipivoxil for 72 to 136 weeks. *Hepatology* 2001;34:316A.

92. Schiff E, Neuhaus P, Tillmann H, Samuel D, Terrault N, Marcellin P, et al. Safety and efficacy of adefovir dipivoxil for the treatment of lamivudine-resistant HBV in patients post-liver transplantation. *Hepatology* 2001;34:446A.

93. Benhamou Y, Bochet M, Thibault V, Vig P, Brosgart CL, Fry J, et al. Safety and efficacy of adefovir dipivoxil for lamivudine-resistant HBV in HIV-infected patients. *Hepatology* 2001;34:319A.

94. Hadziyannis S, et al. Entecavir in patients with chronic hepatitis B failing lamivudine. *Hepatology* 2001;34:340A.

95. Lai CL, Rosmawati M, Lao J, Vlierberghe HV, Anderson FH, Thomas N, Dehertogh D. Entecavir is superiod to lamivudine in reducing hepatitis virus DNA in patients with chronic hepatitis B infection. *Gastroenterology* 2002;123:1831-38.

45

Mechanisms of non-response to interferon in chronic hepatitis B

Sita Naik

The immune response to hepatitis B virus (HBV) encoded antigens is responsible for the clearance of virus as well as for the pathogenesis of the disease. While the humoral antibody response to viral envelope antigens contributes to the clearance of circulating viral particles, the cellular immune responses to the envelope (HBsAg), nucleocapsid (HBcAg, HBeAg) and polymerase antigens eliminate infected cells. The first line of defense against the virus appears to be the production of interferon (IFN) followed by an increased expression of human leukocyte antigen (HLA) class I antigens on the hepatocytes and an elevation in transaminases.[1,2] The viral clearance and liver cell injury during acute disease is mediated by a vigorous, polyclonal HLA class I restricted cytotoxic T-lymphocytes (CTL) response directed against HBcAg and HBeAg displayed on the hepatocyte membranes in association with HLA class I molecules.[3] The HBV-specific cytolytic activity is relatively weak and narrowly focused in patients who fail to clear the virus.[4,5] This is the most widely implicated mechanism for persistence of the virus and is supported by studies which have shown decreased HLA class I expression on the cell membrane of hepatocytes infected by HBV.[6] More recently, the role of non-CTL mediated cytotoxicity and of non-cytolytic mechanisms have gained importance.[7] The principal non-CTL mechanism is hepatocyte apoptosis mediated by TNF-α secreted by the liver infiltrating lymphocytes that form part of the necroinflammatory process.

Interferon-alpha therapy has become the mainstay of treatment in chronic hepatitis B infection. The response rate, however, is less than 50% in most of the studies. The exact mechanism by which IFN mediates its action is not fully understood. The class I IFNs (α and β) exert their direct antiviral effect through the IFN inducible genes, a protein kinase (PKR) and a 2', 5'–oligoadenylate synthetase (2, 5 OAS) as shown in Fig. 1. However, it is clear that this alone cannot explain the efficacy of IFN and part of its action is mediated through immunological mechanisms. This is supported by the results of a large meta-analysis of 40 interferon trials, 13 of which included HIV patients. The IFN response among patients with HBV and HIV coinfection was significantly lower than among those without HIV coinfection.[8] Besides,

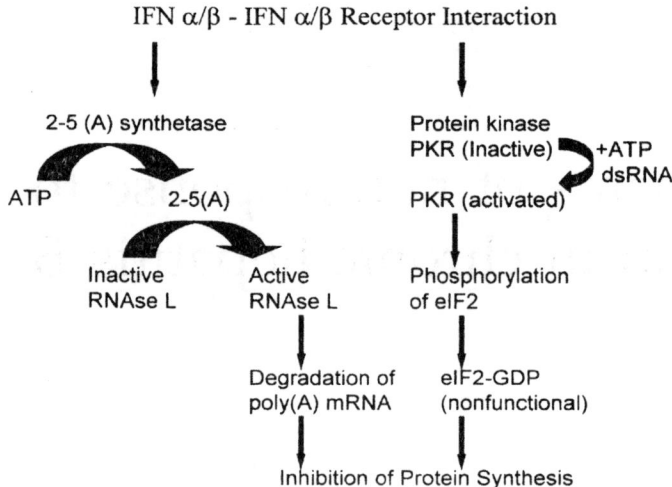

CTL-cytotoxic T-cell, HBV-hepatitis B virus, HLA-human leucocyte antigen, Mo-monocyte, Th-1-T helper 1

Fig. 1. The mechanisms of antiviral action of Interferon (IFN). By interfering with the protein synthesis machinery, IFN prevents viral replication

the direct antiviral proteins, type I IFNs are also potent inducers of HLA class I antigens and interferons in general but more particularly IFNγ augment a wide range of immune functions. It is postulated that the upregulation of class I antigen expression would increase the efficiency of the cytotoxic T-cell response (Fig. 2).

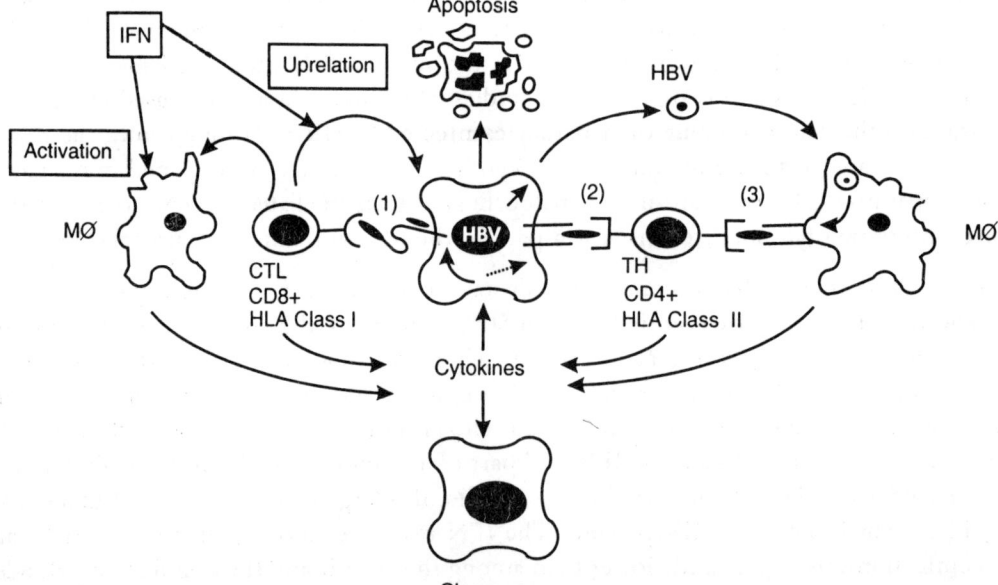

Fig. 2. The immune mechanisms involved in hepatocyte lysis and the level at which Interferon (IFN) may act

Host factors that influence response

Due to its known immunomodulatory functions, Scully et al[9] investigated several components of the immune response prior to and during IFN therapy. Pre-treatment elevated IgM anti-HBe levels were associated with a beneficial response to therapy but there was no correlation between response and pre-treatment CD4/CD8 ratio, natural killer (NK) activity, or lymphocyte proliferation responses. No measurable changes in the immunological parameters were observed in the non-responders to IFN. Significant rise in CD4/CD8 ratio along with fall in CD8 numbers and NK cell activity was observed in responders. The latter changes were most evident at the time of HBV-DNA clearance and could be due to the increased hepatic inflammation during sero-conversion or were induced by IFN itself. An interesting observation was that 6 of the 7 patients who responded to treatment had HLA-DR3. However, response was not clearly related to HLA haplotypes. Other HLA studies also did not find any genetic basis for IFN response.[10]

The most significant immunological function of IFN is induction of HLA class I and II genes and HLA class I expression has been shown to be increased in primary liver cultures treated with IFN.[6] In this study, Lau et al found no correlation between HBV replication rate and HLA class I expression and upregulation of class I was seen around areas of hepatic inflammation, probably as a consequence of IFNγ secreted by activated T-cells. However, the situation is complex since chronic hepatitis B patients have been found to have a hyporeactive state with low endogenous production of IFNα.[11-13] Transfection of HBV genes into cell lines reduces the cellular response to IFN as measured by the development of antiviral state and β_2m production.[14] The virus also has trans-acting function that inhibits interferon transcription.[15, 16] This in turn may be related to the nucleotide level homology between HBV and gene sequences regulating the IFN-induced antiviral system.[17] The opposing action has also been demonstrated – IFNγ and TNFα negatively down regulate hepatitis B gene expression which might favour persistence of the virus by helping in the escape from CTL-mediated viral clearance.[18,19]

In patients with chronic hepatitis B, quantitation of the level of inducible HLA antigens on the peripheral blood mononuclear cells measured by flow cytometry during IFN therapy did not predict treatment response.[20] However, β_2m is an integral part of the HLA class I molecule and a significantly lower rise in circulating β_2m was found in IFN non-responders.[21] Due to the overall futility of these studies, the enthusiasm for identifying an immune marker of non-response to the treatment declined.

Viral factors that influence response

In recent years, the search for predictive markers has shifted to the virus itself. Variations in the Pre-S1 region of the virus genome has not been found to have any influence on the response to IFN therapy although T and B-cell epitopes have been described in this area.[22] An early report on the high frequency of precore mutants in chronic patients with sustained sero-conversion from HBeAg to anti-HBe following IFN therapy suggested that the presence of these mutants prior to therapy might be a predictor of response.[23] The rationale for implicating this region of HBV is sound since the major T-cell epitopes for CTL are located here and any mutations would help the virus in evading the CTL response and support persistence of the virus. However, many reports have not found any correlation between the number of core gene mutations and response to IFN in adults and children with chronic hepatitis B.[24-27] Naoumov et al[28] found substitutions in amino acids 21-27 of the core protein, an HLA-A2 restricted T-cell epitope, in all five of the IFN non-responders that they tested and in none of the responders. However, HLA phenotyping was available only for one patient who had HLA-A2. Other reports of mutations in the core B and T-cell epitopes did not find any correlation with the treatment response.[28,29] Recently Erhardt et al have sequenced the regions of basic core promoter (BCP), core upstream regulatory sequence (CURS) and negative regulatory elements (NRE) of 96 patients with chronic replicative hepatitis B treated with IFNα. Prediction of response was possible on the basis of nt1764 of BCP in 77% of HBeAg+ve and 78% of HBeAg−ve patients.[30] The recent report that HBV genotype C, compared to genotype B, is associated with a higher frequency of core promoter mutation and a lower response to IFN therapy, holds some promise.[31]

Simon et al[32] have shown a significant correlation between the pre-treatment viral load and response to therapy, with response being best in those with low viral load. It has also been suggested that response is best if IFN is given just after a spontaneous decrease in HBV replication as assessed by change in the HBe antigen status.[33] This offers the possibility that therapy can be timed to give the best benefit to the patient.

There is an urgent need to identify reliable predictors of treatment response to interferon, especially in view of the cost of therapy and the unavoidable side-effects. Factors that favor response include active hepatitis, raised serum aminotransferase levels, low serum HBV-DNA, and absence of immunosuppression. Much needs to be done before we have more reliable predictors of response.[34,35] In view of the development of better anti-nucleoside drugs for HBV, interferon in future is likely to have a limited role in the treatment of chronic hepatitis B. The availability of better formulations, like the Pegylated IFN, may decrease the side-effects. *In vitro* predictors for IFN response would then allow rational use of this powerful agent. Of all the markers available to date, viral load and genotyping hold promise. However, excellent kits are available for viral quantitation while genotyping is more complex and difficult to set up. Hence, viral load seems to be the most feasible option and more studies are needed to establish the validity of this parameter.

REFERENCES

1. Heron I, Hokland M, Berg K. Enhanced expression of B_2 microglobulin and HLA antigens on human lymphoid cells by interferon. *Proc Natl Acad Sci USA* 1978;75:6215-9.
2. Nagafuchi Y, Scheuer PJ. Expression of B_2–microglobulin on hepatocytes in acute and chronic type B hepatitis. *Hepatology* 1986;6:20-3.
3. Chisari FV, Ferrari C. Hepatitis B virus immunopathogenesis. *Ann Rev Immunol* 1995;13:29-60.
4. Nayersina R, Fowler P, Guilhot S, Missale G, Cerny A, Schlicht HJ, Vitiello A, et al. HLA-A2-restricted cytotoxic T-lymphocyte responses to multiple hepatitis B surface antigen epitopes during hepatitis B virus infection. *J Immunol* 1993;150:4659-71.
5. Penna A, Chisari FV, Bertoletti A, Missale G, Fowler P, Giuberti T, Fiaccadori F, et al. Cytotoxic T-lymphocytes recognize an HLA-A2-restricted epitope within the hepatitis B virus nucleocapsid antigen. *J Exp Med* 1991;174:1565-70.
6. Lau JYN, Bird GLA, Naoumov NV, Williams R. Hepatic HLA antigen display in chronic hepatitis B virus infection. *Dig Dis Sci* 1993;38:888-95.
7. Guidotti LG, Rochford R, Chung J, Shapiro M, Purcell R, Chisari FV. Viral clearance without destruction of infected cells during acute HBV infection. *Science* 1999;284:825-9.
8. Wong DKH, Cheung AM, O'Rourke K, Naylor CD, Detsky AS, Heathcote J. Effect of alpha-interferon treatment in patients with hepatitis B e antigen positive chronic hepatitis B. A meta-analysis. *Ann Intern Med* 1993;119:812-23.
9. Scully LJ, Brown D, Lloyd C, Shein R, Thomas HC. Immunological studies before and during interferon therapy in chronic HBV infection: Identification of factors predicting responses. *Hepatology* 1990;12:1111-7.
10. Van Huttum J, Schreuder GMT, Schalm SW. HLA antigens in patients with various courses after hepatitis B virus infection. *Hepatology* 1987;7:11-4.
11. Kato Y, Nakagawa H, Kobayashi K, Hattori N, Hatano K. Interferon production by peripheral lymphocytes in HBsAg positive liver disease. *Hepatology* 1982;2:789-90.
12. Ikeda T, Lever AML, Thomas HC. Evidence for a deficiency of interferon production in patients with chronic hepatitis B virus infection acquired in adult life. *Hepatology* 1986;6:962-6.
13. Nouri-Aria KT, Arnold JC, Davison F, Portmann BC, Meager A, Morris AG, Eddleston ALWF, et al. Regulation of interferon-alpha gene activation in acute and chronic HBV infection. *Hepatology* 1991;13:1029-34.
14. Onji M, Lever AML, Saito I, Thoams HC. Defective response to interferon in cells transfected with hepatitis B virus genome. *Hepatology* 1989;9:92-6.
15. Twu J, Schlomemer RH. Transcription of the human beta interferon gene is inhibited by hepatitis B virus. *J Virol* 1989;63:3065-71.
16. Whitten TM, Quets AT, Schloemer RH. Identification of the hepatitis B virus factor that inhibits expression of the beta interferon gene. *J Virol* 1991;65:4699-704.
17. Thomas HC, Pignatelli M, Lever AML. Homology between HBV-DNA and a sequence regulating the interferon–induced antiviral system: possible mechanism of persistent infection *J Med Virol* 1985;19:63-9
18. Romero R, Lavine JE. Cytokine inhibition of the hepatitis B virus core promoter. *Hepatology* 1996;23:17-23.
19. Gilles PN, Fey G, Chisari FV. Tumor necrosis factor alpha negatively regulates hepatitis B virus gene expression in transgenic mice. *J Virol* 1992;66:3955-60.
20. Paul RG, Roodman ST, Campbell CR, Bodicky CJ, Perrillo RP. HLA class I antigen as a measure of response to antiviral therapy of chronic hepatitis B. *Hepatology* 1991;13:820-5.

21. Pignatelli M, Waters J, Brown D, Lever A, Iwarson S, Schaff Z, et al. MHC class I antigens on the hepatocyte membrane during recovery from acute hepatitis B virus infection and during Interferon therapy in chronic hepatitis B virus infection. *Hepatology* 1986;6:349-53.
22. Nakajima E, Minami M, Ochiya T, Kagawa K, Okanoue T. Pre-S1 deleted variants of hepatitis B virus in patients with chronic hepatitis. *J Hepatol* 1994;20:329-35.
23. Takeda K, Akahane Y, Suzuki H, Okamoo H, Tsuda F, Miyakawa Y, Mayumi M. Defects in the precore region of the HBV genome in patients with chronic hepatitis B after sustained sero-conversion from HBeAg to anti-HBe induced spontaneously or with interferon therapy. *Hepatology* 1990;12: 1284-9.
24. Xu J, Brown D, Harrison T, Lin Y, Dusheiko G. Absence of hepatitis B virus precore mutants in patients with chronic hepatitis B responding to interferon-alpha. *J Hepatol* 1992;15:1002-6.
25. Bozkaya H, Ayola B, Lok ASF. High rate of mutations in the hepatitis B core gene during the immune clearance phase of chronic hepatitis B virus infection. *Hepatology* 1996;24:32-7.
26. Shindo M, Okuno T. Genomic variations in precore and cytotoxic T-lymphocyte regions in chronic hepatitis B in relationship to interferon responsiveness. *Liver* 2000;20:136-42.
27. Cabrerizo M, Bartolome J, Otero M, Ruiz-Moreno M, Carreno V. Sequence variation of hepatitis B virus precore open reading frame isolated from serum and liver of children with chronic hepatitis B before and after interferon treatment. *J Med Virol* 1999;58:208-14.
28. Naoumov NV, Thomas MG, Mason AL, Chokshi S, Bodicky CJ, Farzaneh F, Williams R, et al. Genomic variations in the hepatitis B core gene: A possible factor influencing responses to interferon-alpha treatment. *Gastroenterology* 1995;108:505-14.
29. Fattovich G, McIntyre G, Thursz M, Colman K, Giuliano G, Alberti A, Thomas HC, et al. Hepatitis B virus precore core variation and interferon therapy. *Hepatology* 1995;22:1355-62.
30. Erhardt A, Reineke U, Blondin D, Gerlich WH, Adams O, Heintges T, Niederau C, et al. Mutations of the core promoter and response to interferon treatment in chronic replicative hepatitis B. *Hepatology* 2000;31:716-25.
31. Kao JH, Wu NH, Chen PJ, Lai MY, Chen DS. Hepatitis B genotypes and the response to interferon therapy. *J Hepatol* 2000;33:998-1002.
32. Simon K, Rotter K, Zalewska M, Gladysz A. HBV-DNA level in blood serum as a predictor of good response to therapy with interferon-alpha-2b of patients with chronic hepatitis B. *Med Sci Monit* 2000;6:971-5.
33. Heijtink RA, Janssen HL, Hop WC, Osterhaus AD, Schalm SW. Interferon-alpha therapy for chronic hepatitis B: early response related to pre-treatment changes in viral replication. *J Med Virol* 2001;63: 217-9.
34. Cheng AS, Chan HL, Leung NW, Liew CT, To KF, Lai PB, Sung J Jr. et al. Expression of cycloxygenase-2 in chronic hepatitis B and the effects of antiviral therapy. *Aliment Pharmacol Ther* 2002;16:251-60.
35. Guidotti LG, Morris A, Mendez H, Koch R, Silverman RH, Williams BR, Chisari FV. Interferon-regulated pathways that control hepatitis B virus replication in transgenic mice. *J Virol* 2002;76: 2617-21.

46

Nucleoside analogues for the treatment of chronic hepatitis B

Julie C Dent, Mark Atkins

The introduction of vaccination programs against hepatitis B has led to significant reduction in the prevalence of hepatitis B virus (HBV) with subsequent reduction in the incidence of hepatocellular carcinoma in children.[1] Until recently, there remained a large need for an effective drug for patients with chronic hepatitis B (CHB). Interferon may induce HBeAg loss in approximately 33% of patients.[2] However, even to attain this level of efficacy it requires careful selection of patients. These include patients with HBV-DNA below 200 pg/ml and raised serum aminotransferases.[3]

The HBV polymerase provides an obvious target for selective antiviral compounds as it plays a key role in viral replication. It has multiple activities including DNA dependent-DNA synthesis, RNA dependent-DNA synthesis (reverse transcription), and RNase-H activity. A new class of antiviral agents, called nucleoside analogues, are being developed against this target and several are now in clinical development (Table 1).

LAMIVUDINE

Lamivudine is the first of this new class of antiviral agents available for the treatment of

Table 1. Nucleoside analogues for chronic HBV infection

Lamivudine (Heptodin™, Zeffix™, Epivir®-HBV™) – Discontinued
Famciclovir (Famvir®), lobucavir–In development
Adefovir dipivoxil, entecavir (BMS 200-475)
Ganciclovir
FTC, DAPD, L-FMAU
b-L-Fd4C, L-dT, L-dC

chronic hepatitis B. The primary mode of action of lamivudine involves inhibition of viral DNA synthesis. This occurs primarily through incorporation of lamivudine monophosphate molecules into newly synthesised HBV-DNA, resulting in chain termination (Fig. 1). Suppression of viral DNA synthesis by lamivudine reduces the release of virions by infected cells, and may reduce nuclear pool of covalently closed circular DNA (cccDNA), which is the template for transcription of viral gene products.

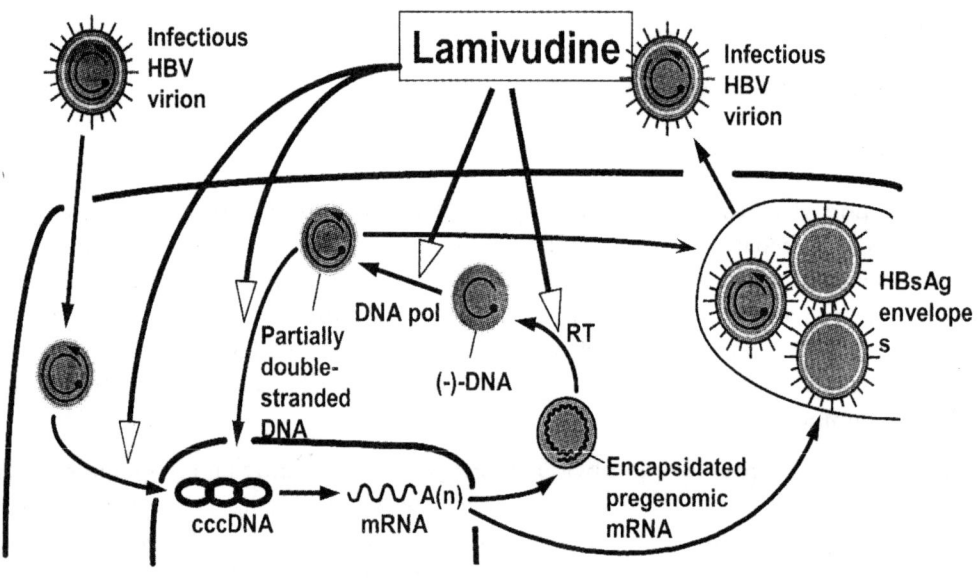

Fig. 1. Mechanisms of action of lamivudine

Pharmacokinetics and Pharmacodynamics

The pharmacokinetics and safety of lamivudine has been studied extensively in animal models and man.[4] Clinical pharmacology studies indicate that lamivudine is associated with excellent tolerability and a satisfactory pharmacokinetic profile. Early phase I studies were carried out in asymptomatic human immunodeficiency virus (HIV)-positive patients. Initial dose-ranging studies in patients with chronic hepatitis B explored the relationship between dose, systemic exposure, changes in serum HBV-DNA concentration, and compared once- with twice-daily dosing. A range of serum concentrations was evaluated, spanning those shown to be active against HBV in preclinical studies.

Lamivudine is rapidly absorbed after oral dosing, reaching maximum serum concentrations within 0.5 to 1.5 hours. The absolute bioavailability of lamivudine is approximately 82% and 68% in adults and children respectively. It is widely distributed in body fluids, with a mean volume of distribution of 1.3 l/kg after intravenous dosing. Lamivudine distributes freely across the placenta in pregnant women. About 70% of an oral dose is eliminated through kidneys as unchanged drug and a further 5% to 10% is eliminated as the trans-sulphoxide metabolite. Dose adjustment is required for patients with moderate to severe renal impairment, and for paediatric patients (Table 2). Clinically significant interactions with other drugs have not been observed.[4]

Table 2. Dose of lamivudine for treatment of chronic hepatitis B in patients with renal impairment

	First dose	Maintenance Dose
Clcr 30-49	100 mg	50 mg OD
Clcr 15-29	100 mg	25 mg OD
Clcr 5-14	35 mg	15 mg OD
Clcr < 5	35 mg	10 mg OD

Dialysis: No data available, Clcr – creatinine clearance

Clinical studies

Lamivudine is the most extensively studied of the nucleoside analogues in HBV infection and is licensed for the treatment of CHB infection in many countries. Extensive clinical studies in patients with CHB have been completed. Over 1500 patients have been included in a range of trials from different ethnic groups, in combination with α-interferon, in the treatment of patients with precore mutant chronic hepatitis B, in interferon non-responders and in patients with HBV-related disease listed for liver transplantation.[5-16] The phase II studies evaluated a range of doses (5–600mg/day). Results from these studies demonstrated that suppression of HBV replication is dose-dependent with maximal suppression (3 to 4 log10 reductions) being achieved at doses of 100 mg once daily.[5,6]

Data from 5 phase III studies have been published. The first phase III Asian study to be reported was a one year double blind trial of lamivudine in 358 Chinese patients with CHB.[7] This study was conducted in different centres in Hong Kong, Taiwan and Singapore. Patients were randomly assigned to receive 25 mg lamivudine, 100 mg lamivudine, or placebo. Patients underwent liver biopsies before entering the study and after completing treatment. In the intent-to-treat analysis, hepatic necro-inflammatory activity improved by two points or more in 56 percent of the patients receiving 100 mg of lamivudine compared to 25% of placebo patients (p<0.001). The 100 mg dose was also associated with a reduced progression

(Fig. 2) of fibrosis compared to placebo (p=0.01). Lamivudine significantly reduced serum ALT, increased HBeAg sero-conversion and reduced HBV-DNA levels compared to placebo. An interesting observation was that patients with higher baseline ALT had the highest sero-conversion rate.[8]

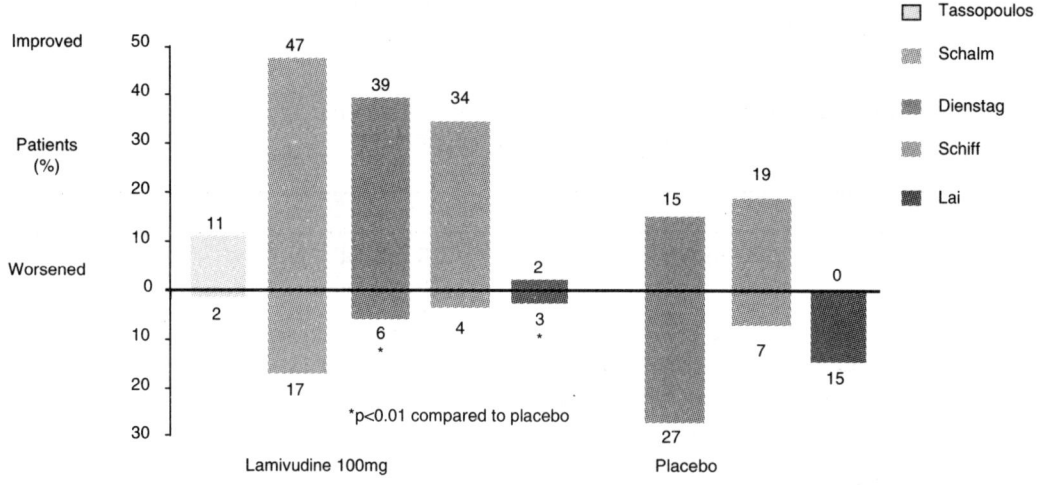

Fig. 2. Effect of lamivudine (100 mg/d) on the progression of fibrosis in patients with CHB

A similar trial was undertaken in the USA on previously untreated patients.[10] Sixty-six patients were randomized to receive 100 mg of lamivudine and 71 to placebo, once daily for 52 weeks. Histological response (≥ 2 point reduction in the Knodell histologic activity index) was seen in 52% of the patients who received lamivudine compared to only 23% response rate in those receiving placebo (p<0.001). In addition, after 52 weeks treatment, patients receiving lamivudine were more likely to experience HBeAg sero-conversion than placebo patients (17% vs. 6% p<0.04). HBV-DNA suppression (44% vs. 16% p<0.001) and ALT normalization (41% vs. 7% p<0.001) were also more common in patients receiving lamivudine than patients receiving placebo. Lamivudine was well-tolerated in both of these studies with no dose-dependent or treatment limiting adverse events.

A cohort of 58 patients, from the original Asian study,[7] were randomized to receive lamivudine for 4 years. Extended treatment resulted in continued improvement in liver histology, viral suppression, normalization of serum ALT, and increased HBeAg sero-conversion. By the end of fourth year, 27/58 (47%) had achieved HBeAg sero-conversion. In those patients with baseline ALT >2×ULN, HBeAg sero-conversion increased to a remarkable 73% (19/26). This also included patients with YMDD variant HBV, the incidence of which increases over time.[8]

The durability of the loss of HBeAg and sero-conversion on lamivudine is being evaluated in a no-treatment follow-up study. In a recent interim analysis, 43 CHB patients with HBeAg sero-conversion after lamivudine in previous trials were evaluated.[11] Patients could be re-treated with lamivudine if they experienced reactivation of HBV replication. The median duration of follow up in this study was 21 months (range 0–30). Eighty-six per cent (37/43) of patients showed durable response that is similar to the durability reported for interferon induced sero-conversion (Fig. 3). It is important to note that 9 patients (21%) also experienced a durable HBsAg sero-conversion. Normal ALTs were recorded at last visit for 65% (28/43) of HBeAg negative and 89% (8/9) of HBsAg negative patients.

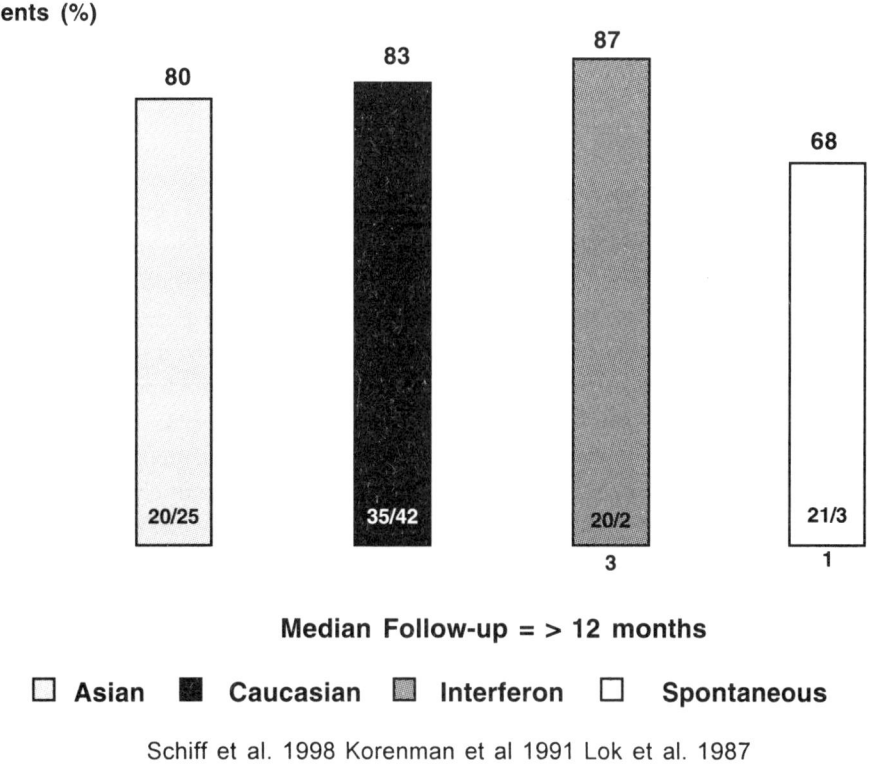

Fig. 3. Durability of HBeAg sero-conversion after lamivudine therapy for one year

Interferon non-responders

Patients who have failed a previous course of interferon pose a difficult management problem. A phase III randomized, partially-blinded study was performed to assess the efficacy and safety of three treatment regimens in patients with CHB who were interferon non-responders.[12] A total of 238 patients were randomized to receive (a) lamivudine 100 mg orally, once daily; (b) placebo orally, once daily; or (c) lamivudine 100 mg orally, once daily for 8 weeks followed by interferon-alpha-2b 10 MU subcutaneously, three times weekly plus lamivudine 100mg orally, once daily for 16 weeks. The primary efficacy measurement was histologic response, as indicated by a 2-point or greater reduction in Knodell histological activity index (HAI) score. Liver biopsies were performed at baseline and at week 52. Endpoints for treatment response included HBeAg loss, HBV-DNA suppression, and ALT normalization at week 52. Histologic response was significantly more common in patients treated with lamivudine (52%) compared to those treated with placebo (25%, $p<0.002$) or the combination therapy (32%, $p<0.01$). HBeAg loss was most common in patients treated with lamivudine (33%) compared to placebo (13%) or the combination (21%). Sustained ALT normalization was also significantly more common in the lamivudine group (44%) compared to placebo (15%, $p<0.001$) or combination (18%, $p<0.005$). These results show that lamivudine is an effective treatment for interferon non-responders and that the anti-viral effect of lamivudine is similar in interferon non-responders to that seen in interferon naive patients.[12]

Lamivudine and interferon in combination

The use of interferon in combination with lamivudine has been investigated in controlled trials. The efficacy and safety of lamivudine and interferon-alpha (IFN) combination treatment was compared to the respective monotherapies in a study on 226 patients in centers from Europe, Australia, Canada, and South Africa.[13] Patients were randomized to receive lamivudine 100mg once daily for 52 weeks, IFN 10 MU three times weekly for 16 weeks, or lamivudine for 8 weeks followed by combination treatment of lamivudine plus IFN for 16 weeks. HBeAg sero-conversion rates at week 52 for lamivudine, IFN, and lamivudine plus IFN were 18%, 19% and 29% and at week 64 were 20%, 22% and 25% respectively with no significant difference between the groups. This study concluded that HBeAg sero-conversion rates for one year of lamivudine and a standard course of IFN are similar. The HBeAg sero-conversion rate for combination treatment although higher did not achieve statistical significance. Further studies to evaluate the benefit of lamivudine and IFN combination (including pegylated interferon) are needed.

HBeAg negative CHB

Precore mutant HBV infection is a significant problem especially in the Asian continent (Fig. 4). These patients generally respond poorly to IFN. A phase III study in patients with

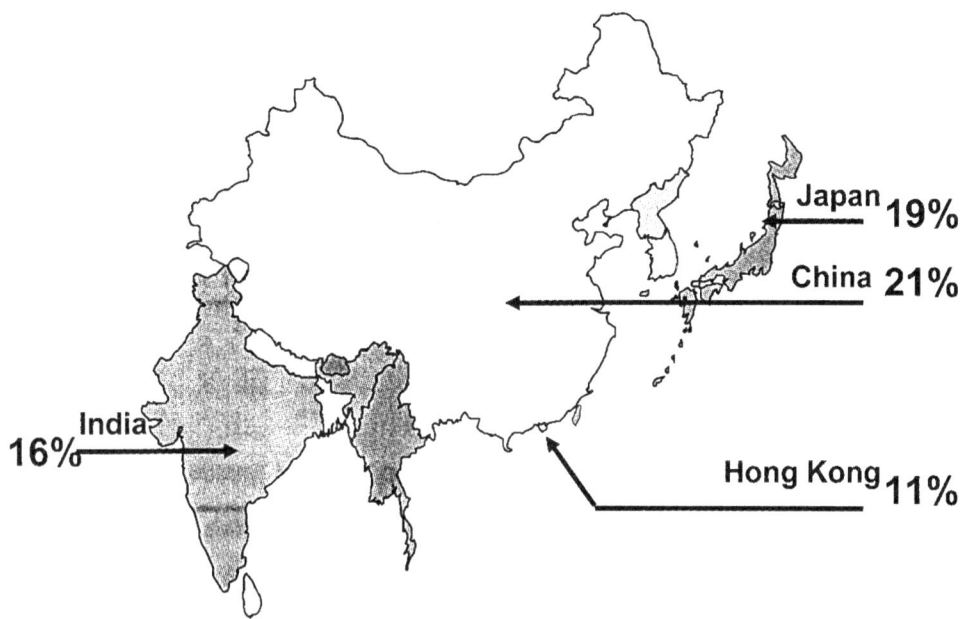

Fig. 4. Prevalence of precore mutant HBV in Asian continent

precore mutant CHB was conducted in centers in Greece, Italy, Spain, Canada and the UK.[14] This study reports the efficacy of lamivudine in anti-HBe positive patients who were HBsAg positive and HBeAg negative and HBV-DNA positive. Patients were randomized to receive lamivudine 100 mg or placebo once daily for 26 weeks. One hundred and twenty-four patients with confirmed CHB were randomized to placebo (64) or lamivudine (60). At week 24, 63% of lamivudine treated group were HBV-DNA negative and had ALT within the normal range compared to 6% of those receiving placebo ($p<0.001$). At week 52, 65% of the lamivudine treated patients were HBV-DNA negative and had ALT within the normal range (Fig. 5). Forty-two percent of the lamivudine group patients with pre- and post-treatment liver biopsies available showed a ≥ 2 point decrease in Knodell necro-inflammatory score at week 52 compared to baseline. Studies evaluating treatment for a longer duration with lamivudine are in progress.

Decompensated liver disease

A significant advantage of nucleoside analogues compared to IFN is that they can be used in patients with decompensated liver disease. In this setting, interferon is contraindicated due to toxicity and an increased risk of graft rejection. Lamivudine has been used successfully in the

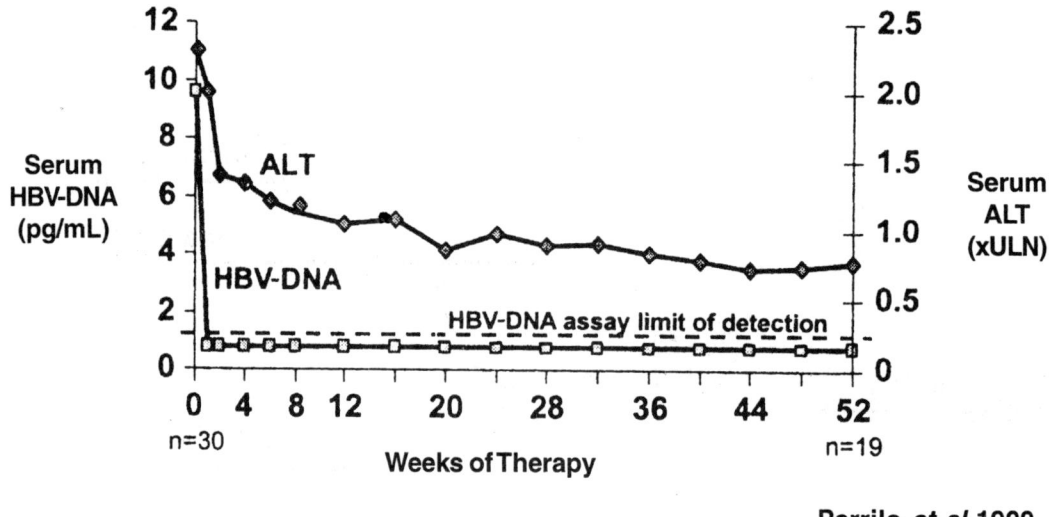

Fig. 5. Effect of lamivudine on HBV-DNA and ALT levels in patients with CHB

setting of liver transplantation and in the treatment of decompensated liver disease.[15, 16] This issue has been discussed at length in the chapter on anti-viral therapy in HBV-related decompensated cirrhosis.

YMDD variant HBV

With prolonged lamivudine treatment, variants emerge in some patients that have a reduced susceptibility to lamivudine *in vitro*. The predominant sequence changes responsible for this are in the YMDD motif of the HBV polymerase. There is *in vitro* and *in vivo* data to show that these variants do not replicate as effectively as wild type HBV and hence cause less severe disease.[17, 18] Although these variants are resistant to lamivudine *in vitro*, clinically, the majority of patients appear to receive benefit, if lamivudine treatment is continued.[6, 8, 12]

In phase III studies, YMDD variants were detected in few chronic hepatitis B patients during the first 6 months of lamivudine therapy. After one year of therapy, YMDD variants were detected in 14 to 32% of patients in different phase III studies.[6, 7, 10, 12] After 2 and 3 years of therapy with lamivudine, YMDD variants were detected in 42% and 52% of Asian patients respectively. During four years of treatment with lamivudine, the majority of patients maintained HBV-DNA and ALT values below the baseline, including those patients with YMDD variant HBV. In addition, 33% of patients with YMDD variants experienced HBeAg seroconversion.[8]

Safety

In phase III studies, lamivudine was well tolerated in all populations studied including those with cirrhosis, decompensated liver disease, and precore mutant HBV infection. The overall incidence of adverse events potentially attributable to lamivudine was similar for all groups. Thus, there is no evidence of drug safety concerns associated with the use of lamivudine.

In report on 999 patients (Fig. 6) treated with lamivudine for up to four years, 35 (3.5%) experienced a liver disease related adverse event, approximately half of these were in patients with YMDD variant HBV, 11/35 experienced a transient episode of decompensation, 7 of whom had YMDD variants; 4 out of the 11 patients experienced HBeAg sero-conversion. Therefore <1% of patients given treatment with lamivudine for many years experienced decompensation in association with the presence of YMDD variant HBV.[19]

Infrequent post-treatment ALT elevations were observed in patients receiving lamivudine,

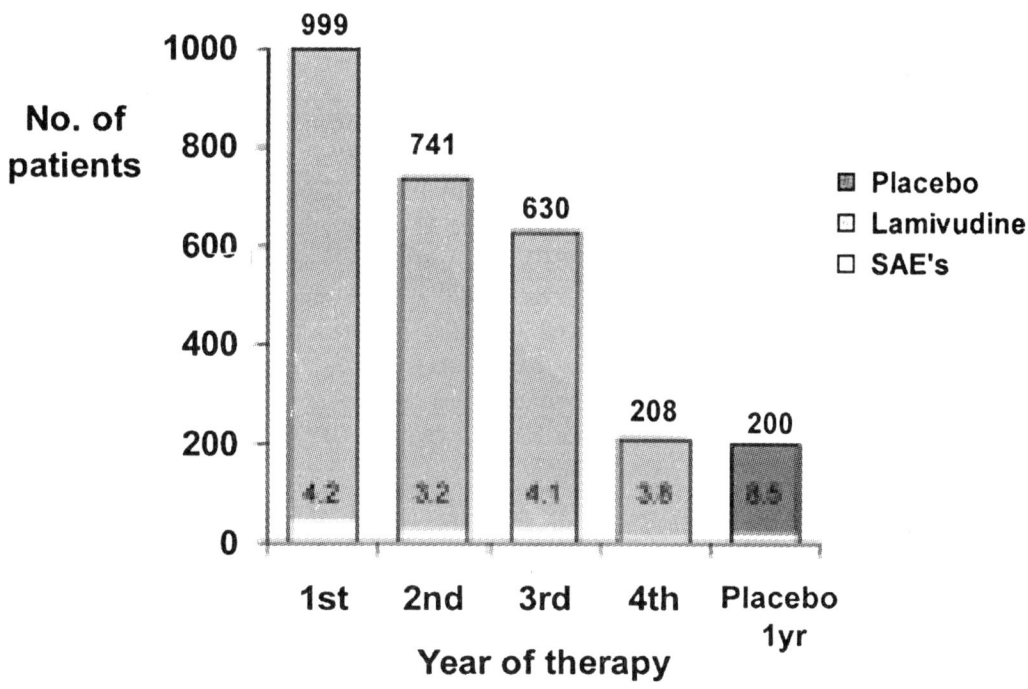

Fig. 6. Occurence of serious adverse events (SAE) after prolonged (4 years) lamivudine therapy

however, a similar low incidence of clinically significant events was observed in patients receiving lamivudine or placebo.

OTHER AGENTS IN DEVELOPMENT

A number of other agents have been investigated or are in development for the treatment of hepatitis B.

Famciclovir

Famciclovir is the orally administered prodrug of penciclovir. It has activity against herpes viruses and is licensed for the treatment of herpes zoster and genital herpes. It has also been shown to be active against HBV and has been evaluated in clinical trials in patients with CHB.

In the largest study reported till date, 333 patients with CHB received 16 weeks treatment with famciclovir at doses of 500 mg, 250 mg, 125 mg or placebo three times a day.[20] In the patients receiving 500 mg of famciclovir, a significant reduction in HBV-DNA levels was demonstrated within 1 week of treatment compared to placebo ($p<0.007$). There was also significantly more sero-conversion in the 500 mg group. Despite these promising early results, famciclovir has proved relatively ineffective and its development for this disease has been stopped.

Adefovir dipivoxil

Adefovir dipivoxil is an oral prodrug of adefovir (formerly known as PMRA), a phosphonate nucleotide analogue of adenosine monophosphate with a broad-spectrum antiviral activity against HIV, CMV and HBV. *In vitro* and *in vivo* activity has been shown against wild type and YMDD variant HBV-DNA polymerases.[21] In phase II trials adefovir treatment has been shown to result in a 4 log10 reduction in HBV-DNA after 12 weeks at doses of 30 mg and 60 mg daily. HBeAg sero-conversion rates were higher at both the doses than in the placebo group.[22, 23] Adefovir has been generally well tolerated in these studies, however, concern regarding its nephrotoxicity has stimulated the evaluation of a smaller (10 mg) dose in the ongoing phase III studies. Recently, adefovir has been reported to reduce HBV-DNA and improve the liver function in 5 patients with YMDD variant HBV.[23]

Entecavir

This nucleoside analogue is a selective inhibitor of HBV replication. It is very potent against Woodchuck HBV with oral dose of only 0.1 mg/kg producing up to a 7 log10 reduction in WHBV levels within 4 weeks of starting treatment. Dose ranging studies in man report a mean log 10 reduction in HBV-DNA of 2.2–2.4 for 0.05–1mg doses over 28 days. There were 2/32 patients who withdrew due to raised ALT and due to mild or moderate headache.[24]

Other agents such as FTC, DAPD and L-FMAU are in the early stages of development.

FUTURE PERSPECTIVES

Although the treatment with lamivudine monotherapy is sufficient for the majority of patients with chronic hepatitis B, selected patients, such as a proportion of those with YMDD variants, liver transplant recipients, and some patients with HBeAg negative disease, may receive added benefit if a combination of treatment was available.[26-28] Using a combination of nucleoside analogues to treat these variants is the logical next step and studies to evaluate this are in progress.

REFERENCES

1. Chang MH, Chen CJ, Lai MS, Hsu HM, Wu TC, Kong MS, Liang DC, et al. Universal hepatitis B vaccination in Taiwan and the incidence of hepatocellular carcinoma in children. *N Engl J Med* 1997;336: 1855-9.
2. Wong DK, Cheung AM, O'Rourke K, Naylor CD, Detsky AS, Heathcote J. Effect of alpha-interferon treatment in patients with hepatitis B e antigen positive chronic hepatitis B. A meta-analysis. *Ann Intern Med* 1993;119:312-23.
3. Perillo RP, Schiff ER, Davis GL, Bodenheimer HC, Jr., Lindsay K, Payne J, Dienstag JL. A randomized, controlled trial of interferon-alpha-2b alone and after perdnisone withdrawal for the treatment of chronic hepatitis B. *N Engl J Med* 1990;323:295-301.
4. Johnson MA, Moore KH, Yuen GJ, Bye A, Pakes GE. Clinical pharmacokinetics of lamivudine. *Clin Pharmacokinet* 1999;36:41-66.
5. Honkoop P, de Man RA, Niesters HG, Main J, Nevens F, Thomas HC, Fevery J, et al. Quantitative HBV-DNA assessment by the limiting-dilution polymerase chain reaction in chronic hepatitis B patients: evidence of continuing viral suppression with longer duration and higher dose of lamivudine therapy. *J Viral Hepat* 1998;5:307-12.
6. Dienstag JL, Perrillo RP, Schiff ER, Bartholomen M, Vicary C, Rubin M. A preliminary trial of lamivudine for chronic hepatitis B. *N Engl J Med* 1995;333:1657-61.
7. Lai CL, Chien RN, Leung NW, Chang TT, Guan R, Tai DI, Ng KY, et al. A one year trial of lamivudine for chronic hepatitis B. *N Engl J Med* 1998;339:61-8.
8. Chang TT, Lai CL, Liaw YF, Leung NWY, Guan R, Lim SG. Enhanced HBeAg sero-conversion rates in Chinese patients on lamivudine. *Hepatology* 1999;30:420A.
9. Chien RN, Liaw YF, Atkins M. Pretherapy ALT level as a determinant for HBeAg sero-conversion during lamivudine therapy in patients with chronic hepatitis B. *Hepatology* 1999;30:770-4.
10. Dienstag J, Schiff ER, Wright TL, Perillo RP, Hann HW, Goodman Z, Crowther L, et al. Lamivudine as initial treatment for chronic hepatitis B in the United States; *N Engl J Med* 1999;341:1256-63.
11. Schiff E, Cianciara J, Karyalcin S, Kowdley K, Woesner M, McMullen S, et al. Durable HBeAg and HBsAg sero-conversions after lamivudine for chronic hepatitis B. *J Hepatol* 2000;32(suppl 2):99 (abstract).
12. Schiff E, Karayalcin S, Grimm I, Perrillo R, Dianstag J, Husa P, Schalm S, et al. A placebo-controlled study of lamivudine and interferon-alpha-2b in patients with CHB who had previously failed interferon therapy. *Hepatology* 1998;28:388A.
13. Schalm SW, Heathcote J, Cianciara J, Farrell G, Sherman M, Willems B, Dhillon A, et al. Lamivudine and alpha-interferon combination treatment of patients with chronic hepatitis B infection: a randomized trial. *Gut* 2000;46:562-8.

14. Tassopoulos NC, Volpes R, Pastore G, Heathcote J, Buti M, Golden RD, Hawley S, et al. Efficacy of lamivudine in patients with hepatitis B e antigen, negative/hepatitis B Virus DNA-positive (precore mutant) chronic hepatitis B. Lamivudine Precore Mutant Study Group. *Hepatology* 1999;29:889-96.
15. Perillo R, Rakela J, Martin P, Levy TNG, Schiff E, Dienstag J, Gish R, et al. Lamivudine for suppression and/or prevention of hepatitis B when given pre/post liver transplantation (OLT). *Hepatology* 1997;26:260A.
16. Villeneuve JP, Condreay LD, Willems B, Pomier-Layranrgues G, Fenyves D, Bilodeau M, Leduc R, et al. Lamivudine treatment for decompensated cirrhosis resulting from chronic hepatitis B. *Hepatology* 2000;31:207-10.
17. Allen M, Deslauriers M, Andrews CW, Tipples GA, Waltens KA, Tyrell DL, Brown N, et al. Identification and biological characterization of mutations in HBV resistant to lamivudine. *Hepatology* 1998;27:1670-7.
18. Melegari M, Scaglioni PP, Wands JR. Hepatitis B virus mutants associated with 3TC and famciclovir administration are replication defective. *Hepatology* 1998;27:628-33.
19. Lai CL, Maddrey C, Marr C, Woessner M, Atkins M. Long-term safety of lamivudine in patients with chronic hepatitis B. *J Gastroenterology and Hepatology* 2000;15(suppl):1208.
20. Trepo C, Jezek P, Atkinson G, Boon R, Young C. Efficacy of famciclovir in chronic hepatitis B: results of a dose finding study. *J Hepatol* 2000;32:1011-8.
21. Xiong X, Flores C, Yang H, Toole JJ, Gibbs CS. Mutations in Hepatitis B DNA polymerase associated with lamivudine resistance do not confer resistance to adefovir. *Hepatology* 1998;28:1669-73.
22. Heathcote J, Jeffers L, Wright T, Sherman M, Perrill R, Sacks S, Carithers R, et al. Loss of serum HBV-DNA and HBeAg i sero-conversion following short-term adefovir therapy in CHB. *Hepatology* 1998;28(suppl):317A.
23. Cullen JM, Li DH, Brown C, Eisenburg EJ, Cundy KC, Wolfe J, Toote J, et al. Antiviral efficacy and pharmacokinetics of oral adefovir dipivoxil inchronically woodchuck hepatitis virus-infected woodchucks. *Antimicrob Agents Chemother* 2001;45:2740-5.
24. Perillo R, Schiff E, Yoshida E, Statler A, Hirsch K, Wright T, Gutfreund K, et al. Adefovir dipivoxil for the treatment of lamivudine resistant hepatitis B mutants. *Hepatology* 2000;32:129-34.
25. DeMan RA, Walters LM, Nevens F, Chua D, Sherman M, Lai CL, Lee Y, et al. Safety and efficacy or oral entecavir given for 28 days in patients with chronic hepatitis B virus infection. *Hepatology* 2001;34:578-82.
26. Locarnini SA, Bartholomeusz A, Delaney WE. Evolving therapies for the treatment of chronic hepatitis B virus infection. *Expert Opin Investing Drugs* 2002;11:169-87.
27. Perrillo RP. How will we use the new antiviral agents for hepatitis B? *Curr Gastroenterol Rep* 2002;4:63-71.
28. Wolters LM, Neisters HG, deMan RA. Nucleoside analogues for chronic hepatitis B. *Eur J Gastroenterol Hepatol* 2001;13:1499-506.

47

Incidence and profile of lamivudine resistance

Deepak N Amarapurkar

Lamivudine, a nucleoside analogue has been found to be effective in the treatment of chronic hepatitis B virus (HBV) infection.[1] Though lamivudine suppresses HBV-DNA levels in more than 95% patients, long lasting viral suppression is seen in only 18 to 20% patients at the end of one year of treatment.[2] This viral suppression is characterized by loss of HBeAg and development of antibodies to 'e' antigen. Recently it has been shown that continuing lamivudine therapy for 2 to 3 years, HBeAg sero-conversion rate may increase beyond 50%.[3] Lamivudine is an oral drug, easy to administer and reasonably safe when compared with traditional interferon therapy. In spite of these advantages, there are two main caveats for the use of lamivudine: first, inability of lamivudine to suppress supercoiled DNA, i.e., cccDNA of HBV and hence high rate of relapse after stopping treatment;[4] and second, development of viral mutation which is resistant to lamivudine.[5-10] Initially it was observed that YMDD mutation developed only in immune suppressed patient,[6] but now it is clearly seen to occur in immunocompetent patients as well.[8] YMDD mutant virus was thought to be replication-deficient, and 'e' antigen sero-conversion was seen by continuing lamivudine therapy after YMDD mutation.[11]

It is quite evident that YMDD mutation is not a clinical curiosity but it can cause flare in HBV-related liver damage[11] and few patients have decompensated and died due to the development of YMDD mutants.[12]

WHAT IS YMDD MUTATION?

YMDD motif is a highly conserved region of all reverse transcriptases and this is a nucleoside binding groove. The wild type amino acid sequence in this region is Tyr-Met-Asp-Asp (YMDD).[9] Substitution of methionine by valine (M522V) or isoleucine (M522I) in the motif has been demonstrated in patients with lamivudine resistance.[6-10] Identical mutation in HIV reverse transcriptases confers resistance to lamivudine. A second mutation (L528M) which results in methionine replacing leucine, 24 amino acid upstream to YMDD motif has been documented in association with M552V and M552I mutations.[13] Recently, alanine 529 to threonine mutant has been demonstrated in patients having YMDD mutants during prolonged lamivudine therapy.[14]

MOLECULAR CHARACTERISTICS OF YMDD MUTATION

YMDD variants do not replicate as effectively as the wild virus. Hence, YMDD variants will be predominant only in the presence of lamivudine treatment and as lamivudine is withdrawn, the wild type virus will predominate again.[10]

YMDD mutation prevents binding and entry of lamivudine in the virus and confers resistance to the drug.[5] Three different types of mutations as described earlier have been reported. L528M mutation[15] confers cross-resistance to famciclovir but no cross-resistance to adefovir has been demonstrated.[16] The EC_{50} of lamivudine increases many folds in primary human hepatocytes transfected with YMDD mutant virus.[17]

CLINICAL CHARACTERISTICS OF YMDD MUTATION

Though YMDD mutations are known to occur between 12 to 116 weeks after initiation of therapy, average time when these mutants appear is 8 to 9 months.[18] Development of mutants is associated with rise in transaminases and rise in HBV-DNA titers.[19] Though there is rise in transaminase and HBV-DNA levels, these levels are less than the pretreatment levels.[11] Discontinuation of lamivudine after YMDD mutation, allows replication of wild type virus which suppress the YMDD mutant virus and soon wild type virus becomes dominant.[10] In patients with YMDD mutants, if lamivudine therapy is continued, sero-conversion of HBeAg to anti-HBe can occur. Transaminase elevation is seen in almost 90 to 95% patients. More than 10 times elevation in ALT and decompensation have been noticed.[11] Few deaths due to decompensation have been reported.[12]

During prolonged treatment (i.e., more than 52 weeks) with lamivudine after YMDD mutation, HBeAg sero-conversion and histological improvement can occur. This improvement is significantly less as compared to the patients without YMDD mutation on continuing lamivudine therapy beyond 52 weeks.[19]

Pre-treatment variables like serum HBV-DNA levels, histological activity index, baseline ALT and body mass index have been directly correlated with YMDD mutation development.[11, 20] Patients who are immunetolerant, who have high levels of serum HBV-DNA are less likely to seroconvert from HBeAg to anti-HBe and high chance of developing YMDD mutation.

Prediction of presence of YMDD mutation after 24 weeks of lamivudine treatment can be done based on certain biochemical and virological characteristics.[21-23] Patients with ALT levels, more than 1.3 times the normal upper limit, HBeAg positive and HBV-DNA levels more than 20 pg/ml had a 99% chance of developing YMDD mutation. In our experience, 20%

patients developed YMDD mutation after 52 week of lamivudine treatment. All the patients with mutant virus were 'e' antigen positive, had elevated ALT levels and HBV-DNA levels more than 20 pg/ml.[21]

INCIDENCE OF YMDD MUTATION

YMDD mutants can appear after 12 weeks upto 116 weeks after initiation of treatment with lamivudine. The average incidence of YMDD mutant is 4% after 9 months of treatment which increases to 14% by 12 months.[24] Pooled data from 4 major studies show that lamivudine resistance develops in 16 to 32% of patients treated with 100 mg of lamivudine for 52 weeks.[21] In our experience, 20% patients developed clinically evident YMDD mutation at the end of 12 months.[25] Preliminary data from New Delhi, India have shown low incidence of YMDD mutation.[26, 27] However, more concrete data are now emerging from India on the prevalence and profile of mutations after lamivudine therapy in patients with chronic hepatitis B.[28]

In the Asian extended study, YMDD variants were detected in 67% of patients at some point of time during 4 years of treatment.[20] Distinct lamivudine-resistant mutants which can replace YMDD mutants can appear during prolonged lamivudine therapy and cause exacerbation. YMDD mutation is a significant problem during prolonged treatment and to overcome this, use of combination of nucleoside analogues or combination of nucleoside analogues with other drugs should be evaluated.

REFERENCES

1. Xie H, Vornohov M, Liolta DC, Korba BA, Schinazie RF, Richman DD, Hosteler KY. Phosphatidyl 2' 3'dedoxy 3'–thiacytidine: Synthesis and activity in hepatitis B and HIV infected cell. *Antiviral Res* 1995;28:113-20.
2. Papatheodoridis GV, Dimou E, Papadimitropoulos V. Nucleoside analogues for chronic hepatitis B: antiviral efficacy and viral resistance. *Am J Gastroenterol* 2002;97:1618-28..
3. Laiw YF, Lai CL, Leung NWY, Chang TT, Guan R, Tai DI, Ng KY, et al. Two year lamivudine therapy in chronic hepatitis B infection: result of placebo-controlled multicentre study in Asia. *Gastroenterology* 1998;114:1289A (abstract).
4. Moraleda G, Saputelli J, Aldrich CE, Avereft D, Condreay L, Mason WS. Lack of effect of antiviral therapy in nondividing hepatocyte cultures on in closed circular DNA of Woodchuck hepatitis virus. *J Virol* 1997;71:9392-9.
5. Hussain M, Lok ASF. Mutation in the hepatitis B virus polymerase gene associated with antiviral treatment for hepatitis B. *J Viral Hepat* 1999;6:183-94.
6. Ling R, Mutimer D, Ahmed M, Boxall EH, Elias E, Dusheiko GM, Harrison TJ. Selection of mutations in hepatitis B virus polymerase during therapy of transplant recipients with lamivudine *Hepatology* 1996;3:711-3.
7. Schalm SW. Clinical implications of lamivudine resistance by HBV. *Lancet* 1997;9044:3-4.
8. Honkoop O, Niesters HG, De Man RA, Osterhans AD, Schalm SW. Lamivudine resistance in immunocompetent chronic hepatitis B. *J Hepatol* 1997;26:1393-5.
9. Tripples GA, Ma MM, Fischer KP, Bain VG, Kneteman NM, Tyrell DZ. Mutation in HBV-RNA dependent DNA polymerase confers resistance to lamivudine *in vivo*. *Hepatology* 1996;3:714-7.

10. Chayama K, Suzuki Y, Kobayashi M, Kobayashi M, Tsubota A, Hashimoto M, Miyano Y, et al. Emergence and take over of YMDD motif mutant hepatitis B virus during long-term lamivudine therapy and retakeover by wild type after cessation of therapy. *Hepatology* 1998;27:1711-6.
11. Liaw YK, Chien RN, Leung NW, Chang TT, Yeh CT, Tsai SL, Chu CM. Acute exacerbation and hepatitis B clearance after emergence of v YMDD motif mutation during lamivudine therapy. *Hepatology* 1999;30:567-72.
12. Malik AH, Lee WM. Hepatitis B Plot thickens. *Hepatology* 1999;30:579-81.
13. Nassal M, Schaller H. Hepatitis B virus replication: an update. *J Viral Hepat* 1996;3:217-26.
14. Yeh CT, Chen RN, Chu CM, Liaw YF. Clearance of the original hepatitis B virus YMDD motif mutants with emergence of distinct lamivudine resistant mutant. During prolonged lamivudine therapy. *Hepatology* 2000;31:1318-26.
15. Tillman HL, Trautwein C, Bock T, Boker KH, Jackel E, Glowienka M, Oldhafer K, et al. Treatment with lamivudine in relation to response under famciclovir and mutation. *J Hepatol* 1999;30:(suppl)77.
16. Xiong X, Flores C, Yang H, Toole JJ, Gibbs CS. Mutation in hepatitis B DNA polymerase associated with resistance to lamivudine do not confer resistance to adefovir in vitro. *Hepatology* 1998;28:1669-73.
17. Bartholomew MM, Jansen RW, Jeffers LJ, Reddy KR, Johnson LC, Bunzendahl H, Condreay LD, et al. Hepatitis B virus resistance to lamivudine given for recurrent infection after orthotopic liver transplant. *Lancet* 1997;349:20-2.
18. Blair J, Faulds D. Lamivudine a review of its therapeutic potentials in chronic hepatitis B. *Drugs* 1999;58:101-41.
19. Liaw YF, Leung NW, Chang TT, Guan R, Tai DI, Ng KY, Chien RN, et al. Effects of extended lamivudine therapy in Asian patients with chronic hepatitis B. Asia Hepatitis Lamivudine Study Group. *Gastroenterology* 2000;119:172-80.
20. Mutimer D, Pillay D, Dragon E, Tang H, Ahmed M, O'Donnell K, Shaw J, et al. High pre-treatment serum hepatitis B titers predict failure of lamivudine prophylaxis and graft reinfection after Liver transplantation. *J Hepatol* 1999;30:715-21.
21. Atkins M, Hunt CM, Brown N, Gray F, Sanathanan L, Woessner M, Lai CL, et al. Clinical Significance of YMDD mutant hepatitis B virus (HBV) in a large cohort of lamivudine treated hepatitis B patients. *Hepatology* 1998;28:319A.
22. Buti M, Cotrina M, Valdes A, Jardi R, Rodriguez-Frias F, Esleban R. Is hepatitis B virus subtype testing useful in predicting virological response and resistance to lamivudine? *J Hepatol* 2002;36:445-6.
23. Buti M, Sanchez F, Cotrina M, Jardi R, Rodriguez F, Esteban R, Guardia J. Quantitative hepatitis B virus DNA testing for the early prediction of the maintenance of response during lamivudine therapy in patients with chronic hepatitis B. *J Infect Dis* 2001;183:1277-80.
24. Lai CL, Chien RN, Leung NW, Chang TT, Gyan R, Tai DI, Ng KY, et al. One year trial of lamivudine for chronic hepatitis B. *N Engl J Med* 1998;339:61-8.
25. Amarapurkar DN, Rao A. Lamivudine in decompensated liver disease due to chronic HBV infection. *J Gastroenterol Hepatol* 2000;15:(suppl)F44.
26. Kapoor D, Guptan RC, Wakil S, Kazim SN, Kaul R, Raisuddin S, Sarin SK, et al. Beneficial effects of lamivudine in hepatitis B related decompensated cirrhosis *J Hepatol* 2000;33:308-12.
27. Singal AK. Lamivudine in HBV-related decompensated cirrhosis: a preliminary study. *J Assoc Phys India* 2003 (submitted for publication).
28. Wakil SM, Kazim SN, Khan LA, Raisuddin S, Parvez MK, Guptan RC, Thakur V, et al. Prevalence and profile of mutations associated with lamivudine therapy in Indian patients with chronic hepatitis B in he surface and polymerase genes of hepatitis B virus. *J Med Virol* 2002;68:311-8.

48

Mechanisms and treatment options for lamivudine resistance

Ching L Lai

YMDD VARIANT HEPATITIS B VIRUS

The major site of mutation of the hepatitis B virus (HBV) associated with lamivudine therapy is the tyrosine-methionine-asparate-aspartate amino acid (YMDD) motif. The YMDD motif is a highly conserved motif in the catalytic domain of the reverse transcriptase (RT)/DNA polymerase and is shared by all hepadnaviruses as well as retroviruses. The variants are characterized by the mutation of the methionine (codon 552) to either valine or isoleucine (YMDD to YVDD or YIDD). There is often a contributing mutation in the "B domain" of the RT where the leucine (codon 528) is mutated to methionine. Other sites of mutation are less commonly found and are of doubtful clinical significance.

The amino acid changes of the YMDD motif, YVDD and YIDD also result in changes in the amino acid in sequence of HBsAg in positions 195 and 196 respectively. Since the immunodominant protective epitope (the "a" determinant from amino acid position 124 to 147) of the surface antigen is situated away from these mutations, it is unlikely that the YMDD variant HBV would affect the immune response.

In the wild-type HBV, the YMDD motif is in a region with high affinity for nucleotides, hence facilitating the formation of the nascent minus strand of the HBV-DNA (Fig. 1a). Lamivudine has an affinity for the RT domain of the virus, probably, because it binds at a pocket formed partly by the methionine in position 552. At the presumed binding site of lamivudine, the side chain of the methionine in position 552 is in van der Waal contact with lamivudine, with a distance of approximately 3Å.[1,2] The presence of lamivudine will suppress the formation of minus strand of HBV-DNA by chain termination and competitive inhibition of the RT activity (Fig. 1b). With the mutation of methionine in the YMDD motif to isoleucine or valine (YMDD to YIDD or YVDD), the length of the amino acid side chain gets shorter. Allen et al, postulates that this increases the size of the binding pocket, thereby attenuating the affinity of lamivudine for the RT domain. Lamivudine, therefore, has little or no inhibitory effect on the replication of the YMDD variant HBV.

However, with the alteration in the configuration of the YMDD region when the methionine in position 552 is mutated, the interaction between nucleotides and the active catalytic site of the RT is also affected, so that viral replication of the YMDD variant HBV is less competent than that of the wild type HBV (Fig. 1c). The marked impairment in the replication competence of HBV bearing the YIDD/YVDD mutations has been demonstrated in transiently

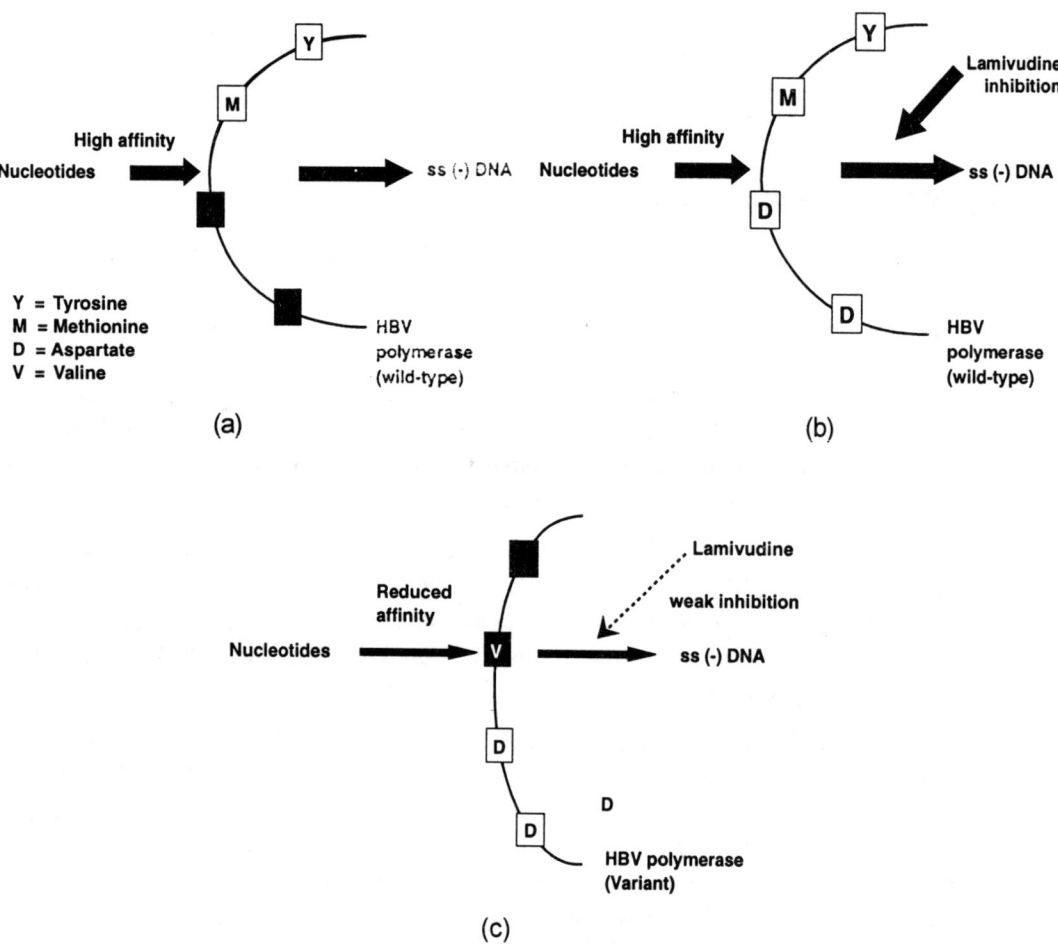

Fig. 1. Diagrammatic representation of the effect of the mutation of the YMDD motif on lamivudine binding and nucleotide affinity.
(Source: Lai CL, Yuen MF, Locarnini S. Treatment of Chronic Hepatitis B. In: Lai CL, Locarnini S, Ed. Hepatitis Virus, IMP, in press)

transfected untreated HCC cell lines, and in HEK 293 human embryo kidney-derived cell lines. These later cell lines require deoxynucleotide depletion with hydroxyurea treatment.[3]

In the multiple centre Asian trial of lamivudine involving 358 patients,[4] 58 Chinese patients continued to receive lamivudine for over 3 years. The incidence of YMDD variant HBV at the end of the first, second, third and fourth years of lamivudine was 16%, 38%, 56% and 67% respectively. Despite the emergence of YMDD variant HBV, the median HBV-DNA level was significantly lower than the pretreatment HBV-DNA level. The median alanine transaminase (ALT) level increased with the development of the variants but remained below the pretreatment level. The lower HBV-DNA levels suggest that the YMDD variant HBV is less replication competent than the wild-type HBV, and the lower ALT levels suggest that the YMDD variant HBV causes less aggressive disease than the wild-type HBV (Fig. 2).

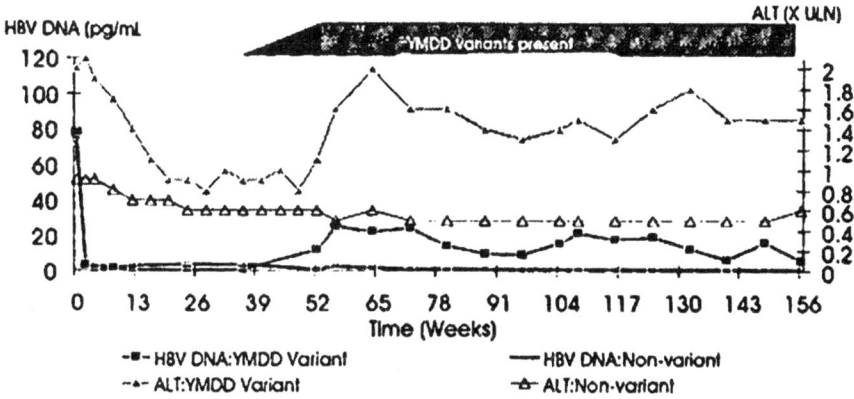

Fig. 2. Median levels for alanine aminotransferase (ALT) and HBV-DNA in patients on long-term lamivudine including 17 patients who have the YMDD variant HBV for at least 3 years and 49 patients without the variant. The ALT levels are expressed as the ratio of the upper limit of the normal range (ULN). (Data from Glaxo Smithkline Laboratories, unpublished.)

Among 81 Chinese patients who had a liver biopsy at the end of third year of lamivudine treatment, 43 patients had YMDD variant HBV, 49% of these patients still had improvement of liver histology while only 23% of patients had worsening of liver histology. The proportion of patients with improvement in histology was similar, irrespective of whether the patients had the YMDD variants for less than one year, for one to two years, or for over two years.

TREATMENT OPTIONS

The majority of patients with normal transaminases may not require treatment other than lamivudine. In patients who develop acute exacerbation after the emergence of YMDD variant, the serum HBV-DNA rises to a peak followed 1–4 weeks later by a peaking in the serum ALT levels. Up to 75% of these patients may develop HBeAg sero-conversion.[5] Other nucleoside analogues are currently under trial for the treatment of chronic hepatitis B. Some of these may be of use in treating the YMDD variant.

The agent most studied to date is adefovir dipivoxil. In a report of 5 patients with the YMDD variant after lamivudine therapy (4 of whom had liver transplantation), 4 patients had a 2–4 $\log_{10}$ reduction in HBV-DNA levels and the fifth patient became negative by quantitative polymerase chain reaction after retransplantation together with hepatitis B immunoglobulin.[6] The main side effect of adefovir dipivoxil is renal toxicity in the form of creatinine elevation or lowering of serum phosphorus. In the 60–120 mg dosage used in previous trials against the human immunodeficiency virus (HIV), these effects are dose-dependent.[7] Trials for HIV-infected patients have been suspended because of these side effects. Currently, a 10 mg dosage is recommended for patients with YMDD variant HBV. The long-term efficacy and toxicity of this low dose of adefovir remains to be elucidated.

There are very few clinical trials on the use of the newer nucleoside analogues in patients with YMDD variants, mainly because most of these agents are still in the relatively early stages of trial. However, there is a reason to believe that at least some of these agents may be efficacious against the YMDD variants. The IC_{50} of entecavir, a guanine nucleoside analogue, against YMDD HBV-DNA polymerase appears to be higher than for the wild-type. B-L-2'-deoxythymidine, the L-enantimer of deoxythymidine, has potent anti-HBV activity and is almost without side effects. Its effects on the YMDD variant are currently being studied. No study has yet been performed using immunomodulators for patients with YMDD variants. It is not known what effects interferon-alpha, in the conventional form or as pegylated interferon, has on the YMDD variants.

CONCLUSIONS

The YMDD variant HBV is less replication competent and less aggressive than the wild-type HBV. Patients who develop the YMDD variants and have acute exacerbations often achieve HBeAg sero-conversion. Though certain novel nucleoside analogues are likely to be effective against these variants, trials are at a comparatively early stage.

The future of therapy for hepatitis B probably lies in combination therapy, of two or more nucleoside analogues or of nucleoside analogues with immunomodulators (Table 1).[8-11] The rapid reduction of HBV-DNA viral load and/or the action of these drugs at different steps

Table 1. Possible agents for combination therapy

Immunomodulators and nucleoside analogues
- *Interferon-α and lamivudine*
  - Preliminary results disappointing. More trials with different timing of interferon-α and lamivudine.
- *Steroid withdrawal and lamivudine*
  - Preliminary results encouraging for patients with low ALT levels. Steroid withdrawal is potentially dangerous and therefore not recommended for routine use.
- *Therapeutic vaccine and lamivudine (under trial)*

Combination of nucleoside analogues*
  - lamivudine
  - adefovir
  - entecavir
  - emtricitabine
  - L-deoxythymidine

* The data on combination of nucleoside analogues are still emerging

of the viral replication cycle may prove to be ultimate treatment for chronic hepatitis B infection.

REFERENCES

1. Allen MI, Deslauriers M, Andrew CW, Tipples GA, Walters KA, Tyrell DLJ, Brown N, et al. Identification and characterization of mutations in hepatitis B virus resistant to lamivudine. *Hepatology* 1998; 27:1670-7.
2. Fisher KP, Gutfreund KS, Tyrrell DL. Lamivudine resistance in hepatitis B: Mechanisms and clinical implications. *Drug Resist Updat* 2001;4:118-28.
3. Mfelegari M, Scaglioni PP, Wands JR. Hepatitis B virus mutants associated with 3TC and famciclovir administration are replication defective. *Hepatology* 1998;27:628-33.
4. Lai CL, Chien RN, Leung NWY, Chang TT, Guan R, Tai DI, Ng KY, et al. A one-year trial of lamivudine for chronic hepatitis B. *N Engl J Med* 1998;339:61-8.
5. Liaw YF, Chien RN, Yeh CT, Tsai SL, Chu CM. Acute exacerbation and hepatitis B virus clearance after emergency of YMDD motif mutation during lamivudine therapy. *Hepatology* 1999;30:567-72.
6. Perrillo R, Schiff E, Yoshida E, Statler A, Hirsch K, Wright T, Gutfreund K, et al. Adefovir dipivoxil for the treatment of lamivudine-resistant hepatitis B mutants. *Hepatology* 2000;32:129-34.
7. Kahn J, Lagakos S, Wulfsohn M, Cherng D, Miller M, Cherrington J, Hardy D, et al. Efficacy and safety of adefovir dipivoxil with anti retro viral therapy. A randomized, controlled trial. *JAMA* 1999;282:2305-12.
8. Shaw T, Locarnini S. Combination chemotherapy for hepatitis B virus: The final solution? *Hepatology* 2000;32:430-2.
9. Tang S, Ho SK, Moniri K, Lai KN, Chai TM. Efficacy of famciclovir in the treatment of lamivudine resistance related to an atypical hepatitis B virus mutant. *Transplantation* 2002;73:148-51.
10. Mutimer D, Feraz-Neto BH, Harrison R, O'Donnell K, Shaw J, Cane P, Prillay D. Acute liver graft failure due to emergence of lamivudine resistant hepatitis B virus: rapid resolution during treatment with adefovir. *Gut* 2001;49:860-3.
11. Bozakaya H, Yurdaydin C, Bozdayi AM, Erkan O, Karyalain S, Uzunalimoglu O. Oral ganciclovir for treatment of lamivudine-resistant hepatitis B virus infection: a pilot study. *Clin Infect Dis* 2002;35:960-5.

49

Steroid priming before interferon therapy for chronic hepatitis B

Debendra N Guhamazumder, Sujit Chaudhuri, Sethu Babu

Chronic hepatitis B virus (HBV) infection is a continuing global public health problem. The aims of therapy of chronic hepatitis B (CHB) are to eradicate the virus, halt necro inflammation, and reduce and/or prevent risk of cirrhosis and development of hepatocellular carcinoma (HCC). Therapy of chronic hepatitis B (CHB) related liver disease remains complex and incomplete even in modern medical practice. Only interferon and lamivudine have been shown to be effective in patients with CHB.

Multiple randomized controlled trials have shown that a 4 to 6 months course of alpha-interferon induces a loss of HBeAg and HBV-DNA from the serum along with a long-term remission in 25–40% of patients.[1] In a meta-analysis of 15 clinical trials, the overall response rate (as measured by the number of patients in whom there was disappearance of HBeAg from serum) was 33% among the patients treated with interferon, as compared with 12% among controls.[2] Two controlled clinical trials in India,[3,4] however, showed higher response rate (50% and 64%) with low-dose, i.e., 3 million units thrice weekly for 4 months when given in properly selected cases. Early studies of interferon therapy in children with chronic hepatitis B in Asia found very low rates of response.[5] However, the majority of these children had normal serum aminotransferase levels, a factor associated with a low rate of response. Later studies indicate that children with chronic hepatitis B and high serum aminotransferase levels respond to interferon at rates similar to those in adults.[6] Various forms of combination therapy have been studied in the hope that additive or synergistic effects of interferon would be noted. One such approach is the combination of corticosteroids with interferon.

The mechanism of liver damage in hepatitis B virus infection is immune-mediated. Immunosuppressive therapy with corticosteroids reduces the immune recognition of infected hepatocytes and reciprocal increase in viral replication and a surge in the HBV-DNA levels. Withdrawal of corticosteroid therapy frequently results in an acute hepatitis-like elevation of serum transaminase levels that are thought to represent an 'immune rebound' against the virus. This enhanced immuologic activity results in transient decline in HBV-DNA and DNA polymerase. The immunologic events after withdrawal of corticosteroids have not been extensively studied and the mechanisms involved are poorly understood. However, corticosteroids enhance the expression of hepatitis B core antigen (HBcAg) and a corticosteroid-induced shift from nuclear to cytoplasmic HBcAg is thought to occur during immune rebound.[7] Theoretically it might permit HBcAg peptides to become associated with cellular membrane and serve as a target for cytotoxic T-cell responses. After a short course of steroid therapy, changes in the host interferon system activity have been studied.[8] There is initial fall of *in vitro* interferon production in peripheral blood lymphocytes during therapy and subsequent recovery of interferon levels on withdrawal of steroids. This change in the host interferon system may appear to promote viral replication in the early phase and the development of acute and transient exacerbation of hepatitis in the post-steroid withdrawal phase, which may lead to HBeAg/anti-HBe sero-conversion in HBeAg positive chronic hepatitis B patients.

Corticosteroids have been tried as monotherapy in chronic hepatitis B, both as a short course therapy[9,10] and as low-dose long-term treatment.[11] These trials showed no beneficial effect with prednisolone therapy. On the contrary, such treatment was found to be harmful particularly in the most severe and advanced cases. Attempts have been made to combine the 'immune rebound' effect of corticosteroids with interferon therapy. Controlled trials have given conflicting results (Table 1). In Perrillo's initial study[12] of prednisolone withdrawal followed by interferon, 44% patients cleared HBeAg compared with 19% of untreated subjects. However, in a large US multi-centric trial comparing the efficacy of interferon alone with corticosteroids priming before interferon, Perrillo et al[13] demonstrated nearly identical rates of HBeAg sero-conversion in the two treatment groups (36% vs. 37%). However, patients with low pre-therapy ALT levels (less than 100 IU per liter) were observed to respond more frequently to the combination regimen as compared to interferon alone (44% vs. 18%). Fevery et al[14] in a similar randomized controlled trial reported that there was no

Table 1. Western data regarding the rate of HBeAg/HBV-DNA clearance by interferon treatment in chronic hepatitis B

	With steroids	Without steroids
Perrillo et al[12]	8/18 (44)	4/21 (19)
Perrillo et al[13]	16/44 (36)	15/41 (37)
Fevery et al[14]	6/15 (40)	4/13 (31)
Krossgaard et al[15]	42/101 (42)	26/99 (26) (p = 0.02)
Gregorio et al[16]	12/34 (35)	12/30 (40)

Figures in parentheses are percentages

improved effect of steroid priming. They observed a tendency to an increased effect of steroid priming in a sub group of patients with ALT level less than 100 IU/l. In a large randomized controlled trial, Krossgaard et al[15] compared the effects of steroid priming in a large number of European patients. In this study, 213 patients were randomized to receive prednisolone or placebo followed by interferon. A significantly higher rate of disappearance of HBeAg was observed in the prednisolone primed group (42% vs. 26%). Prednisolone therapy was more effective in those with higher baseline transaminase values and low HBV-DNA levels. Three of the 22 patients with cirrhosis, one who had received prednisolone, developed hepatic decompensation with a fatal outcome. Gregorio et al[16] examined the efficacy of steroid priming in caucasian children. There was no significant difference between patients with and without steroid pretreatment (35% vs. 40%).

Studies from Asia (Table 2) also showed varying response rates with steroid priming. In the study by Lai et al,[17] 90 asymptomatic HBeAg positive Chinese children, age 2 to 17 years, were randomized to receive recombinant interferon-alpha-2b (5 mIU/m^2 subcutaneously thrice weekly for 16 weeks) 2 weeks after priming with prednisone (0.6 mg/kg/day for 2 weeks, 0.4 mg/kg/day for 2 weeks, 0.2 mg/kg/day for 2 weeks) or placebo tablets or no treatment. All except 8 children (91%) had normal serum ALT levels at entry. A higher proportion of children who received interferon after prednisone priming cleared HBeAg compared to those receiving interferon after placebo priming (13% vs. 3%). However, the response was still far from satisfactory. Children who had elevated pretreatment serum ALT levels responded better. Three (60%) of five treated children with raised serum ALT levels, but only two (4%) of 55 who had normal ALT levels, cleared HBeAg. In another randomized controlled trial in Chinese adults, Lok et al[18] compared the effect of steroid priming in 115 patients with chronic HBV infection who were HBeAg and serum HBV-DNA positive by randomization to one of three groups.[16] Group 1 received oral prednisone in decreasing daily doses of 45 mg, 30 mg, and 15 mg, each for 2 weeks, followed by a 2-week rest, and then 16 weeks of recombinant interferon-alpha-2b in doses of 10 mIU subcutaneously thrice weekly. Group 2 received a 6-week tapered course of placebo tablets followed by a 2-week rest and then 16 weeks of interferon in the same dose regimen. Group 3 received no treatment. Among the interferon-treated patients, prednisone priming did not improve the

Table 2. Asian data regarding the rate of HBeAg/HBV-DNA clearance by interferon treatment in chronic hepatitis B

	With steroids	Without steroids
Lai et al[17]	4/31 (13)	1/29 (3)
Lok et al[18]	9/40 (23)	6/39 (15)
Liaw et al[19]	18/39 (46)	9/37 (24)

Figures in parentheses are percentages

overall response rate (23% vs. 15%). The subgroup of patients with elevated ALT levels had a slightly higher response rate (43% vs. 28%), compared to those who were primed with placebo, but the difference was not statistically significant. In a large study by Liaw et al[19] in Taiwan, 116 male Chinese patients with chronic HBV infection were randomized to receive 4 weeks of prednisolone followed by 2 weeks of no therapy and 12 weeks of IFN-α, placebo and IFN or placebo. After cessation of therapy, clearance of HBeAg was noted in 21% of those who received the combination treatment compared with 5% who received IFN monotherapy throughout the study. Twelve months after cessation of therapy, the response rate had increased to 46% in those who received the combination, 24% in those who received IFN monotherapy and 25% in those who received only placebo. In contrast to the results of previous IFN monotherapy studies, those with low baseline transaminase values (< 200 IU/l) were more likely to respond to the combination approach (48%). In a very recent study from Taiwan, Yeh et al[20] have demonstrated that prednisolone priming modulates the therapeutic effect of IFN to eliminate preferentially the hepatitis B virus pre-core stop mutant.

Cohard et al[21] did a meta-analysis of published data on prednisone priming before interferon therapy in chronic hepatitis B. Two types of meta-analysis were carried out – direct meta-analysis comparing the prednisolone and interferon combination to interferon alone and indirect meta-analysis comparing prednisone and interferon combination to interferon with control results. Direct analysis included seven trials comparing prednisone plus interferon with interferon. No significant differences were observed between the two types of therapy for all the criteria given. However, in patients with low ALT levels, the prednisolone and interferon combination gave significantly better results than interferon alone; HBeAg loss was 48% in comparison to 18.4% with interferon alone. Fifteen trials compared interferon with control values, seven trials of these compared prednisolone plus interferon with control results showing significant improvement in the treated group. Indirect meta-analysis showed that the differences in odds ratios for prednisolone plus interferon / control group and interferon / control group studies were negative for all assessable end points. In conclusion, the use of corticosteroids did not produce any significant increase in the efficacy of interferon treatment with chronic hepatitis B and high initial ALT levels. However, it is possible that corticosteroids increased the HBeAg sero-conversion in the group of patients with low ALT levels.

Recently, role of steroid priming has been evaluated before lamivudine therapy. The HBeAg sero-conversion rate is only 16% after one year of lamivudine monotherapy in large series of Asian patients.[22] Further analysis of this Asian trial by Chien et al[23] has shown that patients with a pretherapy ALT level over five-fold the upper limit of normal (ULN) have a HBeAg sero-conversion rate of 64% which is much higher than a rate of 26% and 5% in patients with a pretherapy ALT of 2 to 5 times of ULN and less than 2 times ULN, respectively ($P<0.001$). To test whether ALT rebound following corticosteroid withdrawal enhances response to lamivudine therapy, a pilot study was conducted by Liaw et al[24] in 30 patients with ALT level less than 5 times ULN. They received 30 mg of prednisolone daily for 3 weeks, 15 mg daily for 1 week, no treatment for 2 weeks and then 150 mg lamivudine daily for 9 months. Clinical rebound with an ALT over 5 times ULN was observed in 20 patients (67%). Of these 20, 12 (60%) showed complete response with normalization of ALT with HBV-DNA clearance and HBeAg sero-conversion. HBeAg sero-conversion was sustained in 70% of patients 3 to 6 months after the end of lamivudine therapy. Immunological assays revealed that the responders showed Th-1 dominant response and higher stimulation index to prednisolone priming. These results suggest that corticosteroid priming induced immune/ALT rebound greatly enhances response to lamivudine therapy in chronic hepatitis B.

In spite of several randomized controlled trials both in the West and in Asia, the role of steroid priming before interferon therapy is still controversial. Recent large scale controlled trials indicate the utility of the combination therapy, but other randomized trials show no significant benefit of steroid priming. Factors that influence the effect of steroid priming may include pretreatment levels of HBV-DNA, serum ALT, activity of hepatitis, dose and duration of steroids, dose, duration and type of IFN, etc.[25, 26] Steroid priming may be useful in a subpopulation of the patients with chronic hepatitis B with ALT level of <100 IU/l. This therapy must be carefully performed due to the potential risk of liver failure. Recent pilot study has shown encouraging results on the role of steroid priming before lamivudine therapy, particularly in patients with low serum ALT levels. Confirmation of this result is necessary by randomized controlled trials.

REFERENCES

1. Hoofnagle JH. Therapy of Viral Hepatitis. *Digestion* 1998;59:563-78.
2. Wong DKH, Cheung AM, O'Rourke K, Naylor CE, Detsky AS, Heathcoat J. Effects of alpha-interferon treatment in patients with hepatitis B e antigen positive chronic hepatitis B: a meta-analysis. *Ann Intern Med* 1993;199:312-23.
3. Sarin SK, Guptan RC, Thakur V, Malhotra S, Malhotra V, Banerjee K, Khandekar P. Efficacy of low-dose alpha-interferon therapy in HBV-related chronic liver disease in Asian Indians: a randomized controlled trial. *J Hepatol* 1996; 24:391-6.
4. Guha Mazumder DN, Chaudhuri S, Konar A, Santra A, Pal B, Sarkar S. Response to low-dose interferon in chronic liver disease due to hepatitis B virus infection *Ind J Gastroenterol* 1998;17:97-9.
5. Lai CL, Lok ASF, Lin HJ, Wu PC, Yeoh EK, Yeung CY. Placebo-controlled trial of recombinant alpha-interferon in Chinese HBsAg-carrier children. *Lancet* 1987;2:877-80.
6. Ruiz-Moreno M, Rua MJ, Molina J, Moraleda G, Moreno A, Garcia-Aguado J, Carreno V. Prospective, randomized controlled trial of interferon-alpha in children with chronic hepatitis B. *Hepatology* 1991; 13:1035-9.
7. Sagnelli E, Manzillo G, Maio G, Pasquale G, Felaco FM, Filippini P, Izzo CM, et al. Serum levels of hepatitis B surface and core antigens during immunosuppressive treatment of HBsAg − positive chronic active hepatitis. *Lancet* 1980;2:395-7.
8. Hirai N, Shimizu M, Morioka T, Hinoue Y, Tanaka N, Kobayashi K, Hattori N, et al. Activities of the interferon system in patients with HBsAg–positive chronic hepatitis B during short-term steroid withdrawal therapy. *Liver* 1988;8:138-45.

9. Rahela J, Redeker AG, Weliky B. Effect of short-term predinsone therapy on aminotransferase levels and hepatitis B markers in chronic type B hepatitis. *Gastroenterology* 1983; 84:956-60.
10. Nair PV, Tong MJ, Stevenson D, Roskamp D, Boone C. Effects of short-term, high-dose prednisone treatment of patients with HBsAg-positive chronic active hepatitis. *Liver* 1985;5:8-12.
11. A trial group of the European Association for Study of the Liver. Steroids in chronic B-hepatitis. A randomized, double-blind, multinational trial on the effect of low-dose, long-term treatment on survival. *Liver* 1986; 6:227-32.
12. Perrillo R, Regenstein FG, Peters MG, De Schryver-Kecskemeti K, Bodicky CJ, Campbell CR, Kuhns MC. Prednisolone withdrawal followed by recombinant alpha-interferon in the treatment of chronic type B hepatitis: a randomized controlled trial. *Ann Intern Med* 1988;109:95-100.
13. Perrillo RP, Schiff ER, Davis GL, Bodenheimer HC, Lindsay K, Payne J, Dienstag JL, et al. A randomized controlled trial of interferon-alpha-2b alone and after prednisolone withdrawal in the treatment of chronic hepatitis B. *N Engl J Med* 1990; 323:295-301.
14. Fevery J, Elewaut A, Michielsen P, Nevens F, Van Eyken P, Adler M, Desmet V. Efficacy of interferon-alpha-2b with or without prednisone withdrawal in the treatment of chronic viral hepatitis B. A prospective double-blind Belgian-Dutch trial. *J Hepatol* 1990;11(suppl):S108-12.
15. Krossgaard K, Marcellin P, Trepo C, Berthelot P, Sanchez-Tapias JM, Bassendine M, Tran A, et al. Prednisolone withdrawal therapy enhances the effect of human lymphoblastoid interferon in chronic hepatitis B. *J Hepatol* 1996;25:803-13.
16. Gregorio CV, Jara P, Hierro L, Diaz C, de la Vega A, Vegnente A, Iorio R, et al. Lymphoblastoid interferon alfa with or without steroid pretreatment in children with chronic hepatitis B: a multicenter controlled trial. *Hepatology* 1996;23:700-07.
17. Lai CL, Lin HJ, Lau JN, Flok AS, Wu PC, Chung HT, Wong LK, et al. Effect of recombinant alpha-2-interferon with or without prednisone in Chinese HBsAg carrier children. *Q J Med* 1991;78:155-63.
18. Lok AS, Wu PC, Lai CL, Lau JY, Leung EK, Wong LS, Ma OC, et al. A controlled tiral of interferon with or without prednisolone priming for chronic hepatitis B. *Gastroenterology* 1992;102:2091-7.
19. Liaw YF, Lin SM, Chen TJ, Chien RN, Sheen IS, Chu CM. Beneficial effect of prednisolone withdrawal followed by human lymphoblastoid interferon on the treatment of chronic type B hepatitis in Asians: a randomized controlled trial. *J Hepatol* 1994;20:175-80.
20. Yeh CT, Sheen IS, Chen TC, Hsieh SY, Chu CM, Liaw YF. Olone modulates the therapeutic effect of interferon to eliminate preferentially the hepatitis B virus precore stop mutant. *J Hepatol* 2000;32: 829-36.
21. Cohard M, Poynard T, Mathurin P, Zarski JP. Prednisone-interferon combination in the treatment of chronic hepatitis B: direct and indirect meta-analysis. *Hepatology* 1994;20:1390-8.
22. Lai CL, Chein RN, Leung NW, Chang TT, Guan R, Tai DI, Ng KT, et al. A one year trial of lamivudine for chronic hepatitis B. *N Engl J Med* 1998;339:61-8.
23. Chien RN, Liaw YL, Atkins M. For the Asian hepatitis lamivudine trial group. Pretherapy alanine aminotransferase level as a determinant for HBeAg sero-conversion during lamivudine therapy in patients with chronic hepatitis B. *Hepatology* 1999;30:770-4.
24. Liaw YF, Tsai SL, Chien RN, Yeh CT, Chu CM. Prednisolone priming enhances Th-1 response and efficiency of subsequent lamivudine therapy in patients with chronic hepatitis B. *Hepatology* 2000;32: 604-9.
25. Yokosuk O. Management of chronic hepatitis B: Role of steroid priming in the treatment of chronic hepatitis B. *J Gastroenterol Hepatol* 2000:15(suppl) E41-5.
26. Akuta N, Suzuki F, Tsubota A, Arase Y, Suzuki Y, Someya T, Kobayashi M. Long-term clinical remission induced by corticosterioid withdrawal therapy (CSWT) in patients with chronic hepatitis B infection: a prospective randomized controlled trial–CSWT with and without follow-up interferon-alpha therapy. *Dig Dis Sci* 2002;47:405-14.

Ribavirin in the management of chronic hepatitis B

V G Mohan Prasad

Interferon-alpha (IFN-alpha) remains the sheet anchor of therapy for chronic hepatitis B today. However, the sero-converstion from HBeAg to anti-HBe happens only in 25–40% of chronic hepatitis B patients treated with interferon-alpha, while the rate of spontaneous remission remains only at 5%.[1] Existence of precore mutation is associated with lower rate of response to interferon-alpha therapy. Even in responders, results were transient.[2] Clearly, better agents or newer approaches are needed to manage chronic hepatitis B.

LAMIVUDINE

Lamivudine (3TC) is well-tolerated, produces a rapid 2 to 3 log reduction in serum HBV-DNA levels in patients with chronic hepatitis B. However, on discontinuing the therapy, HBV-DNA rapidly reappears.[3] Several randomized controlled trials of a 1-year course of lamivudine totaling approximately 1000 patients have been completed by now. Only 17-20% patients show HBeAg sero-conversion, which makes it similar to results of monotherapy with Interferon-alpha.[4,5] While treating precore-mutants, most patients show inhibition of HBV replication and improvement in histology, but almost all of them relapse on discontinuing the therapy.[3] Combination therapy with IFN-alpha and lamivudine does not seem to have any added advantage compared to monotherapy with either agent.[6,7]

When given in a 100 mg daily dose, continuously for 3 years, lamivudine therapy achieved HBeAg sero-conversion in 40% of the 58 Asian patients, but 53% of these patients developed YMDD mutations, indicating that longer the duration of therapy, the frequency of resistant mutants increases.[8]

The long-term clinical significance of lamivudine-resistant mutations is unknown. While on long-term lamivudine therapy, wild type HBV gets suppressed, mutants continue to thrive and immune flares have been reported to be 10-fold more than in those without resistant mutant virus (40% vs. 4%).[9] Severe hepatitis and hepatic decompensation could occur.[10,11]

OTHER AGENTS

While famciclovir, FTC, adefovir dipivoxil have completed or are presently undergoing clinical trials, they are not close to ideal. Famciclovir has week antiviral effects as seen in a large phase III placebo-controlled trial.[12] Efficacy of FTC is only similar to lamivudine.[13] While adefovir dipivoxil may be effective in inhibiting lamivudine-resistant HBV mutants, when used in high doses for long duration, it can be associated with nephrotoxicity.[14]

Most antivirals are effective in viral suppression rather than eradication. This is due to lack of effect on covalently closed circular (ccc) HBV-DNA, which has a long half-life and the loss of ccc DNA is dependent on the elimination of infected hepatocytes.[15] Based on viral kinetic studies, the half-life of infected hepatocytes is estimated to be 10–100 days relatively longer in the immune tolerant patients.[16] Thus viral clearance would require continuous therapy with a potent antiviral agent for a minimum of 1 to 10 years. Costs, adverse events and emergence of drug resistant mutants would not permit such a course.

Immunomodulators

Immunomodulation therapy alone may not be the answer to viral elimination. Patients with chronic HBV infection mount a weak T and B-cell response to a few HBV epitopes, whereas a strong immune response against multiple HBV epitopes would ensure viral clearance as is seen in acute hepatitis B. Current data shows that the present immunomodulation therapy is insufficient to produce an efficient antiviral response and hence is more likely to play role as an adjunct to antiviral therapy. Thus, combination therapy using one or two antivirals and an immunomodulatory agent is needed to improve efficacy and prevent resistance.

Ribavirin

Ribavirin is a broad spectrum, non-interferon inducing virustatic chemotherapeutic agent that demonstrates activity against a broad range of RNA and DNA viruses. Ribavirin is a synthetic antiviral activity after intracellular phosphorylation, without an apparent development of resistance. Primarily ribavirin causes intracellular virustasis of most susceptible viruses, rather than virucidal action or induction of interferon. It plays the role of inhibitor of macrophage pro-inflammatory cytokines and as an immune modulator that preserved the Th-1 and reduced the Th-2 cytokine production.[17] Following are the mechanism of antiviral effect of ribavirin:

(a) Depletion of intracellular pool of GTP via inhibition of inosinate dehydrogenase,
(b) Interruption of viral mRNA synthesis by incorporation of ribavirin metabolites into viral RNA, and
(c) Direct inhibition of the virus encoded RNA polymerase.[18]

Ribavirin and mycophenolic acid are both inhibitors of inosine 5' monophosphate dehydrogenase and cause depletion of intracellular dGTP levels. This action potentiates the antiviral efficacy of guanine-based nucleoside analogues like pencilovir.[19] Ribavirin has a oral bioavailability of 20–50% and 24–39% of the drug is excreted unchanged. Activity requires intracellular phosphorylation. The drug has no protein binding at all. It has a half-life of 2 hours. However, ribavirin is sequestrated in red blood cells with slow release that occurs with a half-life of 6 days, the clinical significance of which is unknown.

Contraindications to usage of ribavirin include pregnancy, hypersensitivity to ribavirin and autoimmune hepatitis.

Adverse effects

The adverse effects are experimental in about 10% patients, usually, while receiving combination with IFN-alpha-2b. These are listed in Table 1.

Table 1. Adverse effects in various trials of ribavirin and interferon combination

CVS	Chest pain
CNS	Dizziness, headache, fatigue, insomnia, depression, impaired concentration and emotional lability
Skin	Alopecia, rash, pruritus
GI	Nausea, anorexia, dyspepsia, vomiting, dysgeusia
Hematological	Anemia, leukopenia
Musculo Skeletal	Myalgia, arthralgia, weakness, rigors
Respiratory	Dyspnea, sinusitis
Miscellaneous	Flu-like syndrome (1 to 10%)
Endocrine	Thyroid test abnormalities

When used as monotherapy for the treatment of chronic hepatitis B, ribavirin brings about virologic and biochemical response in approximately 22% of the patients at the end of therapy.[20, 21] The response rates to combination therapy using interferon-beta in naive patients is also in the same range.[22]

The low response rates with monotherapy necessitated its combination with interferon-alpha. The rationale behind trying this combination is that ribavirin promotes antiviral (Type 1) cytokine expression in human T-cells and thus helps to enhance the antiviral activity of interferon-alpha in the treatment of chronic hepatitis B. Results from a pilot study using the interferon plus ribavirin combination in patients with precore mutant virus infection not responding to interferon show an overall sustained response of 21%.[23] Combination of ribavirin with interferon in chronic hepatitis B e antibody positive patients not only significantly reduced viremia but also induced lasting CD4+ T-cell proliferation and Th-1 cytokine release at the site of infection which might lead to sustained eradication of HBV.[24]

The advantages like tolerability, safety and lack of development of mutants (which is seen commonly with lamivudine) clubbed with the fact that ribavirin suppresses hepatitis B virus replication makes it useful as an adjunctive therapy for chronic hepatitis B. Although the combination of interferon-alpha and ribavirin is safe and well tolerated, the response rates have to be further improved and for this a combination of two or more agents like UDCA and *Phyllanthus amarus* may be considered.

RIBAVIRIN IN CHRONIC HEPATITIS B

The various trials on the use of ribavirin in chronic HBV infection are listed in Tables 2 and 3.

Table 2. Randomized double-blind placebo-controlled trial of ribavirin in chronic HBV infection

Galban-Garcia et al[25]	No. of† patients	ETBR HBeAg	ETVR DNA −ve	ETVR score −ve	Knodell improvement
Placebo (Phase I)	25	0	0	0	13 %
Treatment arm* (Phase II)	25	50%	56%	36%	86.7 %

ETBR – End of treatment biochemical response
ETVR – End of treatment virological response
* Ribavirin 1200 mg/d × 6 months
† Same 25 patients treated with placebo (Phase I) for 6 months and than treated with Ribavirin (Phase II) for next 6 months.

Table 3. Randomized double-blind placebo-controlled trials of ribavirin in chronic HBV infection

Galban-Garcia et al[26]	No. of patients	ETVR HBeAg −ve	ETVR DNA −ve	Knodell score improvement
Placebo	30	6.6%	6.6%	23.3%
Ribavirin 1200 mg/d	30	50%	33.3%	53.3%

Trials of ribavirin with interferon-alpha-2b in chronic hepatitis B e antibody positive patients

Cotonat et el[23] evaluated the efficacy of ribavirin (1200 mg/d) in combination with alpha-interferon (5 mIU three times a week) in patients with anti-HBe +ve status. A total of 24 patients were treated for a period of 12 months and were followed up for a further 12 months period. The results showed that the end of treatment virological response (HBeAg sero-conversion) was seen in 33% along with improvement in Knodell scoring in 50% cases, while a sustained response was achieved in only 21% patients.

Ursodeoxycholic acid

Ursodeoxycholic Acid (UDCA) is an effective agent for the treatment of patients with chronic hepatitis. It has been reported that administration of UDCA changes features of the serum bile acid to be more hydrophilic and that UDCA has a cytoprotective function.[27]

When given as monotherapy for the treatment of chronic hepatitis C, it has been shown to improve transaminase and gamma GT levels and when given in combination with interferon-alpha, it enhances the virological and biochemical efficacy.[28]

Phyllanthus amarus

Phyllanthus amarus is a herb quoted in Indian Ayurvedic literature for more than 2000 years for the treatment of jaundice. *Phyllanthus amarus* inhibits HBV polymerase activity, decreased episomal B virus DNA content and suppressed virus-released into culture medium when tested in HepG2.2.15 cell line. Hepatic HBsAg mRNA levels decreased indicating transcriptional and post-transcriptional down-regulation of trans-gene.[29] *Phyllanthus amarus* also inhibits HBV I enhancer activity which regulates all the four open reading frames of the virus.[30] When 37 HBeAg positive subjects were treated with *Phyllanthus amarus* for 30 days, 59% of patients lost HBsAg when tested 2 to 3 weeks after the therapy compared to 4% in placebo-treated controls, the results being sustained during 9 months follow-up.[31]

Combination therapy

Therapy with interferon-alpha leads to remission of disease in less than one third of patients with chronic hepatitis B. The aim of our pilot study was to assess if the treatment outcome could be improved by adding ribavirin to interferon and other agents.

A total of 21 patients were enrolled, four of them were failure to prior antiviral therapies.. All patients were in the age range of 24 to 70 years, and were HBsAg, HBeAg (except the mutants) and/or HBV-DNA positive with ALT and AST levels of 1.5 to 7 times the upper limit of normal for 6 months or more before induction into the study. Pre-therapy liver biopsies showed chronic active hepatitis in 43 % of patients and compensated cirrhosis in the remaining patients.

Group A had 3 patients who served as controls; Group B had 4 patients who had monotherapy with interferon-alpha-2b; Group C had 5 naïve patients who received interferon with ribavirin and 3 interferon non-responders, who received interferon and ribavirin and another antiviral like lamivudine or famciclovir. Group D had 6 mutants. All 4 groups of patients received refined extract of 3 grams of *Phyllanthus amarus* and 600 mg of UDCA daily throughout the study period.

Results

Of the 3 controls, 1 female cirrhotic lost HBeAg and HBsAg spontaneously while on

Phyllanthus amarus alone over a period of 7 years. The other two had fluctuating levels of enzymes and maintained their viral status during the observation period of upto 3 years.

Group B had 4 patients, all of whom received interferon-alpha-2b thrice weekly as monotherapy. Two patients received IFN 3 mIU, one patient received IFN 5 mIU and the fourth patient received 9 mIU. None of them normalized their ALT or lost the virus.

Group C had four cirrhotics and one patient with chronic hepatitis who were naïve patients put on a combination of interferon 3 mIU three times a week and ribavirin 800 mg per day. All of them lost their HBeAg (100%), 4 out of 5 lost HBV-DNA (80%) and 2 of the 5 who are alive, even lost the HBsAg. Of the 3 patients who died, two died of unrelated causes. The third person who died was positive for HBV-DNA at the end of therapy and died of liver failure three years post-therapy.

Group C also had 3 patients who were interferon non-responders. One patient was put on interferon 3 mIU three times a week with ribavirin 800 mg per day for four months, who completely lost the virus at end of therapy and also lost HBsAg during the follow-up period of 2 years. The other 2 patients were treated with interferon 5 mIU three times a week, ribavirin 1000 mg per day and lamivudine 100 mg per day and both normalized their enzymes at the end of therapy but lost the HBeAg and HBV-DNA during the period of 4 months follow-up on continuing ribavirin and lamivudine. The success rate in this group was 100%.

Group D had 4 patients with HBeAg–negative chronic hepatitis. One of the patients, a 57 years old male cirrhotic treated with interferon and ribavirin in combination, had a good end of therapy biochemical response, but remained positive for HBV-DNA, with enzymes rising over a follow-up period of 4 months. This patient along with two others were put on a combination of Interferon 5 mIU three times a week, ribavirin 1000 mg per day and lamivudine 100 mg per day for 6 months. Only one of the three lost HBV-DNA and normalized the liver enzymes. Of the other two who did not respond, one patient died after 6 months of therapy. A 45-year old male cirrhotic was put on a combination of interferon, ribavirin and famciclovir 100 mg per day who lost the HBV-DNA at the end of therapy, HBV-DNA reappearing 6 months post-therapy. This gives us an end therapy response rate of 50% but sustained response rate of 25% in treating mutants with interferon and even two antivirals. A 52-year old female patient who had HBsAg and HBeAg negative chronic hepatitis successfully lost HBV-DNA under a combination of interferon, lamivudine and ribavirin.

CONCLUSIONS

This pilot study showed poor response in chronic HBV patients who either served as controls or were treated with interferon alone. Naïve patients who received a combination of interferon and ribavirin showed 100% of HBeAg sero-conversion and loss of HBV-DNA to the tune of 80%. Interferon non-responders who were treated with a combination of interferon with two anti-virals showed 100% response (two of the three while continuing on the anti-virals alone for 4 months after the treatment period). The success rates in mutants were disappointing even when two anti-virals were added to interferon. Definitely newer approaches are needed in treating mutant HBV.

REFERENCES

1. Hoofanagle, diBisceglie AM. The treatment of viral hepatitis. *N Engl J Med* 1997;336:347-56.
2. Hadziyannis S, Bramou T, Makris A, Moussoulis G, Zigncol, Pappioanou C. Interferon-alpha-2b – treatment of HBeAg negative/serum HBV-DNA positive chronic active hepatitis type B. *J Hepatol* 1990;11(suppl 1):133-6.
3. Tassopoulos NC, Vopes R, Pastore G, Heathcote J, Buti M, Goodin RP, Hawley S, et al. Efficacy of Lamivudine in patients with Hepatitis B e antigen–negative/HBV-DNA positive (precore mutant) chronic hepatitis B. Lamivudine Precore Mutant Study Group. *Hepatology* 1999;29:889-96.
4. Lai CL, Chein RN, Leung NW, Chang TT, Guan R, Tai Dl, Ng KY, et al. A one year trial of lamivudine for chronic hepatitis B. Asia Hepatitis Lamivudine study Group. *N Engl J Med* 1998;339:61-8.
5. Dienstag JL, Schiff ET, Wright TL, Perrillo RP, Hann HW, Goodman Z, Crowther L, et al. Lamivudine as initial treatment for chronic hepatitis B in United States. *N Engl J Med* 1999;341:1256-63.
6. Heathcote J, Schalm SW, Cianciara J, Farrell G, Feinmann V, Shermann M, Dhillon AP, et al. Lamivudine and Intron A combination treatment in patients with chronic hepatitis B infection. *J Hepatol* 1998;29(suppl 1):43-7.
7. Schiff E, Karalyacin S, Grimm I, Perrillo R, Dienstag J, Husa P, Schalm S, et al. Brown N and the International Lamivudine Investigator Group. A placebo-controlled study of lamivudine and interferon-alpha-2b in patients with chronic hepatitis B who previously failed interferon therapy. *Hepatology* 1998;28:388A.
8. Leung NWY, Lai CL, Chang TT, Guan R, Lee CM, Ng KY, Wu PC, et al. Three year lamivudine therapy in chronic HBV. *J Hepatology* 1999;30(suppl 1):59-64.
9. Liaw YF, Chein RN, Yeh CT, Tsai SL, Chu CM. Acute exacerbation and hepatitis B virus clearance after emergence of YMDD motif mutation during lamivudine therapy. *Hepatology* 1999;30:567-72.
10. Ling R, Mutimer D, Ahmed M, Boxall EH, Eilas E, Dusheiko GM, Harrison TJ. Selection of mutations in the hepatitis B virus polymerase during therapy of transplant recipients with lamivudine. *Hepatology* 1996;24:711-3.
11. Bartholomew MM, Jansen RW, Jaffers LJ, Reddy KR, Johnson LC, Bunzendahl H, Condreay LD, et al. Hepatitis B Virus resistance to lamivudine given for recurrent infection after orthotopic liver transplantation. *Lancet* 1997;349:20-2.
12. deMan RA, Habal F, Marcellin P, Wright R, Rose T, Jurewicz R, Young C. The Famciclovir Hepatitis B study Group. A randomized placebo-controlled study on the efficacy of 12 month famciclovir treatment in patients with chronic HBeAg +ve hepatitis. *J Hepatol* 1999;30(suppl.1):59.
13. Gish RG, Leung NEY, Wright Tl, Tranh H, Robertson AT, Harris JJ, Delehanty JT, et al. Anti-hepatitis B virus (HBV) activity and pharmacokinetics of FTC in a 2 month trial in HBV infected patients. *Gastroenterology*, 1999;116:1216A.
14. Heathcote EJ, Jeffers L, Wright TL, Shermann M, Perrillo R, Sacks S, Carithers R, et al. for the Adefovir Dipivoxil HBV Study Team. Loss of serum HBV-DNA and HBeAg and sero-conversion following short-term (12 weeks) adefovir dipivoxil therapy in chronic hepatitis B: Two placebo-controlled phase II studies. *Hepatology* 1998:28:317A.
15. Moraleda G, Saputelli, J, Aldrich CE, Averett D, Condreay L, Mason WM. Lack of effect of antiviral

therapy in nondividing hepatocyte cultures on the closed circular DNA of woodchuck hepatitis virus. *J Virol* 1997;71:9392-9.
16. Zeuzem S, de Man RA, Honkoop P, Roth WK, Schalm SW, Schmidt JM. Dynamics of hepatitis B virus infection *in vivo*. *J Hepotal* 1997;27:431-6.
17. Ning Q, Brown D, Parodo J. Ribavirin inhibits viral induced macrophage production of tumor necrosis factor, interleukin-1 and procoagulant activity and preserves Th-1 cytokine production, but inhibits Th-2 cytokine response. *Hepatology* 1996;24:355A.
18. Patterson JL, Fernandez–Larson R. Molecular action of ribavirin. *Rev Infect Dis* 1990;12:1132-46.
19. Ying C, De clercq E, Neyts J. Ribavirin and mycophenolic acid potentiate the activity of guanine–and diaminopurine–based nucleoside analogues against hepatitis B virus. *Antiviral Research* 2000;48:2:117-24.
20. Fried MW, Fong TL, Swain MG, Park Y, Beames MP, Banks SM, Hoofnagle JH. Therapy of chronic Hepatitis B with a 6 month course of ribavirin. *J Hepatol* 1994;21:145-50.
21. Jain S, Thomas HC, Oxford JS, Sherlock S. Trial of ribavirin for the treatment of HBsAg positive chronic liver disease. *J Antimicrob Chemother* 1978;4:367-73.
22. Kakumu S, Yoshioka K, Wakita T, Ishikawa T, Takayanagi M, Higashi Y. Pilot study of ribavirin and interferon-beta for chronic hepatitis B. *Hepatology* 1993;18:258-63.
23. Cotonat T, Quiroga JA, Lapez Alcorocho JM, Clouet R, Pardo M, Manzarbeitia F, Carreno V. Pilot study of combination therapy with ribavirin and interferon-alpha for the retreatment of chronic hepatitis B e antibody-positive patients. *Hepatology* 2000;31:502-6.
24. Rico MA, Quiroga JA, Subira D, Castanon S, Esteban JM, Pardo M, Carreno V. Hepatitis B virus – specific T-Cell proliferation and cytokine secretion in chronic hepatitis B e antibody-positive patients treated with ribavirin and interferon-alpha. *Hepatology* 2001;33:295-300.
25. Galban-Garcia E, Vega-Sanchez H, Gra-Oramas B, Doval Hernindez MA, Haedo Castro D, Rolo-Gomez F, Lorenzo Morein I, et al. Role of ribavirin in the treatment of chronic hepatitis B. *J Gastroenterol Hepatol* 2000;23:165-9.
26. Galban-Garcia E, Vega-Sanchez H, Gra-Oramas B, Jorge-Riano JL, Soneiras-Perez S, Haedo-Castro D, Rolo-Gomez F, et al. Efficacy of ribavirin in patients with chronic hepatitis B. *J Gastroenterol* 2000;35:347-52.
27. Higashi K, Saso K, Nomura T. Effect of Ursodeoxycholic acid on serum liver enzymes and bile acid composition of serum and bile inpatients with chronic active hepatitis C. *Hepatology* 1997;26(suppl 1):1778-82.
28. Brunner H, Kopty C, Wiese M. Does additional urso deoxy cholic acid improve the outcome of therapy with interferon-alpha 2b in chronic hepatitis C. *Hepatology* 1997;26(suppl 1):1431-5.
29. Lee CD, Ott M, Thyagarajan SP, Shafritz A, Burk R, Gupta S. Phyllanthus amarus down-regulates hepatitis B virus mRNA Transcription and replication. *Eur J Clin Invest* 1996;26:1069-76.
30. Ott M, Thyagarajan SP, Gupta S. Phyllanthus amarus suppresses hepatitis B virus by interrupting interactions between HBV enhancer I and cellular transcription factors. *Eur J Clin Invest* 1997;27:908-15.
31. Thyagarajan SP, Subramaniam S, Thirunalasundari T, Venkateswaran PS, Bulmberg BS. Effect of *Phyllanthus amarus* on chronic carriers of hepatitis B virus. *Lancet* 1988;2:764-6.

Current status of *Phyllanthus amarus* and other herbal drugs in the treatment of chronic hepatitis B

Sadras P Thyagarajan, Raghu Hari, Sannadi Jayaram, Venkataraman Gopalakrishnan, Preethi Jeyakumar

Nearly 150 phytoconstituents from 101 plants have been claimed to possess hepatoprotective activity.[1,2] Only a few of these hepatoprotective plants as well as their formulations have been pharmacologically evaluated for their efficacy. The constituents of these plants when used clinically are called herbal drugs. In studies done in India and abroad, for hepatoprotective actions of these herbal drugs, only marginal or moderate benefit has been observed. Systematic and detailed investigations have to be done to separate the good ones from the therapeutically useless plants.

The efficacy of very few of these traditional plants against the hepatitis viruses have been studied in the experimental animals. *Phyllanthus amarus*, *Picrorhiza kurroa*, *Glycyrrhiza glabra*, *Eclipta alba* and *Andrographis paniculata* are reported to have activity against the hepatitis B virus.[1,2] "Gomishin" isolated from the Chinese medicinal plant *Schizandra chinensis* is used for the treatment of chronic hepatitis.[3] The plants and its constituents, which exhibit hepatoprotective activity, are described in Table 1.

Even though *Phyllanthus amarus* is shown to be clinically effective, the active constituent is yet to be identified.

METHODS FOR EVALUATION OF EFFICACY OF HEPATOPROTECTIVE PLANTS

Both *in vitro* and *in vivo* test systems are used to assess the hepatoprotective activity of herbal drugs. *In vitro* assays against hepatitis B virus have been proposed by Ono et al, Thyagarajan et al and Lofgren et al. Lofgren et al[5] studied the inhibition of RT enzyme of the duck hepatitis B virus DNA by nucleoside and pyrophosphate analogs. Ono et al[4] standardized the assay to

Table 1. Plants and their constituents having hepatoprotective activity

Plant constituent	Name of the plant
Andrographolide	*Andrographis paniculata*
Silybin	*Silybum marianum*
Picroside I	*Picrorhiza kurroa*
Picroside II	*Picrorhiza kurroa*
Kutkoside	*Picrorhiza kurroa*
Gomishins	*Schizandra chinensis*
Schisandrin A	*Schizandra chinensis*
Glycyrrhizin	*Glycyrrhiza glabra*
Glycyrrhetinic acid	*Glycyrrhiza glabra*
Saikosaponins	*Bupleurum falcatum*
Sarmentosins	*Sedum sarmentosum*
Wuweizisu C	*Schizandra chinensis*
Catechin	*Anacardium occidentalis*
Ursolic acid	*Eucalyptus spp.*
Curcumin	*Curcuma longa*
Fumaric acid	*Sida cordifolia*

study the inhibition of DNA polymerase of hepatitis B virus. A simplified novel assay for the *in vitro* activation of HBsAg has been standardized by Thyagarajan et al.[27]

In vivo models

Toxic chemical induced liver damage by hepatotoxins like CCl_4, paracetamol, thioacetamide, alcohol, D-galactoasamine, allylalcohol, etc. have been administered to induce liver damage in experimental animals. The test substance is administered along with, prior to, or after the toxin treatment. If hepatotoxicity is prevented or reduced, the test substance is considered to be active.

A careful review of the literature on this subject reveals that the extensive research data are restricted mainly to four plants: These include *Silybum marianum, Picrorrhiza kurroa, Glycyrrhiza glabra,* and *Phyllanthus amarus.*

Silybum marianum (Silymarin)

Silybum marianum has been shown to have clinical applications in the treatment of toxic hepatitis, fatty liver, cirrhosis, ischemic injury, radiation hepatitis, and viral hepatitis through its antioxidative, anti-lipid peroxidative, antifibrotic, anti-inflammatory, immunomodulating, and liver regenerating effects.[6]

The following sections summarize the existing literature and data on important herbal plants as potential treatment modalities for acute and chronic liver diseases.

Glycyrrhiza glabra

Glycyrrhizin has been identified as the active principle of *Glycyrrhiza glabra*. Glycyrrhizin has also been found to have anti-viral properties through endogenous interferon induction as well as hepatocytoprotective effect.[7-9] Endogenous interferon induction by glycyrrhizin have been documented both in mice[7] as well as humans.[10] Clinical trials in sub-acute hepatic failure and fulminant hepatic failure using glycyrrhizin have shown some improvement in the patient survival in anecdotal studies. However, antiviral effects in chronic hepatitis B are not significant. Clinical trials using glycyrrhizin among patients with chronic hepatitis due to HCV have documented normalisation or decrease in ALT values.[11-13] Glycyrrhizin has also been shown to slightly inhibit RNA viruses through a hitherto unknown mechanism.[14] Glycyrrhizin is a safe drug with minimal side effects.

Picrorhiza kurroa

Picroside 1 and 2, catapol, kutkoside I, and kutkoside have been identified as major bioactive components of *Picrorhiza kurroa*.[15,16] *Picrorhiza kurroa* (Pk), a known hepatoprotective plant, has been studied in experimental as well as in clinical studies. Basic research has been carried out on the whole plant, picroside 1 alone, and on picroliv which contains picroside 1, catapol, kutkoside I and kutkoside.

Dwivedi et al[17-19] have shown significant hepatoprotective properties of Picroliv using models like monocrotaline induced hepatic damage in rats, thioacetamide induced hepatic damage in rats, and also against carbon-tetrachloride induced liver damage in rats. Shukla et al[20] comparing Picroliv with Silymarin in rat and guinea pig models have shown potent choleretic and anticholestatic functions. Chander et al[21] evaluating the hepatoprotective activity of Picroliv in *Mastomys natalensis* infected with *Plasmodium berghei* have shown significant reduction of biochemical parameters of liver function and decrease in the levels of lipid peroxides and hydroperoxides and facilitated the recovery of superoxide dismutase and glycogen. However, picroliv did not have any effect on the degree of parasitemia.

Mehrotra et al[16] using *in vitro* HBsAg binding assay have shown HBsAg inhibition in Picroliv and its major component, catapol. Pandey et al[22,23] and Atal et al[24] have shown anti-inflammatory and immuno-modulating potentials of *Picrorhiza kurroa* stimulating both cell-mediated and humoral immunity. Jayaram et al[25] in their Ph.D. thesis entitled "Studies on prevention and control of hepatitis B virus infection" have conducted a double blind clinical trial on four groups of subjects with chronic HBV infection (40 subjects in all) who were treated under code with *Phyllanthus amarus*, *Picrorhiza kurroa*, a combination of *P. amarus* and *P. kurroa* with the fourth group being treated with lactose used as a placebo. After six months regimen of treatment with 500 mg oral capsules given thrice daily, the HBsAg clearance rate was 25% in the *P. amarus* treated group, 11.1% in the combination treatment while none cleared in *P. kurroa* alone and placebo treated groups. HBeAg sero-conversion was seen in 57.1% of *P. amarus* treated patients followed by 33% in the combination treatment group, 28.5% of *P. kurroa* group, and 16% in the placebo group.

Phyllanthus amarus

Even though the clinical uses of *P. niruri* and other species, viz. *P. amarus* have been cited for over a century in the Ayurveda and Siddha literatures, studies evaluating its efficacy in the treatment of viral hepatitis have been attempted only during the last 50 years. A logical approach towards identification of the active principles of *P. amarus* is to fractionate the plant extracts and identify biologically active compounds and to chemically characterize them.

The first ever designed *in vitro* study on *Phyllanthus niruri* against any hepatitis virus with HBV as a model was reported by Thyagarajan in 1979[26] from Chennai, India. Subsequently, Thyagarajan et al[27] have shown the whole plant extract of *P. niruri* brought about binding of hepatitis B surface antigen (HBsAg) through several solvents. This plant from Tamilnadu, India was later identified taxonomically by Unander as *P. amarus*. Venkateswaran et al[28] and Blumberg et al[29] from United States in *in vitro* studies using *P. amarus* plant obtained from Chennai, India have shown that the aqueous extracts of the plants bound the surface antigen of HBV and inhibit the DNA polymerase (DNAp) of HBV and woodchuck hepatitis virus (WHV). When administered intraperitoneally to WHV infected woodchucks, acutely infected animals lost the surface antigen and the surface antigen titer dropped in some chronically infected animals. The rate of occurrence of liver cancer was lower in treated animals than in the untreated controls.

Yanagi et al[30] from Japan have reported that aqueous extracts of high dilutions of *P. amarus* collected from South India inhibited HBV DNAp, DNApI, T4-DNAp, the Klenow fragment, and reverse transcriptase of avian mycloblastosis virus. Shead et al[31] from Australia have shown the aqueous extracts to inhibit the endogenous DNAp of DHBV at high dilutions. Niu et al[32] from Australia in collaboration with Thyagarajan from India using *P. amarus* collected from Chennai, Tamilnadu, have shown that the treatment of 4–5 week old ducks congenitally infected with duck hepatitis B virus (DHBV) for 10 weeks transiently reduces viral DNA in the serum. However, there is no effect on the level of HBV-DNA or presence of surface antigen in the liver.

Jayaram et al[33] reported, that the treatment of PLC/PRF/5 (Alexander) cell line with 1 mg/ml concentration of *P. amarus* as a single dose inhibits the HBsAg secretion by the cell lines. Lee et al[34] from USA in collaboration with Thyagarajan have shown that *P. amarus* down-regulates hepatitis B virus mRNA transcription and replication using transgenic mice and transgenic cell lines. Ott et al[35] has shown that the cellular and molecular mechanisms of HBV suppression of *P. amarus* are due to inhibition of interactions between HBV enhancer I and cellular transcription factors.

The biosafety studies on *P. amarus* date back to 1971 when Mokkhasmit et al[36] from Thailand using *P. niruri* (10g/hg) reported it to be non-toxic to mice. Rao[37] from Andhra Pradesh, India reported that 20% aqueous extract of *P. niruri* is effective as an oral pretreatment of 0.2 ml/100 mg body weight against CCl_4 induced hepatotoxicity in rats. Syamasundar et al[38] from Uttar Pradesh, India showed the hexane extracted compounds phyllanthin and hypophyllanthin reduced CCl_4 or galatosamine induced cytotoxicity in cultured rat hepatocytes. Jayaram et al[39] from Chennai, India, using the aqueous extract of dried whole plant showed no chronic toxicity in mice at a dose of 0.2 mg per day per animal for 90 days as revealed by physiological, biochemical, and histopathological parameters. There was also no cytotonic or cytotoxic changes when tested in a tissue culture model using vero cell line. Venkateswaran et al[40] from USA demonstrated its *in vivo* safety using woodchucks as animal models, while Niu et al[33] from Australia have shown *P. amarus* to be non toxic in Pekin ducks chronically infected with duck hepatitis B virus. Jayaram and Thyagarajan[41] studying the effect of *P. amarus* on β-galactosamine induced hepatotoxicity on isolated rat hepatocytes have shown that (a) *P. amarus* by itself is not hepatotoxic to rat hepatocytes, (b) at 1 mg/ml concentration, the aqueous extract was shown to protect isolated rat hepatocytes from β-galatosamine induced hepatotoxicity.[42]

In the traditional medicine systems, there have been several formulatory medicines for the treatment of jaundice in general without taking into consideration their etiology. *P. niruri* is one of the constituents of such these multiherbal preparations containing upto 12 medicinal herbs. Most of the treatment evaluation of such preparations was based only on clinical improvement.

It was in this context, Thyagarajan and his collaborators, conducted two open clinical trials in cases with acute viral hepatitis. Till date, seven clinical trials are available (two of them being double blind trials and the others Phase I/II open trials) in patients with chronic HBV infection (Table 2). Jayanthi et al[43] in a controlled clinical trial in acute viral hepatitis (AVH) using *P. niruri*, on one arm, and other herbal medicines in the other group have shown that *P. niruri* significantly decreases transaminases after two weeks of treatment in patients with HBsAg positive as well as HBsAg negative disease. In a clinical trial on patients with acute viral hepatitis, Geetha et al[43] have shown that (a) *P. amarus* treatment brings about significantly faster biochemical normalcy in both acute hepatitis A and B; (b) there is a higher rate of HBsAg clearance in *P. amarus* treated patients with acute viral hepatitis B, and (c) there are no side effects due to *P. amarus* treatment. In an Indian study done by Narendranathan et al[44] it was observed that *P. amarus* powder did not significantly reduce the duration of jaundice in patients with acute HBV infection.

Thyagarajan et al reported in 1988,[45] 59% HBsAg clearance in the *P. amarus* treated group, as against 4% in the placebo group. In another open trial thus showed 20% HBsAg clearance and 63.6% loss of infectivity indicated by HBeAg sero-conversion.[46] In summary, these trials (Table 2) have shown a mean HBsAg clearance rate of 25.6% and mean HBeAg sero-conversion rate of 55.3%. On the other hand, investigators from other countries like Leelarasamee et al,[47] Wang et al,[48] Milne et al[49, 49a] and Thamilkutil et al[55] have reported the non-reproducibility of treatment efficacy by *P. amarus* grown in their respective countries. A single clinical trial done by Doshi et al[54] in India also failed to reproduce the same beneficial effect. In the light of these studies, it has become necessary to explain the reasons for non-reproducibility of the clinical efficacy of *P. amarus*. It is necessary to conduct further clinical trials independently in different places using the *P. amarus* preparation from Chennai, India (Table 2).

There can be many explanations for the discrepant results. *Phyllanthus amarus*, which belongs

Table 2. Summary of seven clinical trials on subjects with chronic HBV infection using *P. amarus* grown in Tamil Nadu ("University preparation")

Authors (year)	Dose (mg/t.i.d)	Duration	Number treated		HBsAg clearance (%)		HBeAg sero-conversion (%)	
			Test	Placebo	Test	Placebo	Test	Placebo
Published								
Thyagarajan et al (1988)	200	1 m	40	38	59	4	ND	ND
Thyagarajan et al (1990)	250	3 m	20	Nil	20	–	63.6	–
Unpublished								
Samuel B et al (1991)	250	2 m	10	12	20	8.3	37.5	0
Thyagarajan et al (1992)	250	6 m	72	Nil	25	-	54.0	-
Thyagarajan et al (1993)	500	3 m	8	8	25	0	71.4	16.0
Walker E et al (1993-95)	500	4–6 m	26	Nil	11.6	-	45.4	-
Thyagarajan et al (1996-97)	500	6 m	37	Nil	18.9	-	60.0	-
TOTAL			213	58	25.6	3.4	55.3	1.7

ND – Not done

to the family Euphorbiaceae, consists of nearly 400 species. In all the trials conducted earlier, the authors have not clarified that which of the chemo-biologically bio-typed variety of the *Phyllanthus* species was used. It has also been observed that intraspecies variation and intergeographical variation has been observed in *Phyllanthus* species. Therefore, selection of the right species and the chemobiologically fingerprinted biotype of *Phyllanthus* species is of utmost importance in obtaining the enhanced clinical response. Secondly, the dosage given to the patients is important. Leelarasamee et al[47] used a higher dose of 1200 mg per day for the patients, the duration of the treatment was however only for a period of thirty days. Till date, no assay to quantify the half-life of the herbal drug has been reported.

MECHANISM OF ACTION OF PHYLLANTHUS

Thyagarajan et al[27] demonstrated that the extracts of *Phyllanthus amarus* produce consistent inhibition of HBV in *in vitro* studies. The extracts were capable of eliminating the virus from the serum of woodchucks as well. Studies done by Unander et al,[52] Jayaram et al,[33] Yanagi et al,[30] Mehrotra et al,[16] Ogata et al[53] and Shead et al[31] have confirmed that *Phyllanthus amarus* is able to inhibit the HBV virus replication as well as reverse transcriptase and DNA polymerase.

Niu et al[32] were, however, unable to demonstrate any significant reduction of circulating viral DNA in ducks congenitally infected with HBV. Such discrepant findings can be attributed to a combination of factors, like variations in the plant material or animal species, period and place where the botanical samples were collected, age of the plants, and also the part of the plant that was used.

Recently, Ott et al reported the mechanisms of action of *P. amarus* by suppression of HBV by a specific mechanism of interrupting the interaction between HBV enhancer I and cellular transcription factors.[35] The same authors[34] give further support to the antiviral mechanism of action for *P. amarus* extract by demonstrating disruption by the HBV polymerase activity and mRNA transcription, and replication by the active principle of the plant. Although the chemical constituent present in the plants belonging to the genus *Phyllanthus* responsible for its action is not properly defined, it is believed that the hydrolyzed tannins mainly ellagic acid, might account for the beneficial effects of *Phyllanthus*.[55] In another study, hydrolysable tannins isolated from *P. amarus* have been found to be potent inhibitors of rat liver cyclic AMP-dependent protein kinase catalytic subunit, with IC_{50} values ranging from 0.2 to 1.7 υm.[56]

REFERENCES

1. Doreswamy R, Sharma D. Plant drugs for liver diseases management. *Indian Drugs* 1995;32:139-44.
2. Handa SS, Sharma A, Chakraborty KK. Natural products and plants as liver protecting drugs. *Fitoterapia* 1989;57:307-51.

3. Wang M, Lajrange L, Tao J. Hepatoprotective properties of Silybium marianum herbal preparation on ethanol induced liver damage. *Fitoterapia* 1996;67:166-71.
4. Ono K, Nakane H, Meng ZM, Ose Y, Sakai Y, Mizuno M. Differential inhibitory effects of various herb extracts on the activities of reverse transcriptase and various deoxyribonucleic acid (DNA) polymerases. *Chem Pharm Bull (Tokyo)* 1989;37:1810-2.
5. Lofgren B, Nordenfelt E, Oberg B. Inhibition of RNA and DNA dependent duck hepatitis B virus DNA polymerase activity by nucleoside and pyrophosphate analogs. *Antiviral Res* 1989;12:310-4.
6. Luper S. A review of plants used in the treatment of liver disease: Part 1. *Altern Med Rev* 1998;3:410-21.
7. Abe N, Ebina T, Ishida N. Interferon induction by glycyrrhizin an glycyrrheticinic acid in mice. *Microbiol Immunol* 1982;26:535-9.
8. Shiki Y, Shirai K, Saito Y, Yoshida S, Mori Y, Wakashin M. Effect of *glycyrrhizin* of glycyrrhizin on lysis of hepatocyte membranes induced by antiviral cell membrane antibody. *J Gastroenterol Hepatol* 1992;7:12-6.
9. Nagai T, Egashira T, Kudo Y, Yamanka Y, Shimada T. Attenuation of dysfunction in the ischemia reperfused liver by Glycyrrhizin. *Jpn J Pharmacol* 1992;58:209-18.
10. Shinada M, Azuma M, Kawai H, Sazaki K, Yoshida I, Yoshida T, Suzutani T, et al. Enhancement of interferon gamma production in glycyrrhizin treated human peripheral lymphocytes in response to concanavalin A and to surface antigen of hepatitis B virus. *Proc Soc Exp Biol Med* 1986;181:205-10.
11. Fujisawa K, Watanabe H, Kimata K. Therapeutic approach to chronic active hepatitis with gycyrrhizin. *Asian Med J* 1973;23:745-6.
12. Suzuki H, Ohta Y, Takino T, Fujisawa K, Hirayama C. Effects of glycyrrhizin on biological test in patients with chronic hepatitis : a double blind trial. *Asian Med J* 1983;26:423-38.
13. Yasuda K, Hino K, Fujioka S, Kouki K, Fukuhara A, Nashida Y, et al. *Effects of high-dose therapy with stronger neominophagen C (SNMC) on hepatic histigraphy in non-A, non-B chronic active hepatitis.* In: Shikata T, Purcell RH, Vchida T, Eds. Viral hepatitis C, D and E: Elsevier Science Publication, 1991; pp.205-9.
14. Pompei R, Flore O, Marcialis MA, Pani A, Loddo B. Glycyrrhizin acid inhibits virus growth and inactivates virus particles. *Nature* 1979;281:689-90.
15. Vaidya AB, Antarkar DS, Doshi JC, Bhatt AD, Ramesh V, Vora PV, Perissond D, et al. Picrorhiza kurroa (Kutaki) Royle ex Benth as a hepatoprotective agent – experimental and clinical studies. *J Postgrad Med* 1996;42:105-8.
16. Mehrotra P, Rawat S, Kulshreshtha DK, Patnaik GK, Dhawan BN. *In vitro* studies on the effect of certain natural products against hepatitis B virus. *Ind J Med Res* 1990;92:133-8.
17. Dwivedi Y, Rastogi R, Sharma SK, Mehrotra R, Garg NK, Dhawan BN. Picroliv protects against monocrotaline – induced hepatic damage in rats. *Pharmacol Res* 1991;23:399-407.
18. Dwivedi Y, Rastogi R, Sharma SK, Garg NK, Dhawan BN. Picroliv affords protection against thioacetamide-induced hepatic damage in rats. *Plants Med* 1991;57:25-8.
19. Dwivedi Y, Rastogi R, Chander R, Sharma SK, Kapoor NK, Garg NK, Dhawan BN. Hepatoprotective activity of picroliv against carbon tetrachloride induced liver damage in rats. *Ind J Med Res* 1990;92:195-200.
20. Shukla B, Visen PK, Patnaik GK, Dhawan BN. Choleretic effect of picroliv, the hepatoprotective principle of Picrorhiza kurroa. *Planta Med* 1991;57:29-33.
21. Chander R, Dwivedi Y, Rastogi R, Sharma SK, Garg NK, Kapoor NK, Dhawan BN. Evaluation of hepatoprotective activity of picroliv (from Picrorhiza kurroa) in Mastomys natalensis infected with Plasmodium berghei. *Ind J Med Res* 1990;92:34-7.
22. Pandey BL, Das PK. Immunopharmacological studies on Picrorhiza kurroa Royle-Ex-Benth. Part IV: Cellular mechanisms of anti-inflammatory action. *Ind J Physiol Pharmacol* 1989;33:28-30.

23. Pandey BL, Das PK. Immunopharmacological studies on picrorohiza kurroa Royle-Ex-Benth. Part V: Anti-inflammatory action: relation with cell types involved in inflammation. *Ind J Physiol Pharmacol* 1988;32:289-92.
24. Atal CK, Sharma ML, Kaul A, Khajuria A. Immunomodulating agents of plant origin. I: Preliminary screening. *J Ethnopharmacol* 1986;18:133-41.
25. Jayaram S. Studies on prevention and control of Hepatitis B virus infection. Ph.D. Thesis, University of Chennai, June 1992.
26. Thyagarajan SP. Studies on hepatitis B virus infection in Tamil Nadu, laying special emphasis on the immunological and biochemical markers with an assessment on the antiviral properties of certain indigenous drugs. Thyagarajan SP. Ph.D. Thesis, University of Chennai, 1979.
27. Thyagarajan SP, Thiruneelakandan K, Subramaniam S, Sundaravelu T. In vitro activation of HBsAg by Eclipto Alba, Hassk: and Phyllanthus niruri Linn. *Ind J Med Res* 1982;76(suppl):124-30.
28. Venkateswaran PS, Millman I, Blumberg BS. Effect of an extract from P. niruri on Hepatitis B and Woodchuck Hepatitis B virus: in vitro and in vivo studies. *Proc Natl Acad Sci USA* 1987;84:274-78.
29. Blumberg BS, Millman I, Venkateswaran PS, Thyagarajan SP. Hepatitis B virus and primary hepatocellular carcinoma: treatment of HBV carriers with Phyllanthus amarus. Cancer Detection and Prevention 1989:14:195-202. CRC Press, Inc. Bocaraton, FL. USA.
30. Yanagi M, Unoura M, Kobayashi K, Hattori N, Murakami S. *Inhibitory effect of an extract from Phyllanthus niruri on reaction of endogenous HBV-DNA Polymerase and other DNA synthetases*. In: Abstracts of papers presented at the 1989 meeting on Hepatitis B Viruses. September. 25-28, 1989. Cold spring Harbor laboratory, Cold spring Harbor, New York, 1989;77.
31. Shead A, Vickery K, Medurst R, Freiman J, Cossart Y. *Neutralisation but not cure of Duck Hepatitis B by Australian Phyllanthus extracts. Abstracts 602. In:* Scientific program and abstract volume, the 1990 International Symposium on Viral Hepatitis and Liver Diseases, April 4-8, 1990, Houston, Texas.
32. Niu Jianzhang, Yanyan Wang, Ming Qiao, Eric Gowans, Patrick Edwards, Thyagarajan SP, Ian Gust, et al. Effect of Phyllanthus amarus on Duck Hepatitis B virus replication *in vivo. J Med Virol* 1990;32:212-21.
33. Jayaram S, Thyagarajan SP. Inhibition of HBsAg secretion from Alexander cell line by Phyllanthus amarus. *Ind J Pathol Microbiol* 1996;39:211-5.
34. Lee CD, Ott M, Thyagarajan SP. Sharfritz DA, Burk RD, Gupta S. Phyllanthus amarus down regulates hepatitis B virus mRNA transcription and replication. *European J Clin Invest* 1996;26:1069-76.
35. Ott M, Thyagarajan SP, Gupta S. Phyllanthus amarus suppresses Hepatitis B virus by interrupting interactions between HBV enhancer I and cellular transcription factors, European. *J Clin Invest* 1997;27: 908-15.
36. Mokkhasmit M, Swasdimongkol K, Satrawaha P. Study on toxicity of Thai medicinal plants. Bulletin of the Department of Medical Science, 12;36-65. Abstract R – 001 from NAPRALERT, College of Pharmacy, University of Illinois – Chicago, Chicago, IL 1971.
37. Rao YS. Experimental production of Liver damage and its protection with Phyllanthus niruri, Capprris spinosa (both ingredients of Liv-52), in White albino rats. *Probe* 1985;117-9.
38. Syamasunder KV, Singh B, Thakur RS, Hussain A, Kiso Y, Hikino H. Anti hepatotoxic principles of Phyllanthus niruri herbs. *J Ethno Pharmacol* 1985;14:117-9.
39. Jayaram S, Thyagarajan SP, Madanagopalan N. Anti hepatitis B virus properties of Phyllanthus niruri Linn and Eclipta Alba Hassk: In vitro and In vivo safety studies. *Biomedicine* 1987;7:9-16.
40. Venkateswaran PS, Millman I, Blumberg BS. Effect of an extract from P. *niruri* on hepatitis B and woodchuck hepatitis B virus: in vitro and in vivo studies. *Proc Natl Acad Sci USA* 1987;84:274-8.
41. Jayaram S, Udayashankar K, Rajendran P, Thyagarajan SP. Anti hepatotoxicity potentials of Phyllanthus amarus : an in vitro study using isolated rat hepatocyte cultures. *Ind J Med Microbiol* 1994;12:248-51.

42. Jayanthi V, Madanagopalan N, Thyagarajan SP, Balakumar V, Parimalam, Malathi S. Value of Herbal Medicines, Phyllanthus niruri, Eclipta alba, Piper Longus, Thippili (Tamil) and combination of Phyllanthus niruri and Ricinus communis (Icterus-Pharm Products) in acute viral hepatitis. *J Gastroenterol Hepatol* 1988;3:533-4.
43. Geetha J, Manjula R, Malathi S, Usha K, Chari ST, Raghuram K, Thyagarajan SP, et al. Efficacy of "Essential Phospholipid substance" of Soya bean oil and Phyllanthus niruri in acute viral Hepatitis. *J Gen Med* 1992;4:53-8.
44. Narendranathan M, Remla A, Mini PC, Satish P. A trial of Phyllanthus amarus in acute viral hepatitis. *Trop Gastroenterol* 1999;20:164-6.
45. Thyagarajan SP, Thirunalasundari T, Subramanium S, Nammalwar BR, Madanagopalan N, Prabha V. Effect of Phyllanthus niruri on hepatitis B surface antigen carriage: A double blind clinical trial Proceedings of Asian Pacific Associations for the study of the liver – Sixth biennial Scientific meeting, New Delhi 1988;A145.
46. Thyagarajan SP, Jayaram S, Valliammai T, Madanagopalan N, Pal VG, Jayaraman K. Phyllanthus amarus and hepatitis B. *Lancet* 1990;336:949-50.
47. Leelarasamee A, Trakulsomboon S, Maunwongyathi P, Somanabandhu A, Pidctcha P, Motrakool B, Labnak T, et al. Failure of Phyllanthus amarus to eradicate hepatitis B surface antigen from symptomless carriers. *Lancet* 1990;335:1600-1.
48. Wang MX, Meng L, Zhao G, Zhao S, Mai K. Phyllanthus cannot eliminate HBsAg in chronic hepatitis B virus infection. *Hepatology* 1991;21:22.
49. Milne A, Hopkrik N, Lucas CR, Waldon J, Foo Y. Failure of New Zealand hepatitis B carriers to respond to Phyllanthus amarus. *N Z Med J* 1994;107:243.
49a. Mc Culloch M. Broffman M, Gao J, Cofford JM, Jr. Chinese herbal medicine and interferon in the treatment of chronic hepatitis B: a meta-analysis of randomized, controlled trials. *Am J Public Health* 2002;92:1619-28.
50. Thamilikitkul V, Wasuwat S, Kanchanapee P. Efficacy of P. amarus for eradication of hepatitis B virus in chronic carriers. *J Med Assoc Thai* 1991;74:381-5.
51. Doshi JC, Vaidya AB, Antarkar DS, Deolahkar R, Antari DH. A two-stage clinical trial of Phyllanthus amarus in hepatitis B carriers; failure to eradicate the surface antigen. *Ind J Gastroenterol* 1994;13:7-8.
52. Unander DW, Webster GL, Blumberg BS. Records of usage in Phyllanthus (Euphorbiaceae). In sub genera Isocladus, Kirganelia, Cioca and Emblica. *J Ethno Pharmacol* 1990;30:233-64.
53. Ogata T, Higuchi H, Mochida S, Matsumoto H, Kato A, Endo T, Kaji A, et al. HIV-I reverse transcriptase inhibitor from Phyllanthus niruri. *Aids Res Hum retroviruses* 1992;8:1937-44.
54. Wang BE. Treatment of chronic liver diseases with traditional Chinese medicine. *J Gastroenterol Hepatol* 2000;15:E67-70.
55. Zhang JT. New drugs derived from medicinal plants. *Therapie* 2002;57:137-50.
56. Polya GM, Wang BH, Coo LY. Inhibition of signal-regulated protein kinases by plant derived hydrolysable tannins. *Phytochemistry* 1995;38:307-14.

52

Combination therapy for chronic hepatitis B

George K Lau, Xunrong Luo

Chronic hepatitis B virus (HBV) infection is one of the most common viral infections in humans affecting over 300 million individuals, or 5% of the world's population. It is of particular concern in the Asia-Pacific areas where the infection is highly prevalent. Of the chronic HBV patients, around 25–40% will eventually die of liver disease (i.e., cirrhosis with or without hepatocellular carcinoma); the death rate being 50% for male patients and 15% for female patients.[1] To date, in China, only interferon, thymosin-α1 and lamivudine monotherapy have been approved for the treatment of chronic HBV infection. Other treatment modalities currently undergoing investigation include DNA vaccines, therapeutic vaccines,[2,3] antigen-antibody complexes,[4] adoptive immune transfer,[5,6] traditional chinese medicine (TCM)[7,8] and new nucleoside or nucleotide analogues such as adefovir dipivoxil,[9,10] emtricitabine[11] and entacavir.[12] Moreover, in order to enhance therapeutic effect, combination therapy with immunomodulatory agents plus nucleoside analogues[13,14] or dual nucleoside analogues, are being explored. It is likely that in the future, treatment of chronic HBV infection will be tailored made to the individual virological, histological, and clinical profile based on the understanding of the natural history of chronic HBV infection.[14]

NATURAL HISTORY OF CHRONIC HBV INFECTION AND AIM OF TREATMENT

The clinical management of chronic HBV infection is best approached from an understanding of the natural history of the disease[14] (Fig. 1). The natural history of chronic HBV infection in Chinese is characterized by an initial active viral replicative state with minimal liver damage (immune tolerance phase). This period can last for over 2–3 decades. The patient then enters the phase of "immunoelimination" which is associated with decreasing viral burden, fluctuations of serum alanine aminotransferase (ALT) levels ("hepatitic flares"), and the appearance of significant necroinflammatory disease within the liver. A subset of these individuals "clear" HBeAg from the serum and enter into the third phase of the chronic HBV infection state

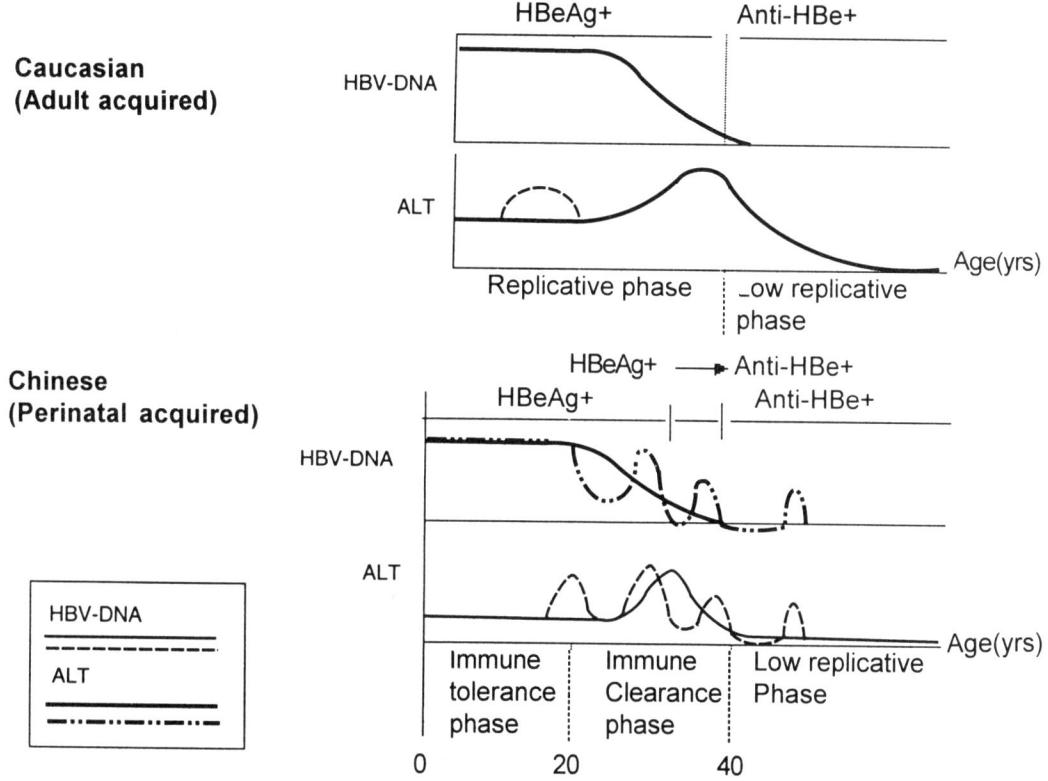

Fig. 1. Natural history of chronic HBV infection in Chinese and caucasian.

known as "latency", typically characterized by persistent HBsAg, very low levels of HBV-DNA (only second-round PCR positive) and essentially normal serum ALT. In contrast, a subgroup of individuals have ongoing liver disease activity and are HBV-DNA positive by at least first-round PCR. This latter group have developed HBeAg negative chronic HBV infection, with persistent ongoing active viral replication, and are usually infected with the pre-core mutant form of HBV.[15] Patients can also present to the liver clinic with clinical cirrhosis and be infected with either "wild-type" HBV (i.e., HBeAg positive) or pre-core mutant HBV (i.e., HBeAg negative).

From immunological studies, the vigour of the cytotoxic T-cell response to HBV is found to be the principal determinant of viral clearance/suppression in HBV infected patients. The T-cell response to the HBV is vigorous, polyclonal, and multispecific in acutely infected patients who successfully clear the virus with loss of HBeAg/HBsAg, and relatively weak and narrowly focussed in chronically infected patients, who remain HBeAg and HBsAg positive.[16] In addition, it is now known that very low levels of HBV-DNA, detectable only by nested polymerase chain reaction (PCR), are present in the serum and peripheral blood mononuclear cells for several decades following complete clinical and serological resolution of diseases. This, together with the presence of CD69+ (marker of recent activation) cytotoxic T-lymphocyte (CTL) in the PBMC of these patients, signifies an active CTL control on actively replicating HBV (at a very low level).[17] Therefore, from the immunological point of view, the aim of the treatment is to restore effective T-cell control, and not elimination of HBV replication; and this has to be achieved with as little irreversible liver damage as possible.[14]

PROBLEMS WITH CURRENT USE OF MONOTHERAPY

In China, interferon (IFN)-α, thymosin-α1, and lamivudine monotherapy have been registered for treatment of chronic HBV infection.

Interferon-α

The use of interferon-α typically is associated with influenza-like reaction with fever, chills, weakness, myalgia and headaches, which begins 6 hours after the first injection and lasts for up to 12 hours and abates with subsequent injections. Other chronic side effects include fatigue, myalgia, headaches, irritability, depression and bone marrow suppression.[18] In addition, the overall response to interferon in Asian patients is unsatisfactory: approximately 15–20% will clear hepatitis B e antigen (HBeAg), but less than 5% will clear hepatitis B surface antigen (HBsAg).[1] The long-term benefit of interferon remains to be determined. In a recent 9-years follow-up study, it was found that IFN treatment resulted in higher and earlier rates of clearing of HBeAg and HBV-DNA by hybridization in Chinese patients with chronic hepatitis B. Very few patients lost HBsAg despite sustained HBeAg clearance. There was no difference in incidence of hepatic complications between patients and controls and between those who did and didn't clear HBeAg.[6] However, in another study conducted in Taiwan, 101 male patients with chronic hepatitis B in a randomized controlled trial were followed up for 1.1 to 11.5 years after the end of therapy. Thirty-four patients received a placebo (control), and 67 patients were treated with IFN. HCC was detected in 1 (1.5%) of the 67 treated patients and 4 (12%) of the 34 untreated patients ($P = .043$). The interval between entry and HCC detection was 3.5 to 8.2 years. The cumulative incidence of HCC development was significantly higher in the control group than in the treated group ($P = .013$).[19]

Thymosin-α1 (Tα1)

Tα1 is a immunomodulatory agent with very good safety profile. In the US phase III multicenter, placebo-controlled, double-blind study, 99 HBsAg positive, HBeAg positive and HBV-DNA positive were randomized to receive Tα1 at the dose of 1.6 mg, subcutaneously two times per week ($n=50$) and placebo ($n=49$) for 6 months and followed at 6-monthly intervals. Twelve (25%) patients treated with Tα1 and 6 (13%) patients given placebo (p<0.11) showed a sustained loss of HBV-DNA with negative HBeAg during the 1 year study or post study follow-up. These results suggest a trend in favour of Tα1. However, before recommending, further evaluation of Tα1 needs to be undertaken in chronic hepatitis B. In a randomized placebo-controlled trial conducted in Taiwan, complete virological response (with clearance of HBeAg and serum HBV-DNA by liquid hybridization) was significantly higher in those who receive Tα1 ($n=32$) for 6 months than the placebo group ($n=32$) (40.6% vs. 9.4%; $p=0.004$), 18 months after entry, although complete response was similar at the end of treatment.[20] In a recent study conducted in China, the safety and efficacy of Tα1 for 6 months was compared with combination of Tα1 and IFN-α (3 MU qd × 10 d then 3 × weekly for 6 months) in the treatment of chronic HBV infection. Loss of HBeAg and HBV-DNA was 27.8 % in either groups at 12 months. No significant side effects were observed in either group.[21] Clearly larger studies have to be conducted to determine its role in the treatment of chronic HBV infection.

Lamivudine

So far, lamivudine is the only nucleoside analogue approved for the treatment of chronic HBV infection. Clinical trials showed that lamivudine monotherapy results in marked suppression of HBV-DNA replication, normalization of serum ALT levels, and improvement in the liver biopsy.[22-25] However, monotherapy with lamivudine is unlikely to be sufficient for eradication of HBV infection in the majority of patients who are chronically infected. With prolonged therapy, a sustained HBeAg sero-conversion rate is achieved in 22%, 29%, 40% and 47% of Chinese patients at weeks 52, 104, 156 and 208 respectively.[26] Moreover, the durability of HBeAg loss and sero-conversion is variable. In the US multicenter study, the HBeAg sero-conversion was sustained in 73% of cases, 16 weeks after treatment.[25] In the Asian study, 73% (11/15) HBeAg sero-conversion was sustained.[27] However, in Korea, the cumulative relapse rate in sero-converters was 63%, 12 months after discontinuation of lamivudine therapy.[28] Larger studies in Asia will be needed to clarify the issue.

In the majority of patients who do not seroconvert, the use of lamivudine for more than 6 months is associated with the emergence of resistant HBV mutants. Two type of mutations have been identified to account for lamivudine resistance.[29] Mutation at codon M552 of the YMDD motif results in substitution of isoleucine for methionine (M552I). An alternative mutation at this site results in substitution of methionine by valine (M552V). The M552V mutation is accompanied by a second mutation at codon 528 that results in substitution of leucine by methionine (L528M). These YMDD variants had been described in both immunosuppressed liver transplantation patients and immunocompetent patients[30-33] who received lamivudine treatment. In the Asian study, YMDD variants increase with longer duration of treatment; 15%, 38%, 49% and 67% in the 1st, 2nd, 3rd and 4th years.[26] The median serum HBV-DNA and ALT levels were below baseline values. The biological significance remains to be determined. There are preliminary data suggesting that YMDD variants is not a benign disease. In Taiwan, 55 patients who received lamivudine therapy over 104 weeks at Chang

Gung Memorial Hospital, were assayed for YMDD variant. Thirty-two of them were found to have the YMDD mutation. They continued lamivudine therapy and were followed up weekly or biweekly if clinically indicated. Thirty (93.7%) of them showed elevation of alanine transaminase (ALT), and 13 (40.6%) experienced acute exacerbation at 4 to 94 weeks (median, 24 weeks) after emergence of the YMDD mutant. The incidence of exacerbation is much higher than 4.3% in patients without the YMDD mutation ($P = .003$). Compared with patients without exacerbation, patients with exacerbation had a significantly higher serum HBV-DNA level after emergence of the YMDD mutant ($P < .005$). Before exacerbation, serum HBV-DNA level was rising to its peak, followed by the peaking of ALT (247-2,010 U/L) 1 to 4 weeks later. Three patients developed hepatic decompensation, but then in association with hepatitis B e antigen (HBeAg) sero-conversion, recovered. Of the 12 evaluable patients, 8 (75%) showed HBeAg sero-conversion, and 3 showed mutant clearance within 1 to 5 months after exacerbation. In contrast, none of the patients without exacerbation showed HBeAg sero-conversion ($P < 0.001$). These results indicate that acute exacerbations may occur after emergence of the YMDD mutation.[34] Histologically, among the 37 patients without variants, 68% showed 2-point reduction in Knodell's scoring while 22% showed deterioration. On the other hand, histology in 45 patients with variants did not demonstrate significant overall deterioration. The results showed that 32% had deterioration of their histology at 1 year and this increased to 47% at 2 years of follow-up.[31] At present, the advice is to continue with lamivudine to avoid reappearance of the wild-type HBV, which is assumed to cause more severe disease. A solution is urgently required for those patients suffering from hepatitis due to variants.

USE OF COMBINATION THERAPY: FUTURE PERSPECTIVES

In patients with human immunodeficiency virus, the use of combination therapy has revolutionized its management.[35, 36] In duck hepatocyte cultures, the combination of penciclovir and lamivudine, has additive or synergistic effect in reducing the DHBV viral load. In addition, penciclovir but not lamivudine was effective in decreasing the production of ccc DNA and the expression of pre-S antigen. In-vitro studies have demonstrated that lamivudine and penciclovir (the active metabolite of famciclovir) act synergistically to inhibit hepatitis B virus (HBV) replication.[37] In a recent phase II trial, 21 Chinese hepatitis B e antigen (HBeAg) positive patients, with detectable HBV-DNA (Digene Hybrid Capture II), were randomized to receive either lamivudine 150 mg per day orally or lamivudine 150 mg per day plus famciclovir 500 mg three times per day orally for 12 weeks, with a follow-up period of at least 16 weeks. Serial serum HBV-DNA levels were determined and a mathematical model with provision for incomplete inhibition of virus production during therapy was applied to analyze the dynamics of viral clearance. The mean antiviral efficacy was significantly greater in patients treated with lamivudine plus famciclovir than those who received lamivudine alone (0.988 ± 0.012 vs. 0.94 ± 0.03, p=0.0012). This suggested that combination of lamivudine and famciclovir was superior to lamivudine monotherapy in inhibiting HBV replication.

Further, studies of longer duration are needed to define whether combination therapy will increase the HBeAg sero-conversion rate and decrease the rate of emergence of lamivudine resistant variants.[38]

On the other hand, combination of nucleoside analogues with immunomodulatory agents has also been explored in human trials.[39-43] In a recent randomized controlled trial in naïve Caucasian with hepatitis B e antigen (HBeAg) and HBV-DNA positive chronic hepatitis B, the effect of combining lamivudine and interferon appeared to be most useful in patients with moderately elevated alanine aminotransferase levels at baseline.[13] In Chinese HBeAg positive immunotolerant patients, use of thymosin-α1 and famciclovir has been shown to enhance antiviral effect as compared to monotherapy with famciclovir alone.[39] Another interesting therapeutic concept is lamivudine therapy after corticosteroid priming. On withdrawal of prednisolone, ALT usually rises and one can expect enhanced HBeAg sero-conversion with lamivudine.[44]

SUMMARY

Chronic HBV infection is a serious health treat in Asia-Pacific region. The introduction of lamivudine has greatly improved the hope of these patients and is undoubtly a milestone in the management of chronic HBV infection. To further improve its therapeutic efficacy, combination with another nucleotide/nucleoside analogues or immunomodulatory agent has to be sorted.

REFERENCES

1. Lok ASF, Wu PC, Lai CL, Lau JYN, Leung EKY, Wong LSK, Ma OCK, et al. A controlled trial of interferon with or without prednisone priming for chronic hepatitis B. *Gastroenterology* 1992;102:2091-7.
2. Pol S, Driss F, Michel ML, Nalpas B, Berthelot P, Brechot C. Specific vaccine therapy in chronic hepatitis B infection. *Lancet* 1994;344:342.
3. Couillin I, Pol S, Mancini M, Driss F, Brechot C, Tiollais P, Michel ML. Specific vaccine therapy in chronic hepatitis B: induction of T-cell proliferative responses specific for envelope antigens. *J Infect Dis* 1999;180:15-26.
4. Wen YM, Xiong SD, Zhang W. Solid matrix-antibody-antigen complex can clear viraemia and antigenaemia in persistent duck hepatitis B virus infection. *J Gen Virol* 1994;75:335-9.
5. Ilan Y, Nagler A, Adler R, Tur-Kaspa R, Slavin S, Shouval D. Ablation of persistent hepatitis B by BMT from a hepatitis B immune donor. *Gastroenterology* 1993;104:1818-21.
6. Lau GKK, Lim WL, Lok ASF. Nine years follow-up after interferon (IFN) treatment for chronic hepatitis B (CHB) in Chinese patients. *Hepatology* 1997; 26:259A.
7. Wang BE. Treatment of chronic liver diseases with traditional Chinese medicine. *J Gastrol Hepatol* 2000;15:E67-70.
8. Blumberg BS, Millman I, Venkateswaran PS, Thyagarajan SP. Hepatitis B virus and primary hepatocellular carcinoma: Treatment of HBV carriers with Phyllanthus amarus. *Vaccine* 1990;8:S86-92.
9. Gilson RJ, Chopar KB, Newell AM, Murray-Lyon IM, Nelson MR, Rice SJ, Tedder RS, et al. A

placebo-controlled phase I/II study of adefovir dipivoxil in patients with chronic hepatitis B virus infection. *J Viral Hepat* 1999;6:387-95.
10. Heathcote EJ, Jeffers L, Wright T, Sherman M, Perrilo R, Sacks S, Carithers R, et al. Loss of serum HBV-DNA and HBeAg and sero-conversion following short-term (12 weeks) adefovir dipivoxil therapy in chronic hepatitis B: two placebo-controlled phase II studies. *Hepatology* 1998;28:317A.
11. Gish R, Leung NWY, Wright TL, Trinh H, Robertson AT, Harris JJ, et al. Anti-hepatitis B virus (HBV) activity and pharmacokinetics of FTC in a 2-month trial in HBV-infected patients. *Gastroenterology* 1999;116:A1216.
12. Innaimo SF, Seifer M, Bisacchi GS, Standring DN, Zahler R, Colonno RJ. Identification of BMS-200475 as a potent and selective inhibitor of hepatitis B virus. *Antimicrob Agents Chemother* 1997;41:1444-8.
13. Schalm SW, Heathcote J, Cianciara J, Farrell G, Sherman M, Willems B, Dhillon A, et al. Lamivudine and alpha-interferon combination treatment of patients with chronic hepatitis B infection: a randomized trial. *Gut* 2000;46:562-8.
14. Lau GKK, ST Yuen, A Kwok, ST Lai, W Lim, Lam SK. Six-months follow-up on 26 weeks trial of Thymosin-α1 plus Famcilcovir in the treatment of Chinese immune tolerant adult patients with chronic hepatitis B. *Gastroenterology* 1999;116:339A.
15. Carman WF, Jacyna MR, Hadziyannis S, Karayiannis P, McGarvey MJ, Makris A, Thomas HC, et al. Mutation preventing formation of hepatitis B e antigen in patients with chronic hepatitis B infection. *Lancet* 1989;2:588-91.
16. Chisari FV, Ferrari C. Hepatitis B virus immunopathogenesis. *Annu Rev Immunol* 1995;13:29-60.
17. Rehermann B, Ferrari C, Pasquinelli C, Chisari FV. The hepatitis B virus persists for decades after patients' recovery from acute viral hepatitis despite active maintenance of a cytotoxic T-lymphocyte response. *Nature Med* 1996;1104-8.
18. Guan R. Interferon monotherapy in chronic hepatitis B. *J Gastrol and Hepatol* 2000;15(suppl):E34-40.
19. Lin SM, Sheen IS, Chien RN, Chu CM, Liaw YF. Long-term beneficial effect of interferon therapy in patients with chronic hepatitis B virus infection. *Hepatology* 1999;29: 971-5.
20. Chien RN, Liaw YF, Chen TC, Yeh CT, Sheen IS. Efficacy of Thymosin-α1 in patients with chronic hepatitis B: a randomized, controlled trial. *Hepatology* 1998;27:1383-7.
21. Lu ZM, Gao J, Yao GB, Ji YY, Wu XH, Zhang QB, Lau GKK and China Thymosin Study Group. A comparative trial of thymosin alone and thymosin plus interferon in the treatment of Chinese patients with chronic hepatitis B (CHB). *Hepatology* 1997;26:426A.
22. Dienstag JL, Perrillo RP, Schiff ER, Bartholomew M, Vicary C, Rubin M. A preliminary trial of lamivudine for chronic hepatitis B infection. *N Eng J Med* 1995;333:1657-61.
23. Nevens F, Main J, Honkoop P, Tyrrell DL, Barber J, Sullivan MT, Fevery J, et al. Lamivudine therapy for chronic hepatitis B: a six-month randomized dose-ranging study. *Gastroenterology* 1997;113:1258-63.
24. Lai CL, Chien RN, Leung NW, Chang TT, Guan R, Tai DI, Ng KY, et al. A one-year trial of lamivudine for chronic hepatitis B. Asia Hepatitis Lamivudine Study Group. *N Engl J Med* 1998;9:3 39:61-8.
25. Dienstag JL, Schiff ER, Wright TL, Perrillo RP, Hann HW, Goodman Z, Crowther L, et al. Lamivudine as initial treatment for chronic hepatitis B in the United States. *N Engl J Med* 1999;21:341:1256-63.
26. Chang TT, Lai CL, Liaw YF, Guan R, Lim SG, Lee CM, Ng KY, et al. Incremental increases in HBeAg sero-conversion and continued ALT normalisation in Asian chronic HBV patients treated with lamivudine for four years. (Glaxo data).
27. Chang TT, Lai CL, Liaw YF, Leung N, Guan R, Lim SG, Lee CM, et al. Enhanced HBeAg sero-conversion rate in Chinese patients on lamivudine. *Hepatology* 1999;30:1038.

28. Song BC, Suh DJ, Lee HC, Chung YH, Lee YS. Sero-conversion after lamivudine is not durable in chronic hepatitis B. *Hepatology* 1999;30:245A.
29. Allen M, Deslauriers M, Andrews C, Tipples G, Walters KA, Tyrrell D, Brown N, et al. Identification and characterization of mutations in hepatitis B virus resistant to lamivudine. *Hepatology* 1998;27:1670-7.
30. Perrillo RP, Rakela J, Dienstag J, Levy G, Martin P, Wright T, Caldwell S, et al. Multicenter study of lamivudine therapy for hepatitis B after liver transplantation. *Hepatology* 1999;29:1581-6.
31. Leung NWY, Lai CL, Chang TT, Guan R, Lee CM, Ng KY, Wu PC, et al. Three year lamivudine therapy in chronic HBV. *J Hepatol* 1999;30:59 (abstract).
32. Bartholomew MM, Jansen RW, Jeffers LJ, Reddy KR, Johnson LC, Bunzendahl H, Condreay LC, et al. Hepatitis B virus resistance to lamivudine given for recurrent infection after orthotopic liver transplantation. *Lancet* 1997;349:20-2.
33. Yoshida EM, Ma MM, Davis JE, Fischer KP, Kneteman NM, Erb SR, Tyrrell DL, et al. Post-liver transplant allograft reinfection with a lamivudine-resistant strain of hepatitis B virus: long-term follow-up. *Can J Gastroenterol* 1998;12:125-9.
34. Liaw YF, Chien RN, Yeh CT, Tsai SL, Chu CM. Acute Exacerbation and Hepatitis B Virus Clearance After Emergence of YMDD Motif mutation during lamivudine Therapy. *Hepatology* 1999;30:567-72.
35. Corey L, Holmes KK. Therapy of human immunodeficiency virus infection-what have we learned? *N Eng J Med* 1996;335:1142-4.
36. De Jong MC, Boucher CAB, Cooper DA, Galasso GJ, Gazzard B, Lange JM, Montaner JS, et al. Summary of the II International Consensus Symposium on combined antiviral therapy and implication for future therapies. *Antiviral Res* 1997;35:65-82.
37. Chen Y, Guo S, Qi Z, Huang A. Experimental Study on the effect of combination therapy with lamivudine and famciclovir against duck hepatitis B virus *in vivo*. *Zhonghua Gan Zang Bing Za Zhi* 2001;9:209-11.
38. Lau GK, Tsiang M, Hou J, Yuen S, Carman WF, Zhang L, Gibbs CS, et al. Combination therapy with lamivudine and famciclovir for chronic hepatitis B infected Chinese: a viral dynamics study. *Hepatology* 2000;34:394-9.
39. Lau GK, Carman WF, Locarnini S, Okuda K, Williams R, Lam SK. Treatment of chronic HBV infection: an Asia-Pacific perspective. *J Gastroenterol Hepatol* 1999;14:3-12.
40. Serfaty L, Thabut D, Zoulim F, Andreani T, Carbonell N, Loria A, Poupan R, et al. Sequential treatment with lamivudine and interferon monotherapies in patients with chronic hepatitis B not responding to interferon alone: results of a pilot study. *Hepatology* 2001;34:573-7.
41. Schlam SW. Lamivudine interferon combination therapy for chronic hepatitis B: further support but no conclusive evidence. *J Hepatol* 2002;35:419-20.
42. Barbaro G, Zechini F, Pellicelli AM, Francavilla R, Scotto G, Becca D, Bruno M, et al. Long-term efficacy of interferon-alpha-2b and lamivudine in combination compared to lamivudine monotherapy in patients with chronic hepatitis B. An Italian Multicenter, randomized trial. *J Hepatol* 2001;35:406-11.
43. Chan HL, Tang JL, Tam W, Sung JJ. The efficacy of thymosin in the treatment of chronic hepatitis B virus infection: a meta-analysis. *Aliment Pharmacol Ther* 2001;15:1899-905.
44. Liaw YF, Tsai SL, Chien RN, Yeh CT, Chu CM. Prednisolone priming enhances Th-1 response and efficacy of subsequent lamivudine therapy in patients with chronic hepatitis B. *Hepatology* 2000;32:604-9.

Gene therapy for hepatitis B

Darius Moradpour, Wolf B Offensperger, Fritz V Weizsäcker, Hubert E Blum

The hepatitis B virus (HBV) infects more than 300 million people worldwide and is a leading cause of chronic hepatitis, liver cirrhosis, and hepatocellular carcinoma.[1] Current therapeutic options include interferon-alpha and nucleoside analogues such as lamivudine.[2,3] Standard interferon-alpha therapy for chronic hepatitis B with 4–6 million units 3 times per week subcutaneously for 4–6 months results in a sustained response in 30–40% of patients (as defined by normalization of serum aminotransferases, sero-conversion from HBeAg to anti-HBe or, loss of HBV-DNA in HBeAg negative or anti-HBe-positive patients). Lamivudine, a well-tolerated oral necleoside analogs, has emerged as an effective alternative.[4] After prolonged lamivudine therapy, HBV-DNA polymerase escape mutants may develop, resulting in reappearance of HBV-DNA in the serum.[5] Apart from lamivudine, other nucleoside analogues, such as adefovir dipioxil, lobucavir, emtricitabine (FTC), tenofovir, and entecavir, BMS-200475, are currently being evaluated for the treatment of chronic hepatitis B. In addition, combination therapy of lamivudine with interferon-alpha or with other nucleoside analogs are being evaluated.[6] Taken together, the efficacy of the current therapeutic options for chronic hepatitis B are still very limited. Alternative therapeutic strategies, therefore, are being explored, including gene therapy.

BIOLOGY OF THE HEPATITIS B VIRUS

The structure and biology of HBV have been described in detail.[7] HBV is a small DNA virus of 42 nm diameter and belongs to a group of hepatotropic DNA viruses (hepadnaviruses) that share common features, such as genomic organization, virion structure, replication strategy, and pattern of gene expression. The *hepadnaviridae* family is divided into the mammalian and avian branches. Mammalian hepadnaviruses include HBV and the hepatitis viruses of the woodchuck (WHV),[8] and the ground squirrel (GSHV),[9] and wooly monkey (WMHBV). Avian hepadnaviruses are more distantly related to HBV and include the duck hepatitis B virus (DHBV), which infects Pekin ducks,[10] and the heron hepatitis B virus (HHBV),[11] and the snow goose hepatitis B virus (SGHBV). HBV consists of an outer envelope and an internal core (nucleocapsid, C) (Fig. 1A). The envelope is composed mainly of hepatitis B surface antigen (HBsAg) which plays a central role in the immunodiagnosis of HBV infection. The nucleocapsid contains hepatitis B core antigen (HBcAg), a DNA polymerase/reverse transcriptase (P), and the viral genome.

The genome consists of an incompletely double-stranded circular DNA molecule of about 3,200 base pairs length and known sequence as well as genetic organization (Fig. 1B). The pre-surface 1 (pre-S1)/pre-surface 2 (pre-S2)/surface genes (S) code for the various HBsAg molecules such as, large, middle, and small hepatitis B surface proteins (LHBs, MHBs, and SHBs). The protein encoded by the pre-core (pre-C)/core (C) gene undergoes post-translational modification to yield hepatitis B e antigen (HBeAg), a marker for viral replication. The core gene codes for HBcAg, the major structural protein of the viral nucleocapsid. The X gene, finally, codes for the hepatitis B x protein, designated HBx, whose physiological role in the viral life cycle is still enigmatic. The viral DNA polymerase/reverse transcriptase is encoded by the polymerase gene (P). Different from all known mammalian DNA viruses, hepadnaviruses replicate *via* reverse transcription of an RNA intermediate,[12] a strategy central to the life cycle of retroviruses. In addition to the known viral genes, several *cis*-acting genetic elements for the fine control of gene expression, RNA packaging, and viral replication have been identified.[13]

GENE THERAPY FOR HEPATITIS B

Viral infections can be viewed as acquired genetic diseases and represent a major potential application of gene therapy.[14-16] In the context of this brief review, gene therapy is defined as the introduction of foreign nucleic acids into cells or tissues with a therapeutic benefit. For

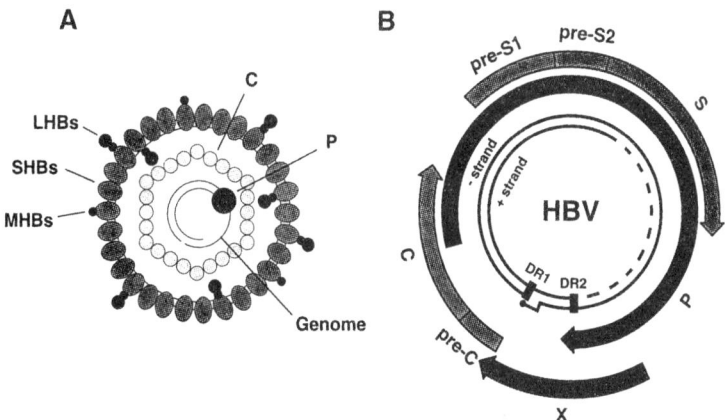

Fig. 1. Structure and genetic organization of HBV

the treatment of HBV infection, several antiviral strategies aimed at blocking viral gene expression or function as well as DNA vaccination and other immunotherapeutic strategies aimed at boosting the humoral and cellular immune response are being explored (Table 1). Antisense oligonucleotides, ribozymes, and dominant negative mutants strongly inhibit viral replication and gene expression in experimental systems *in vitro* and in some animal models *in vivo*. Despite exciting recent developments, a number of issues, such as the efficacy and safety of gene transfer need to be resolved before accepting gene therapy of hepatitis B as a supplement to existing therapeutic and preventive modalities.

Table 1. Gene therapy for hepatitis B

- Ribozymes
- Antisense oligonucleotides
- Interfering peptides or proteins (dominant negative mutants, recombinant antibody fragments)
- DNA vaccination

Antiviral strategies are aimed at one or several steps of the viral life cycle, e.g., attachment of the virus to the cell membrane, internalization and uncoating, viral replication and gene expression, virus assembly, and finally virion export. An attractive genetic antiviral concept is blocking viral gene expression or function (Fig. 2). Several strategies can be explored, e.g. interfering with the transcription of genes by sequestration of transcription factors *via* binding to nucleic acids introduced into or synthesized in the cells (decoy strategy), by binding of single-stranded nucleic acids to double-stranded DNA, forming a triple helix structure, by hybridization of RNA molecules possessing endoribonuclease activity (ribozymes) to target RNA molecules resulting in sequence-specific RNA cleavage, by blocking translation through

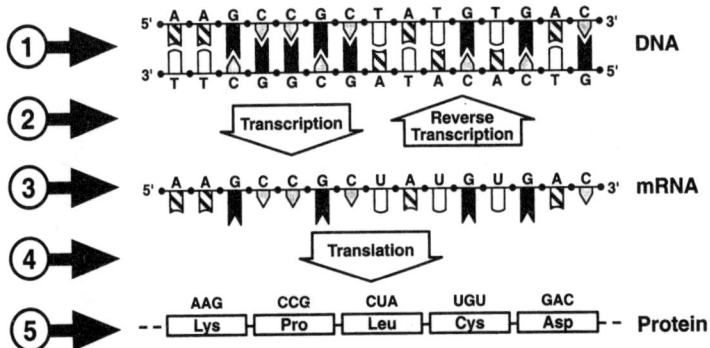

Fig. 2. Strategies aimed at blocking gene expression or function: (1) decoy strategy; (2) triple helix formation (transcription), decoy or antisense strategy (reverse transcription); (3) ribozymes; (4) antisense strategy; (5) interfering peptides or proteins

binding of antisense oligonucleotides to RNA, and by the intracellular synthesis of peptides or proteins that interfere with the assembly and functions of viral proteins (dominant negative mutants).

Ribozymes

Ribozymes ('ribonucleic acid enzymes') were originally discovered as naturally occurring RNA molecules that catalyze the sequence-specific cleavage of RNA and RNA splicing reactions.[17, 18] The catalytic activity is the major attraction of the ribozyme concept because one ribozyme can cleave many target RNAs. The hammerhead ribozyme consists of antisense flanking sequences mediating its binding to the target RNA as well as a conserved catalytic domain. Several studies have shown that hammerhead ribozymes can specifically cleave HBV RNA in cell-free[19, 20] and cellular model systems.[21, 22]

Antisense oligonucleotides

Antisense nucleic acids are designed to specifically bind to RNA, resulting in the formation of RNA-DNA (antisense DNA) or RNA-RNA hybrids (antisense RNA) with an arrest of mRNA translation or RNA reverse transcription.[23-25] Antisense effects can be potentiated by degradation of RNA in RNA-DNA hybrids by cellular RNases H. These nucleases degrade RNA whenever an RNA-DNA hybrid as short as 10 base pairs is formed. While conceptually simple, it is clear now that not all desired as well as undesired effects are caused by the target sequence-specific antisense action of the oligonucleotides.[26, 27] The antisense strategy has been successfully applied to HBV *in vitro*.[28-30] In addition, studies in nude mice,[31] in DHBV-infected Pekin ducks[32, 33] and in WHV-infected woodchucks[34] showed the *in vivo* applicability of this approach. In addition to antisense oligonucleotides, intracellularly expressed antisense RNA transcripts have recently been explored with respect to their antiviral potential *in vitro*.[35]

Interfering peptides or proteins

The intracellular synthesis of interfering peptides or proteins, including recombinant antibody fragments is aimed at the specific interference with the assembly or function of viral structural or nonstructural proteins and represents a type of intracellular immunization.[36] This approach has proven effective for both mammalian and avian hepadnaviruses in cell culture experiments.[37-39] Thus, the fusion of the different polypeptides of various lengths to the carboxyterminus of the viral core protein yields dominant negative mutants that suppress viral replication by more than 90% at an effector to target molecule ratio of 1:10. More recently, intracellular immunization by intracellular expression of single chain antibody fragments against the HBV core and surface proteins has been explored.[40, 41] The potential advantage of interfering peptides or proteins is their relative independence from viral sequence variation, minimizing the risk of selecting or accumulating 'therapy escape' mutants.

DNA vaccination

Based on the observation that plasmid DNA could directly transfect muscle, dendritic and other cells *in vivo*, the potential of expression of plasmids encoding antigenic proteins to induce immune responses by direct injection was explored.[42-44] This method, termed DNA vaccination or genetic immunization, has now been used to elicit protective antibody and cellular immune responses in a wide variety of preclinical animal models for viral, bacterial, and parasitic diseases.[45-47] The mechanism of DNA vaccination is illustrated in Fig. 3. DNA vaccination is particularly useful for the induction of cytotoxic T-cells and may, therefore, have therapeutic potential as well. Proof-of-principle for this concept was recently demonstrated in an animal model of tuberculosis.[48] DNA vaccination for hepatitis B was explored in mice[49-51] and in primates.[52, 53] The protective potential of this strategy has been demonstrated in chimpanzees against HBV,[54] in Pekin ducks against DHBV,[55, 56] and in woodchucks against WHV.[57] Genetic immunization of chimpanzees chronically infected with HBV using a recombinant retroviral vector encoding the HBV core protein revealed that this strategy may be therapeutically beneficial in the treatment of chronic hepatitis B.[58]

SUMMARY AND FUTURE PERSPECTIVES

Chronic hepatitis B can be viewed as an acquired genetic disease that can be treated by genetic antiviral strategies, including among others, antisense oligonucleotides, ribozymes, dominant negative mutants, recombinant antibody fragments, and DNA vaccination. While their therapeutic potential has been clearly demonstrated *in vitro*, experimental studies in

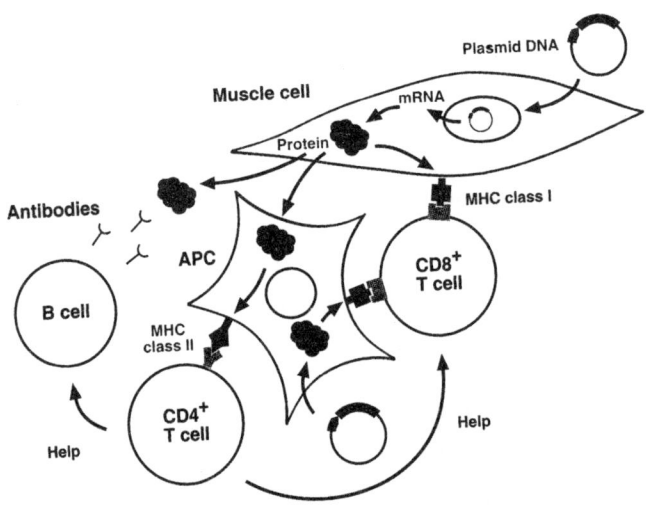

Fig. 3. Mechanism of DNA vaccination

established or novel animal models[59-62] will be central for the evaluation of the major current issues of gene therapy *in vivo*. These include the specificity of gene therapy for the targeted gene, the stability and potential toxicity of the therapeutic nucleic acids or proteins, and their delivery to and regulated expression in infected hepatocytes and non-hepatocytes, the potential development of viral or immune mediated resistance as well as various safety considerations. The understanding of viral as well as host genetic factors affecting the natural course of viral hepatitis will not only provide clues to the pathogenesis of virus-induced liver diseases but will also be the basis for novel therapeutic strategies.[63-69] These strategies, may in the future, complement existing therapeutic modalities, thereby contributing to the prevention and elimination of HBV-associated chronic liver disease, including liver cirrhosis and hepatocellular carcinoma.

REFERENCES

1. Lee WM. Hepatitis B virus infection. *N Engl J Med* 1997;337:1733-45.
2. Hoofnagle JH, Di Bisceglie AM. The treatment of chronic viral hepatitis. *N Engl J Med* 1997;336:347-56.
3. Zoulim F, Trépo C. New antiviral agents for the therapy of chronic hepatitis B virus infection. *Intervirology* 1999;42:125-44.
4. Lai CL, Chien RN, Leung NW, Chang TT, Guan R, Tai DI, Ng KY, et al. A one-year trial of lamivudine for chronic hepatitis B. Asia Hepatitis Lamivudine Study Group. *N Engl J Med* 1998;339:61-8.
5. Zoulim F, Trépo C. Drug therapy for chronic hepatitis B: antiviral efficacy and influence of hepatitis B virus polymerase mutations on the outcome of therapy. *J Hepatol* 1998;29:151-68.
6. Ka-Kit G, Lau K, Tsiang M, Hou J, Yuen S, Carman WF, Zhang L, et al. Combination therapy with lamivudine and famciclovir for chronic hepatitis B-infected Chinese patients: a viral dynamics study. *Hepatology* 2000;32:394-9.
7. Nassal M. Hepatitis B virus replication: novel roles for virus-host interactions. *Intervirology* 1999;42:100-16.
8. Summers J, Smolec JM, Snyder R. A virus similar to human hepatitis B virus associated with hepatitis and hepatoma in woodchucks. *Proc Natl Acad Sci USA* 1978;75:4533-7.
9. Marion PL, Oshiro LS, Regnery DC, Scullard GH, Robinson WS. A virus in Beechey ground squirrels that is related to hepatitis B virus of humans. *Proc Natl Acad Sci USA* 1980;77:2941-5.
10. Mason WS, Seal G, Summers J. Virus of Pekin ducks with structural and biological relatedness to human hepatitis B virus. *J Virol* 1980;36:829-36.
11. Sprengel R, Kaleta EF, Will H. Isolation and characterization of a hepatitis B virus endemic in herons. *J Virol* 1988;62:3832-9.
12. Summers J, Mason WS. Replication of the genome of a hepatitis B-like virus by reverse transcription of an RNA intermediate. *Cell* 1982;29:403-15.
13. Huang J, Liang TJ. A novel hepatitis B virus (HBV) genetic element with Rev response element-like properties that is essential for expression of HBV gene products. *Mol Cell Biol* 1993;13:7476-86.
14. von Weizsäcker F, Wieland S, Köck J, Offensperger WB, Offensperger S, Moradpour D, Blum HE. Gene therapy for chronic viral hepatitis: ribozymes, antisense oligonucleotides, and dominant negative mutants. *Hepatology* 1997;26:251-5.
15. Wands JR, Geissler M, Putlitz JZ, Blum H, Weizsacker FV, Mohr L, Yoon SK, et al. Nucleic acid-

based antiviral and gene therapy of chronic hepatitis B infection. *J Gastroenterol Hepatol* 1997;12: S354-69.
16. Blum HE. Molecular biology and gene therapy in gastroenterology and hepatology. *Eur J Gastroenterol Hepatol* 1999;11:1-7.
17. Haseloff J, Gerlach WL. Simple RNA enzymes with new and highly specific endoribonuclease activities. *Nature* 1988;334:585-91.
18. Scott WG, Klug A. Ribozymes: structure and mechanism in RNA catalysis. *Trends Biochem Sci* 1996;21:220-4.
19. von Weizsäcker F, Blum HE, Wands JR. Cleavage of hepatitis B virus RNA by three ribozymes transcribed from a single DNA template. *Biochem Biophys Res Comm* 1992;189:743-8.
20. Beck J, Nassal M. Efficient hammerhead ribozyme-mediated cleavage of the structured hepatitis B virus encapsidation signal in vitro and in cell extracts, but not in intact cells. *Nucleic Acids Res* 1995;23:4954-62.
21. Welch PJ, Tritz R, Yei S, Barber J, Yu M. Intracellular application of hairpin ribozyme genes against hepatitis B virus. *Gene Ther* 1997;4:736-43.
22. Zu Putlitz J, Yu Q, Burke JM, Wands JR. Combinatorial screening and intracellular antiviral activity of hairpin ribozymes directed against hepatitis B virus. *J Virol* 1999;73:5381-7.
23. Wagner RW. The state of the art in antisense research. *Nat Med* 1995;1:1116-8.
24. Kilkuskie RE, Field AK. Antisense inhibition of virus infections. *Adv Pharmacol* 1997;40:437-82.
25. Offensperger WB, Thoma C, Moradpour D, von Weizsäcker F, Offensperger S, Blum HE. Antisense oligonucleotide therapy of hepadnavirus infection. *Methods Enzymol* 2000;314:524-36.
26. Branch AD. A hitchhiker's guide to antisense and nonantisense biochemical pathways. *Hepatology* 1996;24:1517-29.
27. Branch AD. A good antisense molecule is hard to find. *Trends Biochem Sci* 1998;23:45-50.
28. Blum HE, Galun E., von Weizsäcker F, Wands JR. Inhibition of hepatitis B virus by antisense oligodeoxynucleotides. *Lancet* 1991;337:1230.
29. Wu GY, Wu CH. Specific inhibition of hepatitis B viral gene expression in vitro by targeted antisense oligonucleotides. *J Biol Chem* 1992;267:12436-9.
30. Madon J, Blum HE. Receptor mediated delivery of hepatitis B virus DNA and antisense oligodeoxynucleotides to avian liver cells. *Hepatology* 1996;24:474-81.
31. Yao Z, Zhou Y, Feng X, Chen C, Guo J. In vivo inhibition of hepatitis B viral gene expression by antisense phosphorothioate oligodeoxynucleotides in athymic nude mice. *J Viral Hepat* 1996;3: 19-22.
32. Offensperger W-B, Offensperger S, Walter E, Teubner K, Igloi G, Blum HE, Gerok W. In vivo inhibition of duck hepatitis B virus replication and gene expression by phosphorothioate modified antisense oligodeoxynucleotides. *EMBO J* 1993;12:1257-62.
33. Soni PN, Brown D, Saffie R, Savage K, Moore D, Gregoriadis G, Dusheiko GM. Biodistribution, stability, and antiviral efficacy of liposome-entrapped phosphorothioate antisense oligodeoxynucleotides in ducks for the treatment of chronic duck hepatitis B virus infection. *Hepatology* 1998;28:1402-10.
34. Bartholomew RM, Carmichael EP, Findeis MA, Wu CH, Wu GY. Targeted delivery of antisense DNA in woodchuck hepatitis virus-infected woodchucks. *J Viral Hepat* 1995;2:273-8.
35. zu Putlitz J, Wieland S, Blum HE, Wands JR. Antisense RNA complementary to hepatitis B virus specifically inhibits viral replication. *Gastroenterology* 1998;115:702-13.
36. Baltimore D. Intracellular immunization. *Nature* 1988;335:395-6.
37. Scaglioni PP, Melegari M, Wands JR. Characterization of hepatitis B virus core mutants that inhibit viral replication. *Virology* 1994;205:112-20.
38. Scaglioni PP, Melegari M, Takahashi M, Chowdhury JR, Wands J. Use of dominant negative mutants of the hepadnaviral core protein as antiviral agents. *Hepatology* 1996;24:1010-7.

39. von Weizsäcker F, Wieland S, Blum HE. Inhibition of viral replication by genetically engineered mutants of the duck hepatitis B virus core protein. *Hepatology* 1996;24:294-9.
40. Yamamoto M, Hayashi N, Takehara T, Ueda K, Mita E, Tatsumi T, Sasaki Y, et al. Intracellular single-chain antibody against hepatitis B virus core protein inhibits the replication of hepatitis B virus in cultured cells. *Hepatology* 1999;30:300-7.
41. zu Putlitz J, Skerra A, Wands JR. Intracellular expression of a cloned antibody fragment interferes with hepatitis B virus surface antigen secretion. *Biochem Biophys Res Commun* 1999;255:785-91.
42. Wolff JA, Malone RW, Williams P, Chong W, Acsadi G, Jani A, Felgner PL. Direct gene transfer into mouse muscle in vivo. *Science* 1990;247:1465-8.
43. Tang DC, DeVit M, Johnston SA. Genetic immunization is a simple method for eliciting an immune response. *Nature* 1992;356:152-4.
44. Ulmer JB, Donnelly JJ, Parker SE, Rhodes GH, Felgner PF, Dwarki VJ, Gromkowski SH, et al. Heterologous protection against influenza by injection of DNA encoding a viral protein. *Science* 1993;259:1745-9.
45. Davis HL, Brazolot Millan CL. DNA-based immunization against hepatitis B virus. *Springer Semin Immunopathol* 1997;19:195-209.
46. Donnelly JJ, Ulmer JB, Shiver JW, Liu MA. DNA vaccines. *Annu Rev Immunol* 1997;15:617-48.
47. Weiner DB, Kennedy RC. Genetic vaccines. *Sci Am* 1999;281:50-7.
48. Lowrie DB, Tascon RE, Bonato VL, Lima VM, Faccioli LH, Stavropoulos E, Colston MJ, et al. Therapy of tuberculosis in mice by DNA vaccination. *Nature* 1999;400:269-71.
49. Davis HL, Michel ML, Whalen RG. DNA-based immunization induces continuous secretion of hepatitis B surface antigen and high levels of circulating antibody. *Hum Mol Gen* 1993;2:1847-51.
50. Davis HL, Schirmbeck R, Reimann J, Whalen RG. DNA-mediated immunization in mice induces a potent MHC class I-restricted cytotoxic T-lymphocyte response to the hepatitis B envelope protein. *Hum Gene Ther* 1995;6:1447-56.
51. Chow YH, Huang WL, Chi WK, Chu YD, Tao MH. Improvement of hepatitis B virus DNA vaccines by plasmids coexpressing hepatitis B surface antigen and interleukin-2. *J Virol* 1997;71:169-78.
52. Davis HL, McCluskie MJ, Gerin JL, Purcell RH. DNA vaccine for hepatitis B: evidence for immunogenicity in chimpanzees and comparison with other vaccines. *Proc Natl Acad Sci USA* 1996;93:7213-8.
53. Davis HL, Suparto, II, Weeratna RR, Jumintarto, Iskandriati DD, Chamzah SS, Ma'ruf AA, et al. CpG DNA overcomes hyporesponsiveness to hepatitis B vaccine in orangutans. *Vaccine* 2000;18:1920-4.
54. Prince AM, Whalen R, Brotman B. Successful nucleic acid based immunization of newborn chimpanzees against hepatitis B virus. *Vaccine* 1997;15:916-9.
55. Triyatni M, Jilbert AR, Qiao M, Miller DS, Burrell CJ. Protective efficacy of DNA vaccines against duck hepatitis B virus infection. *J Virol* 1998;72:84-94.
56. Rollier C, Sunyach C, Barraud L, Madani N, Jamard C, Trépo C, Cova L. Protective and therapeutic effect of DNA-based immunization against hepadnavirus large envelope protein. *Gastroenterology* 1999;116:658-65.
57. Lu M, Hilken G, Kruppenbacher J, Kemper T, Schirmbeck R, Reimann J, Roggendorf M. Immunization of woodchucks with plasmids expressing woodchuck hepatitis virus (WHV) core antigen and surface antigen suppresses WHV infection. *J Virol* 1999;73:281-9.
58. Sallberg M, Hughes J, Javadian A, Ronlov G, Hultgren C, Townsend K, Anderson CG, et al. Genetic immunization of chimpanzees chronically infected with the hepatitis B virus, using a recombinant retroviral vector encoding the hepatitis B virus core antigen. *Hum Gene Ther* 1998;9:1719-29.

59. Walter E, Keist R, Niederöst B, Pult I, Blum HE. Hepatitis B virus infection of tupaia hepatocytes in vitro and in vivo. *Hepatology* 1996;24:1-5.
60. Petersen J, Dandri M, Gupta S, Rogler CE. Liver repopulation with xenogenic hepatocytes in B and T-cell-deficient mice leads to chronic hepadnavirus infection and clonal growth of hepatocellular carcinoma. *Proc Natl Acad Sci USA* 1998;95:310-5.
61. Dandri M, Burda MR, Trook E, Pollok JM, Iwanska A, Sommer G, Rogiers X, et al. Repopulation of mouse liver with human hepatocytes and *in vivo* infection with hepatitis B virus. *Hepatology* 2001;33:981-8.
62. Schinazi RF, Ilan E, Black PL, Yao X, Dagan S. Cell-based and animal models for hepatitis B and C viruses. *Antivir Chem Chemother* 1999;10:99-114.
63. Thio CL, Thomas DL, Carrington M. Chronic viral hepatitis and the human genome. *Hepatology* 2000;31:819-27.
64. Cantz T, Ott M, Kubicka S, Manns MP. Gene and immunotherapy of liver diseases. *Internist (Berl)* 2001;42:1357-62,1364-5.
65. Chion HC, Lucas MA, Coffin CC, Banaszczyr MG, Ill CR, Lollo CP. Gene therapy strategies for the treatment of chronic viral hepatitis. *Expert opin Biol Ther* 2001;1:629-39.
66. Michel ML, Pol S, Brechot C, Tiollais P. Immunotherapy of Chronic Hepatitis B by anti HBV vaccine: from present to future. *Vaccine* 2001;19:2395-9.
67. Weeratna RD, Wu T, Efler SM, Zhang L, Davis HL. Designing gene therapy vectors: avoiding immune responses by using tissue specific promoters. *Gene Ther* 2001;8:1872-9.
68. Jenson KD, Kopeckova P, Kopecek J. Antisense oligo nucleotides delivered to the lysosome escapeand actively inhibit the hepatitis B virus. *Bioconjug Chem* 2002;13:975-84.
69. Blum HE. Molecular targets for prevention of hepatocellular carcinoma. *Dig Dis* 2002;20:81-90.

54

Instruments for assessment of impact of treatment of chronic hepatitis B on the quality of life

Rakesh K Kochhar

The World Health Organization's definition of health includes not only the absence of disease but also a complete state of physical, mental, and social well-being. During the last decade, patient-based health outcome research has looked at clinical and economic impact of treatment strategies as there is a shift from the "biomedical model" to the "social-science model" of medicine.[1] The biomedical model is founded on the basic sciences (molecular biology, genetics, physiology, etc.) and its main focus is evaluation of clinical, physiological, and biochemical outcomes. On the other hand, the "social-science model" is based on psychosocial and economic foundation and focuses on patient's overall well-being and ability to function. This model emphasizes patient's health-related quality of life (HRQOL) as its main outcome. HRQOL focuses on self-perceived health and well-being domains. These include assessment of physical function, somatic sensation, psychological status, social interactions, functional capacity, and sense of well-being as influenced by health status.[1] Each one of these is subjective, and is self-reported. Although the traditional clinical outcomes are important end-points for clinicians, they are of little value to patients, who view their disease differently. In this regard, HRQOL parameters assess the disease and the outcome of treatment from the patient's perspective. McNeil et al[2] had reported that a significant proportion of cancer patients were more concerned about quality of life than longevity. Hence, assessment of interventions only in terms of length of life, survival, or mortality is insufficient to characterize the health outcomes about which patients care. It is also important that an intervention be assessed not only regarding its clinical effectiveness but also its cost-effectiveness. This assumes significance as the medical world is moving towards cost-containment.

HEPATITIS B INFECTION

Chronic hepatitis B and C constitute a major proportion of chronic liver disease with considerable impact on individual patients, health care economy and society, all over the world. About 5 million, Americans are chronically infected with hepatitis B or C viruses.[3] The figures for India are alarming. With an average HBsAg prevalence rate of 4.7%, about 42.5 million people in India are infected with the hepatitis B virus.[4]

Although some clinical conditions caused by chronic liver disease have obvious manifestations that are measured by the traditional clinical outcomes (ascites, encephalopathy, hemorrhage, etc.), others have no or little physical findings and are difficult to evaluate, like fatigue, loss of esteem, inability to work, anxiety, depression, etc. It is here that HRQOL assessment can be used in defining the impact of disease, and the outcome of interventions.

INSTRUMENTS TO ASSESS QUALITY OF LIFE

As highlighted earlier, treatment of chronic hepatitis should also be aimed at improving the HRQOL of the patient rather than only the clinical and laboratory parameters. Moreover, the side-effects of the drugs and/or procedures used for treatment also need to be taken into consideration. It is only recently that assessment of HRQOL has gained popularity in patients with chronic hepatitis.

Quality of life is measured by two main indices, generic and specific. Each of these indices is assessed by subjecting the patient to a set of questions, which form a particular instrument. There are a number of generic instruments which are used to evaluate HRQOL in a wide variety of diseases (*see below*). Disease-specific instruments for hepatitis and chronic liver disease have been introduced only recently.[5,6] Some workers use a disease specific module, i.e., a generic questionnaire along with a few questions pertinent to that particular disease.[7]

Because many components of HRQOL cannot be measured directly, they are assessed by a series of questions, which are converted into numerical scores amenable to statistical analysis. How accurately these items reflect the true HRQOL depends on the properties of the instrument used. An instrument must be effective in its evaluative function (to measure changes in HRQOL over time) as well as in its discriminative function (to measure differences between patients at a single point of time).[8]

Attributes of instruments

Effectiveness of an instrument is defined by its three essential attributes : (i) responsiveness, (ii) reliability, and (iii) validity.

Responsiveness

A questionnaire needs to be responsive if it is going to detect important changes in an individual over time, no matter how small the changes may be. The magnitude of the changes in the HRQOL scale should also reflect the magnitude of clinical change or changes in the other scales.[9]

Reliability

Reliability or reproducibility is tested by the repeated application of the test questionnaire to a set of stable patients. On repeated testing, stable patients should score relatively similarly.[10]

Test-retest reliability refers to a different type of reliability. Here, the same patients complete the same instrument on two different occasions before and after a period of time that seldom exceeds 2 weeks.[8] The higher the correlation between the first and second administration of the instrument, the higher is the test-retest reliability.

Validity

Validity refers to an instrument's ability to measure accurately what it is intended to measure.[8] Proving that the instrument is actually measuring what it is designed to measure, is crucial for acceptability of the instrument. In other words, one should be able to draw legitimate conclusions regarding the particular disease or outcome from the instrument. It is important to understand the following types of validity.

Criterion validity It asks, "How well does your HRQOL questionnaire compare with what is commonly accepted as the gold standard?"[10]

Content validity It asks whether the instrument samples the area of interest adequately.[10] Is it comprehensive in its coverage of the disease state and applicable to the disease? It is used to determine whether each of the relevant domains is adequately sampled by the questions. For this, disease-specific questions like "how many bowel movements you have?", emotion-related questions like "do you feel depressed because of your disease?", and social-function questions like "how does your disease affect your ability?", are incorporated.

Construct validity It is the most rigorous method of establishing validity. A construct is a theoretically derived notion of the domains being considered for measurement. By understanding each construct, one can predict how the instrument measuring these constructs should behave, and then compare a newly developed instrument to other related measures to determine if the prediction is confirmed or refuted.[10]

Generic and specific indices to measure quality of life

Generic indices

A generic index evaluates the broad impact of a disease on the patient's well-being.[1,8] It can be applicable to a variety of health states or conditions and it can be used to compare the impact of different disease states or their treatment on HRQOL. Such information is necessary if we are to use HRQOL data to guide us in allocating resources across different groups of patients. One drawback of generic indices is that they lack the responsiveness required to capture small but clinically significant changes occurring as a result of disease progression or treatment.[11]

Generic health measures that have proven useful in studies on hepatitis include the Sickness Impact Profile,[12] the Medical Outcome Study Short Form-36 (SF-36),[13] the Karnofsky performance scale,[14] the Nottingham Health Profile[15] and others. The Sickness Impact Profile was used by Davis et al[12] to demonstrate that the HRQOL of patients with chronic hepatitis C receiving interferon was worse than that of normal controls, and it also failed to show any change in the HRQOL of patients with a clinical response to interferon. Lack of responsiveness of the generic measures used has been attributed as one of the factors to explain these findings. The other possible explanations could be too short a study period to detect a change and side effects of interferon negating any improvement.

Other recent studies have used SF-36 as an instrument to measure the HRQOL of chronic hepatitis patients.[16] The SF-36 questionnaire measures eight multi-item variables (Table 1). The resulting scores are transformed onto a scale of 0 to 100. Carithers and co-workers[16] used the SF-36 questionnaire and supplemented it with one or more items specific to patients with chronic hepatitis C. Data revealed that these patients had lower HRQOL than either the general population or those with hypertension, and similar rating to those with type II diabetes. Bonkovsky et al[17] used the SF-36 scoring system in 642 patients of chronic hepatitis C treated with interferon to conclude that those who achieved sustained virologic response had significant improvement of their HRQOL scores. Recently, Toster et al[18] using SF-36 scores have compared HRQOL of patients with chronic HCV infection to those with chronic HBV infection. In the absence of cirrhosis, patients with chronic HCV infection had significant reductions in their SF-36 scores for all of the modalities tested. Patients with chronic HBV infection, on the other hand, had a reduction in the SF-36 scores that assessed mental functions, but they had no decrease in the score that measured physical symptoms, indicating that the symptoms associated with chronic HCV infection are qualitatively different from those in HBV infection.[18] It also suggested that the physician's perception of HBV infection is more negative than the patients' perception of their own illness.

The SF-36 permits rapid measurements; is reasonably easy to administer, score and interpret; and has been shown to have acceptable construct, criterion, and known-groups validity for

Table 1. Parameters assessed with SF-36 scale

Physical functioning
Role disability (physical)
Bodily pain
General health
Vitality
Social functioning
Role disability (emotional)
General mental health

many disorders. It is also reproducible over time in stable patients, is generally responsive to meaningful interventions and clinical changes. SF-36 is the most frequently used instrument in patients with chronic hepatitis, but as this does not have any liver-specific items. Hence, its applicability in evaluating HRQOL in chronic hepatitis has been questioned. Recently two disease-specific instruments have been validated for chronic hepatitis patients.[5, 6]

Disease-specific HRQOL indices

These indices have the responsiveness to detect small but clinically important changes as the disease progresses or an intervention is carried out.[1, 8, 10] A disease-specific instrument does not allow for comparison of different chronic diseases and requires rigorous methodology for development and testing.[1, 8] Such instruments have been in use for various chronic diseases such as inflammatory bowel disease, rheumatoid arthritis, or chronic lung disease. These instruments may incorporate features of the generic instrument and additional items related to the specific disease (disease-specific module) or have a totally separate questionnaire. Two groups of workers have validated disease–specific instruments for evaluating HRQOL in chronic hepatitis.[5, 6]

The hepatitis quality of life questionnaire (HQLQ) is a brief survey that combines both generic and hepatitis–specific concepts.[5] It supplements SF-36 survey with additional generic scales hypothesized to be sensitive to the HRQOL impact of chronic hepatitis C. These include positive well being, sleep somnolence, and health distress, and disease specific scales health distress due to chronic hepatitis, and limitations because of chronic hepatitis C.

Younossi et al have also developed a disease–specific questionnaire termed as chronic liver disease questionnaire, (CLDQ), incorporating 29 items in 6 domains like fatigue, activity, emotional function, abdominal symptoms, systemic symptoms, and worry.[6] In pretesting, the patients found CLDQ to be clear and easy to complete in 10 minutes. In 133 patients, the CLDQ showed a gradient between patients without cirrhosis, Child's A cirrhosis, and those with Child's B or C cirrhosis. The reliability was moderate at six months, and the instrument was found to be more responsive than the generic SF-36. These two disease–specific indices have been described only recently and there is no data till date on their applicability in assessing intervention in patients with chronic hepatitis B infection.

Looking at the data on HRQOL assessment in patients with chronic hepatitis C, Bonkovsky et al[17] have recently reported that baseline scores of HRQOL cannot be used to predict the likelihood of sustained response to treatment with interferon. The finding that HRQOL scores improved in those patients who had sustained biochemical or virological response supports the concept that the diminished HRQOL in these patients is at least, in part, a consequence of the disease. However, it has been suggested that the post-treatment data should be collected more than once to determine whether improvement in HRQOL persists over time in the responders, and whether any changes occur in non-responders. It should also be assessed whether there is a delayed long-term HRQOL benefit of treatment in non-responding patient. Another important aspect is that HRQOL is likely to deteriorate after interferon therapy, given the adverse event profile of this drug. All these arguments are valid for assessing HRQOL in chronic hepatitis B patients as well.

QUALITY OF LIFE AFTER LIVER TRANSPLANTATION

Liver transplantation has emerged as a life-saving procedure in patients with advanced liver disease. As the clinical outcome of liver transplantation improves, other outcomes (HRQOL and economic) are increasingly being evaluated. A number of studies using different instruments (Table 2) have examined the impact of liver transplantation on the patients ability to return to work as a global assessment of HRQOL. HRQOL of liver transplant candidates is so profoundly disturbed that any generic instrument is likely to show a significant change after transplantation. These generic instruments are not likely to detect smaller changes that are experienced by patients with early stages of chronic liver disease.

Table 2. Instruments used to measure HRQOL after liver transplantation

Sickness impact profile
Medical outcome study Short Form-36
United network organ sharing scoring system
Social behaviour adjustment schedule
National institute of digestive disease and kidney–liver transplant quality of life survey

Utility measures

Utility is defined as the desirability or preference of an individual or society for a given outcome. Utility measures can provide a global index of well-being or utility score. Such measures summarize HRQOL as a single number from a state of full health (1.0) to death (0.0). Two common methods of measuring utility are time trade off and standard gamble.[1, 8] In the time trade-off method, patients trade off years of current state for a shorter life span in full health. The standard gamble asks patients to choose between two alternatives, either continuing in their current health state or a gamble with two possible outcomes, full health or death. A third type of instrument is a multi-attribute utility index such as the quality of well-being scale (QWB). Values for such indices originate from the society rather than from individual patients.

STRATEGIES IN QUALITY OF LIFE RESEARCH

To have meaningful conclusions from HRQOL research, it is important to plan a correct strategy so as to avoid the common pitfalls. The instrument for the assessment of HRQOL should be adequately responsive and a sufficient time after the therapy should be allowed to be sure that one is assessing the impact of therapy rather than the patient's perception of receiving a therapy itself. The instrument should not be administered too frequently (usually no more than every 6 to 12 months) to avoid learning by the patients. Both pre- and post-intervention questionnaires should be included to analyze changes within each subject. Finally, interpretation of results should be made with caution, taking into account various factors like bias and psychopathology and balancing different outcomes like life-years gained, cost, or quality of life.[19]

It is also important to take into account the perception of the patient before actually being informed about the disease. Most patients included in various studies have been told of their emotional state causing anxiety and mood disorders. This may influence the patients to lower their ratings of their own health. It would, thus be interesting to measure HRQOL in recently diagnosed patients, before they receive an explanation of the disease. Repeating the measurement on follow-up before the treatment but after they have been educated, might help sort out the influence of information on health perception. This will become possible when HRQOL instruments become a component of routine health assessment.

REFERENCES

1. Younossi ZM. Economic and quality-of-life measures in the study of viral hepatitis. *Viral Hepatitis Reviews* 1999;5:101-11.
2. McNeil BJ, Weichselbaum R, Pauker SG. Speech and survival. Trade offs between quality and quantity of life in laryngeal cancer. *N Engl J Med* 1981;305:982-7.
3. David G (Guest editor) Hepatitis C. *Clib Liv Dis* 1997;1:494-704.
4. Thyagarajan SP, Jayaram S, Mohanavalli B. *Prevalence of HBV in the general population of India.* In: Hepatitis B in India: Problems and Prevention: Sarin SK, Singal AK, Eds. CBS Publishers & Distributors, New Delhi, 1999; pp. 5-16.
5. Bayliss MS, Gandek B, Bungay KM, Sugano D, Hsu MA, Ware JE. A questionnaire to assess the generic and disease-specific health outcomes of patients with chronic hepatitis C. *Quality of Life Research* 1998;7:39-55.
6. Yunossi ZM, Guyatt G, Kiwi M, Bopariai N, King D. Development of a disease specific questionnaire to measure health related quality of life in patients with chronic liver disease. *Gut* 1999;45:295-300.
7. Cirrincione R, Taliani G, Caproraso N, Mele A. Quality of life assessment in Chronic liver disease. *Hepatogastroenterology* 2002;49:813-6.
8. Younossi ZM, Guyatt G. Quality of life assessments and chronic liver disease. *Am J Gastroenterol* 1998; 93:1037-41.
9. Guyatt G, Bmbardier C, Tugwell P. Measuring disease specific quality of life in clinical trials. *Can Med Assoc J* 1986;134:889-95.
10. Cohen RD. Validation of health-related quality of life instruments. *Hepatology* 1999;29:75-85.
11. Bayliss MS. Methods in outcomes research in hepatology: definitions and domains of quality of life. *Hepatology* 1999;29:35-65.
12. Davis GL, Balart LA, Schiff ER, Lindsay K, Bodenheimer HC Jr., Perrill RP, Carey W, et al. Assessing

health-related quality of life in chronic hepatitis C using the Sickness Impact Profile. *Clin Ther* 1994;16: 334-43.
13. Ware JE, Snow KK, Kosinski M, Gandek B. SF-36 *Health Survey Manual and Interpretation Guide.* Boston, MA: New England Medical Center, The Health Institute, 1993.
14. Karnofsky DA, Burchenal JH. *The clinical evaluation of chemotherapeutic agents against cancer. In* : McLord CM, Ed. Evaluations of chemotherapeutic Agents: New York, Columbia University Press, 1949.
15. Hunt SM, McEwen J, McKenna SP. Measure health status. London, Com Helm, 1986.
16. Carithers R, Sugano D, Bayliss M. Health assessment for chronic HCV: results of qualify of life. *Dig Dis Sci* 1996;41:755-95.
17. Bonkovsky H, Wolky M, and the Consensus Interferon Study Group. Reduction of health-related quality of life in chronic hepatitis C and improvement with interferon therapy. *Hepatology* 1999;29: 264-70.
18. Foster G, Goldin R, Thomas H. Chronic hepatitis C infection causes a significant reduction in quality of life in the absence of cirrhosis. *Hepatology* 1998;27:209-12.
19. Brown RS Jr. Strategies and pitfalls in quality of life research. *Hepatology* 1999;29:S9-12.

Section VII

Management of special groups with chronic hepatitis B

55

Management of chronic hepatitis B in children

Surender K Yachha

Hepatitis B virus (HBV) infection in children assumes importance because of two major reasons: (a) perinatally acquired infection has a tendency to become chronic in approximately 90% of cases and (b) infection acquired during first 5 years of life results in chronicity in 20% to 50% of cases.[1,2] Thus, children with hepatitis B infection contribute in a major way to the total pool of infection in endemic areas.[2] It is now well established that HBV infection is a dynamic disease and an individual may shift from one state to the other.[3] Chronic HBV infection is divided into two groups: (a) without any evidence of liver disease (HBsAg positive for > 6 months, no clinical features of liver disease, normal AST/ALT and normal or minimal abnormal liver histology) and (b) with chronic liver disease as defined by clinical, biochemical, imaging, or histological criteria.[3] Interferon (IFN) and lamivudine (LAM) are the drugs which have been found to be useful in the treatment of chronic HBV infection.

INTERFERON

This drug has been used in children with different dosage schedules and duration with an outcome of variable HBeAg clearance rates (Table 1). Treatment based on consensus statement[2] and several recent articles on IFN treatment in children is summarized.

Whom to treat?

Children more than 2 years of age with ALT elevation twice the normal level or higher, HBeAg +ve, HBV-DNA less than 1000 pg/ml, and biopsy-proven chronic hepatitis B should be treated. Based on experience in European children, the consensus opinion has recommended drug treatment with IFN, above 2 years of age, as the administration of this drug may cause growth retardation during a period when growth is crucial.[2] However, a recently published study showed that the children with chronic hepatitis B infection have a compromised growth even in the absence of IFN treatment.[4] A temporary disruption of growth-

"U-shaped pattern" (both in weight and height for age) were also observed among children treated with IFN.[4] Patients with hepatitis C and/or human immunodeficiency virus (in the absence of thrombocytopenia) coinfection can receive IFN. Careful administration is required in children with metabolic disorders and previous history of febrile seizures. Patients with hepatitis D coinfection, cirrhotic children with features of decompensation, patients with thrombocytopenia caused by hypersplenism, and post-transplant recipients should not be treated with IFN.

Results of treatment

The collective data shows that response to treatment measured by HBeAg and HBV-DNA clearance is achieved in about 30% children (Table 1). A consensus advice based on experience in European children recommended a standard IFN treatment schedule of 5 mIU/m^2 subcutaneously or intramuscularly three times a week for 6 months.

Evaluation of response and monitoring on treatment

Response to IFN treatment is considered when patients clear HBV-DNA, HBeAg seroconverts to anti-HBe and levels of ALT return to normal during treatment or within 6 months after completing treatment. HBsAg clearance occurs less often (6–10%). HBsAg clearance is not regarded as a goal of therapy and liver biopsy is not mandatory to evaluate the response. Table 2 summarizes the proposed schedule for monitoring the patients on IFN therapy. However, in Indian settings where the cost of therapy and special investigations are usually unaffordable, monitoring of proposed antibodies and HBV-DNA may be done only after 6 months of treatment completion to assess the clearance of the virus.

Predictors of response

Controlled trials have shown HBV-DNA level (<100 pg/ml), ALT level twice the normal or higher as the main predictors of response. There are opinions to suggest that high histological activity, old age, and infection acquired postnatally are predictors of good response. HBV infection acquired perinatally produces immune tolerance. These cases therefore, develop higher rate of progression to chronic liver disease, manifest with lack of disease activity despite very high levels of viremia and have a very low rates of interferon-induced or spontaneous HBeAg sero-conversion.[5] One study showed that children infected at birth had a 7% response rate to IFN compared to 72% response for those infected after birth.[6]

Side-effects

IFN is usually well tolerated by children. The most frequent adverse effects during early phase of treatment are fever and flu-like syndrome (>80% of cases), transient weight loss, anorexia (30%), and neutropenia. At a count <1500 neutrophils/cmm, the dose of IFN is

Table 1. Controlled trials of alpha-interferon treatment in white children with chronic hepatitis B

Author	n	Schedule	HBeAg Clearance (%)
Ruiz-Moreno	12	10 mU/m^2 IFN three times weekly × 3 months	25
	12	No treatment	8
Ruiz-Moreno	12	10 mU/m^2 IFN three times weekly × 6 months	58
	12	5 mU/m^2 IFN three times weekly × 6 months	42
	12	No treatment	17
Utili	10	3 mU/m^2 IFN three times weekly × 12 months	30
	10	No treatment	10
Sokal	29	9 mU/m^2 IFN three times weekly × 17 weeks	38
	25	No treatment	8
Utili	22	Prednisone × 4 weeks + 3 mU/m^2 IFN three times weekly × 12 months	41
	21	No treatment	9.5
Barbera	21	7.5 mU/m^2 IFN three times weekly × 6 months	30
	19	3 mU/m^2 IFN three times weekly × 6 months	21
	39	No treatment	13.5
Verrucchi	20	5 mU/m^2 IFN three times weekly × 6 months	40
	14	No treatment	7
Sira	20	Prednisone × 6 weeks + 10 mU/m^2 IFN × 16 weeks	5
	18	10 mU/m^2 IFN × 16 weeks	5.5
	20	No treatment	5
Vajro	13	10 mU/m^2 IFN three times weekly × 12 months	46
	9	Prednisone × 6 weeks + 10 mU/m^2 IFN three times weekly × 12 months	44
	9	No treatment	11
Gregorio	34	Prednisone × 4 weeks + 5 mU/m^2 IFN three times weekly × 12 months	35
	30	10 mU/m^2 IFN × 16 weeks	40
	31	No treatment	13
Sokal	70	6 mU/m^2 IFN three times weekly × 6 months	26
	74	No treatment	11

Table 2. Proposed schedule for monitoring the efficacy and side-effects of treatment

	Days	Months								
	15	1	2	3	4	5	6	9	12	18
Physical examination	Y	Y	Y	Y	Y	Y	Y	Y	Y	Y
Alanine aminotransferase	Y	Y	Y	Y	Y	Y	Y	Y	Y	Y
HBeAg/anti-HBe				Y			Y	Y	Y	Y
Hepatitis B virus-DNA				Y			Y	Y	Y	Y
Blood cell count	Y	Y	Y	Y	Y	Y	Y			
Creatinine		Y								

reduced, while it is withdrawn at a count of <1000 neutrophils/cmm. Other side-effects observed are fatigue, myalgia, headache, hair los, abdominal pain, nausea, anxiety, vomiting, seizures, depression, diarrhea, alteration in taste, etc.

Interferon therapy in Asian children

Trials in Asian children have shown much lower response rates due to perinatal mode of acquisition of infection. Randomized control trials in Chinese children aged 1.5 to 5 years, who were HBeAg and HBV-DNA positive with normal pre-treatment ALT levels (except in two cases) did not show clearance of HBeAg at 12 months.[7] This study reflected that Asian children poorly respond to IFN treatment. Further, randomized controlled studies based on currently available inclusion criteria[2] are required to be done to revalidate this fact. In a study from India, Guptan et al[8] used IFN in 22 children (mean age 8.25±3.6 years) with biopsy proven chronic liver disease, HBeAg and HBV-DNA positive, and elevated ALT more than twice the upper limit. Of the 22 children, 9 had acquired HBV infection by vertical route and the other 13 by horizontal route. IFN resulted in loss of HBeAg and HBV-DNA in 9 cases; 4 developed anti-HBe. At the end of treatment, response was observed in 3/9 (33.3%) in vertically transmitted group and 6/13 (46%) in the horizontal group. This study highlights the fact that response to IFN therapy is similar to what has been observed among adults and is not significantly influenced by the mode of acquisition of hepatitis B virus.

Additional aspects

There is evidence to support the fact that IFN should be used to treat selected children having biopsy-proven chronic hepatitis. Children with moderately elevated serum ALT and low viral load are most likely to respond with HBeAg sero-conversion and this may possibly avoid development of cirrhosis and consequently hepatocellular carcinoma.[9] Opinions do not favor treatment of children having normal transaminase levels, however, this does not imply that chronic HBV infection is always benign. Such patients should be followed up with periodic monitoring of ALT levels.[3] At any given point of time if ALT shows more than two-fold increase (in the absence of any other factor), other investigations should be done to see if the patient qualifies for IFN treatment. Available data has not shown benefit of IFN re-treatment of non-responders initially.

Steroid priming

Patients of chronic HBV infection with relatively low elevation of ALT respond poorly to IFN. Prior to initiation of IFN, these patients may be primed with corticosteroids. Subsequent to withdrawal of corticosteroids "acute hepatitis-like flare" develops (HBV-DNA increases followed by elevation of ALT with corresponding decrease in HBV-DNA). Steroid priming has not been shown to have a beneficial effect in children with chronic HBV infection with normal ALT levels.[10,11] It is, therefore, not yet recommended in children.[1]

Newer developments

Few studies have addressed the issue of long-term effect of interferon in children with chronic hepatitis B.[11-13] A recently published multicenter data on long-term effect of IFN in children with chronic HBV infection[11] needs attention. Results showed that 32% (34/107) of treated children responded to IFN (15% during therapy and 17% during post-treatment follow-up). HBeAg was also lost in 31(29%) non-responders during subsequent years. Kaplan-Meier estimates of cumulative HBeAg clearance rates at five years of follow-up between treated (60%) and untreated (65%) groups were similar. Another interesting observation was that of HBsAg clearance in 25% (4/16) of responders who cleared HBeAg during treatment (early responders) and none of the cases cleared HBsAg in the untreated group. These observations highlight the role of IFN treatment in accelerating natural spontaneous clearance of HBV. The study further substantiated that elevated ALT and HBV-DNA titers more than 1000 pg/ml are predictive factors of IFN response as have been reported by others. This article raised the basic question on recommendations on IFN treatment and generated commentary[9] and views[14] on this subject. It is suggested that IFN treatment perhaps has a role in promoting early clearance of HBeAg which may in the long-term be beneficial in the prevention of cirrhosis and development of hepatocellular carcinoma. Long-term studies are, therefore, required to confirm this in children.[14]

Limitations of treatment

Although interferon has been shown to be beneficial in a subset of p nts with chronic HBV infection, yet, the treatment with this drug is not without major limitations. The most important among these limitations are high cost of IFN, particularly in developing countries. In our personal experience, only 7 children over a period of 8 years could be treated as the majority could not afford the cost despite having fulfilled the criteria for IFN therapy. Several pediatricians in India are unable to treat this subgroup of children due to unaffordable cost (verbal communication), injectable route of administration, uncertainty of response, and side effects.

LAMIVUDINE

This drug is an oral nucleoside analogue that inhibits hepatitis B virus DNA synthesis by chain termination. Studies in adult patients have shown that lamivudine treatment suppresses HBV replication, enhances aminotransferase normalization, and improves liver histology. Treatment with this drug in children lags well behind the data in adults. Dosage and safety of lamivudine in children and adolescents with chronic hepatitis B have been established.[15] The optimal dose for use in children is 3 mg/kg once daily, up to the age of 12 years and after that the adult dose of 100 mg once daily orally should be used. Lamivudine is well tolerated without significant adverse effects or laboratory data changes. Till recently, only a couple of studies of lamivudine in children have been published. Fifty-five children (38 boys, mean age 9.0±3.7 yr.)

with chronic hepatitis B who had not responded to previous recombinant alpha-interferon therapy were treated with lamivudine (dose 3–4 mg/kg/day, maximum 150 mg/day, orally) for 12 months. All these children were positive for HBV-DNA (> 2,000 pg/ml) and HBeAg. At the end of 6 months of treatment, 56.4% patients cleared HBV-DNA and 12.7% of them lost HBeAg and sero-converted to anti-HBe. All children tolerated the therapy without major side-effects.[16] In another study, 54 children (mean age ± SD, 8.0 ± 3.3 years; 9 previously untreated, and 45 non-responders to previous IFN therapy) with chronic HBV infection were treated with lamivudine. At the end of 12 months of lamivudine therapy, 35 children (64.8%) cleared HBV-DNA and 16 (29.6%) had a dramatic fall (>99%) in serum HBV-DNA levels. Only 4 (7.4%) cases cleared HBeAg and of these 3 sero-converted to anti-HBe. ALT values returned to normal in 77.3% patients, decreased by $\geq$ 50% in 13.6% patients.[17] This study has shown that lamivudine treatment of 12 months duration significantly reduces HBV-DNA levels without appreciable sero-conversion of HBeAg. Lamivudine has been shown to increase the efficacy of passive–active immunization in the prevention of perinatal transmission in highly viremic women.[18] No data in children is available to comment on the emergence of YMDD mutations as reported in adults. Lamivudine has also been shown to be beneficial for treatment of chronic HBV infection with decompensated liver disease or immunocompromised status in adults.

SPECIAL PROBLEMS IN INDIA

We have a relatively large pool of HBV infection, a sizeable proportion of chronic liver disease (both adults and children) presenting late to specialists in a decompensated state; and majority of patients cannot afford the cost of IFN therapy. Lamivudine has the advantages of being cheap and ease of administration. In our country, lamivudine has a place for treatment in children with HBV-related decompensated liver disease; and those children with chronic liver disease (high ALT; HBeAg +ve and HBV-DNA +ve) who cannot afford the cost of IFN.[19, 20] The combination therapy is the future of treatment of chronic hepatitis B as in adults. However, the data on combination therapy in children with chronic hepatitis B are still emerging.[21]

REFERENCES

1. Merican I. Management of chronic hepatitis B. Treatment of chronic hepatitis B infection in special groups of patients: decompensated cirrhosis, immunosuppressed and pediatric patients. *J Gastroenterol Hepatol* 2000;15(suppl):E71-8.
2. Jara P, Bortolotti F. Interferon-alpha treatment of chronic hepatitis B in childhood: a consensus advice based on experience in European children. *J Pediatr Gastroenterol Nutr* 1999;29:163-70.
3. Consensus statement hepatitis B and C carrier to cancer. Indian association for study of the liver. *Indian J Gastroenterol* 1999;18 (suppl 1) S16-7.
4. Comanor L, Minor J, Conjeevaram HS, Roberts EA, Alvarez F, Bern EM, Goyens P, et al. Impact of chronic hepatitis B and interferon-alpha therapy on growth of children. *J Viral Hepat* 2001; 8:139-47.

5. Lok AS. Hepatitis B infection: pathogenesis and management. *J Hepatol* 2000;32:89-97.
6. Bruguera M, Amat L, Garcia O, Lambruschini N, Carnicer J, Bergada A, Martin Orte E, et al. Treatment of chronic hepatitis B in children with recombinant alpha-interferon: different response according to age at infection. *J Clin Gastroenterol* 1993:17:296-9.
7. Lai CL, Lok AS, Lin HJ, Wu PC, Yeoh EK, Yeung CY. Placebo-controlled trial of recombinant alpha-2-interferon in Chinese HBsAg carrier children. *Lancet* 1987;2:877-80.
8. Guptan RC, Thakur V, Malhotra V, Sarin SK. Recombinant interferon therapy in Indian children with HBV-related chronic liver disease. *Indian Pediatr* 2002;39462-7.
9. Roberts EA. Why treat chronic hepatitis B in childhood with interferon-alpha. *Gut* 2000;46:591-4.
10. Lai CL, Lin HJ, Lau JN, Flok AS, Wu PC, Chung HT, Wong LK, et al. Effect of recombinant alpha-2-interferon with or without prednisone in Chinese HBsAg carrier children. *Q J Med* 1991;78:155-65.
11. Bortolotti F, Jara P, Barbers C, Gregorio GV, Vegnete A, Zancan L, Hierro L, et al. Long-term effect of alpha-interferon in children with chronic hepatitis B. *Gut* 2000;46:715-8.
12. Kocak N, Saltik IN, Ozen H, Guraken F, Yuce A. Long-term follow-up of interferon responder children with chronic hepatitis. *Gut* 2001;48:740.
13. Camanor L, Minor J, Conjeevaram HS, Roberts REA, Alvarez F. Impact of chronic hepatitis B and interferon-alpha therapy on the growth of children. *J Viral Hepat* 2001;8:139-47.
14. Huang J, Rosenthal P. Is interferon therapy in pediatric chronic hepatitis B infection warranted? *J Pediatr Gastroenterol Nutr* 2000;31:217-8.
15. Sokal EM, Roberts EA, Mieli-Vergani G, McPhillips P, Johnson M, Barber J, Dallow Nm Boxall E, et al. A dose ranging study of the pharmacokinetics, safety, and preliminary efficacy of lamivudine in children and adolescents with chronic hepatitis B. *Antimicrob Agents Chemother* 2000;44:590-7.
16. Kocak N, Saltik IN, Ozen H, Yuce A, Gurakan F. Lamivudine treatment for children with interferon refractory chronic hepatitis B. *Hepatology* 2000;31:545.
17. Kocak N, Ozen H, Saltik IN, Gurakan F, Yuce A. Lamivudine for children with chronic hepatitis B. *Am J Gastroenterol* 2000;95:2989-90.
18. van Nunen AB, deMan RA, Heijtink RA, Niesters HG, Schalm SW. Lamivudine in the last 4 weeks of pregnancy to prevent perinatal transmission in highly viremic chronic hepatitis B patients. *J Hepatol* 2000;32:1040-1.
19. Srivastava A. Clinical trial of lamivudine in children with chronic hepatitis B. *Indian J Gastroenterol* 2002;21:169.
20. Keam SJ, Scott LJ. Lamivudine in children and adolescents with chronic hepatitis B virus infection. *Paediatr Drugs* 2002;4:687-94.
21. Selimoglu MA, Aydogdu S, Unal F, Zeytin Oglu A, Yuce G, Yagci RV. Alpha-interferon and lamivudine combination therapy for chronic hepatitis B in children. *Pediatr Int* 2002;44:404-8.

Management of chronic hepatitis B in patients with end-stage renal disease

Vinay Sakhuja

Chronic hepatitis B virus (HBV) infection was first recognised as a major problem in hemodialysis units in the late 1960s in both Europe and North America and subsequently in other regions as well.[1] After the introduction of infection control measures (segregation of HBsAg positive patients, use of dedicated dialysis machines for HBsAg positive patients, regular serologic screening, etc.), hepatitis B vaccination, and use of erythropoietin, the prevalence of this infection has declined significantly in the West, but continues to be fairly common in the developing world.

HBV INFECTION IN PATIENTS WITH END-STAGE RENAL DISEASE

HBV infection in patients on dialysis

In patients on dialysis, the occurrence of HBV infection correlates with both the number of units of blood transfused as well as the length of time the patient is on hemodialysis.[2] Patients on hemodialysis have a much greater risk of acquiring HBV infection in contrast to those on ambulatory peritoneal dialysis.[3] The infection is frequently asymptomatic in these patients because of the immunosuppressed state.[4] However, in rare instances, a precore mutation may be associated with fulminant hepatitis.[5] Transaminase levels tend to be low even in dialysis patients without liver disease and therefore should not be relied upon for detection of liver disease.[6] As a result, some investigators have suggested that to increase the sensitivity of liver function tests among dialysis patients, lower "normal" values of aminotransferases should be adopted. In one study, the conventional upper limit of normal of 40 IU/l for AST and ALT was changed to 24 IU/l and 17 IU/l, respectively. To detect liver disease resulting from hepatitis B, these altered values enhanced the sensitivity in patients undergoing peritoneal dialysis from about 27 to 72% for AST and from 18 to 64% for ALT.[6a] The authors, therefore, recommended using levels of 24 IU/l and 17 IU/l for AST and ALT, respectively, as the upper limits of normal in dialysis patients. In about 80% of patients, infection is followed by long-term carriage of the virus.[7]

Chronic HBV infection is not an important cause of death on dialysis and survival of HBsAg positive patients is similar to that of HBsAg negative patients.[7,8] This is because the mean delay in the development of HBV-related liver disease exceeds the mean life expectancy of most patients on dialysis.[4] However, as dialysis techniques improve and life expectancy increases, the consequences of chronic HBV infection in this population may become more apparent.

HBV infection in the transplant recipient

Transplant recipients mostly have pre-existing HBV infection acquired while on dialysis but can also get it at the time of transplantation. HBV infection after transplantation is typically asymptomatic.[9] There may be a moderate elevation of transaminases. However, transaminase levels are not a reliable indicator of the activity of liver disease. In rare instances, an HBV pre-core mutant lacking HBeAg expression can induce fibrosing cholestatic hepatitis, a severe liver disease which rapidly progresses to liver failure with a pathologic picture defined by periportal fibrosis, neutrophilic infiltrates, and signs of histologic cholestasis.[10]

The largest study from one centre on 101 HBsAg positive patients who underwent pre-transplant liver biopsies as well as post-transplantation biopsies after a mean interval of 66 months showed that 85% of patients demonstrated histologic deterioration.[11] While 39% had a normal pre-transplant liver biopsy, only 6% showed a normal post-transplant liver biopsy. Chronic active hepatitis and cirrhosis were encountered in 42% and 28% respectively after transplantation. The annual spontaneous disappearance rates of HBsAg, HBeAg, and HBV-DNA were respectively 0.1%, 3% and 3%, lower than those in the general population. Hepatocellular carcinoma developed in 23% of cirrhotics suggesting that the incidence of this malignancy is higher in renal transplant recipients.[11]

Several studies including some from India have shown that the patient and the graft survival are not adversely affected by HBsAg positivity in the first 3–6 years after transplantation.[12-16] However, in the long-term, liver failure and extrahepatic sepsis contribute to a significantly reduced patient survival. Hiesse et al[17] reported a 64% patient survival at 10 years in HBsAg positive patients vs. 80% in HBsAg negative patients. More recently Mathurin et al[18] reported a 10-year survival of 55% in 128 HBsAg positive patients vs. 80% in 490 patients without hepatitis B or C infection.[18] All these studies, however, were done in the pre-lamivudine era.

Influence of pre-transplant liver histology and replication status on risk of progressive liver disease

In a mean follow-up of 4.5±4.3 years, Rao et al[19] did not observe any histologic worsening in patients with only steatosis or chronic portal triaditis on pre-transplant biopsy. In contrast,

26% of those with chronic persistent hepatitis and 64% of those with chronic active hepatitis at initial biopsy died of hepatic failure after transplantation. They also showed that older age and female sex were the other risk factors associated with progressive liver disease. However, even histologically mild disease has the potential to deteriorate under the influence of immunosuppression.[20] It has also been shown that patients with active viral replication prior to transplantation have a poorer survival than those without a replicative HBV.[21] Hepatitis C co-infection may further increase the risk of post-transplant liver disease.[11,22]

Effect of treatment modality (dialysis vs. transplantation) on progression of liver disease

Only two studies have compared the clinical outcome of HBsAg positive patients maintained on dialysis vs. those who had renal transplantation.[20,23] The outcome of 22 transplant recipients treated with azathioprine and steroids was much poorer in comparison to 31 patients maintained on chronic dialysis. Chronic liver disease developed in 100% of transplant recipients compared to 29% of dialysis patients. The overall mortality (64 vs. 19%) and deaths due to liver disease (36 vs. 3%) were much higher in the transplant recipients over a 10-year follow-up.[23]

MANAGEMENT OF HBV INFECTION IN PATIENTS WITH END-STAGE RENAL DISEASE

Evaluation and management on chronic dialysis

There is a paucity of data regarding management of chronic HBV infection in patients with end-stage renal disease. It is uncertain whether alpha-interferon (IFN) would be effective in these patients considering the immunosuppressive effect of uremia. The guidelines for management of these patients are as follows. (a) In those who are positive for HBeAg or HBV-DNA, alanine aminotransferase levels higher than 200U/l, and DNA level lower than 200 pg/ml, IFN in a dose of 5 million units subcutaneously on alternate days should be given for upto 6 months to achieve HBeAg sero-conversion.[24] Lamivudine in a dose of 10–20 mg daily or 50 mg after each dialysis may be given to those with a DNA level higher than 200 pg/ml or those who do not achieve HBeAg sero-conversion after IFN therapy.

Selection of patients for renal transplantation

Assessment of the replication status is important in patients considered for renal transplantation and those with transplantation. Patients positive for HBeAg or HBV-DNA should have a liver biopsy followed by IFN and/or lamivudine therapy.[25-27] The high cost of both interferon and prolonged dialysis coupled with the low efficacy and high frequency of side effects of IFN makes this line of management impractical for most patients in India. Therefore, in the absence of cirrhosis, they should be taken up for transplantation after making these patients HBV-DNA negative with the use of lamivudine before transplantation which should be continued in the post-transplant period also. However, if cost is not a limiting factor, some workers feel that even severe chronic active hepatitis should be a contraindication to transplantation.[26,27]

A liver biopsy should also be done in patients without transminitis or replication markers if a live donor transplant is being considered.[25] While liver biopsy is also worthwhile in those awaiting cadaveric transplants, the timing of such a biopsy depends on the average waiting time for a cadaveric transplant in that center. Patients in whom intensive immunosuppression (e.g. with antilymphocyte antibodies) may be required (spousal transplants or retransplants) should preferably opt for dialysis.

Donor selection

Although HBsAg positive individuals are not suitable for kidney donation, HBsAg positive grafts from live related donors may be transplanted if the recipient is also HBsAg positive.[27] A limited number of transplants have been reported in which positive grafts were transplanted into negative recipients without disease transmission.[28] This should however be done only if the donor is HBeAg negative and the recipient has protective levels of anti-HBs. In addition, hepatitis B immune globulin should also be given to these patients.[27]

Management after renal transplantation

Following transplantation, continued surveillance for reactivation with monitoring of HBeAg and HBV-DNA is necessary so that patients may be considered for antiviral therapy.

Lamivudine

Studies have shown that in patients with viral replication, short-term (6–21 months) administration of lamivudine 100 mg/day was associated with normalization of transaminases, disappearance of HBV-DNA,[29-33] and histologic improvement.[32] The drug was well tolerated and did not affect the metabolism of cyclosporine. However, it requires dose modification in the presence of renal insufficiency. Since withdrawal after DNA clearance was associated with biochemical and virologic relapse, it has to be given indefinitely. However, emergence of resistance due to mutations in the YMDD motif of the hepatitis B polymerase gene may be a limiting factor to long-term therapy.[31] Moreover, the number of patients treated with lamivudine so far is not large. Whether these results would ultimately mean an improved long-term survival and a lower risk of death from chronic liver disease and hepatocellular carcinoma awaits confirmation.

Interferon-α

It may not be safe to use this drug in the setting of kidney transplantation since it has been reported to cause deterioration in graft function not only by inducing acute rejection[34] but also by other mechanisms such as interstitial nephritis and cytokine release.[35]

Post-transplant immunmosuppressive therapy

Immunosuppressive therapy enhances viral replication and accelerates progression of liver disease. Moreover, these patients have a lower immunological reactivity and thus a lower risk of rejection. It is, therefore, preferable to maintain them on the minimum number and dose of immunosuppressive drugs sufficient to prevent rejection.[25,27] Prophylactic use of anti-lymphocyte antibodies should be avoided.[23] Steroid-free immunosuppression may be tried. Since azathioprine also promotes viral replication, cyclosporine monotherapy may be used in these patients. David-Neto et al[36] have shown that withdrawal of azathioprine reduces the risk of severe chronic liver disease in transplant recipients. However, even cyclosporine may have an adverse impact on the outcome of liver disease as shown by Kim et al[37] and Yagisawa et al.[38] No information is available regarding the effects of newer drugs like tacrolimus or mycophenolate on liver disease. Patients with cirrhosis may need a significant reduction in the dose of cyclosporine because of reduced metabolism of the drug. In patients who develop cirrhosis, abdominal ultrasound and tests for serum alfa-fetoprotein should be frequently performed for early detection of hepatocellular carcinoma.

REFERENCES

1. Martin P, Friedman LS. Chronic viral hepatitis and the management of chronic renal failure. *Kidney Int* 1995;47:1231-41.
2. Szmuness W, Prince AM, Grady GF, Mann MK, Levome RW, Friedman EA, Jacobs MJ, et al. Hepatitis B infection: A point prevalence study in 15 US hemodialysis centers. *JAMA* 1974;227:901-6.
3. Neto MC, Draibe SA, Silva AE. Incidence of and risk factors for hepatitis B virus infection among hemodialysis and CAPD patients. *Nephrol Dial Transplant* 1995;10:240-6.
4. Fabrizi F, Martin P. Hepatitis B virus infection in dialysis patients. *Am J Nephrol* 2000; 20:1-11.
5. Tanaka S, Yoshiba N, Iino S, Fukuda M, Nakao H, Tsuda F, Okamoto H, et al. A common-source outbreak of fulminant hepatitis B in hemodialysis patients induced by precore mutant. *Kidney Int* 1995;48:1972-8.
6. Guh JY, Lai YH, Yang CY, Chen SC, Chuang WL, Hsu TC, Chen HC, et al. Impact of decreased serum transaminase levels on the evaluation of viral hepatitis B in hemodialysis patients. *Nephron* 1995;69:459-65.
6a. Hung KY, Lee KC, Yen CJ, Wu KD, Tsai TJ, Chen WY. Revised cut off value of resum amino transfinase in defecting viral hepatitis among CAPD patients: experience from Taiwan, an endemic area for hepatitis B. *Nephron Dial Transplant* 1997;12:180-3.
7. Harnett JD, Parfrey PS, Kennedy M, Zeldis JB, Steinman TI, Guttmann RD. The long-term outcome of hepatitis B infection in hemodialysis patients. *Am J Kidney Dis* 1988;11:210-3.
8. Josselson J, Kyser BA, Weir MR, Sadler JH. Hepatitis B surface antigenemia in a chronic hemodialysis program: lack of influence on morbidity and mortality. *Am J Kidney Dis* 1987;9:456-61.

9. Degos F, Lugassy C, Degott C. Hepatitis B virus and hepatitis B related viral infection in renal transplant recipients. *Gastroenterology* 1988;94:151-6.
10. Fang JWS, Tung FYT, Davis GL, Dolson DJ, Van Thiel DH, Lau JYN. Fibrosing cholestatic hepatitis in a transplant recipient with hepatitis B virus precore mutant. *Gastroenterology* 1993;105:901-4.
11. Fornairon S, Pol S, Legendre C, Carnot F, Bruneel MF, Brechot C, Kreis H. The long-term virologic and pathologic impact of renal transplantation on chronic hepatitis B virus infection. *Transplantation* 1996;62:297-9.
12. Pirson Y, Alexandre GP, Ypersele C. Long-term effect of HBs antigenemia on patient survival after renal transplantation. *N Engl J Med* 1977;296:194-6.
13. Agarwal SK, Dash SC, Tiwari SC. Clinicopathologic course of hepatitis B infection in surface antigen carriers following living related renal transplantation. *Am J Kidney Dis* 1994;24:78-82.
14. Mani MK, Bhaskaran S, Prakash KC. The effect of hepatitis B on a dialysis-transplant program. *Transplantation* 1993;55:1188-90.
15. Roy DM, Thomas PP, Dakshinamurthy KV, Jacob CK, Shastry JCM. Long-term survival in living related donor renal transplant recipients with hepatitis B infection. *Transplantation* 1994;58:118-9.
16. Lee WC, Shu KH, Cheng CH, Wo MJ, Chen CH, Lian JC. Long-term impact of hepatitis B, C virus infection on renal transplantation. *Am J Nephrol* 2001;21:300-6.
17. Hiesse C, Buffet C, Neyrat N, Rieu P, Carpentier B, Etienne JP. Impact of HBs antigenemia on long-term patient survival and causes of death after transplantation. *Clin Transplant* 1992;46:461-7.
18. Mathurin P, Mouquet C, Poynard T, Sylla C. Impact of hepatitis B and C virus on kidney transplantation outcome. *Hepatology* 1999;29:257-63.
19. Rao KV, Anderson WR, Kasiske BL, Dahl DC. Value of liver biopsy in the evaluation and management of chronic liver disease in renal transplant recipients. *Am J Med* 1993;94:241-50.
20. Parfrey PS, Forbes RDC, Hutchinson TA, Kenick S, Farge D, Dauphinee WD, Seely JF, et al. The impact of renal transplantation on the course of hepatitis B liver disease. *Transplantation* 1985;39:610-5.
21. Fairley CK, Mijch A, Gust ID, Nichilson S, Dimitrakakis M, Lucas CR. The increased risk of fatal liver disease in renal transplant patients who are hepatitis B e antigen and/or HBV-DNA positive. *Transplantation* 1991;52:497-500.
22. Zylberberg H, Landau A, Carnot F, Driss F, Chaix ML, Brechot C, Kreis H, et al. Impact of co-infection by hepatitis B virus and hepatitis C virus in renal transplantation. *Transplant Proc* 1998;30:2820-2.
23. Harnett JD, Zeldis JB, Parfrey PS, Kennedy M, Sircar R, Steinmann TI, Gutmann RD. Hepatitis B disease in dialysis and transplant patients. Further epidemiologic and serologic studies. *Transplantation* 1987;44:369-76.
24. Malik AH, Lee WM. Chronic hepatitis B virus infection: Treatment strategies for the next millenium. *Ann Int Med* 2000;132:723-31.
25. Vathsala A. Viral hepatitis in renal transplantation. *Transplant Proc* 1999;31:337-9.
26. Morales JM. Renal transplantation in patients positive for hepatitis B or C. *Transplant Proc* 1998;30:2064-9.
27. Paparella M, Tarantino A, Ponticelli C. How to manage the dialysis patients with chronic viral hepatitis who is considered for renal transplantation. *Nephrol Dial Transplant* 1996;11:2122-4.
28. Okamoto M, Yoshimura N, Nakai I, Nakajima H, Mizuta N, Omori Y, Oka T. Kidney transplantation from a hepatitis B surface antigen positive donor to a HBsAg negative recipient. *Transplant Proc* 1999;31:2869.
29. Rostaing L, Henry S, Cisterne JM, Duffaut M, Ieart J, Durand D. Efficacy and safety of lamivudine

on replication of recurrent hepatitis B after cadaveric renal transplantation. *Transplantation* 1997;64: 1624-6.
30. Jung YO, Lee YS, Yang WS, Han DJ, Park JS, Park SK. Treatment of chronic hepatitis B with lamivudine in renal transplant recipients. *Transplantation* 1998;66:733-7.
31. Goffin E, Horsmans Y, Cornu C, Squifflet JP, Pirson Y. Lamivudine inhibits hepatitis B virus replication in kidney graft recipients. *Transplantation* 1998;66:407-9.
32. Antoine C, Landau A, Menoyo V, Duong JP, Duboust A, Glotz D. Efficacy and safety of lamivudine in renal transplant patients with hepatitis B. *Transplant Proc* 2000;384-5.
33. Samtos FR, Haiashi AR, Arajo MR, Abensur II, Rom o Je Jr. Noronha IL. Lamivudine therapy for hepatitis B in renal transplantation. *Braz J Med Biol Res* 2002;35:199-203.
34. Kramer P, Kate FW, Bijnen AB, Jeekel J, Weimar W. Recombinant leucocyte interferon A induces steroid resistant acute vascular rejection episodes in renal transplant recipients. *Lancet* 1984;1:989-90.
35. Therret E, Pol S, Legendre C, Gagnadoux MF, Cavalcanti R, Kreis M. Low-dose recombinant leucocyte interferon-alpha treatment of hepatitis C viral infection in renal transplant recipients. *Transplantation* 1994;58:625-8.
36. David-Neto E, da Fonseca JA, de Paula FJ, Nahas WC, Sabbaga E, Ianhez LE. Is azathioprine harmful to chronic viral hepatitis in renal transplantation? A long-term study on azathioprine withdrawal. *Transplant Proc* 1999;31:1149-50.
37. Kim YG, Kim S, Lee JH, Kim YK, Han JS, Lee JS, Kim SJ, et al. Renal transplantation in hepatitis B surface antigen positive patients. *Transplant Proc* 1994;26:2143-5.
38. Yagisawa T, Toma H, Tanabe K, Ishikawa N, Tokumoto N, Iguchi Y, Goya N, et al. Long-term outcome of renal transplantation in hepatitis B surface antigen positive patients in cyclosporine era. *Am J Nephrol* 1997;17:440-4.

57

Management of chronic hepatitis B in HIV patients

Gourdas Choudhuri

Infection with human immunodeficiency virus (HIV) and hepatitis B virus (HBV) often coexist in the same patient as the two viruses share similar modes of transmission. Around 10% of patients with HIV infection are co-infected with HBV. With early diagnosis of HIV infection and its improved survival due to effective anti-retroviral treatment, hepatitis B-related liver disease is emerging as a significant health problem in patients with HIV infection.

Acute hepatitis B tends to become chronic more often in HIV patients (80% vs. 10%) indicating an immune dysfunction and defective clearance of the virus. Protection against HBV infection should be provided to patients with HIV by effective use of the hepatitis B vaccine. Higher and frequent doses may be required in HIV patients as their immune response rates are poor. The response to treatment of chronic hepatitis B with interferon-alpha in HIV patients is far poorer (0–10%) than what is achieved in naive patients with HBV infection. Considering the cost, adverse effects, and the poor response with interferon-alpha, there is a lack of optimism with its use in patients with HIV infection.

The nucleoside analogue, lamivudine, has shown promise in this group of patients. Lamivudine is useful in suppressing replication of both HIV and HBV. It has been found to be effective in suppressing HBV replication in 96% of HIV patients with chronic hepatitis B infection. This was associated with clinical, biochemical, as well as histological improvement. The dose of lamivudine required in this special group is higher (300 mg/day), and the duration of treatment is long (until HBe sero-conversion and disappearance of HBV-DNA from blood). Rebound viral replication on discontinuation of treatment and the development of YMDD mutants while on prolonged treatment are the major concerns at the moment.

Chronic hepatitis B (CHB) infection occurs frequently in patients infected with the human immunodeficiency virus (HIV). The two viruses, hepatitis B virus (HBV) and HIV, share the same modes of transmission, are present in the same body fluids, and have similar high-risk groups. Further, they are endemic in the same geographic regions. Before the isolation of the HIV in the late seventies and early eighties, the AIDS epidemic had been linked to HBV, due to the very high prevalence of markers of HBV infection.[1]

The poor prognosis of patients with full-blown AIDS did not justify greater attention to co-infection with HBV a decade or two ago. In recent times, due to a large number of patients being detected to have asymptomatic HIV infection, together with their improved survival with the availability of anti-HIV drug regimen, chronic infection with HBV is emerging as a significant health problem in HIV infected subjects.[2] The epidemiological, clinical, and virological patterns of co-infection with these two viruses and their interaction are now being increasingly recognized, and therapeutic strategies being explored.

HOW COMMON IS THE PROBLEM?

The prevalence rate of HBsAg is about 5% in the global population. Of persons infected with HIV, as many as 10% may show evidence of HBV infection.[3,4] There seems to be a considerable variation in the prevalence rate of HBV infection in HIV infected subjects, perhaps reflecting geographical or ethnic differences. A recent study from the USA reported a rate of 23.7%,[5] while earlier study had shown evidence of HBV infection in as high as 80% of those infected with HIV.[2] The mode of infection with HIV seems to influence the rate of HBV co-infection. Those at highest risk are intravenous drug users (IVDUs). In fact the risk of co-infection with HBV in HIV infected IVDUs is ten times greater than those patients who contracted their HIV infection from infected transfusions.

Table 1. Prevalence of chronic HBV infection in HIV-seropositive patients, according to the risk factor for HIV infection

Group	HBV infection (%)
Homosexuals	10 – 12
Intravenous drug users	10 – 89
Transfusion recipients	1

Influence of HIV on HBV infection

In patients already infected with HIV, acute HBV infection progresses more frequently to chronicity.[6-12] Among homosexuals, for example, acute HBV infection becomes chronic in 20% in those who are HIV infected compared to 6% in those who are not infected with HIV.[1,2] The prevalence of chronic HBsAg carriage increases from 5% in HIV uninfected homosexuals to 12% in those who are HIV infected; the corresponding figures for IVDUs are 3% in HIV antibody-negative and 89% in HIV antibody-positive subjects.[6] These observations point towards a defective immune clearance of HBV in patients infected with HIV. This dysfunction seems to occur even in those with early HIV infection much before an overt immunodeficiency state is reached.

PREVENTION OF HBV INFECTION IN HIV INFECTED PATIENTS

Effective vaccines, prepared from plasma or recombinant technology, have proved extremely useful in preventing HBV infection of groups at high-risk of contracting the infection. HBV infection is effectively prevented in HIV infected patients once protective titers of anti-HBs are achieved. Patients with HIV infection, however, have lower response rates to vaccination than the general population.[1,13] The response rate falls markedly and becomes negligible when the CD4+ cell count starts to decline.

Despite these limitations, hepatitis B vaccination remains a useful strategy for preventing infection with HBV in HIV antibody-positive subjects as well for those at high-risk of contracting either or both of these viral infections, such as homosexuals, commercial sex workers, and IVDUs. A modified schedule of vaccination using higher dose of the vaccine and increased number of injections may be required to achieve protective immunity. Moreover, frequent boosters may be required to maintain the anti-HBs titers above the protective levels (>10 mIU/ml) in these patients. Once adequate levels of antibody are achieved, protection against HBV infection seems to be quite effective.

TREATMENT OF HBV INFECTION IN HIV INFECTED PATIENTS

Interferon

Interferon-alpha (IFN) is a cytokine that has antiviral and immunomodulatory properties and has been in use for the treatment of chronic hepatitis B. Several trials have reported benefit with use of recombinant IFN in reducing necro-inflammation of the liver as well as suppressing and clearing the HBV. Till recently, IFN was, in fact, the only approved drug for this condition. Only one-third to half of the patients treated with IFN have been reported to show response to this drug.

The response to IFN in patients with chronic hepatitis B (CHB) co-infected with HIV has, however, been poor. In a study on 41 patients with CHB, none of those who were seropositive for HIV cleared HBV-DNA.[14] The response rate was a dismal 8% in another study.[15] Somewhat encouraging results were reported from two other studies. In one study on 5 co-infected patients with CD4+ count of about 500/mm^3 and CDC stages II or III treated with interferon 5 mIU three times a week for 6 months, anti-HBe sero-conversion occurred in 2, anti-HBs sero-conversion was observed in one while HBV-DNA disappeared in one. There was documented histological improvement as well.[16] In another recently reported controlled trial, interferon-alpha was given in a dose of 6 mIU three times a week for 6 months to 25 patients of CHB co-infected with HIV who had mean CD4+ count of 480/mm.³ Nine (36%) patients lost HBV-DNA and were considered responders. Antibody to HBe, however, developed in only one while HBsAg disappeared in another. The HBV-DNA loss observed in the anti-HIV positive patients was 2.15 times more with IFN treatment compared to those who did not receive the drug (36% vs. 16.7%). Interestingly, HBV-DNA was not found to correlate with the patient's immune status as the mean CD4+ count was lower in the 9 subjects who lost HBV-DNA compared to those who did not become HBV-DNA negative (283 vs. 454/mm³).[17]

Interferon suppresses HBV replication in HIV positive patients with CHB, although the response rates remain low. The decision to treat CHB aggressively with IFN in this setting will probably be influenced by the relative stages of the 2 diseases and the expected duration of survival. Interferon therapy is expensive and is also associated with significant side effects. Since AIDS predominates as the cause of death in patients with co-infection, some workers argue that the target of treatment should be HIV rather than HBV.[10]

Lamivudine
Mode of action

Lamivudine, the (−) enantiomer of 2'-deoxy-3'thiacytidine, an inhibitor of HIV types 1 and 2 reverse transcriptase, has anti-retroviral activity in HIV infected patients. This drug has also been found to be a potent selective inhibitor of a reverse transcriptase enzyme of HBV that is necessary for its replication. Experimental studies both on HBV transfected cell lines and in chimpanzees have demonstrated the ability of lamivudine in inhibiting viral replication.[4] Several large clinical studies of lamivudine in patients with CHB have shown effective inhibition of viral replication as well as clinical and histological improvement of the liver disease.[18,19] Lamivudine, even when given for long periods, was well tolerated and had a very low incidence of adverse effects.

Replication of HBV requires synthesis of an RNA intermediate that serves as a template for reverse transcription. These RNA molecules are transcribed from a fully double-stranded HBV-DNA template (covalently closed circular DNA), which is believed to persist indefinitely in the nuclei of infected cells. The 5' triphosphate derivative of lamivudine competitively blocks the reverse transcriptase activity of HBV and acts as a chain terminator. Chronic HBV infection is sustained by multiple copies of covalently closed circular DNA (cccDNA) in the nucleus. The pool of cccDNA is maintained by an intracellular conversion pathway to ensure that a stable number of copies of cccDNA exist in equilibrium. Inhibition of HBV replication by lamivudine may result in a decline in the total HBV load through two mechanisms: a combination of diminished production of viable virus (permitting new cells to remain uninfected) with hepatocyte turnover, resulting in a decrease in the number of copies of cccDNA within the infected hepatocyte through inhibition of production of replicative intermediates.

Clinical use

Lamivudine was tried in a dose of 600 mg/day or 600 mg/day followed by 300 mg/day in 40 consecutive patients infected with both HIV and HBV. All patients had progressive HIV disease and HBsAg was documented in the serum for at least one year prior to starting treatment. HBV replication was inhibited as early as 2 months after starting therapy in 86% of patients. After 6 months of treatment, 96.3% had lost serum HBV-DNA, the rate of loss being much higher than that reported with IFN-alpha. Lamivudine was also effective on patients in whom HBV-DNA had not previously cleared from the serum after IFN-alpha therapy.

Response to lamivudine in HIV infected patients may depend on the rate of HBV replication. While serum HBV-DNA levels fell significantly in 96.3% of those with high HBV replication (serum HBV-DNA concentrations >5 pg/ml) after 12 months of treatment, 11.5% still had detectable HBV-DNA in their serum. On the other hand, 100% of those with initially low HBV replication (HBV-DNA concentration <5 pg/ml) had undetectable HBV-DNA in their blood after one year of treatment. Long-term suppression of replication of HBV leads to HBeAg sero-conversion and possibly long-term "cure" in around 20% per year in naïve CHB patients. The only major concern with prolonged use of the drug has been the development of YMDD mutants in as high as 32% of cases. Exacerbation of chronic active hepatitis B in HIV infected patients following development of resistance to or withdrawal of lamivudine has been reported.[4, 20, 21] Data on long-term viral clearance in HIV infected patients is presently scanty, and the duration of lamivudine therapy has not yet been defined.

Several other nucleoside analogues, such as famciclovir and adefovir dipivoxil are in the phase of evaluation for chronic hepatitis B infection. Till such time, the role of lamivudine in treating CHB in HIV infected patients needs further studies by large multi-centric trials especially with regard to dose, duration, and expected outcome.

SUGGESTED APPROACH IN INDIA

AIDS in Asian continent has special features that need to be kept in mind when deciding treatment. The incubation period as well as the survival time after the first clinical manifestation is short. The disease tends to progress more quickly than the Western variety. Most infections are acquired by heterosexual contact; intravenous drug use is an important factor only in the North-East. Also, most patients do not come from affluent homes, do not have adequate health insurance or reimbursement support, and cannot hope to avail expensive treatment free of charge from government hospitals for indefinite period. When HIV infection is detected and the patient is uninfected with HBV, adequate vaccination for HBV should be offered to achieve protective titers of anti-HBs.[22] This should also be prescribed to high-risk groups who are still negative for HIV-antibody such as IVDU, commercial sex workers, homosexuals, and those needing frequent transfusion of blood or blood products.

Co-infection with HBV infection has been shown to be a significant cause of morbidity and liver enzyme elevation in HIV patients.[23,24] If HIV infection is detected early before clinical disease has ensued or CD4+ count has declined, and the patient has co-infection with HBV infection with evidence of ongoing viral replication (detectable HBeAg or HBV-DNA in the serum) and liver inflammation (elevated ALT), anti-viral treatment for HBV should be considered. If there are no constraints on finance, an initial trial of interferon-alpha in high dose and possibly on a daily injection regime may be tried. As very high initial HBV-DNA concentrations are often associated with failure to IFN therapy, such patients may be spared the expense and side effects of IFN therapy. Disappearance of HBeAg and HBV-DNA and the appearance of anti-HBe should be considered the end points of therapy.

Most patients with HIV and HBV co-infection will probably do better with lamivudine treatment given orally. This nucleoside analogue can be used in a wide range of clinical situations, such as (a) early HIV infection or full blown AIDS, (b) high or low HBV replicative states (high or low levels of HBV-DNA concentrations in serum), and (c) naïve patients or those who have failed interferon therapy. While the normal recommended dose of lamivudine for HIV uninfected patients is 100 mg/day, those with co-infection with HIV require a dose of 300 mg per day. The duration of treatment is however long, usually one year or more. Successful virological end point should be development of antibody to HBeAg along with clearance of HBeAg and HBV-DNA from the blood. Withdrawal of lamivudine before complete eradication of the HBV may result in rebound increase in ALT and viremia, while long-term usage may be associated with development of YMDD mutant forms of HBV, whose clinical significance has not yet been adequately studied. Since lamivudine is a component of anti-HIV treatment as well, its use for treating co-infection with HBV seems an easier and more justifiable choice to suppress HBV replication.

The algorithm for management of chronic HBV infection in HIV patients in given in (Fig. 1). In addition to the IFN non-responders, patients who cannot afford IFN and those with decompensated disease are the candidates for lamivudine therapy. Periodic evaluation should

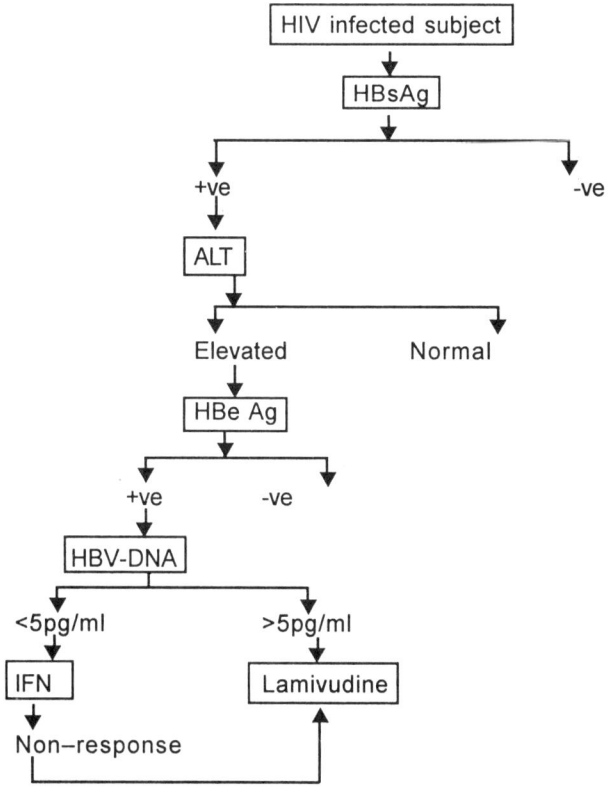

Fig. 1. Algorithm for the management of chronic HBV infection in an HIV patient

include assessment of liver function tests every 3 months and assessment for HBeAg seroconversion every 6 months.

REFERENCES

1. Lunel-fabiani F. *Interactions between Human Immunodeficiency Virus and Hepatitis viruses B, C and D.* In: Sarin SK, Hess G, Eds. Transfusion Associated Hepatitis: Diagnosis, Treatment and Prevention: CBS Publishers & Distributors, New Delhi, 1998; pp.282-94.
2. Hadler JC, Judson FN, O'Malley PM. Outcome of hepatitis B virus infection in homosexual men and its relation to prior immunodeficiency virus infection. *J Infect Dis* 1991;63:454-9.
3. Mc Nair ANB, Main J, Thomas HC. Interactions of the human immunodeficiency virus and the hepatotropic viruses. *Sem Liv Dis* 1992;12:188-96.
4. Benhamou Y, Katlama C, Lunel F, Coutellier A, Dohin E, Hamm N, Tubiana R, et al. Effects of lamivudine on replication of hepatitis B virus in HIV infected men. *Ann Intern Med* 1996;125:705-12.
5. Holland CA, Ma Y, Moscicki B, Durako SJ, Levin L, Wilson CM. Sero-prevalence and risk factors of hepatitis B, hepatitis C, and cytomegalovirus among HIV infected and high-risk uninfected adolescents: findings of the REACH Study. *Sex Transm Dis* 2000;27:296-303.

6. Monno L, Angarano G, Lo Caputo S. *Unfavourable outcome of acute hepatitis B in anti-HIV positive drug addicts. In:* Zuckerman AJ, Ed. Viral Hepatitis and Liver Disease: New York, AR Liss, 1988;pp. 205-6.
7. Bodsworth N, Donovan B, Nightingale BN. The effect of concurrent human immunodeficiency virus infection on chronic hepatitis B: a study of 150 homosexual men. *J Infect Dis* 1989;160:577-82.
8. McDonald JA, Harris S, Waters JA, Thomas HC. Effect of human immunodeficiency virus (HIV) infection on chronic hepatitis B hepatic antigen display. *J Hepatol* 1988;4:337-42.
9. Ockenga J, Stoll M, Tillman HL, Trautwein C, Manns MP, Schmidt RE. Coinfection of hepatitis B and C in HIV infected patients. *Wien Med Wochenschr* 1997;147:439-42.
10. Mai ML, Yim C, O'Rourke K, Heathcote EJ. The interaction of human immunodeficiency virus infection and hepatitis B virus infection in infected homosexual men. *J Clin Gastroenterol* 1996;22: 299-304.
11. Koblin BA, Taylor PE, Rubenstein P, Stevens CE. Effect of duration of Hepatitis B infection of the association between human immunodeficiency virus type-1 and hepatitis B replication. *Hepatology* 1992;15:590-2.
12. Ho D. Viral count in HIV infection. *Science* 1996;272:1124-5.
13. Gesemann M, Sheiermann N, Brokemeyre N. *Clinical evaluation of a recombinant hepatitis B vaccine in HIV infected vs uninfected persons. In:* Zuckerman AJ, Ed. Viral Hepatitis and Liver Disease: New York, AR Liss, 1988;pp.1076-8.
14. McDonald JA, Caruso L, Karayannis P, Scully LJ, Harris JR, Forster GE, Thomas HC. Diminished responsiveness of male homosexual chronic hepatitis B carriers with HTLV-iii antibodies to recombinant alpha-interferon. *Hepatology* 1987;7:19-23.
15. Wong DK, Yim C, Naylor CD, Chen E, Sherman M, Vas S, Wanless IR, et al. Interferon treatment of chronic hepatitis B; randomized trial in a predominantly homosexual male population. *Gastroenterology* 1996;108:165-71.
16. DiMartino V, Lunel F, Cadranel JC, Hoang C, Parlier Y, Le Charpentier Y, Opolon P. Long-term effects of interferon in five HIV positive patients with chronic hepatitis B. *J Viral Hepat* 1996;3:253-66.
17. Zylbergberg H, Jiang J, Pialoux G, Driss F, Carnot F, Dubois F, Brechot C, et al. Alpha-interferon for chronic active hepatitis B in human immunodeficiency virus-infected patients. *Gastroenterol Clin Biol* 1996;20:968-71.
18. Lai CL, Chien RN, Leung NW, Chang TT, Guan R, Tai DI, Ng KY, et al. A one-year trial of lamivudine for chronic hepatitis B. *N Engl J Med* 1998;339:61-8.
19. Dienstag JL, Schiff ER, Wright TL, Perrillo RP, Hann HW, Goodman Z, Crowther L, et al. Lamivudine as initial treatment for chronic hepatitis B in the United States. *N Engl J Med* 1999;341:1256-63.
20. Beesen M, Ives D, Condreay L, Lawrence S, Sherman KE. Chronic active hepatitis B exacerbations in human immunodeficiency virus-infected patients following development of resistance to or withdrawal of lamivudine. *Clin Infect Dis* 1999;28:1032-5.
21. Altfeld M, Rockstroh JK, Addo M, Kupfer B, Pult I, Will H, Spengler U. Reactivation of hepatitis B in a long-term anti-HBs-positive patient with AIDS following lamivudine withdrawal. *J Hepatol* 1998;29:306-9.
22. Welch KJ, Morsa A. Improving screening and vaccination for hepatitis B in patients co-infected with HIV and hepatitis C. *Am J Gastroenterol* 2002;97:2928-9.
23. Gisolf EH, Dreezen C, Danner SA, Weel JLF, Weverling GJ, and the Prometheus Study Group. Risk factors for hepatotoxicity in HIV infected patients receiving ritonavir and saquinavir with or without stavudine. *Clin Infect Dis* 2000;31:1234-9.
24. Sud A, Sing JJ, Dhiman RK, Wanchu A, Singh S, Chawla Y. Hepatitis B virus coinfections in HIV infected patients. *Trop Gastroenterol* 2001;22:90-2.

58

Role of antivirals and immunomodulators in acute hepatitis B

Anuchit Chutaputti

Chronic hepatitis B remains one of the major public health problems in the world. There are more than 350 million people all over the world chronically infected with this virus. About one-third to one-fourth of these chronically infected people are expected to develop progressive liver disease (including cirrhosis and hepatocellular carcinoma).[1,2] An estimated 15–25% of all subjects infected with hepatitis B virus (HBV) will die prematurely from these conditions.[3] The incorporation of hepatitis B vaccine into the universal immunization program for all the neonates has significantly decreased the prevalence of chronic hepatitis B and hepatocellular carcinoma in the adolescent in endemic areas. During the past 20 years, there were many researches to improve the results of therapy for chronic hepatitis B in order to cure or halt the disease progression. The treatment to prevent progression of acute hepatitis B to chronic stage is another strategy which has attracted the attention. This article will review the literature reports about the treatment of acute hepatitis B by focusing in three groups of patients. These are childhood, adulthood and immunocompromised subjects.

ACUTE HEPATITIS B IN CHILDHOOD PERIOD

The infection with HBV acquired in childhood usually becomes chronic. Numerous studies have been conducted to evaluate transmission of HBV from mother to infant during the perinatal period. These studies consistently found that chronic infection follows in a high percentage (80–90%) of infected infants born to hepatitis B e antigen (HBeAg) positive mothers.[4,5] It has been found that the HBV infection in most of the children is asymptomatic, especially boys.[6,7] The incidence of chronic HBV infection was calculated to be 23–46% in prospective studies of initially uninfected Taiwanese children who were less than 6 years of age.[8,9] The study from African children found that the risk of developing chronic HBV infection progressively decreased with age: 54% for age 6–12 months, 25% for age 12–24 months, 15% for age 2–3 years and 6% for age 4–7 years.[6] Another study from Alaska showed that chronic infection developed in 29% of children acquiring HBV infection less than 5 years of age, in 16% of children between 5–9 years of age, and in 7% of children between 10–19 years of age.[7] As most of these infections are asymptomatic, prevention by universal immunization of all the new born children is the only option.

ACUTE HEPATITIS B IN ADULTHOOD PERIOD

The diagnosis of acute hepatitis B and exacerbation of chronic hepatitis B can be problematic in some cases because both groups of patients can produce both IgG and IgM anti-HBc. However, the titer of IgM anti-HBc in acute hepatitis B is frequently higher than in the exacerbation of chronic hepatitis B.[10-12] The radioimmunoassay (RIA) or fully automated microparticle enzyme immunoassay for anti-HBc has higher sensitivity and specificity to distinguish between these two conditions.[13] Maruyama et al found significantly higher levels of free anti-HBe, HBeAg/anti-HBe specific immune complexes and HBsAg/anti-HBs specific immune complex in patients with exacerbation of chronic hepatitis B compared to patients to acute hepatitis B.[14] Furthermore, patients with chronic hepatitis B consistently produce high titer anti-HBc that cross-react with the nucleocapsid of woodchuck hepatitis virus.

Acute hepatitis B in healthy adults leads to chronicity in about 5–10% of patients.[7,15] The chronic stage in adults is more likely to occur following mild or anicteric infection and following infection with a low-dose of HBV.[16] In two studies from Greece, chronic infection developed in one (0.2%) of 507 cases of clinically acute hepatitis and in none of 13 (majority females) infected heterosexual partners of patients who had acute hepatitis B.[17,18] In another study from Italy, about 4% of 150 patients with acute hepatitis B subsequently developed chronic hepatitis B.[19] On a follow-up evaluation for 25–27 years of 100 Swedish patients who got acute hepatitis B during 1969-1972 found that none of them acquired chronic infection.[20] In a study from Taiwan, of the 37 initially healthy uninfected university students, only 2 (2.7%) developed chronic hepatitis B after an acupuncture-associated hepatitis B outbreak.[21]

The occurrence of chronicity in healthy adult population after acute hepatitis B in the prospective studies is now less than 5%, more so in female subjects.[22] HBV infection tends to be symptomatic in 33–50% of cases in the epidemiological studies.[7] These patients will come to seek the medical attention. Unfortunately, at the early phase of acute hepatitis B, there is no definite parameter to predict who will acquire chronic infection. HBV is not directly cytotoxic to the hepatocytes but hepatitis associated with acute HBV infection is caused by immune lysis of infected hepatocytes by natural killer and cytotoxic T-cells. Interferon-alpha can increase natural killer cells activity and enhance human leucocyte antigen (HLA) class I antigen expression on the cytoplasmic membrane of virus-infected hepatocytes.[23,24] Ikeda et al found that approximately 30% of the patients with acute hepatitis B had minimal defect in the ability to produce sufficient interferon-alpha and hence in clearance of HBV.[25] However, the subsequent study from Taiwan failed to demonstrate these defects.[26]

Trepo et al[27] gave interferon 5 million units 3 times a week for 24 weeks in 7 French patients with acute hepatitis B with elevated serum aminotransferase (ALT) level to at least 1.5 times the upper limit of normal between 10 weeks and 6 months and followed up for 1 year comparing to 8 patients who were not given any treatment. Five of the six treated patients had completely eradicated the infection during interferon therapy with the clearance of HBeAg and HBsAg and sero-conversion to anti-HBe and anti-HBs respectively in each case. Tolerance to therapy was satisfactory in all the patients with acceptable mild side effects. Only 2 of the 7 placebo patients had sero-conversion during the placebo period. However, the study did not demonstrate the final serology at the end of one year of follow-up. Tassopoulos et al[28] subsequently reported 100 Greek adults with acute hepatitis B of less than 1 month duration with serum alanine aminotransferase (ALT) concentration of at least 10 times the upper limit of normal, a serum total bilirubin level of at least 5 mg/dl. They were assigned to receive interferon-alpha-2b either 3 or 10 million units three times a week for 3 weeks comparing with placebo. There were no significant differences regarding the aminotransferase and bilirubin levels in the three groups studied. The clearance of viral antigens (HBsAg, HBeAg) did not differ among the three groups. Side effects and bone marrow suppression were more prominent in the treatment groups. A 51-year-old male, receiving 3 million units of interferon, developed stage I hepatic encephalopathy and ascites. Another 25-year-old male, receiving interferon 10 million units developed grade II hepatic encephalopathy without ascites. Weekly clinical evaluation of the patients at each visit showed some amelioration of the symptoms and signs of acute hepatitis in those treated with 3 million units than those treated with 10 million units of interferon or placebo.

Lamivudine, a nucleoside analogue that inhibits viral replication, was used in 2 Caucasian patients, aged 22 and 28 years, who presented with severe cholestasis more than one month after diagnosis of acute hepatitis B. Neither of them was immune compromised. Both complained of severe fatigue, malaise, anorexia, and pruritus for over 2 months. They were treated with lamivudine 300 mg daily for 2 weeks and followed by 100 mg daily for another 4 weeks. After 8 weeks of treatment, both patients showed a significant drop in serum AST, ALT, bilirubin, and improvement in their symptoms. HBV-DNA was undetectable at the fourth month of follow-up period.[29] Less than 1% of patients who get acute hepatitis B will end up with fulminant-liver failure.[30] When patients were in decompensated stage, the HBV-DNA is usually low and, therefore, the use of nucleoside analogue might not alter the course of the disease except in the initial stage of the illness. The use of interferon in this stage is relatively contraindicated because it may stimulate the immune system and can potentially worsen hepatitis. It is very difficult to design any study to have parallel patients to answer this question.

ACUTE HEPATITIS B IN IMMUNE COMPROMIZED HOST

Most of the patients who developed severe or fulminant liver failure from acute hepatitis B are immune compromized such as elderly, patients on immunosuppressive agents or in post-transplantation period. Overall, 25% of acute hepatitis B in the elderly was complicated with fulminant hepatic failure or subacute hepatic failure and 18.4% of them died. The prevalence of fulminant or subacute hepatic failure and the mortality in the elderly were significantly higher than those in the younger patients.[31] There was a report from Israel using lamivudine 100 mg/day in 74 year-old-female with acute hepatitis B of 2 months duration with normal ultrasound of liver and prothrombin time prior to the treatment. Because of high levels of ALT (1185 IU/l) and signs of early encephalopathy, lamivudine was initiated. The transaminases decreased to normal in one month. Two months after the four months course of treatment, HBsAg turned negative.[32] The recent report from Denmark indicated that lamivudine is safe and effective in patients with acute fulminant hepatitis B in immunocompromised host.[33] Lamivudine had been reported in many studies for successful therapy of post-transplant patients with acute hepatitis B.[34-37] In addition, lamivudine has been used more and more with benefit in patients with chemotherapy induced reactivation of HBV infection.[38,39]

CONCLUSION

Specific therapy for acute hepatitis B may be indicated in immune compromised patients who have severe hepatitis which may progress to fulminant liver failure.[40,41] Nucleoside analogues, especially lamivudine, have been used safely and do not interfere with the host immune status, especially in patients who are on immunosuppressive agents or ones with fulminant liver failure with high level of HBV-DNA. Currently, there are no clear data to indicate treatment of immune competent adults with acute hepatitis B as most of them can clear the virus spontaneously.

REFERENCES

1. Zuckerman AJ. More than third of world's population has been infected with hepatitis B virus (letter). *Br Med J* 1999;318:1213.
2. Zuckerman AJ. Progress towards the comprehensive control of hepatitis B. *Gut* 1996;38(suppl 2):S1.
3. Alter M. Epidemiology and disease burden of hepatitis B and C. *Antiviral Ther 1* 1996;(suppl 3): 9-15.
4. Beasley RP, Trepo C, Stevens CE, Szmuness W. The e antigen and vertical transmission of hepatitis B surface antigen. *Am J Epidemiol* 1977;105:94-8.
5. Shiraki K, Yoshihara N, Sakurai M, Eto T, Kawana T. Acute hepatitis B in infants born to carrier mothers with the antibody to hepatitis B e antigen. *J Pediart* 1980;97:768-70.
6. Coursaget P, Yvonnet B, Chotard J, Vincelot P, Sarr M, Diouf C, Chiron JP. Age- and sex-related study of hepatitis B virus chronic carrier state in infants from an endemic area (Senegal). *J Med Virol* 1987;22:1-5.
7. McMahon BJ, Alward WLM, Hall DB, Heyward WL, Bender TR, Francis DP, Maynard JE. Acute hepatitis B virus infection: relation of age to the clinical expression of disease and subsequent development of the carrier state. *J Infect Dis* 1985;151:599-603.
8. Beasley RP, Hwang LY, Lin CC, Leu ML, Stevens CE, Szmuness W, Chen KP. Incidence of hepatitis B virus infections in pre-school children in Taiwan. *J Infect Dis* 1982;146:198-204.

9. Ko YC, Li SC, Yen YY, Yeh SM, Hsieh CC. Horizontal transmission of hepatitis B virus from siblings and intramuscular injection among pre-school children in a familial cohort. *Am J Epidemiol* 1991;133:1015-23.
10. Hoofnagle JH, Seeff LB, Bales ZB, Gerety RJ, Tabor E. *Serologic responses in hepatitis B, In*: Vyas GN, Cohen SN, Schmid R, Eds. Viral hepatitis. Philadelphia: Franklin Institute Press, 1978:219-42.
11. Sjogren M, Hoffnagle JH. Immunoglobulin M antibody to hepatitis B core antigen in patients with chronic type B hepatitis. *Gastroenterology* 1985;89;252-8.
12. Tassopoulos NC, Sjogren MH, Ticehurst JR, Engle RE, Roumeliotou – Karayannis A, Gerin JL, Purcell RH, et al. Significance of IgM antibody to hepatitis B virus infection. *Liver* 1986;6:275-80.
13. Tassopoulos NC, Papatheodoridis GV, Kalantzakis Y, Tzala E, Delladetsima JK, Koutelou MG, Angelopoulou P, et al. Differential diagnosis of acute HBsAg positive hepatitis using IgM anti-HBc by a rapid, fully automated microparticle enzyme immunoassay. *J Hepatol* 1997;26:14-9.
14. Maruyama T, Schodel F, Iino S, Koike K, Yasuda K, Peterson D, Milich DR. Distinguishing between acute and symptomatic chronic hepatitis B virus infection. *Gastroenterology* 1994;106: 1006-15.
15. Tassopoulos NC, Pepatheodoridis GV, Kalantzakis Y, Tzala E, Dalladestima JK, Koutelon MG, Angelopoulou P, et al. Differential diagnosis of acute HBsAg positive hepatitis using IgM anti-HBc by a rapid, fully automated microparticle enzyme immunoassay. *J Hepatol* 1997;26:14-9.
16. Gocke DJ. A prospective study post-transfusion hepatitis: the role of Australia antigen. *JAMA* 1972;219:1165-70.
17. Tassopoulos NC, Papaevangelou GJ, Roumeliotou – Karayannis A, Ticehurst JR, Feinstone SM, Pucell RH. Search for hepatitis B virus DNA in sera from patients with acute type B or non–A, non–B hepatitis. *J Hepatol* 1986;2:410-8.
18. Roumeliotou – Karayannis A, Tassopoulos N, Richardson SC, Kalafatas P, Papaevangelou G. How often does chronic liver disease follow acute hepatitis B adults? *Infection* 1985;13:174-6.
19. Roumeliotou A, Papaevangelou G. Chronic liver disease rarely follows acute hepatitis B in non-immune compromized adults. *Infection* 1992;20:221-3.
20. Blackberg J, Braconier JH, Widell A, Kidd – Ljunggren K. Long-term outcome of acute hepatitis in 1969-72. *Eur J Clin Microbiol Infect Dis* 2000;19:21-6.
21. Kent GP, Brondum J, Keenlyside RA, LaFazia LM, Scott HD. A large outbreak of acupuncture-associated hepatitis B. *Am J Epidemiol* 1988;127:591-8.
22. Lavarini C, Farci P, Chiaberge E, Veglio V, Giacobbi D, Bedarida G, Susani G, et al. IgM antibody against hepatitis B core antigen (IgM anti-HBc): diagnostic and prognostic significance in acute HBsAg positive hepatitis. *Br Med J* 1983;287:1254-6.
23. Chemello L, Mondelli M, Bortolotti M. Natural killer cell activity in patients with acute viral hepatitis. *Clin Exp Immunol* 1986;64:59-64.
24. Pignatelli M, Waters J, Brown D, Lever A, Iwarsons, Schaff Z, Gerety R, et al. HLA class I antigens on hepatocyle membrane: Increased expression during acute hepatitis and interferon therapy of chronic hepatitis B. *Hepatology* 1986;6:349-53.
25. Ikeda T, Lever AML, Thomas HC. Evidence for a deficiency of interferon-alpha production in patients with chronic HBV infection acquired in adult life. *Hepatology* 1986;6:962-5.
26. Chu Cm, Sheen IS, Yeh CT, Hsieh SY, Tsai SL, Liaw YF. Serum levels of interferon-alpha and -gamma in acute and chronic hepatitis B virus infection. *Dig Dis Sci* 1995;40:2107-12.
27. Trepo C, Chemin I, Petit MA, Chossegros P, Zoulim F, Chevallier P, Sepetjan M, et al. Possible prevention of chronic hepatitis B by early interferon therapy. *J Hepatol* 1990;11(suppl):S95-9.
28. Tassopoulos NC, Koutelou MG, Polychronaki H, Paraloglou–Ioannides M, Hadziyannis SJ. Recombinant interferon-alpha therapy for acute hepatitis B: a randomized, double-blind placebo-controlled trial. *J Viral Hepat* 1997;4:387-94.

29. Hassanein T, Haer ME, Monson P, Chatifield S Hwang. Lamivudine improves the cholestatic phase of acute hepatitis B infection. *Hepatology* 1998;28:2257-8.
30. Stroffolini Y, Ragni P, Moiraghi A, Balocchini E, Santonastasi F, Gallo G, Marzolini A, et al. Case fatality rate of acute hepatitis in Italy: results from a 10 year surveillance. *Scand J Infect Dis* 1997;29:87-9.
31. Lin SM. Acute viral hepatitis in the elderly. *Mang Keng I Hsueh Tsa Chih* 1993;16:14-8.
32. Reshef R, Sbeit W, Tur-Kaspa R. Lamivudine in the treatment of acute hepatitis B. *N Engl J Med* 2000;343:1123-4.
33. Santanton OT, Mazzola M, Pastore G. Lamivudine is safe and effective in fulminant hepatitis B. *J Hepatol* 1999;30:551.
34. Dulai G, Higa L, Kobashigawa J, Martin P. Successful use of lamivudine for severe acute hepatitis B virus infection in a cardiac transplant recipient (letter). *Transplantation* 1999;15;67:1288-9.
35. Herrero JI, Quiroga J, Sangro B, Sola I, Riezu Boj JI, Pardo F, Prieto J. Effectiveness of lamivudine in treatment of acute recurrent hepatitis B after liver transplantation. *Dis-Dis Sci*. 1998;43:1186-9.
36. Senecal D, Pichon E, Dubosis F, Delain M, Linassier C, Colombat P. Acute hepatitis B after autologous stem cell transplantation in man previously infected by hepatitis B virus. *Bone Marrow Transplant* 1999;24:1243-4.
37. Andreone P, Caraceni P, Grazi GL, Belli L, Milandri GL, Ercolani G, Jovine E, et al. Lamivudine treatment for acute hepatitis B after liver transplantation. *J Hepatol* 1998;29:985-9.
38. Rayes N, Seehofer D, Bechstein WO, Muller AR, Berg T, Neutaus R, Neuhaus P. Long-term results of famciclovir for recurrent or de novo hepatitis B virus infection after liver transplantation. *Clin Transplant* 1999;13:447-52.
39. Ahmed A, Keeffe EB. Lamivudine therapy for chemotherapy–induced reactivation of hepatitis B virus infection. *Am J Gastroenterol* 1999;94:249-51.
40. Haznedar R, Yagci M. Lamivudine therapy for acute hepatitis B infection following peripheral blood stem cell transplantation. *Am J Hematol* 2002;69:151.
41. Nakhoul F, Gelman R, Khankin E, Baouch Y. Lamivudine therapy for severe acute hepatitis B virus infection after renal transplantation: case report and literature review. *Transplant Proc* 2001;33:2948-9.

Antivirals in hepatitis B virus related decompensated cirrhosis

Radha K Dhiman, Sameer Taneja, Ashwani K Singal

Prognosis of HBsAg positive cirrhosis remains dismal.[1] Orthotopic liver transplantation is a good treatment modality for cirrhosis. In hepatitis B virus (HBV) infected patients there is a rapid development of recurrent active liver disease in the post-transplantation period.[2,3] Pre- and post-transplantation suppression of viral activity improves the prognosis. Whether suppression of viral activity in decompensated cirrhosis can reverse the decompensation and prolong the survival outside the transplant setting till recently remained unanswered.

AIM OF ANTIVIRAL THERAPY

Once decompensated, HBV-related cirrhotics have 5-year survival of less than 15% as compared to 84% in compensated cirrhosis.[1] Suppression of viral activity in patients with decompensated cirrhotics may improve the patient clinical status and hence survival. Interferon has been the mainstay of chronic hepatitis B treatment since its introduction but the development of nucleoside analogues has revolutionized the treatment policies. However, there are no controlled studies for both these modalities in decompensated cirrhosis.

INTERFERON IN DECOMPENSATED CIRRHOSIS

It has been seen that response to interferon can be accompanied by an acute exacerbation of hepatic injury and this can be life-threatening.[4] However, decompensated cirrhotics have low level of circulating HBV-DNA. Based on these pros and cons, interferon has been tried in low-doses ranging from 0.5 mIU to 3.0 mIU per day (Table 1).[4-9]

Results from these studies were not very encouraging. In Child's C cirrhosis, the risks associated with interferon therapy was unacceptable.[6] Though, Child's A and B patients tolerated the therapy better, side effects were common necessitating frequent dose reductions. The response to interferon treatment was seen mainly in Child's A cirrhosis. A survival advantage was not demonstrated because the trials were uncontrolled. However, in cases where inter-

Table 1. Interferon in HBV-related decompensated cirrhosis

Author	Interferon	n	Duration	Response	IFN dose
Perillo	IFN α-2b	26	24 weeks	100/33/0	low dose
Nevens	IFN α-2b	7	10-28 weeks	e Ag–ve –4/7	low dose
Hoofnagle	IFN α-2b	31	16 weeks	DNA eAg–ve 10/31	low dose
Hassanein	IFN α-2b	19	8 weeks	DNA–ve 10/19, eAg–ve 4/10	low dose
Marcellin	IFN α-2b	15	3-48 months	10/15	low dose
Tetervenkov	IFN α-2b	8	24 weeks	8/8	low dose

feron induced sustained loss of serum HBV-DNA, there was a striking clinical improvement indicating that suppression of viral replication even in decompensated cirrhotics can probably prolong survival.

NUCLEOSIDE ANALOGUES

Recently, several new antivirals have been developed for the treatment of HBV infection. Lamivudine is the most widely studied of these agents. Lamivudine reduces serum HBV-DNA to undetectable levels within a few weeks in almost 100% of cases.[10] Sero-conversion as good as interferon therapy has been achieved at 2 years.[11,12] Histological and biochemical improvement occurs in even those patients who do not seroconvert.[13] Therapy is well tolerated and adverse effects are negligible. It has also shown to improve the life expectancy, quality of life (QOL) for a small overall increase in health care costs.[14] The treatment with lamivudine is expected to reduce and delay the progression of chronic hepatitis B. Although the occurrence of HCC is shown to be reduced in animal studies,[15] it still has not been shown conclusively in humans.

Rationale of use of lamivudine

As compared to interferon, use of lamivudine is not associated with exacerbation of liver injury as its action is not dependent on host immune status. Therefore it has been tried in decompensated cirrhosis in transplant setting to prevent reinfection of the graft.[16-18] Results have been very encouraging. Reinfection has been prevented in more than 75% of cases as evidenced by negative serum HBeAg, HBsAg, HBV-DNA and negative post-transplant liver biopsies for HBV-DNA.[18] The therapy was well tolerated with no side effects. These results and the beneficial effects of lamivudine (Table 2) provided the impetus for trials of lamivudine in decompensated cirrhosis outside the transplant settings.

Lamivudine in decompensated cirrhosis

Reports of lamivudine in decompensated cirrhosis outside transplant settings have come up

Table 2. Beneficial effects of lamivudine

Suppression of HBV-DNA and sero-conversion to anti-HBe
Significant improvement in clinical and biochemical status of liver functions
Reduction of the number of hospital admissions for complications of liver disease
Improvement in the QOL
Well tolerated therapy and no side-effects
Improvement in liver function and Child's score. Can avoid transplant also in a few patients
Improvement in pharmacoeconomics

---

recently (Table 3).[19-26] Almost all of these patients who received therapy for more than 6 months showed improvement in Child's score, serum albumin, bilirubin, and transaminases. Improvement was not dependent on the Child's status at enrolment (Figs. 1 and 2). No side effects or flare ups were seen. Kapoor et al[20] demonstrated a reduction in morbidity and the number of hospitalizations for complications of liver disease. They also demonstrated an improvement in quality of life. Both trials included HBeAg negative patients with HBV-DNA positivity. Results were equally good in these patients. Sero-conversion rates achieved was 46% by Villenuve et al[19] at 19 months, 30% by Kapoor et al[20] at 17.9 months and 28.5% by Singal et al at 12 months.[25] This appears to be higher than that seen in compensated cirrhotics.

Though Kapoor et al[20] did not encounter any mortality during the mean follow-up of one and a half years they lost 4 patients to follow-up before completing 6 months of therapy. In the study of Villeneuve et al,[19] 5 patients died before completing 6 months and 7 had to be transplanted. Hence only 65.7% could continue therapy till the benefits of lamivudine appeared. On further follow-up after 6 months, 2 more patients died of liver failure and one had to be transplanted. Hence 20 of 35 (57.1%) were alive and doing well without transplant at a mean follow-up of 19 months.

Most of these studies are uncontrolled. Recently Yao et al[23] analyzed the outcome of lamivudine treatment in 23 consecutive patients with severely decompensated HBV-related cirrhosis defined as Child's score of ≥ 10 and compared with a historical untreated control group of 23 patients matched for age, gender, and baseline Child's score. Significant clinical response, defined as a decrease in Child's score of ≥ 3 points was seen in 14 / 23 (60.9%) of treated vs. none of the controls ($p < 0.001$). Orthotopic liver transplantation (OLT) was needed in 34.8% of treated patients vs. 73.9% of controls ($p = 0.04$). Excluding transplanted patients, there were no deaths in the treated group vs. 6 deaths in the control group ($p=0.009$). These data suggest that lamivudine may also confer a survival advantage.

Therefore, these studies have definitely demonstrated a beneficial effect of lamivudine with improvement in signs of hepatic decompensation, morbidity and quality of life. In some

Table 3. Summary of trials of lamivudine in HBV-related decompensated cirrhosis

Author, Reference, (number of patients enrolled)	Patients completing at least 6 months	Deaths/ transplant/ lost	Baseline characteristics					Outcome		
			HBV-DNA pg/ml before 6 months	HBeAg +ve n (%)	Loss of HBV-DNA n (%)	Sero- conversion n (%)	Improvement in Child score by >2 points n (%)	Deaths/ transplant after 6 months	YMDD muta- tion
Villeneuve et al[19] (35)	23 (66%)	5/7/0	840 ± 253	13 (57)	20 (87)	6 (46)	22 (96)	2/1	3
Kapoor et al[20] (22)	18 (82%)	0/0/4	258 (30-3100)	10 (56)	15 (83)	3 (30)	9 (50)	0	1
Yao et al[21] (13) abstract	11 (85%)	0/2/0	15-9634	7 (64)	11 (100)	3 (42.86)	9/13 (69)	0	—
Perrillo et al[22] (27)	24 (89%)	—	19/27 +ve	20 (74)	12/19 (63)	10(50)	—	6/0	2
Yao et al[23] (23)	23	0/8/0	ND	ND	—	—	14/23 (61)	0/8	2
Da Silva et al[24] (14)	14	—	ND	9	14 (100)	—	10/14 (71)	—	3
Singal et al[25] (18)	15	1/0/2	9/9	7/9	8/8 (100)	2/8 (29)	12/14 (86)	0/0	1

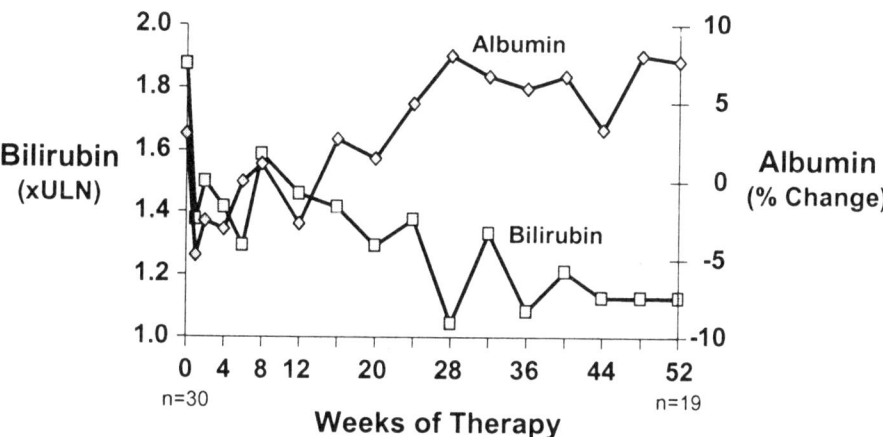

Fig. 1. Effect of lamivudine on liver function and Child's scoring in patients with HBV-related decompensated cirrhotics[22]

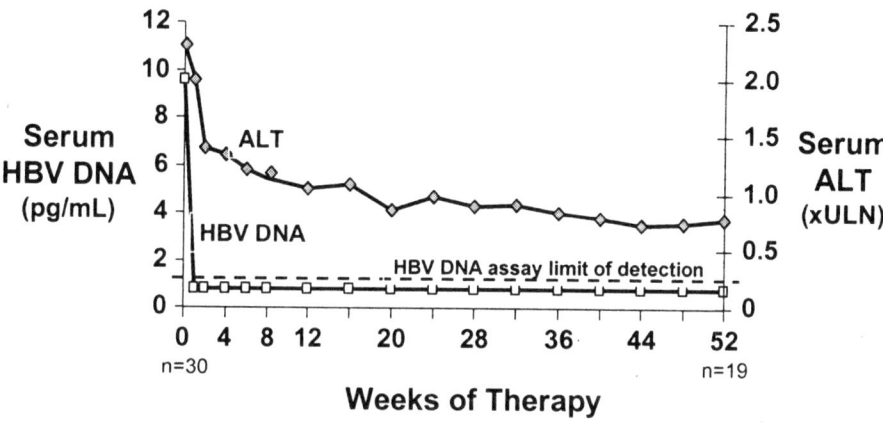

Fig. 2. Effect of lamivudine on ALT and HBV-DNA levels in patients with HBV-related decompensated cirrhotics[22]

patients, treatment with lamivudine may obviate or delay the need for transplantation. Probably there is also a survival advantage because of prolonged period of pre-transplant survival.

Appearance of mutant virus and strategies for future

Villeneuve et al[19] demonstrated a cumulative resistance rate of 10% and 25% at 12 years respectively. This was confirmed to be due to mutations at YMDD motif. Kapoor et al[20] on the other hand demonstrated a resistance rate of 17%, of which only 6% being due to YMDD mutation. Two novel mutations were demonstrated in the rest of the resistant patients. Yao et al[23] demonstrated resistance in 2 (8.6%) out of 23 patients treated. Two problems may be expected in these resistant patients.

Repeat flare-up of disease

This was not seen in any of these studies. However, there was no further improvement in Child's score after the development of resistance. A recently reported compilation of the experience with resistant HBV mutants in four international multicenter trials of lamivudine confirmed that patients with such resistant infections still exhibited significant histologic and biochemical improvement compared with untreated controls.[26,27] Continuation of lamivudine monotherapy, therefore, is prudent even in the face of viral breakthrough, except in the rare instances in which aminotransferase elevations similar to or greater than pre-treatment levels develop.

Problems with transplant

Once the mutant virus takes over, patient becomes HBV-DNA positive and this is a contraindication for transplant at many centers. However, data are now emerging on the role of the liver transplantation for hepatitis B patients with lamivudine induced resistance and mutations.[28] As the timing of mutation is unpredictable, patient may soon revert to the original state. Lamivudine is not the only drug which has shown activity against HBV. Famciclovir has been shown to effectively suppress HBV-DNA.[28] Lobucavir and adefovir dipivoxil have completed phase II trials with good results.[29,30] In *in vitro* studies, adefovir dipivoxil and lobucavir have been shown to maintain efficacy in patients resistant to lamivudine.[31] However, famciclovir usually fails to overcome resistance to lamivudine.[32] Resistance of HBV to lobucavir and adefovir dipivoxil has not yet been observed, but duration of treatment with these agents has been limited. Whether monotherapy with either of these agents or combination with lamivudine can prevent emergence of resistance remains to be seen, but many authorities predict that combination antiviral therapy will emerge as the regimen of choice for treating chronic hepatitis B.[33–36]

REFERENCES

1. De Jongh FE, Janssen HLA, De Man Ra, Hop WCJ, Sclam SW, Van Blankenstein M. Survival and prognostic indicators in hepatitis B surface antigen-positive cirrhosis of the liver. *Gastroenterology* 1992;103:1630-5.
2. Todo S, demetros AJ, Van Theil D, Teperman L, Fung JJ, Starzl TE. Orthotopic liver transplantation for patients with hepatitis B virus related liver disease. *Hepatology* 1991;13:619-26.

3. O'Grady JG, Smith HM, Davies SE, Daniels HM, Donaldson PT, Tan KC, Portman B, et al. Hepatitis B virus reinfection after orthotopic liver transplantation. Serological and clinical implications. *J Hepatol* 1992;14:104.
4. Hoofnagle JH, Peters M, Mullen KD, Jones DB, Rustgi V, Di Biscegille A, Hallahan C, et al. Randomised controlled trials of recombinant human alpha-interferon in patients with chronic hepatitis B. *Gastroenterology* 1988;95:1318-25.
5. Nevens F, Goubau P, Van Eyken P, Desmyter V, Fevery J. Treatment of decompensated viral hepatitis B-induced cirrhosis with low-doses of interferon-alpha. *Liver* 1993;13:15-9.
6. Perillo R, Tamburro C, Regenstein F, Balart L, Bodenheimer H, Silva M, Schiff E, et al. Low-dose titrable interferon-alpha in decompensated liver disease caused by chronic infection with hepatitis B virus. *Gastroenterology* 1995;109:908-16.
7. Hassanein T, Colantani A, DeMaria N, Van Thiel DH. Interferon-alpha-2b improves short-term survival in patients transplanted for chronic liver failure caused by hepatitis B. *J Viral Hepat* 1996;3:333-40.
8. Marcellin P, Giuily N, Loriot MA, Durand F, Samuel D, Bettan L, Degott C, et al. Prolonged interferon-alpha therapy of hepatitis B virus – related decompensated cirrhosis. *J Viral Hepat* 1997;4(suppl 1):21-6.
9. Tchervenkov JI, Tector AJ, Barkun JS, Sherker A, Forbes CD, Elias N, Cantarovich M, et al. Rcurrence free long-term survival after liver transplantation for hepatitis B using interferon-alpha pre-transplant and hepatitis B immune globulin post-transplant. *Ann Surg* 1997;226:356-68.
10. Dienstag JL, Perillo RP, Schiff ER, Bartholomew M, Vicary C, Rubin M. A preliminary trial of lamivudine for chronic hepatitis B infection. *N Engl J Med* 1995;333:1657-61.
11. Dienstag JL, Schiff ER, Mitchell M, Casey DE Jr, Gitlin N, Lissoos T, Gelb LD, et al. Extended lamivudine retreatment for chronic hepatitis B: maintenance of viral suppression after discontinuation of therapy. *Hepatology* 1999;30:1082-7.
12. Liaw YF, Lai CL, Leung NWY, Chang TT, Cuan R, Tai DI, Ng KY, et al. Two year lamivudine therapy in chronic hepatitis B infection: Results of a placebo-controlled multi-center study in Asia. *Gastroenterology* 1998;114:A1289 (abstract).
13. Lai CL, Chien RN, Leung NWY, Chang TT, Guan R, Tai DI, Ng KY, et al. A one year trial of lamivudine for chronic hepatitis B. *N Engl J Med* 1998;339:61-8.
14. Crowley SJ, Tognarini D, Desmond PV, Lees M. Cost effectiveness analysis of lamivudine for the treatment of chronic hepatitis B. *Pharmacoeconomics* 2000;17:409-27.
15. Peek SF, Toshkov IA, Erb HN, Schinazi RF, Korba BE, Cote PJ. 3' Thiacytidine (3TC) delays development of hepatocellular carcinoma in woodchucks with experimental induced chronic woodchuck hepatitis virus (WHV) infection :preliminary results of a life time study. *Hepatology* 1997;26:368A (abstract).
16. Van Thiel DH, Freidlander L, Kania RJ, Molloy PJ, Hassanein T, Wahlstrom E, Faruki H. Lamivudine treatment of advanced and decompensated liver disease due to hepatitis B. *Hepatogastroenterology* 1997;44:808-12.
17. Grellier L, Mutimer D, Ahmed M, Brown D, Burroughs AK, Rolles K, Mc Master P, et al. Lamivudine prophylaxis against reinfection in liver transplantation for hepatitis B cirrhosis. *Lancet* 1996;348:1212-5.
18. Bain VG, Kneteman NM, Ma MM, Gutfreund K, Shapiro JA, Fisher K, Tipples G, et al. Efficacy of lamivudine in chronic hepatitis B patients with active viral replication and decompensated cirrhosis undergoing liver transplantation. *Transplantation* 1996;62:1456-62.
19. Villeneuve JP, ondreay LD, Williams B, Layregues GP, Fanyves D, Bilodeau M, Leduc R, et al. Lamivudine treatment for decompensated cirrhosis resulting from chronic hepatitis B. *Hepatology* 2000;31:207-10.

20. Kapoor D, Guptan RC, Wakil SM, Kazim SN, Kaul R, Agarwal SR, Raisuddin S, et al. Beneficial effects of lamivudine in hepatitis B virus related decompensated cirrhosis. *J Hepatol* 2000;33:308-12.
21. Yao FYK Fracis, Babb NM. Lamivudine reverses severe hepatic decompensation due to replicating hepatitis B infection with cirrhosis. *J Hepatol* 2000;33:301-7 (abstract).
22. Perillio RP, Schiff ER, Dienstag JL, Gish RG, Dickson RC, Adams PC, Brown NA, et al. Lamivudine for suppression of viral replication in patients with decompensated chronic hepatitis B. *Hepatology* 1999;30:301A (abstract).
23. Yao FY, Terrault NA, freise C, Maslow L, Bass NM. Lamivudine treatment is beneficial in patients with severely decompensated cirrhosis and actively replicating hepatitis B infection awaiting liver transplantation: a comparative study using a matched, untreated cohort. *Hepatology* 2001;34:411-6.
24. DaSilva LC, Pinho JR, Sitnik R, Da Fronseca LE, Carrilho FJ. Efficiency and tolerability of long-term therapy using high lamivudine doses for the treatment of chronic hepatitis B. *J Gastroenterol* 2001;36: 476-85.
25. Singal AK. Lamivudine in HBV-related decompensated cirrhosis: a preliminary study. *J Assoc Phys India* 2003 (submitted for publication).
26. Fontana RJ, Hann HW, Perrillo RP, Vierling JM, Wright T, Rahela J, Anschuetz G, et al. Determinants of early motality in patients with decompensated chronic hepatitis B treated with antiviral theraphy. *Gastroenterology* 2002;39:787-90.
27. Saito T, Shinzaa H, Sugahara K, Okumoto K, Togashi H, Kawata S. Lamivudine and rapid regeneration of the atrophic liver in decompensated cirrhosis due to hepatitis B. *Am J Gastroenterol* 2002;97:493-5.
28. Scehofer D, Rayes N, Stein muller T, Neuhaus R, Berg T, Muller A, Neuhaus P. Liver transplantation in hepatitis B patients with preoperative resistance formation during lamivudine treatment. *Transplant Proc* 2002;34:2274-5.
29. Atkins M, Hunt CM, Brown N, Gray F, Sanathanan L, Woessner M, Lai CL, et al. Clinical significance of YMDD mutant HBV in a large cohort of lamivudine treated hepatitis B patients. *Hepatology* 1998;28:319A (abstract).
30. Main J, Brown JL, Howells C, Galassini R, Crossey M, Karayiannis P, Georgiou P, et al. A double-blind placebo-controlled study to assess the effect of famciclovir on virus replication in patients with chronic hepatitis B virus infection. *J Viral Hepat* 1996;3:211-5.
31. Heathcote EJ, Jeffers L, Wright T, Sherman M, Perillo RP, Sacks S, Carithers R, et al. The adefovir dipivoxil study team. Loss of serum HBV-DNA and HBeAg and sero-conversion following short-term (12 weeks) adefovir dipivoxil therapy in chronic hepatitis B: two placebo-controlled phase II studies. *Hepatology* 1998;28:317A (abstract).
32. Heathcote EJ, Chan R, Hutchison J, Lee WM, Sherman M, Utkeiwicz V, De Hertogh D. The labucavir HBV study group. A phase II multi-center study of oral lobucavir for treatment of chronic hepatitis B. *Hepatology* 1998;28:318A (abstract).
33. Ono-Nita SK, Kato N, Shiratori Y, Lan KH, Yoshida H, Kato J, Carrlho FJ, et al. Susceptibility of lamivudine resistant hepatitis B virus to other antivirals; adefovir dipivoxil and lobucavir. *Hepatology* 1998;28:165A (abstract).
34. Jaecket E, Tillman HL, Krueger M, Schmidt H, Boeker K, Trautwein C, Nashan B, et al. Resistance against nucleoside analogues in patients after liver transplantation for hepatitis B cirrhosis. *Hepatology* 1998;28: 235A (abstract).
35. Merle P, Trepo C. Therapeutic management of hepatitis B related cirrhosis. *J Viral Hepat* 2001;8: 391-9.
36. Consensus Statements: Indian Association for Study of Liver. *Indian J Gastroenterol* 2000;20 (suppl 3): C54-66.

60

Hepatitis B virus infection and liver transplantation

Subramanian Venkataraman, Shajan Peter, George M Chandy

The average estimated HBsAg prevalence in India is about 4% with a total pool of approximately 42.5 million people chronically infected with hepatitis B virus (HBV). This places India in the intermediate range for hepatitis B endemicity. Among the 400 million subjects with chronic infection worldwide, India alone represents 9% of the total pool.[1] HBV is reported to be responsible for 70% of cases of chronic hepatitis, 80% of cirrhosis of liver and about 60% of hepatocellular carcinoma in India.[1]

Hepatitis B virus infection is the commonest cause of liver disease worldwide and forms an important indication for liver transplantation. Liver transplantation is the only accepted treatment for end stage liver disease with the promise of a cure. However, early results of liver transplantation for HBV-induced liver disease were poor, with rapid HBV allograft infection leading to 50% mortality rate in the first 3 years after transplantation.[2,3] This compared unfavourably with the 70–80% survival rate for an unselected population of patients undergoing liver transplantation.[4,5] Efforts to improve the outcome of liver transplantation in HBV infected patients have mainly focused on strategies to prevent reinfection. Several new therapies like passive immunization with hepatitis B immune globulin (HBIg) and use of antivirals like lamivudine are improving the outcome in this group of patients.

Currently, there are reports of success in the area of liver transplantation from a few centres in India. The need for transplantation for chronic hepatitis B is likely to be enormous and a uniform consensus about indications, techniques, and antiviral therapies needs to be worked out.

NATURAL HISTORY

Liver transplantation in patients with chronic hepatitis B is fraught with problems. Since the causative agent is not eradicated, infection of the allograft is a virtual certainty in the absence of prophylactic interventions.[6] Acute and chronic liver diseases related to HBV remain the main indications for liver transplantation.

The major reason for patient death or graft failure among these patients is hepatitis B recurrence in the graft. HBV reinfection is related to the presence of active replication before liver transplantation, and is higher in patients with chronic liver disease, than in those with fulminant hepatitis.[7] In a series of 333 patients from 17 different European centres, risk of reinfection defined by the presence of hepatitis B surface antigen (HBsAg) in the serum was highest in patients with HBV-related cirrhosis, lowest in patients with fulminant hepatitis B, and intermediate for patients with associated hepatitis D virus co-infection.[7] Within the subgroup of HBV-related cirrhosis, the risk of reinfection was also related to the level of viral replication before transplantation. Eighty-three percent of patients who were hepatitis B e antigen (HBeAg) and HBV-DNA positive developed recurrent infection compared to 58% of patients who were negative for both the markers.[7]

Retransplantation generally does not change the natural history of infection. In a report by Crippin et al,[8] of 20 patients retransplanted for recurrent HBV infection, there was only one long-term survivor. Sepsis was the most common cause of death in the first 60 days but recurrent HBV infection was responsible for most of the deaths after 60 days.[8]

PATHOGENESIS OF HBV INFECTION IN LIVER TRANSPLANT PATIENTS

Infection with HBV after liver transplantation is primarily because of recurrence of a host infection, occasionally because of transmission of HBV from the donor, and rarely because of transmission of HBV from infected blood products. Patients with recurrence of host infection generally have a poor prognosis and present with significant elevation of aminotransferases with the serum being positive for HBV-DNA.[9] Recurrence of infection after transplantation can be divided clinically into three phases.[3] In the early incubation phase, which is approximately 90 days, recurrence may not be apparent clinically but may be detectable in the serological tests. In the second phase which lasts up to 12 months, it is much more accelerated, with clinical serological, biochemical and histological evidence of hepatitis B. Finally, there is an established plateau phase.[3]

Most liver transplant recipients who are HBsAg positive after transplantation have evidence of histological disease, and, in general, the histological features are fairly similar to those seen in non-transplant patients.[10] The initial histological findings are consistent with acute hepatitis and include both lobular reactivity and necrosis with a positive hepatitis B core antigen (HBcAg). Acute re-infection progresses through a phase of lobular reactivity followed by chronic active hepatitis.[10] The rate of histological progression is accelerated in most patients, with cirrhosis developing within 2 years of transplantation. Rarely, patients who become reinfected develop fibrosing cholestatic hepatitis (FCH) with a rapidly progressive clinical course, and, usually a fatal outcome.[11] Fibrosing cholestatic hepatitis is typified by the presence of periportal and perisinusoidal fibrosis, ballooning of hepatocytes with cell loss, pronounced cholestasis and a paucity of inflammatory activity. Liver injury in FCH is probably due to the direct cytopathic effect of the virus, as suggested by the high cytoplasmic expression of the viral antigens by immunohistochemical stains.[10, 11]

The pathogenesis of liver damage due to HBV in the post-transplant patient is still a nebulous haze. In the immunocompetent patient, an immune response targeted at the hepatitis B core antigen on the hepatocyte surface is probably the primary mechanism of liver injury. Cytotoxic T-cells which express identical antigens to the class I HLA antigens on the hepatocytes expressing the viral peptides, interact to trigger an immune mediated response that results in tissue injury. In contrast, since the HLA antigens of the donor liver and recipient are mismatched, the effectiveness of cytotoxic T-cell response in liver injury is suspect. Direct cytopathic effects of HBV have been shown in transgenic mice, which overproduces $preS_1$.[12] There is inhibition of secretion of HBsAg from the endoplasmic reticulum possibly related to the large amounts of $preS_1$, leading to the accumulation of viral proteins, which are directly injurious to liver cells. These effects are best paralleled by the findings of FCH in humans.[11]

Specific viral mutations are also considered important in the post-transplant HBV infection. Precore mutants with failure of HBeAg production have been noted to have a particularly aggressive clinical course.[13] Mutations in the 'a' determinant of surface gene have been associated with failure of HBIg prophylaxis.[14, 15] It appears that mutations in the S-gene are induced and selected by immune pressure exerted by HBIg.[15] Diminished recognition of variant proteins correlated with failure of HBIg to prevent infection of the liver graft with antigenically altered variant HBV. Patients infected with 'escape' variants s144 or s145 showed a worse clinical outcome compared with other patients on high-dose HBIg prophylaxis (44% vs. 25% graft failure).[15]

HBV infection in liver transplant recipients without prior serological evidence of HBV infection has been referred to as *de novo* infections. In most situations, these infections are due to transmission of HBV from a donor positive for hepatitis B core antibody and rarely from seronegative donors, who harbour and transmit an occult HBV infection.[16, 17] *De novo* infections are usually associated with only modest elevations of aminotransferases and the majority are discovered incidentally by routine post-transplant screening. These patients are usually HBeAg positive and HBV-DNA positive but generally have low HBV-DNA titers, and 5-year survival rates are acceptable.[17]

INDICATIONS FOR TRANSPLANTATION

Chronic hepatitis B

Indications for transplantation are based on the current understanding of natural history of

HBV-related cirrhosis. Patients with Child's B cirrhosis have a 2-year survival of 50–70%[18, 19] in comparison to those with Child's A cirrhosis, who have a very good median survival rate of 80–90%.[20] Since the survival rate of patients with Child's A cirrhosis are comparable to those who undergo liver transplantation, this is not an indication for transplantation.

Timing for transplantation has usually been defined very broadly in general terms. In the United States, minimal listing criteria have been adopted with respect to allocation of liver donations.[21] These criteria are: Child's score ≥ 7, an episode of portal hypertensive bleed, and an episode of spontaneous bacterial peritonitis.

However, it should be noted that these criteria only enable the patient to be enrolled in the organ-sharing network. Transplantation is done only when the patient deteriorates to Child's C status. However, patients who enlist earlier when they are relatively healthy, get priority in allocation of organs. This system may not be suitable for all the situations. Alternative systems with a list of clinical scenarios suitable for transplantation need to be developed. McCaughan has recently proposed one such criteria.[22] These criteria are: Child's score ≥ 9, diuretic "resistant" ascites, recurrent portal hypertensive bleeding not responding to endoscopic therapy, recurrent portal systemic encephalopathy, episode of spontaneous bacterial peritonitis, and development of a less than 5-cm hepatocellular carcinoma.

Fulminant hepatitis B

Indications for transplantation in patients with fulminant and subfulminant hepatitis are still evolving. A number of criteria have been proposed and have been adopted by various transplant centers. The King's College criteria base the need for transplantation on etiology as the most important prognostic factor[23] while the Clichy Paul-Brousse group lay stress on factor V levels.[24] The Chicago group considers criteria like the need for fresh frozen plasma administration to maintain prothrombin time and deterioration of patient's condition during the first 24-48 hours following admission.[25] Van-Theil has suggested that all patients with fulminant hepatic failure should be listed for transplantation and a final decision should be taken only when a suitable organ is available.[26] It is well known that in Asia, many patients with acute hepatitis on underlying chronic HBV infection can present as fulminant or subfulminant hepatitis. A study from Taiwan reported that 63% of patients presenting with FHF like picture had underlying chronic liver disease.[27] These patients have poor clinical outcomes as compared to those patients in fulminant hepatic failure with *de novo* HBV infection. Thus, criteria for western centres may not be appropriate for such a group. Tan[28] considers prothrombin time, level of bilirubin, and degree of encephalopathy to be the most critical parameters. He also found hypoglycemia, acidosis, and increased ammonia levels to be useful parameters in deciding on transplantation. Acharya et al[29] suggested that older age, pro-thrombin time prolongation and cerebral edema may be more appropriate criteria for Indian patients.

THERAPEUTIC STRATEGIES FOR THE MANAGEMENT OF HBV INFECTION IN LIVER TRANSPLANT PATIENTS

Patient selection

The rate of recurrent HBV infection is dependent on the level of viral replication before transplantation.[7] Thus, patients without detectable HBeAg or HBV-DNA have a lower risk of infection and are considered better transplant candidates than patients with actively replicating virus.[30] Although patient selection based on pre-transplant replicative state is still followed by many transplant centres, newer therapeutic regimens may obviate this need. Coexisting HCC is not common in this group but lesions larger than 5 cm in diameter have a very poor prognosis and are not considered for liver transplantation.[31]

Modification of immunosuppression

Activation of a corticosteroid responsive promoter region in the HBV genome has been proposed to lead to increased viral replication and can explain the deleterious effects of steroids in patients with HBV infection.[32,33] Many transplant programs routinely scale down the dose of steroids in liver transplants with HBV infection. This strategy does not increase the risk of rejection.[34] With the more widespread adoption of newer treatment strategies, the doses of immunosuppressants may have less of a role to play in recurrent infection.

Passive immunoprophylaxis

The effectiveness of hepatitis B immunoglobulin (HBIg) in reducing the rate of HBV reinfection has been amply demonstrated.[7,9,35] In a large multicentre trial from Europe, the rate of recurrent HBV infection after 3 years was only 30% in patients receiving long-term HBIg (for at least 6 months) compared with 66% in those who received no prophylaxis.[7] Usually HBIg is given during the anhepatic phase daily for the first week after transplantation. Subsequent schedules vary from center to center. Most centers utilize the titer of anti-hepatitis B surface antigen (anti-HBs) in the serum to determine the frequency of HBIg administration. HBIg given at intervals sufficient to achieve anti-HBs titers of 100–500 IU/l, has reduced the overall recurrence rate to 20–50%.[9,36,37] The patients represented at the higher level of this range are those with markers of active viral replication before transplantation. Some centers give a fixed monthly schedule after an initial week of infusion without monitoring anti-HBs with an acceptable recurrence rate of 17% at 2 years.[38]

Though the beneficial effects of long-term HBIg administration have become widely accepted, there is no consensus on the ideal duration of HBIg therapy. With the treatment schedules available, the rate of recurrence of HBV infection in the graft is significantly less.[7] However, infections are still possible at 12 months post-transplant. The finding of HBV-DNA in the peripheral mononuclear blood beyond 12 months of effective HBV prophylaxis suggests an indefinite risk of reinfection.[39] As a consequence, many liver transplant centers are currently administering lifelong HBIg therapy. Those institutions which use a fixed dose regimen, often vary the dosing interval. For example, a typical fixed dose may be 10,000 IU per week and then monthly. Alternatively, high-risk patients may receive upto 40,000 IU, whereas, low-risk patients may receive 10,000 IU per week since there are large differences in the half-life of the immune globulin between individual patients.[6] Some investigators believe that dosing must be individualized to maintain stable serum titers.[40] Despite the unequivocal evidence of efficacy of HBIg treatment, cost and availability limit their use, especially in higher doses. The US FDA has not approved injection of large doses of HBIg and there is concern about elevated mercury levels due to the thimerosal in the preparation.[41] More recent data seems to indicate that HBIg with lamivudine is more efficacious in the post-transplant period than HBIg alone.[42] The high cost and logistics have recently led to an approach using HBIg only for the first six months in the post-transplant period and continuing later with lamivudine alone to make a cost effective regimen.[42] However, the recent demonstration of low-dose intramuscular HBIg with lamivudine, especially in patients with precore mutations, makes this the most logistically achievable regimen in the developing world.[43]

Mutations in the 'a' determinant of the surface gene have been associated with failure of HBIg prophylaxis.[14] Hepatitis B surface 'escape' mutants are probably selected by passive immunoprophylaxis and result in poorer outcomes.[14,44] Newer HBIg called OMRI-Hep-B (Hepatect) has been shown to induce longer lasting circulating anti-HBs compared to conventional HBIg preparations. Its prolonged half-life reduces the cost by extending the interval between repeat injections.[45]

Antiviral therapy

Antiviral therapies can be used as (a) pre-emptive therapy to prevent graft-reinfection after liver transplantation and (b) post-transplant therapy in patients with overt HBV recurrence, to stabilize graft function and control disease progression.

Interferon-α

Interferon-α has been used with mixed results in both pre- and post-transplant situations. There is some data to suggest that low-dose interferon-α can be used safely in advanced liver disease.[46] In a controlled trial, pre-emptive interferon-α failed to reduce the rate of HBV infection.[47] However, recurrence rates were lower in treated patients than in those with ongoing viral replication. Patients with lower levels of HBV-DNA had a better response to interferon-α. Although HBV-DNA disappeared in approximately one-third of the treated patients, significant side-effects or decompensation of liver disease required cessation of therapy in 50% of these patients.[47] There have been studies showing that the use of interferon in the pre-transplant period leads to stabilization of liver disease and postponement of transplantation.[47,48]

Poor tolerability has been a major limitation, resulting in frequent dosage reduction. This ultimately reduces the antiviral efficacy. In addition to concerns about its tolerability, interferon-α has been found to be relatively ineffective when infection is reestablished in the graft.[49] In a series of 14 liver transplant patients with recurrent HBV, HBV-DNA but not serum alanine amino transferase concentrations, fell with interferon therapy.[49] There is a theoretical risk that interferon-α in liver transplant patients may enhance HLA expression on bile duct epithelial cells and predispose to rejection. The magnitude of this risk is controversial.[47, 49, 50]

Nucleoside analogue therapy

It is now recognized that nucleoside analogue therapy is effective for the treatment of chronic hepatitis B infection. It can be used to prevent HBV infection as well as to treat hepatitis B after liver transplantation. Nucleoside analogues are potent inhibitors of HBV replication and have the potential to substantially improve the outcome of patients with chronic hepatitis B undergoing liver transplantation.[51, 52] Ganciclovir was the first nucleoside analogue to be used after liver transplantation. It reduced HBV-DNA levels in patients with recurrent and *de novo* infection.[53] This response was not sustained and was associated with several side effects. Recent reports have, however, claimed better results.[54] Currently, ganciclovir is only used for HBV recurrence after failure of first line management.

Famciclovir was the first orally administered nucleoside analogue shown to be effective in suppressing viral replication in patients with HBV infection after liver transplantation.[55] In long-term follow-up studies, viral replication increased in 13 out of the 17 initial responders to Famciclovir.[56] A more recent pilot study on six patients with both recurrent and *de novo* HBV infection in the post-transplant period treated with long-term famciclovir reported disappointing results.[57] Virological clearance was observed in only two patients and none of them had a complete biochemical response. These data suggest that famciclovir given as a single agent has limited utility.

Lamivudine given for 52 weeks, on the other hand induces a rapid decline in HBV-DNA levels and has been found to be safe and efficacious in a multicentre study.[58] In this study, lamivudine suppressed HBV-DNA in nearly two-third of the study group with disappearance of hepatitis B e antigen in approximately one-third of patients. Lamivudine used as a single agent reduces the rate of HBV recurrence in the post-transplant period to approximately 20%.[58, 59] Asian patients with chronic hepatitis B undergoing liver transplantation using lamivudine prophylaxis had reported only one instance of breakthrough HBV infection among 31 patients followed up for a median of 16 months.[60] Of these 31 patients, 5 died of causes unrelated to HBV infection early in post-transplant period. Other recently reported trials, however, reveal less impressive results.[61, 62] The Lamivudine North American Transplant Group study on 47 patients who were followed up for 156 weeks after the liver transplantation reported recurrence of HBV infection in 9 out of 22 patients.[61] In another study on 8 patients positive for HBV-DNA treated with lamivudine before the transplantation, it was shown that only three patients had undetectable HBV-DNA after the treatment. On the other hand, liver histology worsened in 5 and was unchanged in 2 patients after treatment.[62]

The major initial limitation to the use of lamivudine therapy is the emergence of drug-resistant variants. Emergence of drug-resistant species, is time dependent[63] and associated with resumption of viral replication and recurrent hepatitis.[64] In the post-transplant setting, YMDD variants have been identified in around 60% of patients treated with lamivudine for longer than 6 months. Such breakthroughs were associated with death or liver failure in upto 50% of patients.[43, 65] Adefovir dipevoxil has been shown to be of benefit in patients who develop resistance to lamivudine.[66]

Combination therapy

The main limitation to the use of nucleoside analogues has been the development of resistance when used for prolonged periods. The use of synergistic combinations that rapidly reduce viral DNA levels have been postulated to reduce the frequency of drug resistance similar to therapy for HIV.[67] Combination therapy with famciclovir and lamivudine has been shown to significantly inhibit formation of drug-resistant covalently closed circular DNA in duck hepatitis B infections.[68] This benefit is lost in humans as there is an accelerated emergence of YMDD resistant variants. The addition of HBIg to lamivudine therapy has been shown to completely prevent HBV reinfection of the allograft.[43, 64, 69, 70] Using a very low-dose HBIg (intramuscular preparation) along with lamivudine seems to be a more practical approach in a country like ours compared with the current high-dose IV regimen. Anti-HBs titers of around 50–100 IU/l have been achieved by this approach and patients remain negative for serum HBV-DNA by PCR.[43]

A new prophylactic strategy has been developed aimed at discontinuation of HBIg treatment after 18 months of administration by giving double dose recombinant hepatitis B vaccine to liver transplant recipients with non-replicative pre-transplant HBV infection. This was found to be effective in inducing protective (>10 IU/ml) serum anti-HBs titers in 82% of patients.[71] Post-transplant HBV vaccination may be a useful cost-effective strategy in the prophylaxis of HBV recurrence allowing the discontinuation of life-long HBIg treatments.

Emerging therapies

Because of high rates of recurrence and mortality, retransplantation for recurrent HBV is a relative contraindication in many centres. However, after the advent of specific antiviral therapies for recurrent HBV infection and post-transplant prophylaxis, the Paul-Brousse group showed significant improvement in survival rates for retransplantation in recurrent HBV infection.[72, 73]

Newer strategies to prevent recurrent hepatitis B that are under consideration include: adoptive transfer of immunity through bone marrow transplantation or lymphocyte transplant of HBV specific cytotoxic T-lymphocytes, xenotransplantation and gene therapy to render donor organs resistant to HBV.[74] Third generation nucleoside analogues that are even more inhibitory to HBV than existing agents are currently in phase II/III studies.[75]

REFERENCES

1. Tandon BN, Acharya SK, Tandon A. Epidemiology of hepatitis B virus infection in India. *Gut* 1996;38 (suppl 2):S56-9.
2. Freeman RB, Sanchez H, Lewis WD, Sherbume B, Dzik WH, Khetty U, Hing S, et al. Serologic and DNA follow-up data from HBsAg-positive patients treated with orthotopic liver transplantation. *Transplantation* 1991;51:793-7.
3. O'Grady JG, Smith HM, Davies SE, Daniels HM, Donaldson PT, Tan KC, Portman B, et al. Hepatitis B virus reinfection after orthotopic liver transplantation. Serological and clinical implications. *J Hepatol* 1992;14:104-11.
4. Krom RA, Wiesner RH, Rettke SR, Ludwig J, Southern PA, Hermans PE, Taswell HF. The first 100 liver transplantations at the Mayo Clinic. *Mayo Clin Proc* 1989;64:84-94.
5. Starzl TE, Todo S, Tzakis AG, Gordon RD, Makowka L, Stieber A, Podesta L, et al. Liver transplantation: an unfinished product. *Transplant Proc* 1989;2197-200.
6. Pruett T. Primary transplant treatment of hepatitis B: hepatitis B immunoglobulin (passive immunization). Liver *Transpl Surg* 1997;3(5 suppl 1): S13-5.
7. Samuel D, Muller R, Alexander G, Fassati L, Ducot B, Benhamou JP, Bismuth H. Liver transplantation in European patients with the hepatitis B surface antigen. *N Engl J Med* 1993;329:1842-7.
8. Crippin J, Foster B, Carlen S, Borcich A, Bodenheimer H Jr. Retransplantation in hepatitis B—a multicenter experience. *Transplantation* 1994;57:823-6.
9. Konig V, Hopf U, Neuhaus P, Bauditz J, Schmidt CA, Blumhardt G, Bechstein WO, et al. Long-term follow-up of hepatitis B virus-infected recipients after orthotopic liver transplantation. *Transplantation* 1994;58:553-9.
10. Demetris AJ, Todo S, Van Thiel DH, Fung JJ, Iwaki Y, Sysyn G, Ming W, et al. Evolution of hepatitis B virus liver disease after hepatic replacement. Practical and theoretical considerations. *Am J Pathol* 1990;137:667-76.
11. Davies SE, Portmann BC, O'Grady JG, Aldis PM, Cgaggar K, Alexander GJ, Williams R. Hepatic histological findings after transplantation for chronic hepatitis B virus infection, including a unique pattern of fibrosing cholestatic hepatitis. *Hepatology* 1991;13:150-7.
12. Chisari FV, Filippi P, Buras J, McLachlan A, Popper H, Pinkert CA, Palmiter RD, et al. Structural and pathological effects of synthesis of hepatitis B virus large envelope polypeptide in transgenic mice. *Proc Natl Acad Sci USA* 1987;84:6909-13.
13. Angus PW, Locarnini SA, McCaughan GW, Jones RM, McMillanm JS, Bowden DS. Hepatitis B virus precore mutant infection is associated with severe recurrent disease after liver transplantation. *Hepatology* 1995;21:14-8.
14. Terrault NA, Zhou S, McCory RW, Pruett TL, Lake JR, Roberts JP, Ascher NL. Incidence and clinical consequences of surface and polymerase gene mutations in liver transplant recipients on hepatitis B immunoglobulin. *Hepatology* 1998;28:555-61.
15. Protzer-Knolle U, Naumann U, Bartenschlager R, Berg T, Hopf U, Meyer zum Buschenfelde KH, Neuhaus P, et al. Hepatitis B virus with antigenically altered hepatitis B surface antigen is selected by high-dose hepatitis B immune globulin after liver transplantation. *Hepatology* 1998;27:254-63.

16. Chazouilleres O, Mamish D, Kim M, Carey K, Ferrell L, Roberts JP, Ascher NL, et al. "Occult" hepatitis B virus as source of infection in liver transplant recipients. *Lancet* 1994;343:142-6.
17. Douglas DD, Rakela J, Wright TL, Krom RA, Wiesner RH. The clinical course of transplantation-associated de novo hepatitis B infection in the liver transplant recipient. *Liver Transpl Surg* 1997;3:105-11.
18. Propst A, Propst T, Zangerl G, Ofner D, Judmaier G, Vogel W. Prognosis and life expectancy in chronic liver disease. *Dig Dis Sci* 1995;40:1805-15.
19. Fattovich G, Giustina G, Schalm SW, Hadziyannis S, Sanchez-Tapias J, Almasio P, Christensen E, et al. Occurrence of hepatocellular carcinoma and decompensation in western European patients with cirrhosis type B. The EUROHEP Study Group on Hepatitis B Virus and Cirrhosis. *Hepatology* 1995;21:77-82.
20. Realdi G, Fattovich G, Hadziyannis S, Schalm SW, Almasio P, Sanchez-Tapias J, Christensen E, et al. Survival and prognostic factors in 366 patients with compensated cirrhosis type B: a multicenter study. The Investigators of the European Concerted Action on Viral Hepatitis (EUROHEP). *J Hepatol* 1994;21:656-66.
21. Lucey MR, Brown KA, Everson GT, Fung JJ, Gish R, Keefe EB, Kneteman NM, et al. Minimal criteria for placement of adults on the liver transplant waiting list: a report of a national conference organized by the American Society of Transplant Physicians and the American Association for the Study of Liver Diseases. *Transplantation* 1998;66:956-62.
22. McCaughan GW. Indications for liver transplantation for chronic viral hepatitis and therapies for controlling hepatitis B virus infection before and after transplantation. *J Gastroenterol Hepatol* 2000:15(suppl):E172-4.
23. O'Grady JG, Alexander GJ, Hayllar KM, Williams R. Early indicators of prognosis in fulminant hepatic failure. *Gastroenterology* 1989;97:439-45.
24. Bernuau J, Samuel D, Durand F. Criteria for emergency liver transplantation in patients with acute viral hepatitis and Factor V below 50% of normal: a prospective study. *Hepatology* 1991;14:49A.
25. Emond JC, Aran PP, Whitington PF, Broelsch CE, Baker AL. Liver transplantation in the management of fulminant hepatic failure. *Gastroenterology* 1989;96:1583-8.
26. Van Thiel DH. When should a decision to proceed with transplantation actually be made in cases of fulminant or subfulminant hepatic failure: at admission to hospital or when a donor organ is made available? *J Hepatol* 1993;17:1-2.
27. Chu CM, Sheen IS, Liaw YF. The aetiology of acute hepatitis in Taiwan: acute hepatitis superimposed on HBsAg carrier state as the main aetiology of acute hepatitis in areas with high HBsAg carrier rate. *Infection* 1988;16:233-7.
28. Tan KC. Fulminant hepatitis B in patients with chronic HBV infection. *J Gastroenterol Hepatol* 2000;15(suppl):E178-80.
29. Acharya SK, Dasarathy S, Kumer TL, Sushma S, Prasanna KS, Tandon A, Sreenivas V, et al. Fulminant hepatitis in a tropical population: clinical course, cause, and early predictors of outcome. *Hepatology* 1996;23:1448-55.
30. Muller R, Samuel D, Fassati LR, Benhamou JP, Bismuth H, Alexander GJ. 'EUROHEP' consensus report on the management of liver transplantation for hepatitis B virus infection. European Concerted Action on Viral Hepatitis. *J Hepatol* 1994;21:1140-3.
31. Mazzaferro V, Regalia E, Doci R, Andreola S, Pulvirenti A, Bozzetti F, Montalto F, et al. Liver transplantation for the treatment of small hepatocellular carcinomas in patients with cirrhosis. *N Engl J Med* 1996;334:693-9.
32. Lam KC, Lai CL, Trepo C, Wu PC. Deleterious effect of prednisolone in HBsAg-positive chronic active hepatitis. *N Engl J Med* 1981;304:380-6.

33. Tur-Kaspa R, Burk RD, Shaul Y, Shafritz DA. Hepatitis B virus DNA contains a glucocorticoid-responsive element. *Proc Natl Acad Sci USA* 1986;83:1627-31.
34. Gish RG, Keeffe EB, Lim J, Brooks LJ, Esquivel CO. Survival after liver transplantation for chronic hepatitis B using reduced immunosuppression. *J Hepatol* 1995;22:257-62.
35. McGory RW, Ishitani MB, Oliveira WM, Stevenson WC, McCullough CS, Dickson RC, Caldwell SH, et al. Improved outcome of orthotopic liver transplantation for chronic hepatitis B cirrhosis with aggressive passive immunization. *Transplantation* 1996;61:1358-64.
36. Samuel D, Bismuth A, Mathieu D, Arulnaden JL, Reynes M, Benhamou JP, Brechot C, et al. Passive immunoprophylaxis after liver transplantation in HBsAg-positive patients. *Lancet* 1991;337:813-5.
37. Rimoldi P, Belli LS, Rondinara GF, Alberti A, DeCarlis L, Minola E, Pirotta V, et al. Recurrent HBV/HDV infections under different immunoprophylaxis protocols. *Transplant Proc* 1993;25:2675-6.
38. Terrault NA, Zhou S, Combs C, Hahn JA, Lake JR, Roberts JP, Ascher NL, et al. Prophylaxis in liver transplant recipients using a fixed dosing schedule of hepatitis B immunoglobulin. *Hepatology* 1996; 24:1327-33.
39. Feray C, Zignego AL, Samuel D, Bismuth A, Reynes M, Tiollais P, Bismuth H, et al. Persistent hepatitis B virus infection of mononuclear blood cells without concomitant liver infection. The liver transplantation model. *Transplantation* 1990;49:1155-8.
40. Sawyer RG, McGory RW, Gaffey MJ, McCullough CC, Shephard BL, Houlgrave CW, Ryan TS, et al. Improved clinical outcome with liver transplantation for hepatitis B-induced chronic liver failure using passive immunization. *Ann Surg* 1998;227:841-50.
41. Lowell JA, Burgess S, Shenoy S, Curci JA, Peters M, Howard TK. Mercury poisoning associated with high-dose hepatitis B immune globulin administration after liver transplantation for chronic hepatitis B. *Liver Transpl Surg* 1996;2:475-8.
42. Markowitz JS, Martin P, Conrad AJ, Marekmann JF, Seu P, Yersiz H, Goss JA, et al. Prophylaxis against hepatitis B recurrence following liver transplantation using combination lamivudine and hepatitis B immune globulin. *Hepatology* 1998;28:585-9.
43. McCaughan GW, Spencer J, Koorey D, Bowden S, Bartholomeusz A, Littlejohn M, Verran D, Chui AK, et al. Lamivudine therapy in patients undergoing liver transplantation for hepatitis B virus pre-core mutant-associated infection: high resistance rates in treatment of recurrence but universal prevention if used as prophylaxis with very low-dose hepatitis B immune globulin. *Liver Transpl Surg* 1999;5:512-9.
44. Shields PL, Owsianka A, Carman WF, Boxall E, Hubscher SG, Shaw J, O'Donnell K, et al. Selection of hepatitis B surface "escape" mutants during passive immune prophylaxis following liver transplantation: potential impact of genetic changes on polymerase protein function. *Gut* 1999;45:306-9.
45. Adler R, Safadi R, Caraco Y, Rowe M, Etzioni A, Ashur Y, Shouval D. Comparison of immune reactivity and pharmacokinetics of two hepatitis B immune globulins in patients after liver transplantation. *Hepatology* 1999;29:1299-305.
46. Perrillo R, Tamburro C, Regenstein F, Balart L, Bodenheimer H, Silva M, Schiff E, et al. Low-dose, titratable interferon-alpha in decompensated liver disease caused by chronic infection with hepatitis B virus. *Gastroenterology* 1995;109:908-16.
47. Marcellin P, Samuel D, Areias J, Loriot MA, Arulnaden JL, Gigou M, David MF, et al. Pre-transplantation interferon treatment and recurrence of hepatitis B virus infection after liver transplantation for hepatitis B-related end-stage liver disease. *Hepatology* 1994;19:6-12.
48. Hoofnagle JH, Di Bisceglie AM, Waggoner JG, Park Y. Interferon-alpha for patients with clinically apparent cirrhosis due to chronic hepatitis B. *Gastroenterology* 1993;104:1116-21.
49. Terrault NA, Holland CC, Ferrell L, Hahn JA, Lake JR, Roberts JP, Ascher NL, et al. Interferon-alpha for recurrent hepatitis B infection after liver transplantation. *Liver Transpl Surg* 1996;2:132-8.

50. Kovarik J, Mayer G, Pohanka E, Schwarz M, Traindl O, Graf H, Smolen J. Adverse effect of low-dose prophylactic human recombinant leukocyte interferon-alpha treatment in renal transplant recipients. Cytomegalovirus infection prophylaxis leading to an increased incidence of irreversible rejections. *Transplantation* 1988;45:402-5.
51. Malkan G, Cattral MS, Humar A, Al Asghar H, Greig PD, Hemming AW, Levy GA, et al. Lamivudine for hepatitis B in liver transplantation: a single-center experience. *Transplantation.* 2000;69:1403-7.
52. Perrillo R, Rakela J, Dienstag J, Levy G, Martin P, Wright T, Caldwell S, et al. Multicenter study of lamivudine therapy for hepatitis B after liver transplantation. Lamivudine Transplant Group. *Hepatology* 1999;29:1581-6.
53. Gish RG, Lau JY, Brooks L, Fang JW, Steady SL, Imperial JC, Garcia-Kennedy R, et al. Ganciclovir treatment of hepatitis B virus infection in liver transplant recipients. *Hepatology* 1996;23:1-7.
54. Roche B, Samuel D, Gigou M, Feray C, Virot V, Majno P, Serraf L, et al. Long-term ganciclovir therapy for hepatitis B virus infection after liver transplantation. *J Hepatol* 1999;31:584-92.
55. Boker KH, Ringe B, Kruger M, Pichlmayr R, Manns MP. Prostaglandin E plus famciclovir—a new concept for the treatment of severe hepatitis B after liver transplantation. *Transplantation* 1994;57:1706-8.
56. Rayes N, Seehofer D, Bechstein WO, Muller AR, Berg T, Neuhaus R, Neuhaus P. Long-term results of famciclovir for recurrent or de novo hepatitis B virus infection after liver transplantation. *Clin Transplant* 1999;13:447-52.
58. Perrillo R, Rakela J, Martin P, Levy GW, Schiff E, Dienstag J, Gish R, et al. Lamivudine for suppression and/or prevention of hepatitis B when given pre/post transplantation. *Hepatology* 1997;26:260A.
59. Grellier L, Mutimer D, Ahmed M, Brown D, Burroughs AK, Rolles K, McMaster P, et al. Lamivudine prophylaxis against reinfection in liver transplantation for hepatitis B cirrhosis. *Lancet* 1996;348:1212-5.
60. Lo CM, Cheung ST, Lai CL, Liu CL, Ng IO, Yuen MF, Fan ST, Wong J. Liver transplantation in Asian patients with chronic hepatitis B using lamivudine prophylaxis. *Ann Sur* 2001;233:276-81.
61. Perrilo RP, Wright T, Rakela J, Levy G, Schiff E, Gish R, Martin P, et al. A multicenter United Sates—Candian trail to assess lamivudine monotherapy before and after liver transplantation for chronic hepatitis B. *Hepatology* 2001;33:424-32.
62. Ben-Ari Z, Mor E, Shapira Z, Tur-Kaspa R. Long-term experience with lamivudine therapy for hepatitis B virus infection after liver transplantation. *Liver Transpl* 2001;7:113-7.
63. Leung NWY, Lai CL, Change TT, Guan R, Lee CM, Ng KY, Wu PC, et al. Three-year lamivudine therapy in chronic HBV. *J Hepatol* 1999;30(suppl):59.
64. Mutimer D, Pillay D, Shields P, Cane P, Ratcliffe D, Martin B, Buchan S, et al. Outcome of lamivudine resistant hepatitis B virus infection in the liver transplant recipient. *Gut.* 2000;46:107-13.
65. McCaughan GW, Koorey D, Spencer J, Spencer J, Verran D, Chui AKK, Shell AGR, Jones R, et al. Prophylactic lamivudine with very low-dose HBIg prevents HBV recurrence post liver transplant. *Hepatology* 1998;28:263A.
66. Perrillo R, Schiff E, Yoshida E, Statler A, Hirsch K, Wright T. Gutfreune K, et al. Adefovir dipivoxil for the treatment of lamivudine-resistant hepatitis B mutants. *Hepatology* 2000;32:129-34.
67. O'Brien WA. Resistance against Reverse Transcriptase Inhibitors. *Clin Infect Dis* 2000;30:S185-92.
68. Colledge D, Locarnini S, Shaw T. Synergistic inhibition of hepadnaviral replication by lamivudine in combination with penciclovir *in vitro*. *Hepatology* 1997;26:216-25.
69. Markowitz JS, Martin P, Conrad AJ, Markmann JF, Seu P, Y Yersiz H, Goss A, et al. Prophylaxis against hepatitis B recurrence following liver transplantation using combination lamivudine and hepatitis B immune globulin. *Hepatology* 1998;28:585-9.

70. Yoshida EM, Erb SR, Partovi N, Scudamore CH, Chung SW, Frigheeo L, Eggen HJ, et al. Liver transplantation for chronic hepatitis B infection with the use of combination lamivudine and low-dose hepatitis B immune globulin. *Liver Transpl Surg* 1999;5:520-5.
71. Sanchez-Fueyo A, Rimola A, Grande L, Costa J, Mas A, Nivasa M, Crrera J, et al. Hepatitis B immunoglobulin discontinuation followed by hepatitis B virus vaccination: A new strategy in the prophylaxis of hepatitis B virus recurrence after liver transplantation. *Hepatology* 2000;31:496-501.
72. Roche B, Samuel D, Feray C, Majno P, Gigou M, Reynes M, Bismuth H. Retransplantation of the liver for recurrent hepatitis B virus infection: the Paul Brousse experience. *Liver Transpl Surg* 1999;5:166-74.
73. Terrault NA. Treatment of recurrent hepatitis B infection in liver transplant recipients. *Liver Transpl* 2002;8(suppl 1):S74-81.
74. Peters MG, Shouval D, Bonham A, Vierling JM, Lok AS. Post-transplantation: future therapies. *Semin Liver Dis* 2000;20(suppl 1):19-24.
75. Perrillo RP, Kruger M, Sievers T, Lake JR. Post-transplantation: emerging and future therapies. *Semin Liver Dis* 2000;20(suppl 1):13-7.

61

Nutrition in the management of acute and chronic liver disease

Yogendra K Joshi, Namrata Singh, Nandini Saxena

During the past few decades role of nutrition has been recognized as a determinant for prognosis in patients with acute and chronic liver diseases. Nutrition also plays a key role in the management of liver diseases. While there is a limited role of nutrition in the management of acute liver disease, it is one of the important strategies in the management of patients with chronic liver disease.

NUTRITION IN ACUTE LIVER DISEASES

Acute viral hepatitis is fairly common in developing countries. Water-borne infection by hepatitis A and hepatitis E viruses is commoner than blood-borne viruses like hepatitis B and C. However, the latter group has chronic sequalae and may lead to cirrhosis of the liver and liver cancer. Hepatitis A is more prevalent in pediatric age group and has mild clinical course leading to almost complete recovery without any chronic sequelae. Hepatitis E is more common in adults and may have moderately severe clinical course and even mortality (1–2%) and this infection also does not lead to chronic sequelae. Hepatitis B and C on the other hand may have a prolonged course and also have a high chance of occurrence of chronic infection, 5–10% and 60–80% respectively.

Studies conducted during the first half of the century to observe the effect of good diet on the recovery from hepatitis (mainly during the epidemics) did not show any significant difference in the recovery period between the treatment and control groups. This could have been because of provision of high carbohydrate diets and inadequate amount of protein supplements. As it is evident from the clinical course, acute hepatitis A and E hardly require any specific dietary modification or nutritional supplements as most of the patients recover within a time period of 4–6 weeks. During this period, most of the patients can take a normal diet with or without symptomatic treatment. However, in case of acute hepatitis B, especially with prolonged course, dietary modification and nutritional supplement may be necessary in order to maintain protein intake and to enhance liver cell regeneration.

Acute viral hepatitis induces the same metabolic effects as any other acute inflammatory systemic disease with an acute phase response. The effect of nutritional support depends on the duration of the acute liver disease and also presence of any underlying chronic liver disease, which may have already compromised the patient's nutritional status. Thus under normal circumstances, no specific diet restriction or supplementation seems necessary. The only challenge is in the circumstances of severe anorexia and nausea where it may be difficult to administer and retain food stuffs. Some believe that a high protein diet is beneficial. Because nausea and anorexia are often less apparent in the morning, it is useful to meet the calorie requirement at this time and to give the rest of the diet in frequent small meals during the day. This may be accomplished with the aid of an increased enteral liquid formula. Fatty foods may not be restricted and extra vitamins supplement is unnecessary unless a specific deficiency already exists. Fluid and electrolytes may be required if the patient continues to vomit and is unable to retain anything orally.

Specific nutrition supplements with adequate calories and protein may be necessary in patients with persistent symptoms like nausea, vomiting, and also prolonged acute phase, as it happens more frequently in cases of acute hepatitis B infection. It is well known that resolution of hepatitis B may take quite a long time especially in diabetics, elderly, and patients with poor oral intake. In case of oral intolerance, it is necessary to provide adequate calories by parenteral nutrition support. Protein restriction usually is not recommended and at least 0.8 to 1 gm per kg/day of protein should be given in the diet.

NUTRITION IN CHRONIC LIVER DISEASE

Malnutrition in chronic liver disease is better defined as protein energy malnutrition (PEM) because both these deficiencies frequently coexist.[1,2] The prevalence and severity of PEM are related to the clinical stage of acute or chronic liver disease. By anthropometric criteria, PEM may be present in 20% of patients with well-compensated liver cirrhosis and in more than 60% of patients with decompemsated chronic liver disease.[3] The causes of malnutrition in liver disease are listed in Table 1.

In India, a recent study done at the GB Pant Hospital, Sarin et al, have shown that protein depletion is common in both alcoholic as well as non-alcoholic cirrhosis, being more pronounced in the latter group.[4] At the All India Institute of Medical Sciences,[5] we found that energy and protein malnutrition was present in 57% and 89% patients with chronic liver disease, respectively. The presence of muscle wasting indicates an advanced stage of malnutrition and is associated with poor survival.[6] Thus, PEM is common in chronic liver disease and positively correlated with functional severity of the liver injury.

Table 1. Causes of malnutrition in patients with liver disease

---
Inadequate dietary intake
Decreased quantity of food intake
Malabsorption and/or maldigestion
Altered nutrient metabolism due to liver disease
Decreased hepatic storage
Increased nutrient losses, frequent large volume paracentesis
Increased nutrient requirements (hypermetabolism)
Drugs

CONSEQUENCES OF PEM

Effect on liver morphology

PEM may affect liver morphology in animals though this has not been demonstrated to any convincing degree in humans. Rats deprived of essential nutrients, develop liver fibrosis. Occasionally, fibrosis is also observed in the liver of children with kwashiorkor. In both cases, fibrosis is readily reversed by the administration of an adequate diet.

Effect on liver function

In patients with cirrhosis, an association between nutritional status and quantitative liver functions, viz., galactose elimination capacity and caffeine clearance, has been observed.[7] Studies evaluating effect of nutritional supplementation in patients with cirrhosis showed that nutritional supplementation improved qualitative liver function tests, e.g. antipyrine,[8] aminopyrine,[9] as well as galactose elimination capacity.[10]

PEM impairs liver function but rarely causes morphological alterations. Qualitative liver function tests can be used as global indicators of functional impairment but they can not help in distinguishing whether the liver dysfunction is because of associated malnutrition or resulting from the disease itself.

Association of PEM with clinical course

PEM is associated with an unfavorable clinical outcome. In cirrhotic patients generally, there is an association between nutritional status and mortality.[2] Furthermore, within Child's groups A and B, the association between nutritional status and mortality is quite apparent.[6] Malnutrition when defined by low dietary intake is associated with high mortality. Malnutrition has also been shown to be an independent predictor of both the first bleeding episode and survival in patients with cirrhosis and esophageal varices.[11] Malnutrition is also associated with the presence of ascites.[2] Pre-operative nutritional status is related to post-operative morbidity and mortality in patients with cirrhosis especially after liver transplantation.

In controlled clinical trials, the rate of response to treatment for complications like ascites, GI bleeding, infection, etc. is better if nutritional supplementation is provided compared to controls, i.e. without nutritional supplementations.[8, 12-15] Malnutrition negatively affects the clinical outcome in terms of survival and the occurrence of complications. The relative contribution of either the PEM-associated liver dysfunction or PEM-associated malfunction of extrahepatic tissues on the clinical outcome cannot readily be differentiated. Apart from improvement of the nutritional status and/or liver function, a beneficial effect of nutritional intervention should be demonstrated on the basis of clinical outcome.

RATIONALE FOR NUTRITIONAL SUPPORT

Child and Turcotte[16] first identified undernutrition as an important risk factor for adverse outcome after surgery (porta caval shunt) in patients with cirrhosis. Poor nutritional status has been repeatedly shown to be a predictor of complications in liver disease including encephalopathy, spontaneous bacterial peritonitis and variceal hemorrhage. More recently, malnutrition has been identified as having predictive value for adverse outcome during acute alcoholic hepatitis and after liver transplantation.[17, 18] Nutritional parameters have been proved to be independent predictors of survival in both compensated[11] and decompensated[19, 20] patients with chronic liver disease. Nutritional assessment should be considered as an important tool in the therapeutic management of patients with acute and chronic liver diseases of varying etiology. The various methods for nutritional assessment are shown in Tables 2 and 3.

Table 2. Methods to detect nutritional deficiency or malnutrition

Anthropometry	Ideal body weight
	Percentage of ideal body weight
	Triceps skinfold thickness
	Midarm muscle circumference
Biochemical	Serum-albumin, prealbumin
	transferrin, hemoglobin
	Immunological – total lymphocyte count
	Urinary indices – creatinine height index
Clinical	Clinical examination of various organs and systems

Goals of nutritional support

The various goals of nutritional support[21] are as follows:

(a) to provide adequate energy and protein in order to facilitate hepatic cell regeneration as an increased number of functioning hepatocytes will improve the liver metabolism and nutritional status,

(b) to decrease ammonia production from endogenous or exogenous protein catabolism,

Table 3. Standards for arm muscle circumference and triceps skin-fold thickness

	Standard	Lower 5th percentile	Percent of standard represented by 5th percentile
Upper arm muscle circumference (mm)			
Male	270	220	81
Female	213	177	83
Triceps skinfold thickness (mm)			
Male	11	4	36
Female	19	9	47

Adapted from Hardy, JE (Ed). *Hardy Textbook of Surgery* 2nd edn, JB Lippincott, Philadelphia, 1988

(c) to correct vitamin/mineral deficiencies, and
(d) to prevent potential complications that may occur as a result of inappropriate nutritional support, e.g., hypoglycemia or hyperglycemia, hypertriglyceridemia, hepatic encephalopathy, fluid overload, electrolyte imbalance, and death.

Nutrient requirements

The dietary any requirements are depicted in Table 4.

Energy requirements

For most patients with chronic liver disease, the daily caloric need equals resting energy expenditure (REE) × 1.2 to 1.4 (factor for stress and activity) which in general practice is

Table 4. Daily requirements of macronutrients in patients with chronic liver disease (CLD)

Energy	Resting energy expenditure (REE)(kcal/day)	Males : $66 + (13.7 \times W) + (5 \times 4) - (6.8 \times A)$ Females : $65.5 + (9.6 \times W) + (1.7 \times H) - (4.7 \times A)$ where W = weight in kg, H = height in cm and A = age in years
	Daily caloric needs	REE × 1.2 – 1.4 or
Fat		25–30 kcal/kg body wt 30–35% of total energy
Protein		1.2–1.3 gm/kg body wt
Carbohydrate		Remainder of caloric requirement

equivalent to 25–30 kcal/kg body weight. In a six-week refeeding study[22, 23] with an ordinary diet in patients with cirrhosis, an average intake of about 40 kcal/kg/day allowed for REE, energy spent on physical activity, and the energy required for synthesis of lean body mass and fat mass. Thus for a nutrition plan aiming at repletion as in case of extensive undernutrition, energy intake should be 40–50 kcal/kg body weight. Under conditions of metabolic stress such as postoperative period, sepsis, gastrointestinal bleeding, and hepatic failure, the energy required to maintain equilibrium is considerably higher (35 to 45 nonprotein kcal/kg of estimated dry body weight/day).

Non-protein calories: carbohydrates and fats

Administration of adequate non-protein calories is critical for the efficient use of protein sources, particularly when protein is restricted. Provision of excess calories as carbohydrates should be avoided as it may promote hepatic lipogenesis, liver dysfunction, and increased carbon-dioxide production, leading to increased breathing.[24, 25] Ideally, 30–35% of total caloric intake should be given as fat. In case of malabsorption, medium-chain triglycerides should be instituted, but for a short period of time, as essential fatty acid deficiency may develop in prolonged absence of long chain fatty acids from the diet.

Protein requirement

Patients with acute and chronic liver disease have high protein requirements. In literature, the recommendations for required protein intake to achieve positive nitrogen balance,[22, 26, 27] ranges from 0.6 gm to 1 gm/kg day. An intake of 1.2–1.3 g/kg/d would thus assure positive nitrogen balance in most of the patients with chronic liver disease. It is not possible on clinical grounds alone to identify patients requiring aggressive nutritional supplementation. Therefore, in clinical practice, the adequacy of intake should be estimated by calculating nitrogen balance at a protein intake of 1 g/kg per day.[22, 23] Patients in negative balance at this intake need additional amounts of protein to achieve positive nitrogen balance and are at risk of developing protein deficiency especially with poor dietary intake.

On the basis of available literature, patients with compensated cirrhosis appear to have increased protein requirement of 1.2 g/kg/d to maintain nitrogen balance[22, 26, 28] as compared to 0.8 g/kg/d in normal individuals. The reasons for this phenomenon are not clear, but increased protein requirement seems to be due to increased whole body protein degradation which in turn may be due to low plasma levels of IGF-1.[23, 29] According to the studies available, malnourished patients who have an inadequate dietary intake are at risk of fatal complications of liver cirrhosis (infections, bleeding, ascites, etc.) and, hence should receive nutritional support. In these patients low grade encephalopathy (grades I-II) should not be considered a contraindication to nutritional support including an adequate protein supply. In all the patients with encephalopathy, other precipitating causes should be excluded before considering the protein intolerance. Transient protein restriction can be instituted but after a few days adequate nutrition should be reinstituted. If encephalopathy improves, protein intake can be liberalized slowly by increments of 0.2 g/kg per day to a final goal of 1.2–1.5 g/kg/day. In proven protein intolerant patients, oral branched chain amino acid (BCAA) enriched hepatic formula may be helpful in achieving an adequate nitrogen intake.

Protein in hepatic encephalopathy in cirrhotic patients: then and now

In the early 1950's it was shown that some patients with cirrhosis given "nitrogeneous substances" including excess dietary protein developed hepatic "precoma".[30] These largely uncontrolled observations led to the introduction of dietary protein restriction to treat hepatic encephalopathy. Recent studies have shown that protein requirements in fact are increased in these patients,[22] that high protein diets are well tolerated, and that their use, particularly in patients who are malnourished, is associated with sustained improvement in mental and physical health.[8, 31] The ESPEN guidelines for nutrition in liver disease has recommended that traditional protein restriction should be abandoned in patients with hepatic encephalopathy in the light of availability of other effective treatment modalities.[32]

The practice of protein restriction in patients with low grade hepatic encephalopathy is empirically based on the evidence that administration of proteins increases encephalopathy. However, it has never been proven in a controlled study that restriction of proteins improves the mental state of these encephalopathic patients. Unnecessary protein restriction may only produce negative nitrogen balance, and therefore must be avoided. In situations of stress such as alcoholic hepatitis or decompensated disease with complications (sepsis, infection, GI bleed, severe ascites), at least 1.5 g protein/kg/day should be provided.

Fluid, electrolyte and micronutrient requirement

Fluid and electrolyte requirements should be calculated on the basis of regular monitoring, especially in patients with decompensated disease and those on diuretics. The parameters to be monitored include: intake/output, sodium, potassium, blood urea, and serum creatinine. Micronutrient (zinc, selenium, vitamin E, etc.) supplementation is essential in order to overcome pre-existing deficiency and continuous losses. The physical signs of nutritional deficiency for vitamins and important minerals are mentioned in Table 5.

Means of nutritional support

Oral diet

In general, patients with liver disease tolerate a normal diet. The majority of patients especially with acute hepatitis do not need any dietary restriction. A decrease in dietary fat may be useful to reduce symptoms of steatorrhea, but it is associated with the risk of inadequate energy intake and is not supported by appropriate clinical trials. Salt restriction is of potential value in patients with ascites not responding to diuretic treatment. Supplementation is necessary

Table 5. Physical signs of nutritional deficiency

	Signs	Deficiencies
Hair	Alopecia	Protein-calorie malnutrition
	Brittle	Biotin
	Color	Zinc
	Dryness	Vitamins E and A
	Easy pluckability	Zinc (?)
Skin	Acneiform lesions	Vitamin A
	Follicular keratosis	Vitamin A
	Xerosis (dry skin)	Vitamin A
	Ecchymosis	Vitamin C or K
	Intradermal petechiae	Vitamin C or K
	Erythema	Niacin
	Hyperpigmentation	Niacin
	Scrotal dermatitis	Niacin
Eyes	Angular palplebritis	Vitamin B_2
	Bitot's spots	Vitamin A
	Conjunctival xerosis	Vitamin A
Mouth	Angular stomatitis	Vitamin B_{12}
	Atrophic papillae	Niacin
	Bleeding gums	Vitamin C
	Cheilosis	Vitamin B_2
	Glossitis	Niacin, Folate, Vitamin B_{12}
	Magenta tongue	Vitamin B_2
Extremities	Genu valgum or varum	Vitamin D
	Loss of deep tendon reflexes of the lower extremities	Vitamins B_1 and B_{12}

Adapted from Bernard MA, Jacobs DO, Rombeau JL. *Nutrition and metabolic support of hospitalized patients*, Philadephia, WB Saunders, 1986.

only when daily requirement of energy, protein, electrolytes, trace elements, or vitamins are not met by daily intake.

Nutritional intervention

Nutritional status can be influenced by manipulation in the delivery of macro- and micronutrients with regard to composition and quality to ensure an adequate supply with nutritious substrates. Second, the regulation of substrate metabolism may be modified by the use of special substrate and/or mediators or hormones. In another strategy, poor nutrient intake due to low appetite could be corrected by measures regulating the apetite via central mechanisms. Effective treatment of anorexia certainly would have a major impact on the nutritional status and prognosis.[33] All the patients who are not eating enough to cover their estimated caloric needs should be offered systematic dietary surveillance, advice, and therapy with an aim to provide adequate nutrient intake. The various ways of nutritional intervention in these patients are as follows.

Eating pattern

A modified eating pattern with four to seven small meals including at least one late evening meal improves nitrogen economy and substrate utilisation in stable cirrhotic patients.[34, 35]

Dietary supplements

Oral supplementation may provide the patient with the desired amount of a particular substrate, while permitting the continuation of normal diet. Short-term supplementation with BCAA enables protein-intolerant patients with cirrhosis to attain positive nitrogen balance without increasing the risk of encephalopathy.[36, 37] Long-term BCAA supplementation seems to be associated with better nitrogen accretion and liver function, however anthropometric measures may not improve.[38] The guidelines for daily dietary feeding have been given by the American College of Gastroenterology (ACG) in patients with alcoholic liver disease.[39] These should be applicable to all the patients with chronic liver disease and malnutrition (Table 6).

Table 6. ACG guidelines for daily dietary feeding in alcoholic liver disease

Protein=1.0–1.5 kg BW*
Total calories= 1.2–1.4 × resting energy expenditure with a minimum of 30 kcal/kg BW* 50–55 percent as carbohydrate (preferably as complex carbohydrates) 30–35 percent as fat; preferably high in unsaturated and with adequate essential fatty acids
Nutrition should be given enterally by voluntary oral intake and/or by small-bore feeding tube; PPN** is second choice, TPN*** is last choice
Salt and water intake should be adjusted for patient's fluid volume and electrolyte status
Liberal multivitamins and minerals
Specialized BCAA† enriched supplements not usually necessary as most patients tolerate standard AA supplements
Reserve BCAA† formulations for patients who cannot tolerate the necessary amount of standard AA (which maintain nitrogen balance) without precipitating encephalopathy Avoid supplements providing only BCAA†; they do not maintain nitrogen balance Conditionally essential AA as well all essential AA are needed Conditionally essential AA are those that normally can be synthesized from other precursors, but they cannot be synthesized in cirrhotic patients. These include choline, cystine, taurin, and tyrosine

* BW   body weight
 ** PPN partial parenteral nutrition
*** TPN total parenteral nutrition
   † BCAA branched chain amino acids
     AA   amino acids

Artificial feeding

Many malnourished cirrhotic patients are anorexic and cannot meet their nutrient requirements by oral intake "ad lib". This has been demonstrated in trials when artificial feeding by using liquid formulae proved more effective in providing adequate amounts of nutrients than normal oral nutrition "ad lib". Intervention by enteral nutrition using liquid formulae to supplement oral intake is associated with improved liver function and in turn a better survival.[8, 12, 34] This could be achieved by the following methods.

Tube feeding The decision when to initiate tube feeding is debated. While tube feeding yields superior results over 'ad lib' oral feeding due to voluntary nutrition intake, others are hesitant because of the risk of variceal bleeding. From the evidence of published trials, however, there is no suggestion that enteral tube feeding increases the incidence of variceal bleeding. In any case, patients must not be fasted and thus the introduction of tube feeding should not be delayed. The enteral feeding could be intermittent or continuous.[8, 12] Liquid enteral formulae for cirrhotic patients should preferably be of high energy density (1.5 kcal/ml) with a low sodium content so that they can be used in patients with fluid retention.

Parenteral nutrition It is not required in cases of acute hepatitis. It should be reserved for those who are not capable or not willing to accept oral supplement or enteral tube feeding and those with deeper grades of encephalopathy.

Liver adapted amino acid solutions Solutions with an increased content of BCAA (40–50%) and reduced amounts of aromatic amino acids and methionine have been introduced for the treatment of patients with liver disease.[40] While they may have some value in the treatment of hepatic encephalopathy, they have no documented effect on the nutritional status.

REFERENCES

1. Mendenhall CL, Anderson S, Weenser RE, Goldberg SJ, Crolie KA. Protein calorie malnutrition associated with alcoholic hepatitis. *Am J Med* 1984:76:211-21.
2. Lautz HU, Selberg O, Korber J, Burger M, Muller MJ. Protein calorie malnutrition in liver cirrhosis. *Clin Invest* 1992;70:478-86.
3. Italian multicentre cooperative project on nutrition in liver cirrhosis, nutritional status in cirrhosis. *J Hepatol* 1994:21:317-25.
4. Sarin, SK, Dhingra N, Bansal A, Malhotra S, Guptan, RC. Dietary and nutritional abnormalities in alcoholic liver disease: a comparison with chronic alcoholics without liver disease. *Am J Gastroenterol* 1997;92:777-83.
5. Singh, N, Saxena, N, Joshi, YK, Garg, PK, Tandon, R. Evaluation of nutritional status by using anthropometry in patients with chronic liver disease. Abstract published in 16th International Congress of Nutrition July 27–August 1, 1997, Montreal, Canada 133.
6. Merli M Riggio O, Dally L, PINC. What is the impact of malnutrition on survival in liver cirrhosis. *Hepatotology* 1996;23:1041-6.
7. Conn, HO. *Cirrhosis. In:* Schiff L, Schiff E, Eds. Diseases of the Liver: Philadelphia: Lippincott, 1982; pp. 864-5.

8. Kearns PJ, Young H, Garcia G, Blaschke T, O'Hanlon G, Rinki M, Sucher K. Accelerated improvement of alcoholic liver disease with enteral nutrition. *Gastroenterology* 1992;102:200-05.
9. O'Keefe SJ, El-Zayadi AR, Carraher TE, Davis M, Williams R. Malnutrition and immunoincompetence in patients with liver disease. *Lancet* 1980;11:615-7.
10. Achord JL. A prospective randomized clinical trial of peripheral amino acid glucose supplementation in acute alcoholic hepatitis. *Am J Gastroenterol* 1987;82:871-5.
11. Moller S, Bendtsen E, Christensen E. Prognostic variable in patients with cirrhosis and oesophageal varices without prior bleeding. *J Hepatol* 1994;21:940-6.
12. Bunout D, Aicardi V, irsch S, Peterman M, Kelly M, Silva G, Garay P, et al. Nutritional support in hospitalized patients with alcoholic liver disease. *Am J Clin Nutr* 1989;43:615-21.
13. Cabre E, Gonzalez-Huix F, Abad-Lacruz A, Esteve M, Acero D, Fernandez-Banars F, Xiol X, et al. Effect of total enteral nutrition on the short-term outcome of severely malnourished-cirrhotics. A randomized controlled trial. *Gastroenterology* 1990;98: 715-20.
14. Mezey E, Cabelleria J, Mitchell MC, Pares A, Herlong HF, Rodes J. Effect of parenteral amino acid supplementation on short-term and long-term outcome in severe alcoholic hepatitis: a randomized controlled trial. *Hepatology* 1991;14:1090-6.
15. Nasrallah SM, Galambos JT. Amino acid therapy of alcoholic hepatitis. *Lancet* 1980;ii:1276-7.
16. Child CG, Turcotte JG. *Surgery and portal hypertension. In:* Child CG, Ed. The liver and portal hypertension: Philadelphia: Saunders, 1964; pp 50-64.
17. Mendenhall CL, Tosch T, Weesner RE, Garcia-Pont P, Goldberg SJ, Kierman T, Seef LB, et al. VA cooperative study on alcoholic hepatitis II: prognostic significance of protein-calorie malnutrition. *Am J Clin Nutr* 1986;43:213-8.
18. Shaw BW, Wood WP, Gordon RD, Iwasuki S, Gillquist WP, Starzl TE. Influence of selected patient variables and operative blood loss on six-month survival following liver transplantation. *Semin Liver Dis* 1985;5:385-93.
19. Llach J, Gines P, Arroyo V, Rimola A, Tito L, Badalamenti S, Jimenez W, et al. Prognostic value of arterial pressure, endogenous vasoactive systems, and renal function in cirrhotic patients admitted to the hospital for the treatment of ascites. *Gastroenterology* 1988;94:482-7.
20. Abad Lacruz A, Cabre E, Gonzalez-Huix F, Fernandez Banares F, Esteve M, Planas R, Llovet JM, et al. Routine tests of renal function, alcoholism, and nutrition improve the prognostic accuracy of Child-Pugh score in non-bleeding advanced cirrhotics. *Am J Gastroenterol* 1993;88:382-7.
21. ASPEN Board of Directors: Guidelines for the use of parenteral and enteral nutrition in adult and pediatric patients. *J Parent Ent Nutr* 1993;17(suppl):SA1-52.
22. Nielsen K, Kondrup J, Martinsea I, Dossing H, Larsson P, Stilling B, Jenssen MG, et al. Long-term oral refeeding of patients with cirrhosis of the liver. *Br J Nutr* 1995;74:557-67.
23. Kondrup J, Nielsen K, Juul A. Effect of long-term refeeding on protein metabolism in patients with cirrhosis of the liver. *Br J Nutr* 1997;77:197-212.
24. Elwyn DH, Kinney JM, Askanazi J. Energy expenditure in surgical patients. *Surg Clin North Am* 1981;61:545-55.
25. Elwyn DH. Nutritional requirements of adult surgical patients. *Crit Care Med* 1980;8:9-20.
26. Swart, GR, van den Berg, JWO, Wattimena JLD, Rietveld T, Van Vuure JK, Frenkel M. Elevated protein requirement in cirrhosis of the liver investigated by whole body protein turnover studies. *Clin Science* 1988;75:101-7.
27. Nielsen K, Kondrup J, Martinsen L, Stilling B, Wikman B. Nutritional assessment and adequacy of dietary intake in hospitalized patients with alcoholic liver cirrhosis. *Br J Nutr* 1993;69:665-79.
28. Swart GR, van den Berg JWO, van Vunre JK, Tietveld T, Wattmena DI, Frenkel M. Minimum protein requirements in liver cirrhosis determined by nitrogen balance measurements at three levels of protein intake. *Clin Nutr* 1989;8:329-36.

29. Kondrup J, Nielsen K, Juul A. Effect of long-term refeeding on protein metabolism in patients with cirrhosis of liver. *Br J Nutr* 1997;77:192-212.
30. Phillips GB, Schwartz R, Gabuzda GJ, Jr, Davidson CS. The syndrome of impending hepatic coma in patients with cirrhosis of the liver given certain nitrogenous substances. *N Engl J Med* 1952;247:239-46.
31. Morgan TR, Moritz TE, Mendenhall CL, Haas R, VA. Cooperative Study Group #275. Protein consumption and hepatic encephalopathy in alcoholic hepatitis *J Am Coll Nutr* 1995;14:152-8.
32. Plauth M, Merli M, Kondrup J, Weimann A, Ferenci P, Miller MJ, and ESPEN Consensus Group. ESPEN guidelines for nutrition in liver disease and transplantation. *Clin Nutr* 1997;16:43-55.
33. Mendenhall CL, Moritz TE, Roselle GA, Morgan TR, Nemchausky BA, Tamburro CH, Schiff ER, et al. A study of oral nutritional support with oxandrolone in malnourished patients with alcoholic hepatitis results of a department of veterans affairs cooperative study. *Hepatology* 1993;17:564-76.
34. Swart GR, Zillikens MC, van Vuure JK, van den Berg JW. Effect of late evening meal on nitrogen balance in patients with cirrhosis of the liver. *Br Med J* 1989;299:1202-3.
35. Verbocket vand de Venne, WPHG. Westerp KR, van Hock B, Swart GR. Energy expenditure and substrate metabolism in patients with cirrhosis of the liver effects of the pattern of food intake. *Gut* 1995;36:110-6.
36. Horst D, Grace ND, Conn HO. Comparison of dietary protein with an oral, branched chain enriched aminoacid supplement in chronic portal-systemic encephalopathy: a randomized controlled trial. *Hepatology* 1984;4:279-87.
37. Egberts EH, Schomerus H, Hamster W, Jurgens P. Branched chain amino acids in the treatment of latent portosystemic encephalopathy. A double-blind placebo-controlled crossover study. *Gastroenterology* 1985;88:887-95.
38. Marchesini G, Dioguardi FS, Bianchi GP. Long-term oral branched chain amino acid treatment in chronic hepatic encephalopathy. A randomized double-blind casein controlled trial. *J Hepatol* 1990;11:92-101.
39. McCullough AJ, O'Connor JF. Alcoholic liver disease: proposed recommendations for the American College of Gastroenterology. *Am J Gastroenterol* 1998;93:2022-36.
40. Freund H, Dienstag J, Lehrich J. Infusion of branched-chain enriched amino acid solution in patients with hepatic encephalopathy. *Ann Surg* 1982;196:209-20.

Abstracts

An epidemiological scoring system for predicting response to interferon-alfa in chronic hepatitis B. K Chakravartty, S Mukherjee, T Maitra, KN Jalan. Kothan Medical Centre, Calcutta.

Prevalence of hepatitis B (HBV and HCV) in patients with hematological malignancies. RC Guptan, V Thakur, SR Agarwal, V Raina, SK Sarin. Department of Gastroenterology, GB Pant Hospital, and AIIMS, New Delhi.

Seroprevalence of Hepatitis B and C markers in hospitalized patients with severe alcoholic liver disease. D Kapoor, A Misra, S Saigal, R Chandra, V Thakur, SK Sarin. Department of Gastroenterology, GB Pant Hospital, New Delhi.

Interferon-alpha-2b (Intron-A) for decompensated liver disease caused by hepatitis B virus infection. A Kumar, SK Thakur, SR Meta, KV Singh, VA Narayanan. Department of Gastroenterology, Army Hospital R and R, New Delhi.

Aetiology of acute viral hepatitis (AVH) in Madurai (South India). P Advaitham and SP Thyagarajan. Department of Gastroenterology, Madurai Medical College, and Department of Microbiology, PG Institute of Basic Medical Sciences, Madras.

Single blind randomized controlled trial to study the efficacy of two recombinant hepatitis B vaccines in healthy adults. N Joshi, A Kumar, DV Sreenivas, YR Nagarjuna Kumar. Department of Gastroenterology, Nizam's Institute of Medical Sciences, Hyderabad.

Fulminant hepatic failure – clinical profile, aetiology and outcome. E Ramanjaneyulu, Sudha, GSK Reddy, R Thyagarajan, KP Rao, B Prabhakar, Asha, R Reddy, S Sharma, SI Hassan, Indira, B Pratap.

Profile of hepatitis B virus (HBV) related chronic liver disease in Indian pediatric population. M Madhura, A Misra, A Govil, RC Guptan, R Chandra, GS Lamba, SK Sarin. Department of Gastroenterology, GB Pant Hospital, New Delhi.

Development and prospect of present and future recombinant hepatitis B vaccines in India. KM Ella, M Kuppuswamy, D Srinivasan. Bharat Biotech Intl Ltd., Hyderabad, and University of Wisconsin-Madison, USA.

Experience with a new indigenous recombinant DNA hepatitis B vaccine. P Abraham, FP Mistry, MR Bapat, TS Narayanan, PV Bhandarkar. Department of Gastroenterology, KEM Hospital, Mumbai.

Acute hepatitis due to dual infection with hepatitis B and C (HCV): comparison of the profile with acute hepatitis B and C. RC Ruptan, V Thakur, SK Sarin. Department of Gastroenterology, GB Pant Hospital, New Delhi.

Prevalence of hepatitis B surface mutants in patients with 'cryptogenic cirrhosis'. M Kabrawala, S Radhakrishnan, P Abraham, G Sridharan, G Chandy. Departments of Gastrointestinal Sciences and Clinical Virology, Christian Medical College and Hospital, Vellore.

Efficacy and safety of first indigenous recombinant hepatitis B vaccine in healthy volunteers: a pilot study. A Kumar, N Joshi, DV Sreenivas, S Palan, YR Nagarjuna Kumar. Nizam's Institute of Medical Sciences, Hyderabad.

Effect of recombinant interferon-alpha-2B (Intron-A) on asymptomatic, replicating Asian Indian adults HBsAg carriers with normal transaminases. A Kumar, AN Malviya, M Jaiprakash, AK Misuriya. Departments of Gastroenterology and Pathology, Army Hospital R and R, New Delhi.

HBsAg prevalence in blood donors in Jaipur. S Nijhawan, RR Rai, D Sharma, HB Saxena. Departments of Gastroenterology and Blood Bank, SMS Medical College, Jaipur.

Hepatocellular carcinoma–clinicoradiological profile. GN Ramesh, M Philip, Zacharias P, RJ Mukkada, J Mathews, T Philip, P Augustine. Digestive Disease Centre, PVS Memorial Hospital, Cochin.

Prevalence of hepatitis B infection and disease in contacts of chronic liver disease patients: analysis of wild versus precore mutant HBV infection. V Thakur, RC Guptan, V Malhotra, SK Sarin. Departments of Gastroenterology and Pathology, GB Pant Hospital, New Delhi.

Indian Journal of Gastroenterology 1998; 17(Suppl. 1)

Enhanced responsiveness to recombinant hepatitis B vaccination in hemodialysis patients with GM-CSF. D Kapoor. Department of Gastroenterology, GB Pant Hospital, New Delhi.

Hepatocellular carcinoma in India: an analysis of possible etiological factors. SK Sarin, RC Gupta, V Thankur, S Saigal, BC Das, V Malhotra. Departments of Gastroenterology and Pathology, GB Pant Hospital, ICPO, New Delhi.

Alpha-interferon therapy in chronic hepatitis due to dual infection with hepatitis B and C. RC Guptan, V Thakur, V Raina, SK Sarin. Department of Gastroenterology, GB Pant Hospital, and Department of Medical Oncology, AIIMS, New Delhi.

Anti-HBs status of high risk health care workers. R Pokharna, S Nijhawan, RR Rai. Department of Gastroenterology, SMS Hospital, Jaipur.

Prevalence of hepatitis B and C virus amongst surgeons and dentists. RR Rai, R Pokharna, S Nijhawan. Department of Gastroenterology, SMS Hospital, Jaipur.

Impaired response of alpha-interferon in patients with an inapparent hepatitis B and hepatitis C virus co-infection. S Mukherjee, K Chakravartty, TK Maitra, KN Jalan. Kothari Medical Centre, Calcutta.

Immunization with low-dose of indigenous recombinant hepatitis B vaccine (Shanvac B) in neonates and infants; safety and efficacy profile. MN Rao, N Joshi, S Babu, VS Raj, A Kumar, CM Habibullah. Owaisi Hospital for Medical Research, Nizam's Institute of Medical Sciences, CDR Hospitals, Hyderabad.

Intrafamilial spread of HBV and HCV in India. NP Bohidar, SK Panda, SK Acharya. Departments of Gastroenterology and Pathology, AIIMS, New Delhi.

High seroprevalence and clinical significance of hepatitis B and C in alcoholic liver disease patients — a prospective analysis of 210 patients. S Saigal, D Kapoor, N Tandon, SK Sarin. Department of Gastroenterology, GB Pant Hospital, New Delhi.

High prevalence of significant chronic liver disease in the contacts of HBV-related chronic liver disease patients. V Thakur, RC Guptan, V Malhotra, SK Sarin. Departments of Gastroenterology and Pathology, GB Pant Hospital, New Delhi.

Influence of an indigenous low iron diet on iron stores in chronic liver disease patients. N Tandon, V Thakur, RC Guptan, SK Sarin. Department of Gastroenterology, GB Pant Hospital, Delhi.

Screening of hepatitis surface antigen (HBsAg) and antibodies to hepatitis D virus in patients with liver diseases. B Aruna, SJ Khundmiri, MN Khaja, N Farees, CM Habibullah. Centre for liver diseases, Owaisi Hospital and Research Centre, Kanchanbagh, Hyderabad.

Hepatitis B and C infection in uremics. SJ Khundmiri, MN Khaja, N Farees, M Hussain, S Krishanan, CM Habibullah. Center for Liver Diseases and Department of Nephrology, Owaisi Hospital and Research Centre, Kanchanbagh, Hyderabad.

Prevalence of HBV and HCV infection in patients with various liver disorders in Andhra Pradesh, south India. MN Khaja, SJ Khundmiri, N Farees, B Aruna, M Hussain, CM Habibullah, Centre for Liver Diseases, Owaisi Hospital and Research Center, Kanchanbagh, Hyderabad.

Fulminant hepatic failure in pregnancy. S Nageswar Rao, BS Sharma, VVR Reddy, T Rao, KP Rao, SI Hassan, Prabhakar, Uma Devi, S Kumar, S Ramana, B Pratap. Department of Gastroenterology, Osmania General Hospital, Hyderabad.

Follow-up of patients with chronic hepatitis B or C mixed B+C on Interferon (IFN) a therapy in a service hospital. Col KV Singh, WG Cdr AK Pujahari, P Manoharan. Department of Gastroenterology, CH (AF), Bangalore.

Sero-protection at one year with the new indigenous recombinant hepatitis B vaccine (Shanvac B) in healthy adults. N Joshi, A Kumar, DV Sreenivas, S Palan, YR Nagarjuna Kumar. Department of Gastroenterology, Nizam's Institute of Medical Sciences, Hyderabad.

Prevalence of hepatitis B markers in hospital nursing staff. RG Shirhatti, P Sawant, S Vispute, S Dhadphale, V Patrawala, K Vyas, HS Das. LTMMC and LTMGH, Sion, Mumbai.

Analyses of point mutation within the hepatitis B virus precore gene in chronic HBV patients in India. SN Kazim, V Thakur, K Banerjee, SE Hasnain, SK Sarin. Department of Gastroenterology, GB Pant Hospital, and Eukaryotic Gene Expression Laboratory, National Institute of Immunology, New Delhi.

The outcome of hepatitis 'B' virus infection in HIV positive patients. Wg Cdr B Singh, Col HS Pruthi, Lt. Col R Chaudhry, Col. SK Sayal. Command Hospital, Armed Forces Medical College, Pune.

How can we improve case finding in HBV/HCV related chronic hepatitis? CE Eapen, G Chandy. Department of Gastrointestinal Sciences, Christian Medical College and Hospital, Vellore.

Indian Journal of Gastroenterology 1999; 18 (Suppl 1)

Spectrum of hepatitis B infection in family contacts. S Nijhawan, RR Rai, R Pokharna, S Nepalia, P Puri, R Singh, SMS Medical College, Jaipur.

HBsAg positivity rate among voluntary and replacement donors in the IRCS blood bank. SK Chaudhuri, Director, Blood Bank, IRCS, New Delhi.

Epidemiology of HBV infection in the general population: Impact or rural–urban difference and socio-economic factors. Abhijit Chowdhury, Amal Santra, Sujit Chaudhuri, Prabir Banerjee and DN Guha Mazumdar. Department of Gastroenterology, Institute of Postgraduate Medical Education and Research, Calcutta.

Precore mutants of HBV and the clinical outcome in chronic liver disease. Sujit Chaudhuri, Bhaskar Bikash Pal, Abhijit Chowdhury, Amal Santra Prabir Banerjee and DN Guha Mazumdar. Department of Gastroenterology, Institute of Postgraduate Medical Education and Research, Calcutta.

Antibody response to hepatitis B vaccine in thalassemic children. Harjeet Singh, Mandakini Pradhan and Sita Naik. Departments of Immunology and Genetics, Sanjay Gandhi Postgraduate Institute of Medical Sciences, Lucknow, Uttar Pradesh.

Prevalence of hepatitis B virus markers in high-risk health care workers. R Pokharna. RR Rai, S Nijhawan. Department of Gastroenterology, SMS Hospital, Jaipur.

Modulation of tumor necrosis factor–α production by hepatitis B virus in human monocytic cell line, THP-1. R Govinarajan and Sita Naik. Department of Immunology, Sanjay Gandhi Postgraduate Institute of Medical Sciences, Lucknow, Uttar Pradesh.

Familial clustering of HBV infection in India. R Chakrabarty, A Chowdhury,[2] S Chaudhuri,[2] PN De,[1] S Chatterjee,[1] D Chattopadhyay[1] and MS Chakraborty.[1] I.C.M.R. Virus Unit, Calcutta and I.P.G.M.E. & R., Calcutta.

The prevalence of hepatitis D in hepatitis B patients—a hospital based study. UK Chattopadhyay, D Pal. All India Institute of Hygiene & Public Health, Calcutta.

HBsAg carrier rate amongst (15–45 years) married women in an urban slum of Delhi. Preliminary communication from RTI project. Suneela Garg,* Nandini Sharma,* R Saha,* Preena Bhalla,** Uma Sareen.*** Departments of *PSM, **Microbiology, and ***Obstetrics & Gynaecology, Maulana Azad Medical College, New Delhi.

Hepatitis B carrier—a study of possible routes of acquiring the infection. SK Thakur, RM Gupta, MKK Rao, SK Dham. Army Hospital RR, Delhi Cantt and Armed Forces Medical College, Pune.

Natural history of chronic hepatitis B—a follow-up of untreated cases. SK Thakur, PS Reddy, H Subramanya. Departments of Gastroenterology and Pathology, Army Hospital Research and Referral, Delhi Cantt.

Chronic hepatitis B: a 7 years histological follow-up of interferon treated patients. SK Thakur, PS Reddy, H Subramanya, SK Dham. Departments of Gastroenterology and Pathology, Army Hospital Research and Referral, Delhi Cantt.

Effect of Jigrine in HBV infected acute viral hepatitis patients. MM Hussain, SP Singh, SJ Khundmiri, N Farees, MN Khaja and CM Habibullah. Centre For Liver Diseases, Owaisi Hospital and Research Centre, Hyderabad.

Efficacy of the first indigenously developed recombinant vaccine against hepatitis B virus in Indian subjects. Naiana Joshi, Ajit Kumar, Nagaraja Rao, M Girish Narayan, Nagarjuna Kumar YR and Sethu Babu. Department of Gastroenterology, Nizam's Institute of Medical Sciences, Owaisi Medical Research Centre, Osmania General Hospital, CDR Hospitals, Hyderabad.

A multicentric open labelled evaluation of immunogenicity (seroprotection rate) and reactogenicity of a recombinant DNA hepatitis B vaccine of Cuban origin when administered in a two dose schedule. Kaushal Madan, Anil Jain, P Jandwani, RK Gupta, P Kar, US Mathur,* Department of Medicine, Maulana Azad Medical College, New Delhi, and *SMS Medical College Hospital, Jaipur.

Abstract

Hepatitis B virus DNA in asymptomatic carriers: relationship with HBeAg/anti HBe and titer status. R Hari, KVK Mohan, KG Murugavel, SP Thyagarajan. Department of Microbiology, Dr. ALM PGffiMS, Taramani, Madras.

Evaluation of risk factors: In HBV infected chronic hepatitis patients. MN Khaja, SJ Khundmiri, MM Hussain, N Farees, DN Reddy,* CM Habibullah. Centre for Liver Diseases, Owaisi Hospital and Research Centre, Hyderabad; * Asian Institute of Gastroenterology, Medinova Hospital, Hyderabad.

Incidence of HBsAg positivity among various population subsets in the armed forces. M Jaiprakash, SK Thakur, MKK Rao. Departments of Gastroenterology and Armed Forces Transfusion Centre, Army Hospital R & R, Delhi Cantt.

Immunohistochemistry for core and surface antigens in chronic hepatitis. RR Sharma, RK Vashist, RK Dhiman, Y Chawla. Departments of Pathology and Hepatology, Postgraduate Institute of Medical Education & Research, Chandigarh.

Poor response to low-dose interferon therapy in chronic liver disease due to hepatitis B virus infection in Indian patients. G Choudhuri, VA Saraswat, S Lakhtakia, SK Dadhich, P Mehrotra, SR Naik. Department of Gastroenterology, SGPGIMS, Lucknow.

Effect of *Phyllanthus amarus*, an Indian medicinal plant on healthy carriers of hepatitis B virus: results of six clinical trials-1990-96. Thyagarajan SP,[1] Jayaram S,[1] Panneerselvam A,[1] Valliammai T,[1] Benajamin Samuel,[2] Sheila Cameron,[3] and Eric Walker,[3] [1]Dept. of Microbiology, Dr. ALM PGIBMS, University of Madras, Chennai, India; [2]Dept. of Nephrology, CMC Hospital, Vellore, India; and [3]Scottish Centre for Infection & Environmental Health & Ruchill Hospital, Glasgow, UK.

Retrospective analysis of children below the age of 2 years and pregnant women for HBsAg positivity. MS Chadha, NS Shaikh, VA Arankalle. National Institute of Virology (Indian Council of Medical Research), Pune.

Prevalence of precore HBV mutants among HBsAg carriers. SS Gandhe, MS Chadha, VA Arankalle. Hepatitis Division, National Institute of Virology (Indian Council of Medical Research), Pune.

HBSAg positivity among urban and rural populations of Pune (1982-1998). VA Arankalle, MS Chadha, SS Gandhe. Hepatitis Division, National Institute of Virology (Indian Council of Medical Research), Pune.

Five year follow-up of HBsAg carriers. VA Arankalle, MS Chadha LP Chobe. Hepatitis Division, National Institute of Virology (Indian Council of Medical Research), Pune.

Correlation of hepatitis B markers with serum enzymes and histopathology in various liver diseases. M Vasenwala,* A Malik,** M Manuja,* MY Rabbani. Departments of *Pathology, **Microbiology and Medicine, JN Medical College, AMU, Aligarh.

Indian Journal of Gastroenterol 1999; 18 (Suppl. 2)

Transactivation of human cytomegalovirus promoter by hepatitis B virus: A possible mechanism of viral pathogenesis. R Govindarajan, S Dwivedi, SR Naik, S Naik. Departments of Immunology and Gastroenterology, Sanjay Gandhi Postgraduate Institute of Medical Sciences, Lucknow.

Enhanced immunogenic and therapeutic effect of recombinant hepatitis B vaccine in exposed family contacts of chronic liver disease patients. V Thakur, RC Guptan, SK Sarin. Department of Gastroenterology, GB Pant Hospital, New Delhi.

Novel mutations in the surface gene of hepatitis B virus in Indian patients. SN Kazim, SM Wakil, LA Khan, V Thakur, SK Sarin. Department of Gastroenterology, GB Pant Hospital, New Delhi. Department of Biosciences, Jamia Millia University, New Delhi, Eukaryotic Gene Expression Laboratory, National Institute of Immunology, New Delhi and Department of Medical Elementology and Toxicology, Jamia Hamdard University, New Delhi.

Demographic, biochemical and serological profile of incidentally detected asymptomatic HBsAg positive subjects. SR Agarwal, D Kapoor, A Tharakan, SK Sarin. Department of Gastroenterology, GB Pant Hospital, New Delhi.

Interferon therapy in chronic hepatitis—preliminary report. Ramachandran, A John, S Ashraf, S Devi. Department of Gastroenterology, Calicut Medical College, Calicut.

Hepatitis B and C viral markers in patients of cirrhosis of liver. Virendra Singh, DK Bhasin, RK Kochhar, K Singh. Department of Gastroenterology, Post Graduate Institute of Medical Education and Research, Chandigarh.

Interferon (IFN) alpha therapy vs. combination (IFN-alplha+lamivudine) therapy in chronic hepatitis B—a pilot study. KV Singh, AK Pujari, R Dogra. Department of Gastroenterology, Command Hospital (Southern Command), Pune.

Indian Journal Gasteroenterol 2000; 19 (Suppl. 2)

Replicating viral markers in chronic HBV infection. Lt. Col VK Gupta, Lt. Col P Puri. Department of Gastroenterology, Command Hospital, (CC), Lucknow.

Profile and significance of HBV genotypes and spectrum of chronic liver disease in Indian continent. V Thakur, RC Guptan, SN Kazim, V Malhotra, SK Sarin. Departments of Gastroenterology and Pathology, GB Pant Hospital, New Delhi.

Hepatitis B immunization in low birth weight infants: effect of an additional dose. S Ganguly, NK Arora, S Agadi, M Deo, AK Deorari, M Irshad, R Kohli, A Kriplani. S Mittal, VK Paul, S Takkar, H Chellani, RN Salhan, S Salhan, MS Prasad. Department of Pediatrics and Departments of Obstetrics and Gynecology, AIIMS, and Safdarjung Hospital, New Delhi.

Safety and efficacy of a new indigenous recombinant DNA hepatitis B vaccine in screened high-risk population. S Subash, S Malathy, Mohammed Ali. Departments of Digestive Health and Diseases, Govt. Peripheral Hospital, Anna Nagar, Chennai, and Kilpauk Medical College, Chennai.

Prevalence, incidence and outcome of hepatitis B and C virus infection in patients with end-stage renal disease before and after renal transplantation. H Gadhikar, P Bhandarkar, P Abraham, AF Almeida. Departments of Gastroenterology and Nephrology, KEM Hospital, Mumbai.

Effects of different doses of interferon-alpha-2b in chronic hepatitis B infection in eastern regional railway hospital. S Pal, FD Sarkar, S Sengupta, R Mukherjee. BR Singh Hospital, Calcutta.

Study to see the possible source(s) of hepatitis B virus infection in eastern regional railway referral hospital. S Pal, D Sarkar, A Sen, G Dasgupta, BR Singh Hospital Eastern Railway, Calcutta.

Prevalence of HBV, HCV, HIV antibodies among 15,600 voluntary blood donors from all over Kerala. N Bindu, N Geetha, M Preethi, A Kale, P Nair. Division of Gastroenterology and Liver Disease, Amrita Institute of Medical Sciences, Kochi, Kerala.

Abstract

Hepatitis B vaccination rates among medical, dental and nursing students at medical college: results of a survey. SP Singh, GC Mishra, AK Mittal, PK Thatoi. Departments of Gastroenterology and Medicine, SCB Medical College, Cuttack.

A study of HBV markers among the first degree relatives of chronic HBsAg carriers. N Joshi, A Kumar, YR Nagarjuna Kumar, E Ramanjaneyulu. Department of Gastroenterology, Nizam's Institute of Medical Sciences, Hyderabad.

Hepatitis B and C viral markers in patients with extrahepatic portal venous obstruction (EHPVO). AK Sharma, BR Thapa, U Poddar, CK Naik, K Singh, Division of Pediatric Gastroenterology, GE Virology and Biochemistry. Department of Gastroenterology, PGIMER, Chandigarh.

Lamivudine/ribavarin therapy for reactivation of HBV/HCV diseases related to immuno-suppression for non-hepatic diseases. P Nair, SD Lee. Division of Gastroenterology and Liver Disease, Amrita Institute of Medical Sciences, Kochi, Kerala, and National Taiwan University, Taipei, Republic of Taiwan.

Severe acute HBV infection—rapid resolution with oral lamivudine. P Nair, P Zacharias, A John. Division of Gastroenterology and Liver Disease, Amrita Institute of Medical Sciences, Kochi, Kerala.

Hepatitis B carrier: clinical, biochemical, virological, histopathological and immunocytochemical profile. A Mukhopadhya, VS Richard, LR Padankatti, B Ramakrishna, GM Chandy. Departments of Gastrointestinal Sciences and Pathology, Christian Medical College and Hospital, Vellore.

Prevalence of hepatitis serological markers in high risk population. J Ubaldhos, Arun, S Rajinikanth, U Srinivas, A Murali, MS Revathy, KR Palaniswamy. Department of Medical Gastroenterology, Govt. Stanley Medical College, Chennai.

Correlation between serum – ascites albumin concentration gradient and endoscopic parameters of portal hypertension. K Narayanasamy, SJ Kumar, T Pugazhendhi, B Ramathilakam, G Ramar. Department of Gastroenterology, Madras Medical College and RI, Chennai.

Initial and 12 months post-vaccination antibody titres following a new indigenous recombinant DNA hepatitis-B vaccine. S Subash, N Dinakaran, S Malathy, Mohammad Ali, P Padmanabhan. Department of Digestive Health and Diseases, Govt. Peripheral Hospital and Kilpauk Medical College, Chennai.

Profile of hepatitis B e antigen-negative chronic hepatitis B. DN Amarapurkar, R Baijal, PP Kulsreshtha, S Agal, MR Chakraborty, SS Pramanik. Department of Gastroenterology, Bombay Hospital, and Jagjivanram Hospital, Mumbai.

HBsAg carrier rate in voluntary donors of armed forces personnel. A. Mohanty, BM Dash. Departments of Medicine and Pathology, 92 Base Hospital, C/o 56 APO.

Liver disease in asymptomatic HBsAg positive patients. Lt Col P Puri, Lt Col VK Gupta. Department of Gastroenterology, Command Hospital, (CC), Lucknow.

Lamivudine in hepatitis B virus related subacute hepatic failure. D Krishnadas, M Hariharan, M Narendranathan. Department of Gastroenterology, Medical College Hospital, Trivandrum.

Quantitative study of hepatitis B virus DNA in sera, saliva, masculine ejaculum or feminine vaginal secretion of patients with chronic hepatitis B virus infection. W Kai, L Xinwen, L Yanqing, Y Tao. Department of Internal Medicine, Affiliated Hospital of Shandong Medical University, Peoples Republic of China.

Changing spectrum of sporadic acute viral hepatitis in children. U Poddar, BR Thapa, A Prasad, K Singh. Division of Pediatric Gastroenterology. Department of Gastroenterology, Postgraduate Institute of Medical Education and Research, Chandigarh.

Replicative status of asymptomatic chronic hepatitis B virus infection. S Chaudhuri, A Chowdhury, GK Dhali, A Santra, R Chakraborty, J Mukherjee, J Dasgupta, SG Maity. Department of Gastroenterology, Institute of Post Graduate Medical Education and Research, Calcutta and ICMR Virus Study Group, Salt Lake, Calcutta.

Authentic base-pairing in the lower stem of epsilon hairpin is a strong evidence to its structural integrity and probably to the selection of HBe negative variants of HBV. MK Parvez, V Thakur, SN Kazim, RC Guptan, SE Hasnain, SK Sarin. Department of Gastroenterology, GB Pant Hospital, New Delhi, and Centre for DNA Fingerprinting and Diagnostics, Hyderabad.

Recombinant interferon in Indian children with HBV related chronic liver disease: a comparison of horizontally vs. vertically acquired infection. RC Guptan, V Thakur, V Malhotra, SK Sarin. Department of Gastroenterology and Pathology, GB Pant Hospital, New Delhi.

Indian Journal of Gastroenterol 2000; 19 (Suppl. 3)

Random survey of HBsAg positivity in asymptomatic population of Sikkim. R Kotwal, CZ Rinchhen, Y Verma. Departments of Gastroenterology and Pathology, STNM Referral Hospital, Gangtok, Sikkim.

Random estimation of HBsAg marker for hepatitis B in asymptomatic population in Gangtok. R Kotwal, CZ Rinchhen, Y Verma. Departments of Gastroenterology and Pathology, STNM Referral Hospital, Gangtok, Sikkim.

Hepatitis B marker HBsAg among the *safai karamchari* of Housing and Urban Department of Sikkim. R Kotwal, CZ Rinchhen, Y Verma. Departments of Gastroenterology and Pathology, STNM Referral Hospital, Gangtok, Sikkim.

Prevalence of HBsAg positivity among urban antenatal females. R Kotwal, CZ Rinchhen, Y Verma. Departments of Gastroenterology and Pathology, STNM Referral Hospital, Gangtok, Sikkim.

Prevalence of HBsAg positivity in rural antenatal females in primary health center in Sikkim. R Kotwal, CZ Rinchhen, Y Verma. Departments of Gastroenterology and Pathology, STNM Referral Hospital, Gangtok, Sikkim.

Prevalence of HBsAg in population referred to a hospital in North Delhi. AK Singal, V Kaur. Departments of Gastroenterology and Pathology, Tirth Ram Shah Hospital, Delhi.

Hepatitis B vaccination in pregnant women: cost-effective approach towards vaccination. A Patwardhan, P Jamjute. Departments of Pediatrics and Gynecology, Getwell Hospital, Mhow, Indore.

Prevalence of hepatitis B virus co-infection and human immunodeficient virus in north India. A Suri, J Singh, RK Dhiman, P Bambery, S Singh, Y Chawla. Departments of Internal Medicine and Hepatology, Postgraduate Institute of Medical Education and Research, Chandigarh.

Some critical issues in the epidemiology of hepatitis B in India. A Phadke, A Kale, Cehat, Pune.

Prevalence of hepatitis B virus infection in acute viral hepatitis in southern Tamilnadu. M Prasad, A Shetty, R Thomas, V Nathan, A Devraj. Departments of Medical Gastroenterology and Microbiology, KG Hospital, Coimbatore.

Prevalence of hepatitis B virus infection in a rural population of southern Tamilnadu. M Prasad, A Shetty, R Thomas, V Nathan, A Devraj. Departments of Medical Gastroenterology and Microbiology, KG Hospital, Coimbatore.

Prevalence of hepatitis B virus infection among voluntary blood donors in southern Tamilnadu. M Prasad, A Shetty, R Thomas, V Nathan, A Devraj. Departments of Medical Gastroenterology and Microbiology, KG Hospital, Coimbatore.

Detection of HBV, HCV and HIV in high-risk patients using rapid test kits. VL Malhotra, A Lakshmy, L Mahajan, L Grover, G Mehta. Department of Microbiology, Lady Hardinge Medical College, New Delhi.

Ten-year serological follow-up of hepatitis B vaccine recipients. MS Chadha, VA Arankalle. National Institute of Virology, Pune.

Efficacy of granulocyte macrophage colony stimulating factor (GMCSF) and lamivudine combination therapy with recombinant interferon in non-responders to interferon in HBV-related chronic liver disease. RC Guptan, V Thakur, SK Sarin. Department of Gastroenterology, GB Pant Hospital, New Delhi.

Seroconversion following recombinant hepatitis B vaccination in adult volunteers. IJ Gandhoke, S Gupta, Suman Gupta, S Khare, KK Datta. National Institute of Communicable Diseases, Delhi.

Controlling perinatally acquired hepatitis B by selective immunization – cost-benefit implications. JM Puliyel, F Abbas, RD Thomas, A Rajkumar, N Gupta. Departments of Pediatrics and Microbiology, St. Stephens Hospital, Delhi.

Indian Journal of Gastroenterol March 2001; 20(Suppl. 1)

Feasibility of goat hepatocytes in the transplantation of hepatic liver failure model system (rat). V Vijayalakshmi, B Naseem, M Aejaz Habeeb, M Chandrashekhar, SSYH Quadri, CM Habibullah. Center for Liver Disease, Owaisi Hospital and Research Center, Kanchanbagh, Hyderabad; National Institute of Nutrition, Tarnaka, Hyderabad.

Emergence and molecular characterisation of lamivudine induced mutations. SN Kazim, S Salma, RC Guptan, V Thakur, SK Sarin. Department of Gastroenterology, GB Pant Hospital, New Delhi.

Truncated HBx—a marker of chronic HBV infection? SP Raykar, P Jagannath, DN Amarapurkar, S Bhatia, NH Merchant, SV Chiplunkar. Immunology Division, Cancer Research Institute, Tata Memorial Center; Tata Memorial Hospital; Bombay Hospital and Medical Research Center; BYL Nair Hospital, Mumbai.

Hepatitis B and hepatitis C infection contribute majority of cases of cryptogenic and alcoholic liver cirrhosis. Neeti Agarwal, Sita Naik, Dinesh Kini, Sanjay K Somani, Harjeet Singh, Rakesh Aggarwal, Gour Choudhuri, Vivek A Saraswat, Subhash R Naik. Departments of Gastroenterology and Immunology, Sanjay Gandhi Postgraduate Institute of Medical Sciences, Lucknow.

Efficacy of low-dose and high-dose of interferon in the treatment of hepatitis B related chronic liver disease. Lt. Col. AK Seth, Col. SK Nema, Lt. Col. S Kakkar, Col. RN Diwan. Command Hospital (East), Alipore Road, Calcutta.

Lamivudine for control of acute hepatitis B infection during cancer chemotherapy: preliminary results. KM Mohandas, S Mehta, V Dhir, SD Bhanavali, R Gopal, SH Advani. Division of Diseases and Clinical Nutrition and Department of Medical Oncology, Tata Memorial Hospital, Mumbai.

Evidence for reservoir of hepatitis E virus in Indian swine. Rakesh Aggarwal, Parvez Akhtar, Sita Naik, Subhash R Naik. Departments of Gastroenterology and Immunology, Sanjay Gandhi Postgraduate Institute of Medical Sciences, Lucknow.

Prevalence of precore/core HBV mutants among north Indian patients with acute liver failure (ALF). V Chaudhuri, A Saxena, SK Acharya, SK Panda. Departments of Pathology and Gastroenterology, All India Institute of Medical Sciences, New Delhi.

A comparative trial of low-dose versus conventional dose of recombinant hepatitis B vaccine in young adults. Surinder Rana, RK Gupta, Sanjay Singh, Deepika R Sharma, P Kar. Department of Medicine, Maulana Azad Medical College, New Delhi; Panacea Biotech, New Delhi.

Could HLA be a predictor for non-response to recombinant hepatitis B vaccination?–A study from north India. Kunal Das, RK Gupta, Richa Dewan, Surinder Rana, P Kar. Department of Medicine, Maulana Azad Medical College and LNJP Hospital, New Delhi.

Seroprevalance of hepatitis A in patients with chronic liver disease–preliminary study. Nirmal Kumar, BC Sharma, Anand Dotihal. Department of Gastroenterology, GB Pant Hospital, New Delhi.

Adult to adult living donor right lobe liver transplantation in India: the success and future. MR Rajasekar, AS Soin, D Vijayarajakumari. Indraprastha Apollo Hospital, New Delhi.

Unusual manifestations and co-infections in acute hepatitis in children. SA Bhave, AR Baydekar, SA Bapat, AN Pandit, SS Chitamber, VA Arankalle. Liver Unit, KEM Hospital, Pune and Hepatitis Section, National Institute of Virology, Pune.

Efficacy of lamivudine therapy in hepatitis B related decompensated liver cirrhosis. VA Saraswat, S Somani, SK Dadhich, VV Raj. Department of Gastroenterology, Sanjay Gandhi Postgraduate Institute of Medical Sciences, Rae Bareli Road, Lucknow.

Prevalence of HBV and HCV infection in alcoholic liver disease. SS Pramanik, PP Kulshreshtha, S Agal, R Baijal, M Chakraborty. Gastroenterology Center, Jagjivan Ram Hospital, Mumbai.

Profile of hepatocellular carcinoma. Deepak N Amarapurkar, Haribhakti Seba Das, Sandeep Punamiya. Departments of Gastroenterology and Radiology, Bombay Hospital and Research Center, Mumbai.

Computer database prediction of a probable HBV core (HBC) protein binding site in the pregenomic RNA-epsilon hairpin. Md Khalid Parvez, Ankur Goyal, Shiv Kumar Sarin. Department of Gastroenterology, GB Pant Hospital, New Delhi.

Inability of lamivudine to suppress transmission of hepatitis B virus from mother to infant. SN Kazim, V Thakur, RC Guptan, V Malhotra, SK Sarin. Departments of Gastroenterology and Pathology, GB Pant Hospital, New Delhi.

Predictors of response to interferon and ribavirin therapy in chronic hepatitis VC patients in India. A Goyal, RC Guptan, V Thakur, P Sakhuja, V Malhotra, SK Sarin. Departments of Gastroenterology and Pathology, GB Pant Hospital, New Delhi.

Horizontal transmission of hepatitis B virus surface mutant 'G145R' in an unrelated third degree household contact. V Thakur, SN Kazim, RC Guptan, SF Basir, SK Sarin. Department of Gastroenterology, GB Pant Hospital, New Delhi, and Department of Biosciences, Jamia Millia Islamia, New Delhi.

Indian Journal of Gastroenterol 2001; 20 (Suppl. 2)

The role of therapeutic vaccination in replicative carriers of hepatitis B virus and its effect on the hepatitis B virus genome and cytokine profile. A. Rajan, S. Rana, BC Das, RK Gupta, D Chattopadhya, P Kar. Department of Medicine, Maulana Azad Medical College, Institute of Cytology and Preventive Oncology (ICMR), National Institute of Communicable Diseases, New Delhi.

Community based epidemiological study of hepatitis B virus (HBV) infection. A. Chowdhury, A Santra, S Pal, R Chakraborty, GK Dhali, S Chaudhuri, SG Maity, S Bhattacharya, DN Guha Mazumdar. Department of Gastroenterology, Institute of Post Graduate Medical Education and Research, Kolkata, ICMR, Virus Unit, Kolkata, and National Institute of Cholera and Enteric Diseases, Kolkata.

Lamivudine pulse therapy in patients with positive HBeAg and normal ALT: is it beneficial? BS Sandhu, M Jain, J Singh, SK Sarin. Department of Gastroenterology, GB Pant Hospital, New Delhi.

Detection of precore mutant of hepatitis B in patients of AVH and FH using ligase chain reaction and its clinical implications. SS Rana, U Kailash, BC Das, RK Gupta, A Rajan, M Mukherjee, P Kar. Department of Medicine, ICPO (ICMR), MAM College, New Delhi, Functional Genomic Unit, Centre for Biochemical Technology (CSIR), New Delhi.

Profile of asymptomatic chronic HBV infection in India – End of the 'carrier' saga? R Chandra, D Kapoor, SR Agarwal, V Malhotra, P Sakhuja, SK Sarin. Departments of Gastroenterology and Pathology, GB Pant Hospital, New Delhi.

Molecular epidemiology of HBV and transmission pattern in close family contacts of HBV related chronic liver disease patients. V Thakur, RC Guptan, SN Kazim, SK Sarin. Department of Gastroenterology, GB Pant Hospital, New Delhi.

Natural history of anti-HBe positive chronic hepatitis B – a prospective study. J Sharma, M Ramchandani, SR Agarwal, J Singh, BC Sharma, V Thakur, SK Sarin. Department of Gastroenterology, GB Pant Hospital, New Delhi.

Treatment of subacutre hepatitis with lamivudine and intravenous glycyrrhizin: a pilot study. A Tandon, BN Tandon, RA Bhujwala. Pushpawati Singhania Research Institute, New Delhi; Metro Liver and Digestive Diseases Centre, NOIDA.

Lamivudine in hepatitis B - related decompensated cirrhosis. VA Saraswat, SK Somani, R Aggarwal. Department of Gastroenterology, Sanjay Gandhi Post-graduate Institute of Medical Sciences, Lucknow.

Hepatitis B virus markers in children living in urban slums of Chandigarh. S Lal, A Sharma, CK Nain, K Singh. Department of Superspeciality of Gastroenterology, PGIMER, Chandigarh.

Prevalence of hepatitis B and C viral infection among alcoholic patients with liver disease. AK Sharma, SK Sinha, CK Nain, PK Sethi, V Singh, K Singh. Department of Gastroenterology, PGIMER, Chandigarh.

Absence of intra-familial spread of hepatitis E virus infection in sporadic setting. SK Somani, R Aggarwal, S Naik, SR Naik. Departments of Gastroenterology and Immunology, Sanjay Gandhi Post-graduate Institute of Medical Sciences, Lucknow.

Efficacy of half-dose (10 microgram) recombinant hepatitis B vaccine in adults. RB Jakareddy, NV Pai, PC Dalai, GR Verma, P Abraham. Department of Gastroenterology, KEM Hospital, Mumbai.

Role of HBV and HCV in chronic renal failure on dialysis – Experience in a tertiary care hospital. N Joshi, A Kumar, E Ramanjaneyulu, KV Dakshina Murthy. Departments of Gastroenterology and Nephrology, Nizam's Institute of Medical Sciences, Hyderabad.

Epidemiology of HBV and HCV in hepatocellular carcinoma in Hyderabad. N Joshi, MSR Sudha Rani, E Ramanjaneyulu, A Kumar. Department of Gastroenterology, Nizam's Institute of Medical Sciences, Hyderabad.

Intra familial transmission of hepatitis B. RR Rai, MP Sharma, NK Jain, S Nijhawan, A Mathur. Department of Gastroenterology, SMS Hospital, Jaipur.

Routes of transmission hepatitis B and C virus as detected in a tertiary centre in eastern India. S Pal, PK Banerjee, G Ray, J Mukherjee, A Pal. Institute of Post-graduate Medical Education and Research (IPGMER), SSKM Hospital, Calcutta.

Clinical profile, aetiology and prognostic indicators in fulminant hepatic failure in children. AV Vikranth Bapu, BB Raju, S Malathi, SP Thiagarajan. Departments of Pediatric Gastroenterology, ICH and HC and Microbiology, PGIBMS, Chennai.

Histologic spectrum of chronic hepatitis in precore mutants and wild type hepatitis B virus infection. P Sakhuja, V Malhotra, R Gondal, SK Sarin, V Thakur. Departments of Gastroenterology and Pathology, GB Pant Hospital, New Delhi.

Response of lamivudine monotherapy in hepatitis B. D Amarapurkar, HS Das, N Patel. Department of Gastroenterology, Bombay Hospital and Research Centre, Mumbai.

Hepatitis B virus markers in patients with HBsAg negative chronic hepatitis C. S Sharma, B Masih, A Sharma, A Duseja, Y Chawla. Department of Hepatology, PGIMER, Chandigarh.

Treatment of chronic hepatitis due to hepatitis B virus infection with interferon-alpha: cost-effective in the Indian setting. R Aggarwal, UC Ghoshal, SR Naik. Department of Gastroenterology, Sanjay Gandhi Post-graduate Institute of Medical Sciences, Lucknow.

Natural history of asymptomatic chronic HBsAg carriers. GR Verma, J Sharma, MR Bapat, P Abraham. Department of Gastroenterology, KEM Hospital, Mumbai.

Efficacy of indigenous (Shanvac-B) recombinant DNA hepatitis B vaccine in health care workers. V Thakur, RC Guptan, SK Sarin. Department of Gastroenterology, GB Pant Hospital, New Delhi.

Short course lamivudine in acute hepatitis B infection: a pilot study. SK Acharya, R Singh, B Bhatkal, SK Panda, S Dutta Gupta. Departments of Gastroenterology and Pathology, AIIMS, New Delhi.

Frequency of hepatitis B virus and its surface mutant infection in north Indian general population. H Singh, RL Singh, R Aggarwal, SR Naik, S Naik. Departments of Immunology and Gastroenterology, Sanjay Gandhi Post-graduate Institute of Medical Sciences, Lucknow; Department of Biochemistry, Dr. RML Awadh University, Faizabad.

Effect of one year lamivudine therapy in chronic HBV infection. S Chaudhuri, A Chowdhury, GK Dhali, A Santra, R Chakraborty. Department of Gastroenterology, Institute of Post-graduate Medical Education and Research, Kolkata; ICMR, Virus Unit, Kolkata.

Interferon and lamivudine combination versus lamivudine alone in the treatment of anti-HBe positive chronic hepatitis B. RC Guptan, V Thakur, RC Garg, V Malhotra, SK Sarin. Departments of Gastroenterology and Pathology, GB Pant Hospital, New Delhi.

Abstract

Efficacy of lamivudine in hepatitis B related chronic liver disease in India. K Chetri, TS Negi, G Choudhuri. Department of Gastroenterology, Sanjay Gandhi Post-graduate Institute of Medical Sciences, Lucknow.

Frequency of precore and surface mutants in HBV-related chronic liver diseases and in incidentally detected asymptomatic HBsAg positive subjects (IDAHS). N Joshi, A Kumar, YR Nagarjuna Kumar, E Ramanjaneyulu, N Chandra, MN Khaja, M Tandon, S Babu. Department of Gastroenterology, Nizam's Institute of Medical Sciences, OMRC, CDR Hospital, Sai Vani Hospital, Hyderabad.

Epidemiology of HBV and HCV in hepatocellular carcinoma in Hyderabad. N Joshi, MSR Sudha Rani, E Ramanjaneyulu, A Kumar. Department of Gastroenterology, Nizam's Institute of Medical Sciences, Hyderabad.

Role of HBV and HCV in chronic renal failure on dialysis—Experience in a tertiary care hospital. N Joshi, E Ramanjaneyulu, A Kumar. Departments of Gastroenterology and Nephrology, Nizam's Institute of Medical Sciences, Hyderabad.

Epidemiology of HBV and HCV in hepatocellular carcinoma in Hyderabad. N Joshi, MSR Sudha Rani, E Ramanjaneyulu, A Kumar. Department of Gastroenterology, Nizam's Institute of Medical Sciences, Hyderabad.

Hepatitis B virus infection in an institution for mentally retarded and efficacy of lamivudine in chronic hepatitis B amongst these patients. RR Rai, NK Jain, MP Sharma, L Shimpi, S Nijhawan, A Mathur. Department of Gastroenterology, SMS Hospital, Jaipur.

Antibody titers in hepatitis B vaccines at six months following vaccination. S Nijhawan, L Shimpi, MP Sharma, A Mathur, RR Rai. Department of Gastroenterology, SMS Hospital, Jaipur.

Intrafamilial transmission of hepatitis B. RR Rai, MP Sharma, NK Jain, A Mathur, S Nijhawan. Department of Gastroenterology, SMS Hospital, Jaipur.

List of Abstracts submitted for March 2002 meeting, Delhi

Prevelence of hepatitis B and C markers amongst alcoholic population. AC Anand, HS Pruthi, N Kekre, MKK Rao. Department of Gastroenterology, Command Hospital (WC), Chandimandir; and Department of Medicine and Microbiology, Armed Forces Medical College, Pune.

A study of sero-prevalence of HBV markers and evaluation of clinical safety and immunogenicity of r-DNA vaccine (Shanvac-B) in hemophiliacs. N Joshi, YR Nagarjuna Kumar, VR Srinivasan, S Babu, A Kumar. Departments of Gastroenterology and Medicine, Nizam's Institute of Medical Sciences, Hyderabad.

Antibody response to indigenous recombinant hepatitis B vaccine (Shanvac-B) in a mass vaccination programme. N Joshi, YR Nargarjuna Kumar, N Chandra, A Kumar. Department of Gastroenterology, Nizam's Institute of Medical Sciences, Hyderabad.

Modes of acquisition of hepatitis B virus infection children with chronic HBV infection in India. BN Soma, A Mishra, RC Guptan, SK Sarin. Department of Gastroenterology, GB Pant Hospital, New Delhi.

Cost-effectiveness of inclusion of hepatitis B (HB) vaccine in India's national immunization program using a decision analysis approach. Rakesh Aggarwal, Uday C Ghoshal, SR Naik. Department of Gastroenterology, Sanjay Gandhi PG Institute of Medical Sciences, Lucknow.

An open label study of lamivudine response for hepatitis B virus infection in renal transplant recipients: A single center study from India. Sanjay K Agarwal, Sanjay Gupta, D Bhowmik, SC Dash, SC Tiwari, S Guleria, SN Mehta. Departments of Nephrology and Surgery, AIIMS, New Delhi.

A prospective evaluation of patients presenting with asymptomatic transaminases to a liver clinic at a tertiary level health care center in north India. Yogesh Batra, Kaushal Madan, Kuldeep Kaur, S Hazari, V Chaudhuri, S Duttagupta, SK Panda and SK Acharya. Department of Gastroenterology and Pathology, AIIMS, New Delhi.

Aetiology of acute liver failure in India in a tertiary medical center in north India over a ten year period. Yogesh Batra, Kaushal Madan, Kuldeep Kaur*, S Hazari*, V Chaudhuri*, S Duttagupta*, SK Panda* and SK Acharya*. Departments of Gastroenterology and Pathology, AIIMS, New Delhi.

Population based epidemiological study of acute viral hepatitis (AVH) and correlation with contaminated sewage and drinking water. Kunal Das, BC Das, RK Gupta, P Kar. Department of Medicine, Molecular Oncology division, Institute of Cytology and Preventive Oncology (ICMR), MAMC and Associated LNJP Hospital, New Delhi.

A comparative study of seasonal incidence of malaria and hepatitis B to find out any link between the two. MK Ghoda, Rajasthan Hospital, Ahmedabad.

Evaluation of vertical and horizontal transmission of hepatitis B in early childhood. Vikas Jain, Urmila Jhamb, Anita Chakravarty, S K Mittal. Departments of Pediatrics and Microbiology, MAMC & Associated LNJP Hospital, New Delhi.

Prevalence of HBsAg among urban and rural antenatal females in Sikkim. Raj Kotwal, CZ Rinchhen, Yogesh Verma. Departments of Gastroenterology and Pathology, STNM Hospital, Gangtok, Sikkim.

Hepatitis B surface antigen (HBsAg) positivity rate among blood donors in Sikkim. Raj Kotwal, DS Hamal. Departments on Gastroenterology and blood Transfusion Medicine, STNM Hospital Gangtok, Sikkim.

Hepatitis B marker HBsAg among the safai karmcharies (lowest socioeconomic group in society) of housing and urban department of Sikkim. Raj Kotwal, CZ Rinchhen, Yogesh Verma. Departments of Gastroenterology and Pathology, STNM Hospital, Gangtok, Sikkim.

Introduction of hepatitis B vaccine into routine immunization in Sikkim since 14th August 2001. Raj Kotwal. Department of Health, Government of Sikkim, Gangtok.

Life style and other risk factors for hepatitis B virus carrier status in Kerala, India: a case control study. KB Leena, KT Shenoy. Department of Gastroenterology, Medical College Hospital, Trivandrum.

Fulminant hepatic failure—etiology and outcome in a north Indian referral hospital. Neelam Mohan, K Chugh, A Sachdev, A Raina, D Gupta. Department of Pediatrics, Sir Ganga Ram Hospital, New Delhi.

Acute flares in chronic hepatitis B infection (CHB). DN Amrapurkar, N Patel. Bombay Hospital, Mumbai.

Histological and immunohistochemical study of asymptomatic hepatitis B carriers. B Ramakrishna, A Mukhopadhya, GM Chandy. Departments of Pathology and Gastrointestinal Sciences, Christian Medical College and Hospital, Vellore.

Histological features of liver biopsy in patients with dual hepatitis B and C virus infection. P Sakhuja, V Malhotra, R Gondal, SK Sarin. Departments of Pathology and Gastroenterology, GB Pant Hospital, New Delhi.

Spectrum of acute hepatitis in adults in a tertiary referral centre in north India. Arora A, Saigal S, Kumar M, Sud R and Sama SK. Departments of Gastroenterology and Hepatology, Sir Ganga Ram Hospital, New Delhi.

Clinical profile, demographic characteristics, aetiologcal profile and treatment of hepatocellular carcinoma in India: A 12-year experience. Satyanarayan, B Nandi, K Madan, Y Batra, S Hazari, V Chaudhuri, S Duttagupta SK Panda, SK Acharya. Departments of Gastroenterology and Pathology, AIIMS, New Delhi.

Delta virus prevalence in HBV infected children. AK Sharma, CK Nain, V Singh, BR Thapa, K Singh. Department of Gastroenterology, Post Graduate Institute of Medical Education and Research, Chandigarh.

Prevalence of hepatitis B and C in chronic renal failure patients. MR Ajmal, I Shukla, SF Haque, J Ismail, N Sharma. Jawaharlal Nehru Medical College Hospital, Aligarh Muslim University, Aligarh.

Prevalence of hepatitis B and C virus markers in patients of cirrhosis of liver. I Shukla, MR Ajmal, J Ismail, N Sharma. Jawaharlal Nehru Medical College Hospital, Aligarh Muslim University, Aligarh.

Hepatitis B virus (HBV) DNA in healthy blood donors. Ajay Duseja, Sanjeev Sharma, PG Subramanian, Nitin, S K Agnihotri, YK Chawla. Departments of Hepatology and Transfusion Medicine, Postgraduate Institute of Medical Education and Research, Chandigarh.

Unusual sexually transmitted sporadic outbreak of hepatitis B in Kerala, India: need for preventive strategy. KT Shenoy, KB Leena. Medical College, Trivandrum.

Profile of hepatocellular carcinoma in Gizan region of Saudi Arabia. AK Singal, Nabeel Tadros. Departments of Gastroenterology and Pathology, King Fahd Central Hospital, Gizan, Kingdom of Saudi Arabia.

Follow-up of asymptomatic HBsAg positive individuals detected incidentally during blood donation. AK Singal. Department of Gastroenterology, Tirath Ram Shah Hospital, Delhi.

Higher efficacy of 'sequential' therapy of lamivudine and interferon compared to lamivudine monotherapy in HBeAg positive, chronic hepatitis B patients. SN Kazim, RC Guptan, SM Wakil, S Kumar, SK Sarin. Department of Gastroenterology, GB Pant Hospital, New Delhi.

Profile of chronic HBV infection in children: an Indian perspective. SK Satpathy, R Chauhan, SK Sarin. Department of Gastroenterology, GB Pant Hospital, New Delhi.

Estimation of anti-HBs titres in health care workers following hepatitis B vaccination. Yogesh Verma, MR Kotwal, STNM Hospital, Gangtok, Sikkim.

Preliminary evaluation of lamivudine in the treatment of subacute hepatic failure due to hepatitis 'B' virus. RP Wadhwa, R Ardhanari. Department of Gastroenterology, Meenakshi Mission Hospital and Research Centre, Madurai.

Study on the transmisssion pattern of hepatitis B virus in asymptomatic pregnant women. E Dhevahi, Parthiban[1], HK Nayak[2], Rajalakshmi[3], Geetha[3], D Guptae[2], SP Thyagarajan[1]. Department of Microbiology, Dr. ALMPGIBMS, University of Madras Chennai;[1] National Institute of Epidemiology, Chennai[2] Department of Neonatology, Obstetrics and Gynaecology, Chennai[3].

HBV infection in HIV/AIDS patients. Saravanan S[1], Uma S[1], Joyee AG[1], Murugavel KG[2], Balakrishnan P[2], Kumarasamy N[2], Suniti Solomon[2], Thyagarajan SP[1]. Department of Microbiology, Dr. ALMPGIBMS, Taramani, Chennai; YRG CARE, Chennai.

Comparative evaluation of the immunogenicity and safety of a new recombinant hepatitis B vaccine with two other commercially available recombinant hepatitis B vaccines. V Vijayakumar, R Hari, R Parthiban, B Krishnamohan, SP Thyagarajan. Department of Microbiology, Dr. ALM PGIBMS, University of Madras, Chennai.

Short term follow-up of hepatitis B and C virus infected renal transplant recipients. PP Varma, AK Seth, A Nagpal, SR Gadela, AC Anand. Departments of Gastroenterology and Nephrology, Army Hospital R & R, New Delhi.

Hepatitis C virus infection is commoner than hepatitis B virus infection in renal transplant recipients. Anand AC, Nagpal A, Varma PP, Seth AK, Narula AS. Department of Gastroenterology, Army Hospital R & R, New Delhi.

Familial clustering of HBV infection: study of one family. Govind Verma, Prakash Dalai, Pravin Rathi, Philip Abraham. Department of Gastroenterology, KEM Hospital, Mumbai.

Spectrum of chronic liver disease in the close family contacts of HBV related chronic liver disease patients. V Thakur, RC Guptan, V Malhotra, SK Sarin. Departments of Gastroenterology and Pathology, GB Pant Hospital, New Delhi.

Response to interferon therapy in chronic hepatitis B infection: a prospective study. TNL Mazumdar, S Sengupta, DK Mitra, M Banerjee. Departments of Gastroenterology and Pathology, Caltutta; and Medical Research Institute, Calcutta.

Histological profile and long-term follow-up of chronic HBV infection with normal ALT levels. AC Anand. N Kekre, M Anand, A Saha, P Puri. Department of Gastroenterology, Command Hospital (WC), Chandimandir.

Prevalence of HBsAg and abnormal liver function test results in thalassemia: a preliminary report. TK Ghosh, UC Ghoshal, R Ghose, U Ghoshal, CR Maity. Departments of Pathology and Biochemistry, Burdwan Medical College, Burdwan; Department of Gastroenterology, Institute of Post Graduate Medical Education and Research and SSKM hospital, Calcutta, and Thalassemia Welfare Society, Burdwan.

HBsAg carrier rate in voluntary blood donors of Kashmir. NA Bhat, SA Kadla, NA Masoodi, MY Wani, I Ahmad, MA Kamili. Department of Medicine, SMHS Hospital, Govt. Medical College, Srinagar, Kashmir.

Alpha-feto protein as a prognostic factor in acute liver failure. D Krishnadas, V Vijayakumr, AG Priyadarsini, M Hariharan. Departments of Gastroenterology and Department of Medicine, Medical College and Hospital, Trivandrum.

Profile of hepatocellular carcinoma in eastern India. VM Dayal, A Kumar, KM Prasad, HP Sharma, P Kumar, HS Rai, A Xess, SK Shahi. Departments of Gastroenterology, Pathology, Radiology and Immunology, Indira Gandhi Institute of Medical Sciences, Patna.

Hepatitis B immunization of hospital nursing staff—intradermal vs. intra-muscular dose. P Sawant, S Vispute, RG Shirhatti, N Borse, S Shetty, K Vyas, HS Das, S Dhadphale, V Patrawala. LTMMC and LTMGH, Sion, Mumbai.

Incidence of hepatitis B virus infection amongst the inpatients and voluntary blood donors from a referral centre in east Godavari district of Andhra Pradesh. JD Ray, K Vengala Rao. Departments of Gastroenterology and Department of Biochemistry, Swatantra Hospitals, Rajahmundry.

Can HBx protein induce apoptosis or modulate TNF-induced apoptosis in transfected cells? R Govindarajan, S Dwivedi, SR Naik, S Naik. Departments of Immunology and Gastroenterology, Sanjay Gandhi Post Graduate Institute of Medical Sciences, Lucknow.

Lamivudine in decompensated HBV related cirrhosis: a pilot study. SK Dadhich, VA Saraswat. Department of Gastroenterology, Sanjay Gandhi Postgraduate Institute of Medical Sciences, Lucknow.

Interferon theraphy in patients with hepatitis B infection: CMCH experience. A Mukhopadhya, S Paul, GM Chandy. Departments of Gastroenterology and Hepatology, Christian Medical College, Vellore.

Seroepidemiology of hepatitis B and hepatitis C in a rural population in West Bengal. A Chowdhury, A Santra, S Chaudhuri, R Chakraborty, DN Guha Mazumder. Department of Gastroenterology, Institute of Post Graduate Medical Education and Research, Calcutta, and Indian Council of Medical Research Virus Group, Calcutta.

Five year follow-up study of low doe IFN therapy in Asian Indians with HBV related chronic liver disease. RC Guptan, V Thakur, V Malhotra, SK Sarin. Department of Gastroenterology, GB Pant Hospital, New Delhi.

Hepatitis B and C viral markers in patients of cirrhosis of liver. V Singh, DK Bhasin, R Kochhar, K Singh. Department of Gastroenterology, Post Graduate Institute of Medical Education and Research, Chandigarh.

List of abstracts published in Indian Journal of Gastroenterology November 2002 (Volume 21, Suppl. 1)

Profile of perinatally acquired HBV infection in India. SK Satapathy, R Chauhan, V Thakur, P Sakhuja, V Malhotra, SK Sarin. GB Pant Hospital, New Delhi.

Molecular characterization of S-gene mutants of hepatitis B virus in India: Naturally occurring and lamivudine induced: a molecular analysis. Syed K Nazim, Salma M Wakil, Shiv K Sarin. Department of Gastroenterology, GB Pant Hospital, New Delhi.

Prevention and management of hepatitis B in India: results of a national survey. AK Singhal, Anjana Singhal*, DK Shukla,** SK Sarin,*** Department of Gastroenterology, Tirath Ram Shah Hospital, Department of Anaesthesia* and Paediatrics,** Sanjay Gandhi Memorial Hospital, Department of Gastroenterology, GB Pant Hospital***, New Delhi.

Effects of long-term lamivudine therapy in patients with e negative chronic hepatitis B (e-CHB). Kazim SN, Wakil SM, Guptan RC, Kumar S, Thakur V, Sakhuja P*, Malhotra V*, Sarin SK. Department of Gastroenterology and Pathology*, GB Pant Hospital, New Delhi.

Asymptomatic HBV carriers: histological profile and long-term follow-up. Anand AC, Paul MS, Nagpal A, Anand M, Dhot PS. Department of Gastroenterology, Army Hospital R & R, New Delhi.

Molecular characteristic based epidemiology of chronic hepatitis B virus infection. Sanjai D, Sugunan VS, Prasanth V, Dawney Zachariah, Narendranathan M. Rajib Gandhi center for Biotechnology & Department of Gastroenterology, Medical College, Thruvananthapurarn, Kerala.

Occult HBV markers in cryptogenic chronic liver disease–a retrospective analysis. Anil John, Rajib Mehta, Sadasivan S, Deepak S, Prem Nair, Balakrishnan V, Digestive Diseases Institute, Amritha Institute of Medical Sciences, Elamakkara, Cochin, Kerala.

Prevalence of hepatitis B virus (HBV) and hepatitis C virus (HCV) infection in alcoholics and non-alcoholic Indian patients with liver disorders. Nafaeesa, Khaja MN, Chandra M, Hussain MM, Aejaz MA, Habibullah CM. Center for Liver Research and Diagnostics, Decan College of Medical Sciences and allied Hospitals, Hyderabad.

Hepatitis B virus infection–An in vitro model. Taher-uz-Zaman, MN Khaja. AA Khan, SJ Hussain and CM Habibullah. Central Research Institute of Unani Medicine, Hyderabad & Center for Liver Research and Diagnostics, Owaisi Hospital & Research Center, Hyderabad.

Evaluation of antibody titers four years after primary vaccination with recombinant hepatitis B vaccine (Shanvac-B). Nnyana Joshi, Ajit Kumar, Kavitha Singh; Praful Bhad. Department of Gastroenterology, Nizam's Institute of Medical Sciences. Shantha Biotechnics Pvt. Ltd, Hyderbad.

Clinical utility of HBV genotype to predict outcome of lamivudine therapy in patients with chronic hepatitis (CHB). Thakur V, Rehman S, Guptan RC, Kazim SN, Kumar S, Malhotra V*, Sarin SK. Department of Gastroenterology and Pathology*, GB Pant Hospital, New Delhi.

Clinical presentation and therapeutic outcome of HBV related CLD. Subrat Pal, J Mukherjee, G Ray and AK Banerjee. IPGMER and SSKM Hospital, Kolkata.

Index

Activated CTL response 84, 473
Acute hepatitis
   antivirals in 574
   epidemic 151
   fulminant 100, 155, 291
   reactivation (*See HBV reactivation*)
   subacute hepatic failure 101, 155
Adefovir dipivoxil 477, 486
Aflatoxin-B1 239, 247
   carcinogenic potential of 239, 247
   hepatocellular carcinoma and 235, 239, 247
   interaction with HBV infection 239
Alanine aminotransferase
   in acute hepatitis 196
   in chronic hepatitis 102
   in IDAHS 95
   in hepatic flare 282, 495
   in reactivation 163
   role in evaluation for treatment 450
   therapy response and 450, 451
Alcohol
   in liver transplantation 290
   percutaneous injection in tumor 283, 284
Alcoholic liver disease 151, 403, 606
Alpha-feto protein
   diagnosis 282
   for HCC screening 252, 267 (*See also screening for HCC*)
   response to therapy 278
Alpha-interferons (*See Interferons*)
Alpha-1 antitrypsin 293, 294
   deficiency 293
ALT (*See alanine aminotransferase*)
Animal models 239, 534
   transgenic mouse models 534

Antenatal
   screening for HBV 26
Anti-HBc (anticore antibody) 197
   isolated anti-HBc 208
Anti-Hbe (antibody to e antigen) 197
   in HBV reactivation 163
   in HBV mutants 104, 206
   in seroconversion 206, 453, 523, 580
   relation with ALT 95, 104
   relation with histology 219
Anti-HBs
   as marker 196
   post-vaccination screening 370, 373, 384, 392
   protective levels of 373, 416 (*See also screening*)
   response to vaccination, kinetics of 370, 392
Anti-HCV antibodies 54, 103, 156, 407
Antiviral therapy (*See specific antiviral agents*)
   of chronic hepatitis B 453, 458
   of decompensated cirrhotics 578
Apoptosis 85, 219
Arthritis
   in hepatitis B (*See also extra hepatic manifestations*) 114
Asymptomatic HBsAg positive subjects
   incidentally detected (*See also IDAHS*)
      definition of 93
      follow-up of 102, 227
      profile of 95, 227
Australia antigen (*See also hepatitis B surface antigen*) 193

b DNA (*See also branched chain DNA assay*) 200, 201
Biopsy
   in acute hepatitis 218
   in chronic hepatitis 215

histological activity index 221
  in hepatocellular carcinoma 223, 270
Blood/ blood products
  and HBV transmission (*See also post-transfusion hepatitis*) 16, 59, 72
  screening for HBsAg 61
Blood donors 67
  commercial, transfusion-associated hepatitis in 59
  professional 59
  voluntary 67
Branched chain DNA assay 200, 201
Breast feeding
  and HBV transmission 17
Bridging hepatic necrosis 221

Carbohydrates
  in liver disease 603
  requirement 602
Carcinogens (*See Hepatocarcinogenesis*)
Carcinoma
  hepatocellular (*See HCC*)
Cellular genes 237, 241
Chemoembolization 284
  in HCC (*See treatment of HCC*)
Chemotherapy systemic
  in hepatocellular cancer 283
  reactivation and 164, 165
  HBsAg screening before 166
Child's grade in cirrhosis 580
Childhood cirrhosis 294
Childhood immunization program 26, 421, 429
Children and infants
  alpha-1 antitrypsin deficiency 293, 294
  biliary atresia in 290
  EPI in 26, 421, 429
  hepatitis B in (*See also Hepatitis B in children and infants*) 25, 37, 73, 154
  hepatocellular carcinoma 244, 263, 553
  post-exposure prophylaxis in 415
  transmission of HBV in 25, 37
  treatment of HBV in 551, 553
Chronic HBV infection
  biopsy in 215
  diagnosis of 197, 206, 208
  spectrum of disease
    ALT 102
    with liver disease 103, 104, 107, 140
    without liver disease 95

Chronic liver disease
  acute on chronic 148
    diagnosis of 156
    etiology 149
    nutrition in 598, 606
    reactivation of 163
    transplantation in (*See also liver transplantation*) 290
    vaccination in (*See also Vaccination*) 401, 405, 407
Chronic active hepatitis (*See also under specific viruses*)
  grading of 216
  histological activity index in 221
  persistent 215
  piecemeal necrosis 222
  staging of 222
  treatment of 453
Cirrhosis of liver
  antiviral therapy in
  compensated 453
  decompensated 577, 578
  HBV-related 102
  HCC and 246, 250
  transplantation
    in hepatitis B 277, 295, 587
    pre-transplant assessment in 291
    recurrence of HBV 293, 589
Commercial sex workers 9
Computerized tomography (CT) scan
  and angiography in HCC 256
  helical 257
  lipoidal Ct scan in HCC 257, 282
  portography arterial in 256
Corticosteroids
  reactivation and 164, 165
  steroid priming 499
  transplantation and 292
CPH (chronic persistent hepatitis) 215
Cryoglobulinemia
  diagnosis of 121
  in HBV 112, 121
Cryoprecipitates
  and HBV transmission 75
Cycloxygenase 266
Cyclosporin A
  in liver transplantation 292
  in reactivation 164
Cytotoxic T-Lymphocytes 84, 473

Delta agent 100, 149
Des-gamma-carboxy prothrombin (DCP)
 role in screening for HCC 253, 268
DNA
 HBV (*See also Hepatitis B virus DNA*) 140
  in chronic HBV infection 95, 101, 204
  covalently closed circular 236, 478
  in HCC 236
  in IFN therapy 134, 454
  integration of 236
  in lamivudine therapy 456, 484, 580
  in perinatal transmission 23, 435
  measurement of 200
  replication of 129
  serum 61, 203
  tissue 208
  vaccination 534
DNA polymerase 137, 175, 236
Donors
 in liver transplantation 288, 289
  in children 293
  criteria for 290
  living related 292
  timing for surgery 290
Doppler ultrasound 254, 256, 269
Drug abuse
 hepatitis B in 53
 intravenous 52
Dual infection 103, 156

ELISA 198, 199
Endoscopes
 accessories 323
  disinfection 323
  reprocessing 323
  reusable 324
 glutaraldehyde and (*See also Glutaraldehyde*) 307, 321, 322, 325
 reprocessing 324, 325
 transmission of HBV 307, 321
Embolization 284
Emergency surgery 338
Entecavir 427, 464
Equipments 305
Expanded program on immunization (EPI)
 antenatal screening 26
 in children 361, 421, 428
 ideal schedule in 26, 420
 polyvalent vaccine in 421

Famciclovir
 for chronic HBV infection 477, 486
 in combination therapy 526
 for reactivation 166
 FCH (*See Fibrosing cholestatic hepatitis*) 136, 586
Fibrosing cholestatic hepatitis 136, 586
Fibrosis
 in chronic hepatitis 222
 in cirrhosis 221
 progression of 221
 reversibility of 226, 480
Fulminant hepatitis
 liver failure in, etiology of 100, 149

Gamma interferon 473
Ganciclovir 165, 477
Gene therapy 531
Genotypes 175
GMCSF (*See also hemodialysis and vaccination*) 393
Graft 292
Ground glass appearance
 in hepatitis B 218

Health care workers 17, 300, 342, 375, 378, 379, 383
Hematological malignancies 72
Hemodialysis
 and transmission of HBV 328, 556
  ALT in 556
  outcome in 557, 558
  treatment of 558
 and vaccination
  response 391
  schedule 394
  role of GMCSF (*See also GMCSF*) 393
  role of levamisole 394
Hemophiliacs
 transmission of HBV in 74
Hepadna viruses 175, 530
Hepatic angiography 255, 269, 282
Hepatic encephalopathy 155, 291, 604
Hepatic fibrosis
 Knodell's score 221
Hepatic steatosis 219
Hepatitis B virus (HBV)
 acute infection with 99, 152, 196, 203, 571, 598
 aflatoxin exposure and 239, 247
 antigens
  core 195

e 195
surface antigen (*See also HBsAg*) 194
  positive mothers 7, 23, 30
  negative 61, 208
anti-HBc 197
assays
  branched chain DNA (b DNA) 200
  hybridization 201
  polymerase chain reaction 201
  positivity
    asymptomatic 93, 102, 204
    in family contacts 9, 48, 49
    HBeAg status 8
    in high-risk groups 8, 9
    histology 215
    host factors 83
    IDAHS 93, 102, 204
    management policy 450
    mothers 7, 23, 30
    pool 42
    prevalence 4, 5
    with liver disease 100, 102, 104, 108
    viral factors 88
chronic HBV infection
  with liver disease 100, 102, 104, 108
  without liver disease 93, 102, 204
chronic hepatitis (*See chronic hepatitis*)
  clinical course of 196, 197
  cytotoxic T-lymphocytes 84, 473
  extrahepatic manifestations 112
  natural history
    acute on chronic 155
    dynamic changes of serum markers 523
    immune clearence phase 523
    immune tolerance phase 523
    pathogenesis 86
    reactivation 163
    seroconversion to anti-Hbe 523
    spectrum of disease 100
    superinfection
      with HAV 149, 151
      with HEV 149, 151
      with HDV 149
      with HCV 149, 150
  co-infection with
    HCV 54, 103, 109, 224
    HDV 224
    HIV 54, 225, 564

diagnosis of
  molecular methods 200
  serological assays (*See also hepatitis B virus assays*) 197
DNA of
  assays procedures for 200
  covalently closed circular (CCC) 236, 478
    for diagnosis 203
    hybridization analysis 200, 201
      in follow-up of chronic HBV infection 450
      in natural history 523
      in vaccine escape mutans 438
      integration, in hepatocellular carcinoma 236
      PCR detection 201, 203
      response of, to interferon therapy 206, 452, 454, 551, 578
      response of, to lamivudine therapy 206, 452, 456, 551, 580
    DNA Polymerase 137, 175, 236
endemicity of 10
extrahepatic manifestations 112
epidemiology
  general population 4, 5
  in acute hepatitis 101
  in blood donors 8
  in children 35, 549, 571
  in chronic liver disease 102, 103
  in drug users 53
  in health care personnel 9, 382
  in hematological disorders 9, 72
  in neonates 25
  in pregnant women 7, 23, 30
genome 128, 177, 195
histology
  bridging hepatic necrosis 221
  histological activity index 220
  in IDAHS 96, 227
  Knodell's scoring system 221
  metavir scoring 221
  modified HAI 222
host interaction 83
immunodeficiency virus (HIV), HBV coinfection with 225, 564
immunization for
  expanded program (*See also EPI*) 25, 361, 421, 428
  mass 360
  universal 421

pilot study 428, 508
immunoglobulin
  hepatitis B immunoglobulin (HBIG) 26, 415, 416, 422, 436, 590
integration 236
lamivudine in
  acute hepatitis 573, 574
  children 553
  combination therapy 526, 590
  decompensated cirrhotics 578, 580
  HBeAg negative 461, 483
  HBeAg positive 456, 481
  post-transplant 591
  YMDD mutant 484, 489, 494
mutants of (*See also variants*)
  BCP mutations 131
  surface mutants 136, 437
    a determinant 437
    epidemiology 438, 439
    G 145 A mutant 438
    liver disease 106, 139
    lamivudine induced 484, 489, 494
    polymerase mutants 137
    precore 130
    prevalence zones 483
  reactivation
    BMT and 165, 166
    cancer chemotherapy and 161
    definition 162
    diagnosis of 162
    HBV-DNA 163
    HBV variants 165
    IgM hepatitis B core antigen 163
    immunosuppressed and 161
    prevention 166
    spontaneous 163
    treatment
      lamivudine 165
      famciclovir 163, 165
      penciclovir 165
  seroconversion
    anti-Hbe 453, 523, 551, 580
    anti-HBs 196, 355, 375, 384, 392, 453
  transmission of
    breast feeding 17
    horizontal 32
    intrafamilial 46
    insects and 18
    in utero 434
    needle-stick, by 16
    perinatal 17, 24, 30
      in HBeAg positive mothers 24, 30
      in HBeAg negative mothers 24, 30
    sexual 19
    transfusion related 16
    vertical 30
  therapy (*See also specific*)
    antisense oligonucleotides 532
    antivirals
      adefovir dipivoxil 463
      famciclovir 463
      lamivudine
        in chronic hepatitis B infection 457, 480
        in combination with interferon 462, 527
        in combination with nucleoside analogues 465, 526
        in combination with HBIg 590
        in decompensated liver disease 580
        in HBV reactivation 164, 165
        in post transplant reinfection 591
        prevention of HCC, and 265
        seroconversion to anti-Hbe 453, 523, 551, 580
        YMDD mutants 481, 489, 494
      nucleoside analogues (*See individual antivirals*)
        penciclovir 165
        resistance 484, 489, 494
    combination therapies 462, 465, 526, 527
    gene therapy 530
    HBeAg seroconversion 423, 523, 551, 580
    immunotherapy
      therapeutic vaccine 535
      thymosin alpha-1 524
      interferon-alpha
    in chronic hepatitis B 453, 524, 549, 578
    in HCC prevention 264
    ribozymes 533
    vaccine
      combination 26, 421
      DNA 535
      escape mutant 438
      plasma derived 351
      polyvalent 26, 421

pre-S1 351
pre-S2 351
recombinant 355
screening
  prevaccination 364
  postvaccination 373
  therapeutic 535
  quality assurance 353
vaccination, for
  adolescents 361
  high-risk babies 415
  impact on disease burden 263, 425, 426
  impact on incidence of HCC 264
  strategies in India 360
  universal childhood vaccination program 421
  pre-vaccination screening 364
  post-vaccination screening 373

Hepatitis C virus
  dual infection 103, 109, 224
    anti-HCV antibodies 54, 103, 156, 407
    histology in 224
    screening before therapy 448
  in HCC
    HBsAg negative HCC 208
    cofactor 108
  occult hepatitis B 18, 208
  screening before therapy 448

Hepatitis B core antigen (HBcAg) 195
  antibody to
    and HBsAg screening 65, 208
    in organ donor screening 18
    and reactivation 163
  in core promoter mutations 130
  and liver biopsy 157, 586

Hepatitis B e antigen (HBeAg)
  seropositivity of
    in children 523, 552
    in chronic HBV infection 93, 100, 102, 104, 108
    in core promoter mutations 130
    in interferon therapy 453, 524, 549, 578
    in non-replicating phase 523
    in pre-core mutations 130
    in replicative phase 523
    perinatal transmission and 24, 30
    relation with ALT 95, 102
    relation with HAI 96, 227
    relation with HCC 108

Hepatitis B Genes
  core 195
    mutations 133
  core promoter region
    mutations of 130
  in HCC 235
  mutations of 127
  precore / core 130
  pre S/S 136
  replication of 129
    mutations of 127
    in recombinant vaccines 352
  structure and organization of X 237
    mutations 135

Hepatitis B immunoglobulin
  after needle-stick 416
  in children 415
  with lamivudine 590

Hepatitis B surface antibody (anti-HBs)
  seroprotective titers 368
  in vaccination follow-up 373

Hepatitis B surface antigen
  prevalence rate
    in general population 4, 5
      geographical distribution 5
    in children 35, 549, 571
    in chronic liver disease 102, 103
    in HCC 108
    in HIV patients 54, 225, 564
    in injecting drug users 53
    immunohistochemical staining of 157
    in interferon therapy 453, 524, 549, 578
    in non replicative phase 523
    in organ donation 18
    in pregnant women 7, 23, 30
    in patients with hematological disorders 9, 72
    post-transfusion hepatitis, and 58
    positivity of ELISA for 198, 199
    recombinant vaccines, and 355
    s gene mutations, and 136, 437
    tests for HBV-DNA, and 200

Hepatocarcinogenesis
  aflatoxin-B1 239, 247
  alcohol 108, 235
  growth factors
  HBV 237

Index

HBV integration 236
HDV coinfection
immunopathogenesis 224
  HBx
    molecular pathogenesis 237
  p 53
    tumor suppressor gene 224, 239
  viral (*See specific viral agents*)
Hepatocellular carcinoma
  diagnosis of
    alpha-feto protein 282
    CT arterial portography 256
    CT hepatic angiography 255, 269, 282
    CT scan
      dual phase 255
      helical 257
      lipiodol 257
      hepatic angiography 255, 269, 282
    MRI 255
    MRI angiography 255
    radionuclide scintigraphy 257
    tumor markers
      des-gamma carboxy prothrombin 253, 268
      fucosidase 253
      pivka-II 253
  epidemiology of
    age distribution 247
    geographic distribution
      in Asia 245
      in India 245, 246
      prevalence 244
      registry data 245
      time trends 246
  HBV-related 108, 246, 295
  HBV integration 236
  HBx 135, 196, 237
  prevention
    antiviral therapy 264, 265
    chemotherapy and 265
    HBV vaccination, and 264
  risk factors 258
  screening modalities
    alpha-feto protein 252, 267
    cost-effectiveness 259, 270
    ultrasound 254, 268
  thrombosis in 283
  treatment of
    chemoembolization in 284
    chemotherapy 283
    combination therapy 283
    gene therapy 531
    hepatic resection in 271, 275
    liver transplantation in 271, 277, 287, 585
    newer modalities 281
    percutaneous ethanol injection 283, 284
    radiation therapy 284
    resection 271, 275
    surgery 271, 275
    tamoxifen 283
    transcatheter arterial embolization (TAE) 271, 284
    TAE-PEI combination 284
    TAIE 285
Hepatocytes
  enlargement of 218
  ballooning degeneration of 218
  in chronic hepatitis 215
Hospital waste disposal 311
Herbal drugs 512

IDAHS 93, 102, 204
Imaging techniques
  advanced 256
  CT 255, 256, 258, 282
  MRI 255, 257
  US 254, 268
  CTAP 256
  lipoidal CT 257
  screening for HCC, and 250, 269
Immunoglobulins
  IgG 208
    anti-HBs 196
    anti-HBc 197, 208
  IgM 197
Immune globulin prophylaxis 415, 416, 590
Immune response against HBV 84
Immunotolerance 523
Immunization, (*See Vaccines*)
Indian Association for Study of the Liver 449
Indomethacin 266
Interferons
  for HBV infection 453, 524, 549, 578
    adverse effects 451
    dosage schedule 453
    ideal patient 450
    monitoring 451

prednisolone priming 499
selection criteria
for HBV infection 451
response rate for 454
serological response to 452
Interlukins 87
Intrafamilial/household transmission of HBV 9, 46, 49
Intravenous drug addicts 53

Knodell's scoring 221

Lamivudine
histological improvement 226, 480
in chronic hepatitis B 456, 461, 481, 483, 553, 573, 574, 578, 580
in combination with IFN 526, 590
in HBV reactivation 165
in post transplant reinfection 591
in precore mutant 461, 483
seroconversion to anti-Hbe 456, 481
YMDD mutants 484, 489, 494
Levamisole 394
Liver biopsy (See also histology)
baseline, before treatment 215
for follow-up 225
in chronic hepatitis 215
interpretation of
Knodell 221
metavir 221
post-treatment, in clinical trials 225, 226
scoring, semiquantitative 222
with normal ALT 93, 227
Liver cancer, primary (See hepatocellular carcinoma)
Liver cirrhosis (See cirrhosis of liver)
Liver transplantation
for HBV infection 277, 295, 587
chronic 290
for HBV reinfection
post-transplant antiviral treatment and 591
pre-transplant antiviral treatment and 590
prevention 590

Magnetic resonance imaging (MRI) 255, 257, 269
angiography 255
Maternal infant transmission 7, 17, 23, 30, 434
perinatal 24, 30

Needle-stick injuries 416
Nucleoside analogues
for chronic HBV infection 456, 462, 477, 580
in HBV reactivation 164, 165
in post transplant reinfection 591
in precore mutants 461, 483

Organ transplantation, HCV transmission and 18

Parenteral transmission (See blood/blood products)
Passive immunization
against HBV 415, 416
with anti-HBs, after liver transplantation 590
PCR (See Polymerase chain reaction) 201
Penciclovir 165
Percutaneous ethanol injection (PEI) 283, 284
Piecemeal necrosis 222
Perinatal transmission (vertical) 36
PIVKA-II 253, 268
Polyarteritis 114
Polymerase chain reaction (PCR)
HBV-DNA assay, and 201
HBV-DNA detection 203
HCVRNA detection 208, 209
Polyprenoic acid 266
Precore mutant, of hepatitis B virus 104, 130, 206, 458
Preventive strategies
for HCC 262
for reinfection after transplantation 590
Primary liver cancer (See Hepatocellular carcinoma)
P53 tumor suppressor gene 224, 239

Quality of life 296
instruments to measure 539

Radiation therapy, for hepatocellular carcinoma 284
Renal transplantation, and HBV 558, 559
histological severity 557, 558
natural history 556
therapy 559
Ribavirin
for HBV infection 505, 507
with interferon (See also Combination therapy) 509
Ribozymes 533

Semen
HBV in 19

Index

Seroconversion, anti-Hbe 453, 523, 551, 580
Serologic tests
   for acute HBV infection 196
   for HBV infection 198, 207
Sexual transmission 19
Solution hybridization assay 200, 201
SPIO-MRI 257
Staining 157, 218
Steroids
   before interferon 499
   transplantation and 292
   reactivation and 164, 165
Sulindac 266

TAE (transcatheter arterial embolization), for hepato-cellular carcinoma 284
TAH (*See transfusion associated hepatitis*)
Tamoxifen in HCC 283
Thalassemics 9, 73
TH-1 response 87
Thymosins 524
Tissue diagnosis 270
Transmission
   breast feeding 17
   horizontal 32
   intrafamilial spread 46
   intrauterine 434
   perinatal (*See perinatal transmission*)
   sexual (*See sexual transmission*)
   vertical (*See perinatal transmission*)
Transplantation
   hepatitis B screening in 295
   cadaver 289, 291
   complications in 292
   CT in 289
   contraindications 290, 589
   donors in 289
   in hepatitis B 295, 585
      in adults 290
      in children 290, 293
      in HIV coinfection 290
      in YMDD mutations 582
      recurrent infection 586, 587
         prevention of 589, 293
         treatment of 590, 591
   in HCC 295
   in India 287, 288, 297
   long term treatment in 591, 592
   MRI in 289
   organ transplant act 289
   orthotopic 287, 290
   retransplantation 592
   timing of 290
   results of 293, 296
Truck drivers 9
Tumors
   HCC (*See Hepatocellular carcinoma*)
Tumor suppressor gene 224, 239

Vaccination
   hepatitis A
      in chronic liver disease 401, 402
      dosage schedule in 402
      efficacy of 401, 402
      pre-vaccination screening 402
      in India 398, 402
   hepatitis B
      adverse reactions to 356
      in children and infants 264, 360, 415, 421, 425, 426
      combined with other vaccines 26, 421
      DNA in 535
      duration and protection in 370, 392
      efficacy of 355
      escape mutants in 438
      global programs 421
      in HIV patients 374, 565
      immunogenecity of 355
      indications for 360
      non-responsiveness in 356
      plasma derived 351
      post-exposure 415, 416
      pregnancy and 436
      pre-S vaccines 352
      quality assurance 353
      recombinant preparations 355
      s-gene mutations and 437
      T-cells in 433
      vaccine failure and 431

Hepatitis B in India
Prevention and Management

About the Book

Along with increasing awareness on hepatitis B, immense knowledge and information has been added in the last decade, particularly on the treatment of chronic hepatitis B. This book *Hepatitis B in India: Prevention and Management*, conceived on the occasion of the second National Single Theme Symposium on "Hepatitis B in India: Therapeutic Options and Prevention Strategies" under the auspices of INASL in September 2000, is an honest endeavour of the editors to create an updated and comprehensive manual on hepatitis B, especially in the Indian context.

The contributions have been made by the leading experts from all over India. In addition, a few areas in which not much national work is available, have been covered well by the experts from abroad. The chapters included in this manual which give new dimension to the book are on transmission of hepatitis B in children and neonates, in family contacts, and in injecting drug users; reactivation of hepatitis B; acute on chronic liver disease; HBV genotypes; viral kinetics; screening and prevention of HCC; liver transplantation; HBV mutants; pre- and post-vaccination screening and the need for boosters; economic burden of hepatitis B in India; ideal schedule for vaccinating newborns in EPI in India; vaccine failure, etc. One major highlight of the book is the section on hospital policies in reference to hepatitis B patients. Issues like "routine screening for HBV before surgery" and "policy for HBsAg positive health care worker" are timely and crucial in the Indian scenario.

The major thrust has been given to the treatment of chronic hepatitis B. Areas such as combination therapy, steroid priming before interferon, role of herbal drugs and ribavirin have been dealt in detail. The problems of monotherapy, especially YMDD mutations and lamivudine resistance, newer therapeutic non-surgical options for HCC have been incorporated. Treatment of hepatitis B in special cases like children, patients with CRF, HIV coinfection and post-transplant recurrent hepatitis B and use of antivirals in acute hepatitis have been discussed extensively. In addition, two separate chapters on the nutritional supplementation and the instruments to assess the impact of treatment on the quality of life are the other features of the book.

The editors feel that this manual shall be found useful by the students, clinicians, epidemiologists, basic scientists and the policy makers at large, not only in India but elsewhere also.